The SAGES Manual of Strategy and Leadership

Shaneeta M. Johnson
Alia P. Qureshi
Andrew T. Schlussel
David Renton • Daniel B. Jones
Editors

The SAGES Manual of Strategy and Leadership

Springer

Editors
Shaneeta M. Johnson
Department of Surgery,
Morehouse School of Medicine
Satcher Health Leadership
Institute, Morehouse School of
Medicine
Atlanta, GA, USA

Andrew T. Schlussel
Department of Surgery
HCA Florida Jacksonville
Surgical Specialists
Jacksonville, FL, USA

Daniel B. Jones
Department of Surgery
Rutgers New Jersey Medical
School
Newark, NJ, USA

Alia P. Qureshi
Department of Surgery
Oregon Health Sciences
University
Portland, OR, USA

David Renton
Department of Surgery
OSU East Hospital, Ohio State
University
Columbus, OH, USA

ISBN 978-3-031-62358-5 ISBN 978-3-031-62359-2 (eBook)
https://doi.org/10.1007/978-3-031-62359-2

This Springer imprint is published by the registered company Springer Nature Switzerland AG
The registered company address is: Gewerbestrasse 11, 6330 Cham, Switzerland

Foreword 1

In the dynamic landscape of our modern surgical world, the art of strategy and the essence of leadership have never been more critical. It is the organizations and leaders who master strategic development and execution, inspire and galvanize their teams towards shared goals and visions, and who exhibit resilience and adaptability that stand the greatest chance of achieving enduring success and impact.

The Society of American Gastrointestinal and Endoscopic Surgeons (SAGES) embodies a legacy of pioneering leadership and innovation in surgery. Since its inception in 1981, SAGES has been at the forefront of minimally invasive surgery, steered by visionary leadership who have championed educational excellence and groundbreaking innovation. These have included the creation of the Fundamentals of Laparoscopic Surgery and Fundamentals of Endoscopic Surgery Examinations, now integral components of the American Board of Surgery's certification process. In recent years, SAGES has expanded its offerings globally, developing a sustainable model for training and implementing laparoscopic skill training through the Global Laparoscopic Advancement Program (GLAP) in Low and Middle Income Countries (LMICs). GLAP was designed to be implemented as a partnership with local institutions or societies to ensure the GLAP curriculum fits in the local framework for laparoscopic skills training and that local sites can eventually administer GLAP courses themselves.

The tapestry of SAGES' leadership reflects a rich diversity, with four innovative female presidents—Jo Buskye (2010), Aurora Pryor (2019), Liane Feldman (2021), and Patricia Sylla (2023)—two black presidents—Kenneth Forde (1983) and Patricia Sylla (2023), with Horacio Asbun as the first Hispanic president (2021), and the trailblazing Patricia Sylla as the first black female president (2023). This evolution mirrors the organization's commitment to embracing diverse perspectives and experiences.

This manual is intended to equip the practicing surgeon with the vital competencies of effective leadership and strategic acumen. Within these pages, preeminent surgeons share a comprehensive blueprint for acquiring and refining the essential skills to attain and improve the necessary strategy and leadership skills for success.

As an organizational leader, there is no greater source of satisfaction than to have the opportunity to promote and inspire the next generation of surgical leaders who will need to confront and respond to the rapid changes that may threaten access to equitable, affordable, and high-quality care for our patients. SAGES was born out of a group of innovators advocating for the right of surgeons to adopt and be trained in endoscopy at a time when surgeon endoscopists were actively discouraged from pursuing this field. It is my sincere hope that our current and budding leaders, who aspire to lead OR teams, specialty and multi-specialty groups, clinical research teams, quality or sustainability initiatives, operations or administrative teams, divisions, hospitals, or systems, will find this manual helpful in growing and refining leadership skills with particular attention to the mission of advocating for equitable, sustainable high quality care for our patients.

We dedicate this manual to Dr. Kenneth A. Forde (1933–2019), the visionary and iconic SAGES co-founder and second SAGES President, who devoted his career to developing surgical endoscopy and advocating for surgeons' right to perform and be trained in endoscopy in order to better serve our patients.

Sincerely,

Department of Surgery & Satcher Health Leadership Institute
Morehouse School of Medicine,
Atlanta, GA, USA
Shaneeta M. Johnson

Division of Colorectal Surgery,
Icahn Mount Sinai School of Medicine
NY, USA
Patricia Sylla

Foreword 2

SAGES: In the Beginning

My odyssey and love affair with SAGES began in early 1980 when I received a letter from Dr. Gerald Marks, a noted colorectal surgeon in Philadelphia, inviting me to a meeting to discuss the future of flexible gastrointestinal endoscopy performed by surgeons. Jerry had actually begun to ruminate several years previously over the need for a gastrointestinal endoscopic society dedicated to the clinical work and education of surgeons. Some of the prime motivators for the creation of such an organization were prevailing issues affecting many surgeons wishing to perform GI endoscopy on their own patients. Surgeons did not find it easy to secure endoscopic privileges and to have access to hospital endoscopic suites controlled by gastroenterologists. Many community surgeons wanting to include flexible endoscopy in their practices also experienced, as did I, the threat of having referrals curtailed by their colleagues in gastroenterology. The numbers of endoscopic cases required in the privileging of surgical endoscopists were out of line compared with those required of gastroenterologists. Additionally, there was an absence of both will and interest in any surgical organization to create pathways for clinical involvement and to advocate for surgical endoscopists. Thus, the need for such and organization was ripe.

Jerry's letter invited a small group of surgeons to meet in the Peachtree Plaza Hotel in Atlanta to discuss and formally propose an organization that would support the needs of surgical endoscopists and to both advocate for and educate surgeons wishing to participate. Beginning with this early meeting, the group embraced the concept that guidelines for the safe and effective use of gastrointestinal endoscopy should be a primary undertaking. While there would yet be several years before an annual educational conference was launched, we, as founders of SAGES, believed that education and research would serve as our North-Star. In addition, although the acronym SAGES included the term "American", we felt that the need to serve as an international organization, open to surgeons throughout the world would be of great benefit to all surgeons.

Throughout the 1980s and 1990s, SAGES grew in complexity through the leadership of creative Boards of Directors and an incredibly talented administrative team led by the exceptionally gifted Barbara Saltzman Berci. Her devotion in these early years served as the glue and stabilizing factor that guaranteed our organization's success. Also, during the late 1980s, the leadership recognized the value of having a peer-reviewed journal dedicated to endoscopic education and dissemination of new knowledge. At the First World Congress on Surgical Endoscopy held in Berlin in 1988, the Springer-generated publication, *Surgical Endoscopy*, was launched and included the scientific papers from that first world congress. The creation of the Journal also consummated the goal of having SAGES as the leadership surgical organization supporting surgical endoscopy.

For me, working with superb and talented leaders in those early days of SAGES was my greatest privilege. Appropriately, Jerry Marks served as the first president and, through his vision and tenacity, effectively navigated SAGES through its first 2 years (1981–1983). It was natural that Dr. Kenneth Forde would take over the mantle in 1983–1984. Ken's stentorian presence alone guaranteed that SAGES would be on a trajectory of greatness. Ken was also emblematic of a tradition followed by many SAGES past-presidents: the term of one's presidency was only a prelude to many years of serving in other capacities and contributing to our organization. During the remainder of the 1980s, I was fortunate to garner leadership skills from a superb array of SAGES presidents: Tom Dent (1984–1985), Jim Lind (1985–1986), John Coller (1986–1987), Ted Schrock (1987–1988), Joe Bowden

(1988–1989), Lee Smith (1989–1990), and Jeff Ponsky (1990–1992).

It was one of the highlights of my surgical career to follow this outstanding cast of surgical leaders as SAGES president in 1992–1993. This was indeed an inflexion point for the organization. Just a couple of years previously, laparoscopic cholecystectomy had burst onto the scene creating shockwaves both in the United States and internationally. Thankfully, our SAGES leadership understood the need to embrace this non-flexible technology and to create a meaningful home for all surgeons who would gravitate to minimal access surgical techniques. This period in the growth of SAGES certainly was not all a "bed of roses"! Journal articles, as well as broadcast and print media, decried the abbreviated learning paradigms of these new surgical approaches and resultant heightened morbidity and mortality that ensued following the launch of laparoscopic approaches to the biliary system. As SAGES president during these chaotic times, I benefitted and matured greatly by serving as the spokesperson for our organization when interviews from various media sources were requested. It was also a period of exponential growth in our organization, not only in membership, but in the complexity regarding our educational efforts and relationships with other surgical organizations. Those early 1990s paved the way for many of the creative concepts spawned by SAGES leadership over the ensuing three decades.

One of the most valuable gifts offered by any organization is the opportunity to contribute and to grow into a leadership position. This is the message that must be shared with all young surgeons embarking on either a community practice or academic career. There is no doubt that for me, leadership roles in SAGES contributed directly into opportunities that have led to a career as a division chief, residency director, departmental chair and opportunities to lead other surgical organizations. These valuable opportunities must not be taken lightly. Every circumstance in my career hearkens back to the opportunities that were afforded to me through SAGES membership. Although not all have the good fortune of growing with an organization from its beginning, everyone can have the opportunity to volunteer, to learn from colleagues and to ascend to leadership positions. It is a further SAGES-related privilege to contribute to this monograph that highlights the benefits of learning leadership skills in a variety of organizational and healthcare settings. Leadership is a skill that is honed with practice and devotion. The contributors to this monograph have offered a variety of guidelines emanating from their own leadership experiences.

From those few surgeons who met in Atlanta in 1980 to the current 7000-plus members throughout the world, it was my greatest privilege to be "in the room" where SAGES was created. Watching the growth and increasing complexity of our organization and having the opportunity to contribute and lead have been the joys of my surgical career. The last four decades are surely only a preview of the amazing leadership opportunities yet to evolve from SAGES.

Frederick L. Greene

Carolinas Medical Center,
Charlotte, NC, USA

Cancer Data Services, Levine Cancer
Institute, Charlotte, NC, USA

Foreword 3

Leadership Tips for Surgeons

Most societies are a meritocracy, whereby people are selected for leadership based on their ability. In the *SAGES Manual of Strategy and Leadership*, the authors address unconscious bias and other factors that may play a role in who does and does not become the leader of the organization.

My advice to MIS Fellows aspiring to leadership include the following:

1. Be yourself. Every surgeon is a leader in and out of the OR. Every day, you set a vision, you communicate, and you execute a plan as part of a team.
2. Join a committee. Sometimes the committees are open, and you just show up. Other times, you need to be selected. If you are interested, let folks know. Remember, there are more people wanting to serve on committees than there are open spots; someone needs to be kicked off the committee for every person added to a committee.
3. Once on a committee, engage, speak up, and volunteer. If you get the opportunity to lead an initiative or project, embrace the opportunity. But never ever say you will do something and fail to deliver or deliver late. Under promise and over deliver. Attendance is taken; the easiest way to be tossed off a committee is by not showing up repeatedly.

4. When asked who would you like to run to be a Vice Chair of a Committee, raise your hand. Good Vice Chairs get selected to be Chairs of Committees.
5. Chairs are evaluated not on what they do but on what their committee does as a team.
6. Chairs are asked to identify leaders who could be a Vice Chair, next Chair, or Board member.
7. After two terms as Committee Chair, you may be selected to join the Board. Attendance and prompt email votes are expected. Being tardy and late to vote are sure ways to be bounced from leadership. No one has the bandwidth to send you multiple emails for your input.
8. Leadership is expected to donate something to the Foundation. How much you give is totally up to you.
9. Leadership is expected to do journal reviews. If asked, do them well and promptly.
10. Being the Program Chair for the Annual meeting is a good way to get noticed. If interested, speak to the President-elect and share your interest. The President-elect is more likely to ask someone who wants the job than to ask someone who may not have the bandwidth. It is a big commitment to the organization. With two to three cochairs, it is not a sure thing the program chair will become President one day. But everyone recognizes the tremendous work that goes into making the annual meeting a success. You also gain the loyalty of the President, who likely will have some say in the future.
11. Becoming President is less predictable. Often, to be considered, the successful candidate has contributed in measurable ways. Leading successful teams (committees and task forces) is paramount [1].
12. Many considered for senior leadership positions already hold leadership positions at their home institutions. Most surgeons have earned an MBA, MPH, or Master's in Healthcare Leadership and Management.
13. A little luck helps [2].
14. Have fun.

References

1. Jones DB. On championship TEAMS. Association for Surgical Education (ASE) 34th presidential address, April 25, 2015. Am J Surg. 2016;211(2):309–14.
2. Jones DB. It's better to be lucky. Society of American Gastrointestinal and Endoscopic Surgeons (SAGES) presidential address, April 13, 2018. Surg Endosc. 2018;32:3001–3008.

SAGES, Los Angeles,
CA, USA
Daniel B. Jones

Preface

The SAGES Manual of Strategy and Leadership is a comprehensive text providing strategy and leadership principles for all levels of practice and mastery. Leading surgeons across the United States and globally have contributed their expertise to provide a roadmap for surgical leadership skill acquisition and career development. The SAGES Diversity, Leadership, and Professional Development (DLPD) Committee laid the groundwork for this manual and principally contributed to its fruition.

This book will equip the new and practicing surgeon with the skills and expertise to lead practices and organizations. It will serve as a roadmap to engage the surgeon in leadership development skills and knowledge acquisition to progress further within healthcare leadership. It is intended for practicing surgeons who are interested in healthcare leadership. In this manual, the authors address a gap in the development of surgeons into surgical leaders. It will prepare the surgeon to comprehensively master surgical leadership, including developing a practice, developing a national reputation, leading a healthcare organization, and fostering a culture of change within an organization or institution.

In the realm of leadership for healthcare practices and organizations, a scarcity of accessible references or books exists. Very few references or books on this topic provide the practicing surgeon with a roadmap for acquiring skills and expertise for leadership of practices and organizations. This manual aims to bridge this gap by presenting a comprehensive roadmap for practicing surgeons. It commences with chapters dedicated to self-leadership, exploring topics such as determining the type of practice, career advancements across systems, and defining the scope of practice. Subsequently, the manual delves into mastering the art of leading others. It encompasses managing the work environment, policy and administration, and fostering engagement and consensus building. The concluding chapters focus on leading systems. These chapters discuss the creation of efficient systems and organizational structures, along with aspects crucial to delivering quality healthcare.

I extend my heartfelt gratitude to the esteemed surgeon leaders and diligent DLPD committee members for their contributions.

This work is affectionately dedicated to my family, who have nurtured my passion for education, leadership, and purpose from my earliest days. To my nieces and nephews—Kaylee, Anna, and Liam—and to my parents, Cynthia and Lionel, your unwavering support has been my guiding light. Additionally, this book honors the surgical residents I have had the privilege to mentor and all those who aspire to leave a lasting mark on the world of surgery and healthcare.

Atlanta, GA, USA Shaneeta M. Johnson

SAGES Past Presidents

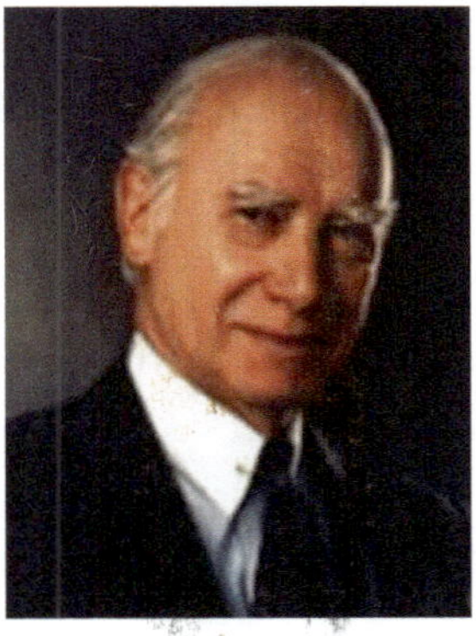

Gerald Marks, MD
1981–1982

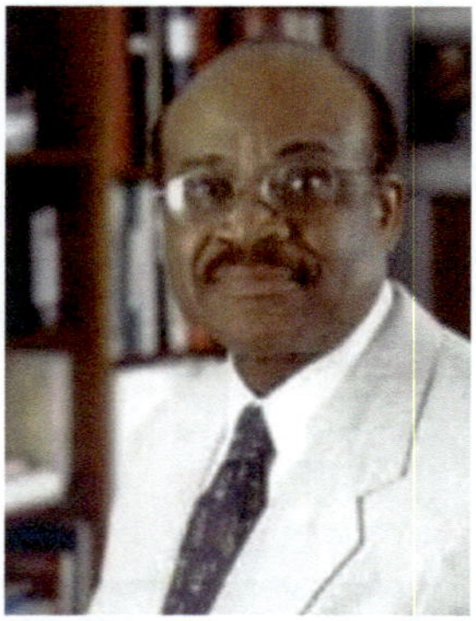

Kenneth A. Forde, MD
1983

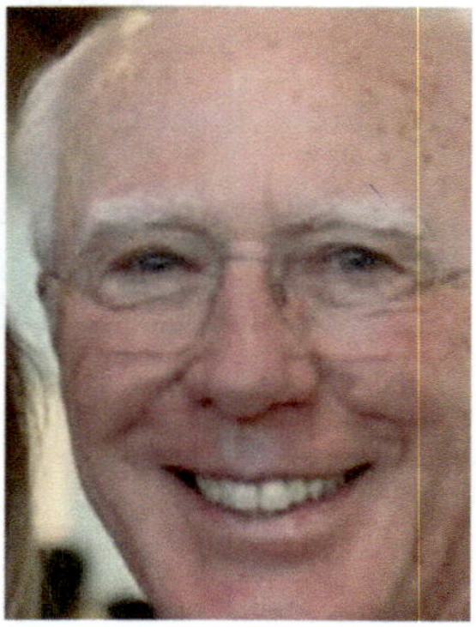

Thomas L. Dent, MD
1984–1985

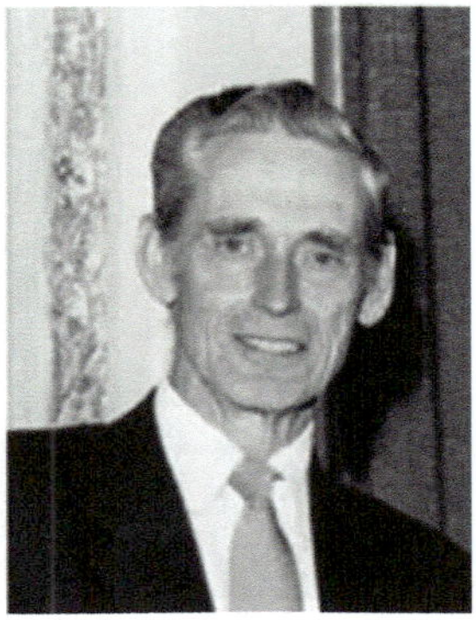

James F. Lind, MD
1985

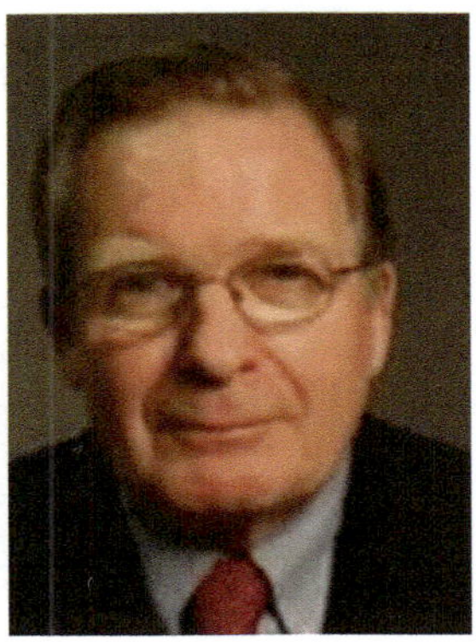

John A. Coller, MD
1986

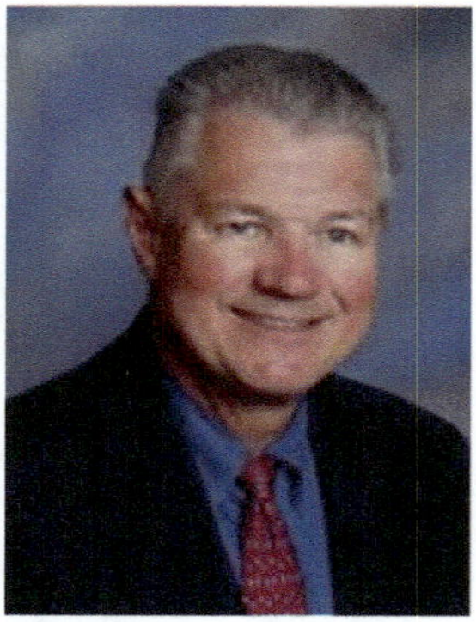

***Theodore R. Schrock, MD**
1987

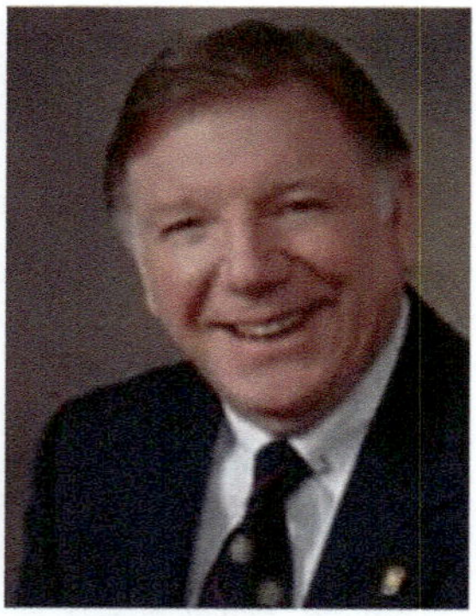

Joe A. Bowden, MD
1988

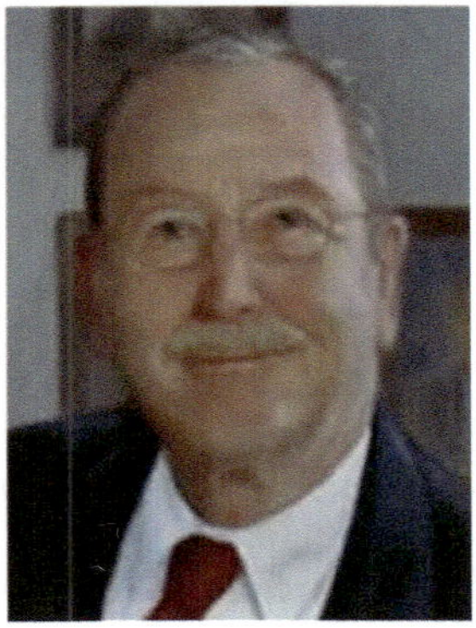

Lee E. Smith, MD
1989

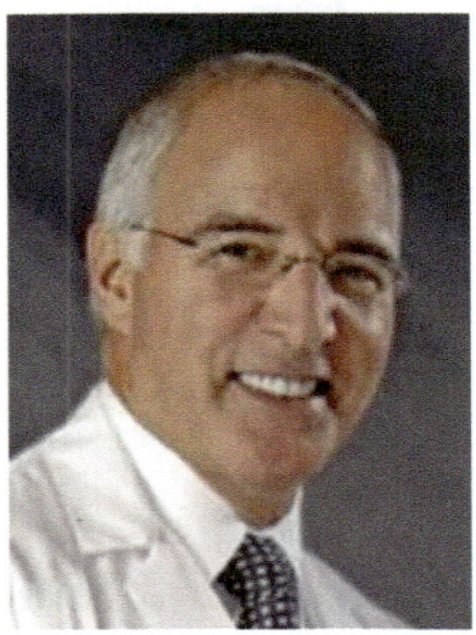

Jeffrey L. Ponsky, MD
1990–1991

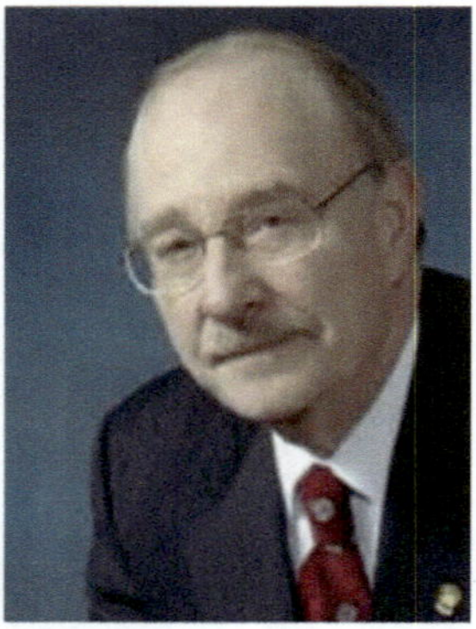

Frederick L. Greene, MD
1992–1993

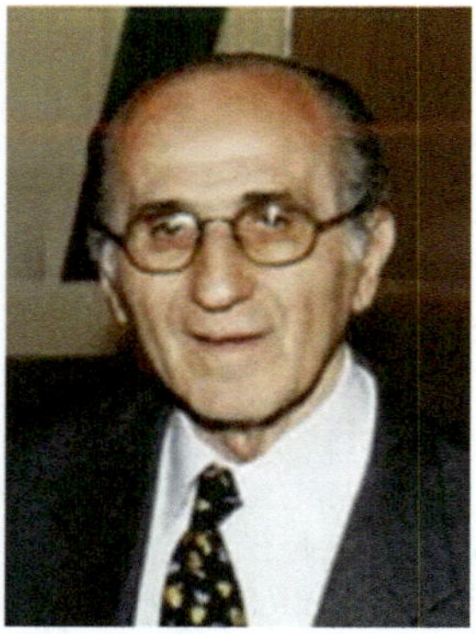

George Berci, MD
1993–1994

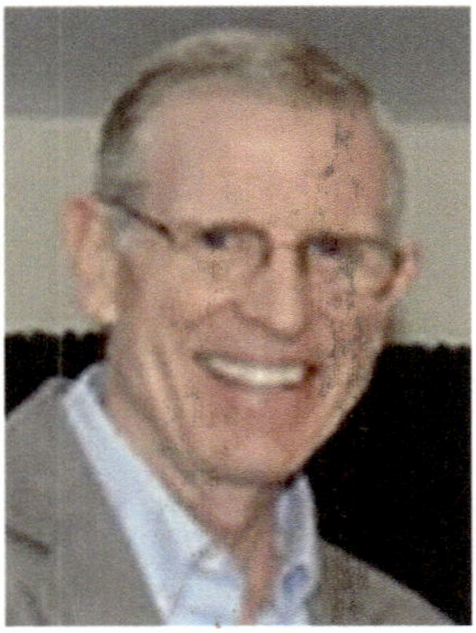

Bruce V. MacFadyen Jr, MD
1994–1995

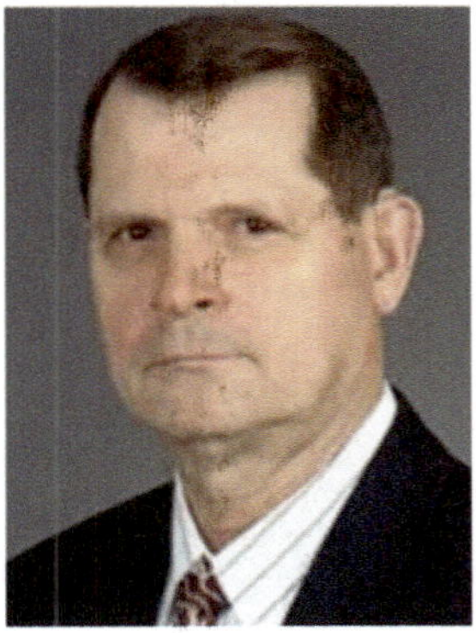

Richard M. Satava, MD
1995–1996

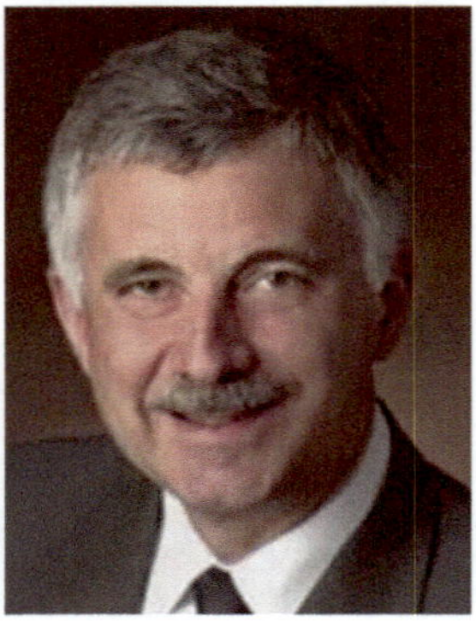

Greg V. Stiegmann, MD
1996–1997

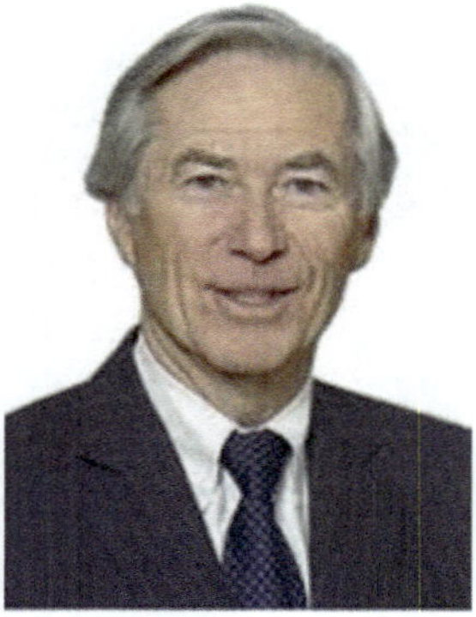

Desmond H. Birkett, MD
1997–1998

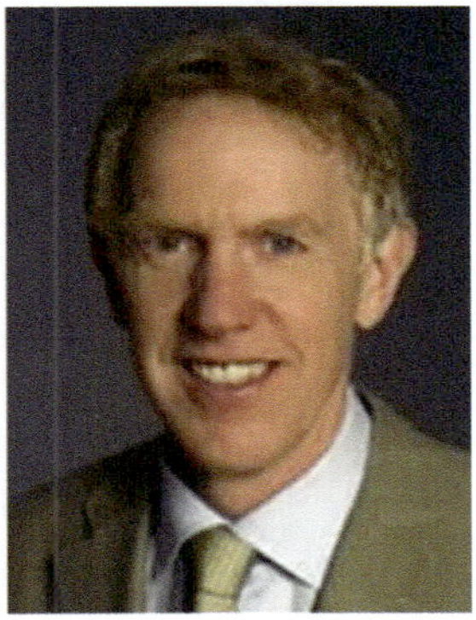

John Hunter, MD
1998–1999

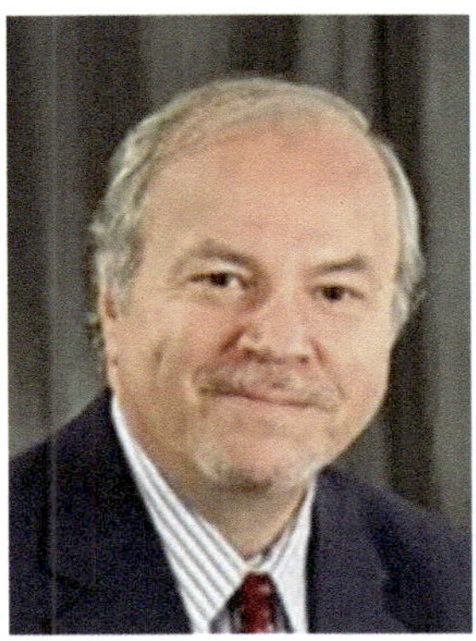

Jeffrey H. Peters, MD
1999–2000

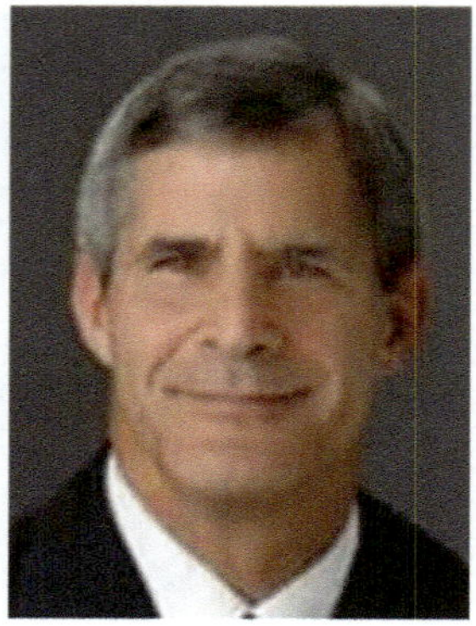

Nathaniel J. Soper, MD
2000–2001

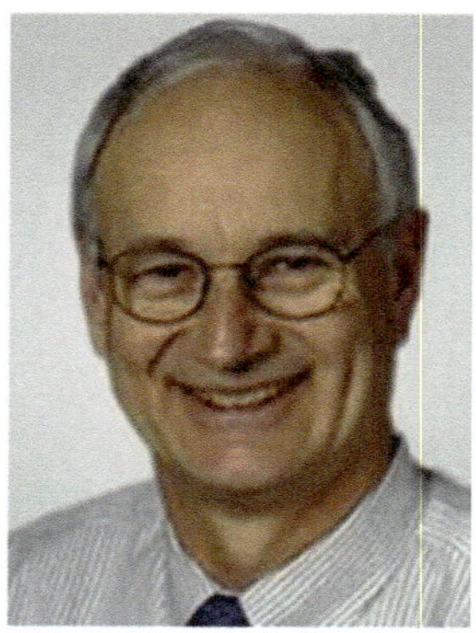

L. William Traverso, MD
2001–2002

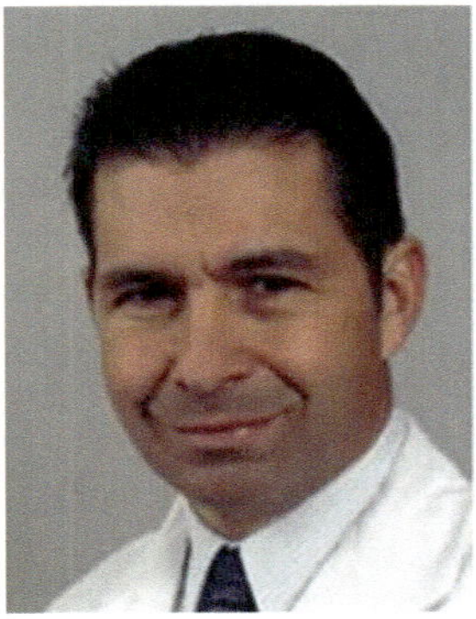

Bruce D. Schirmer, MD
2002–2003

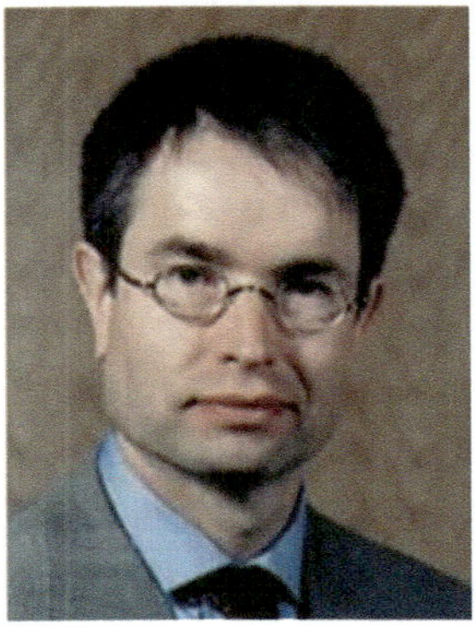

Lee L. Swanstrom, MD
2003–2004

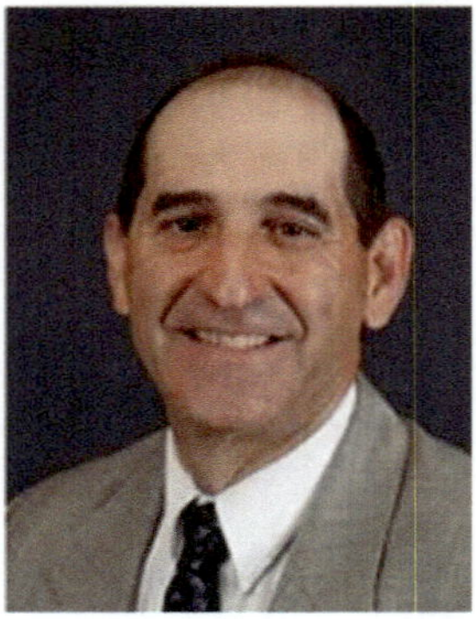

David W. Rattner, MD
2004–2005

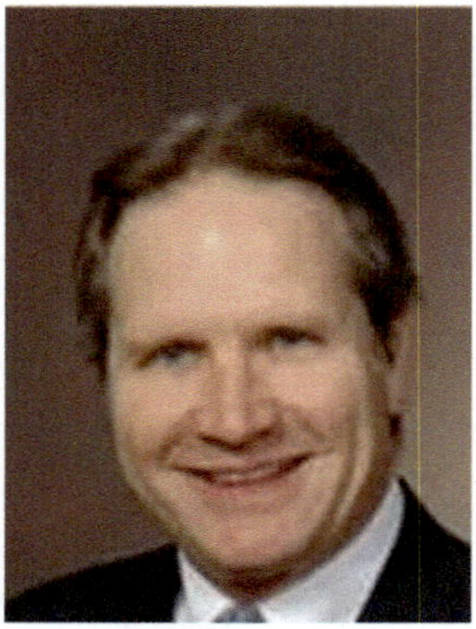

Daniel J. Deziel, MD
2005–2006

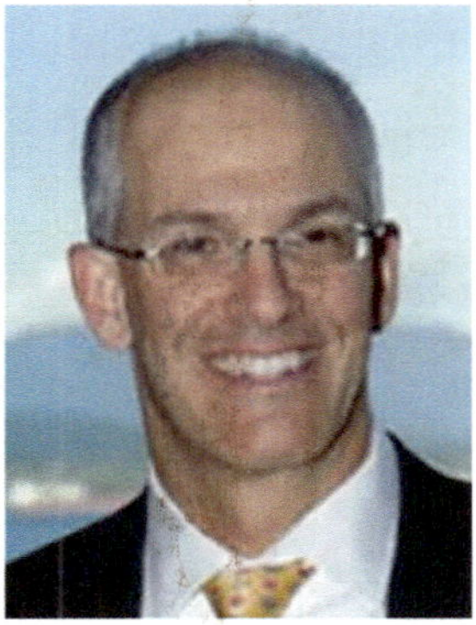

Steven D. Wexner, MD
2006–2007

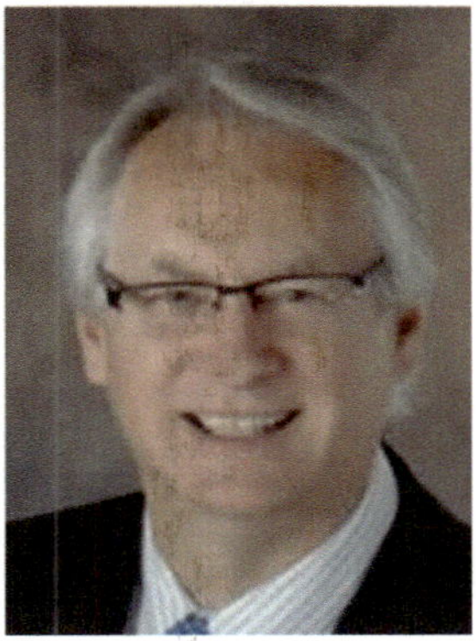

Steve Eubanks, MD
2007–2008

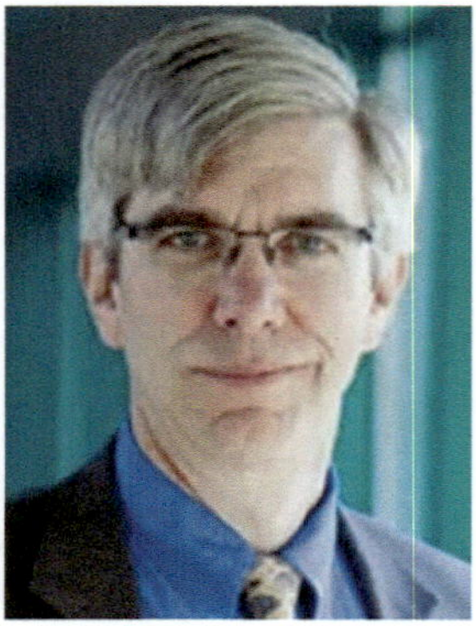

Mark A. Talamini, MD
2008–2009

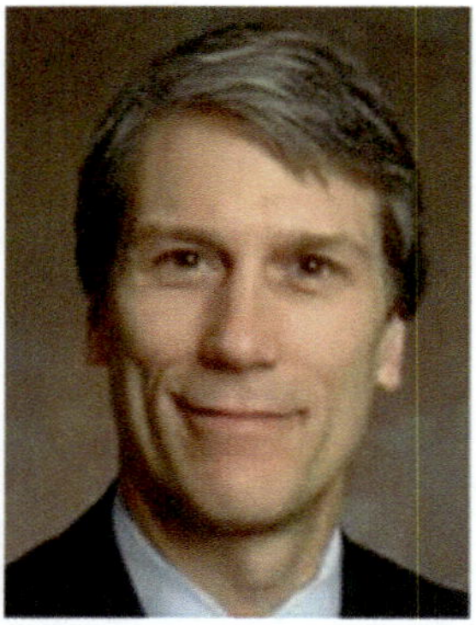

C. Daniel Smith, MD
2009–2010

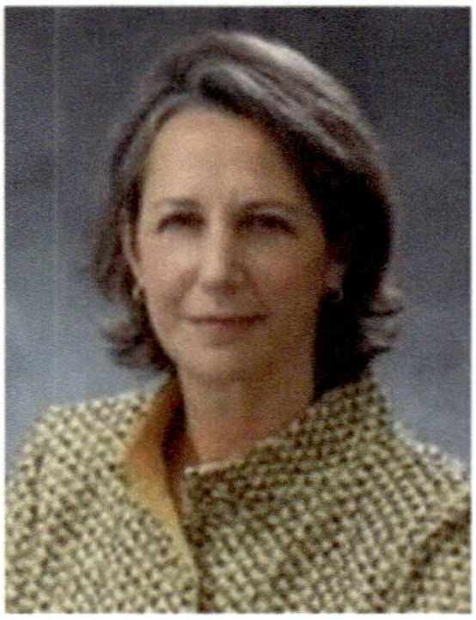

Jo Buyske, MD
2010–2011

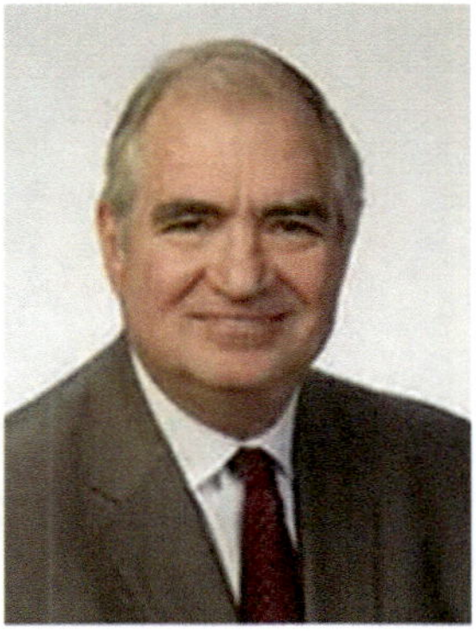

Steve Schwaitzberg, MD
2011–2012

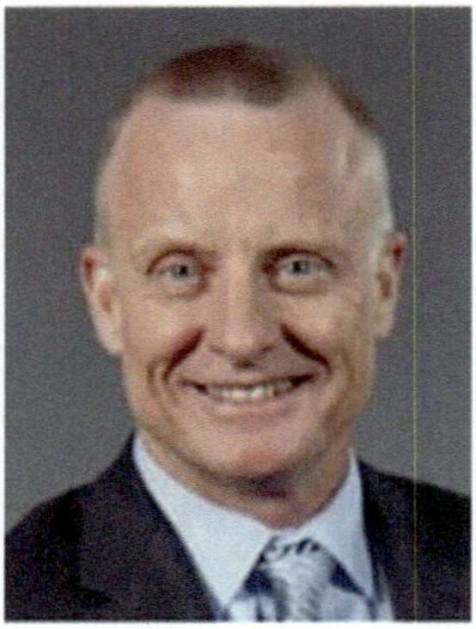

W. Scott Melvin, MD
2012–2013

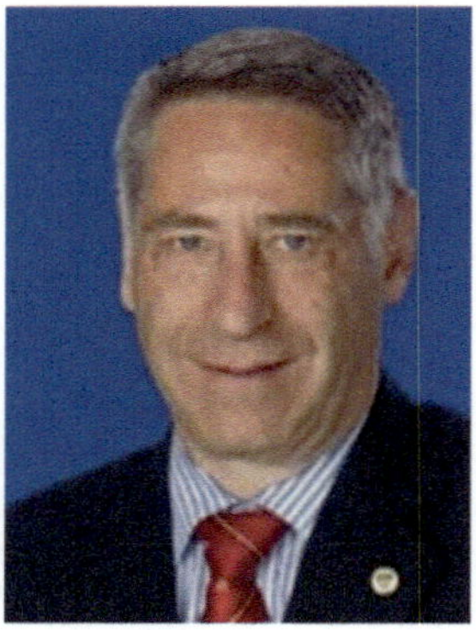

Gerald M. Fried, MD
2013–2014

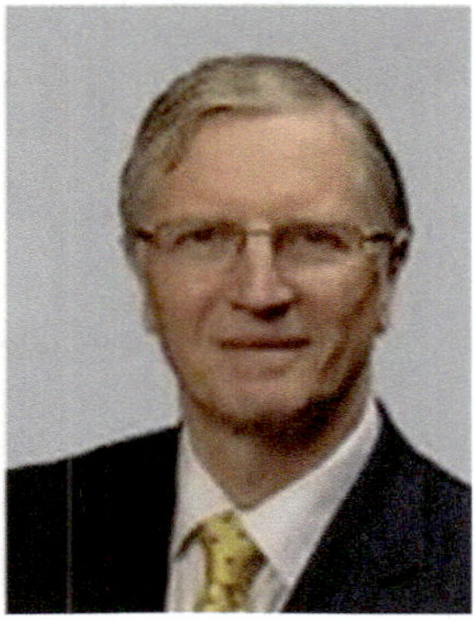

L. Michael Brunt, MD
2014–2015

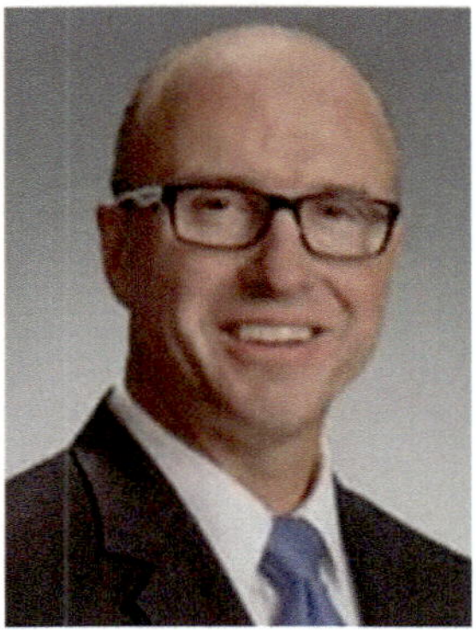

Brian J. Dunkin, MD
2015–2016

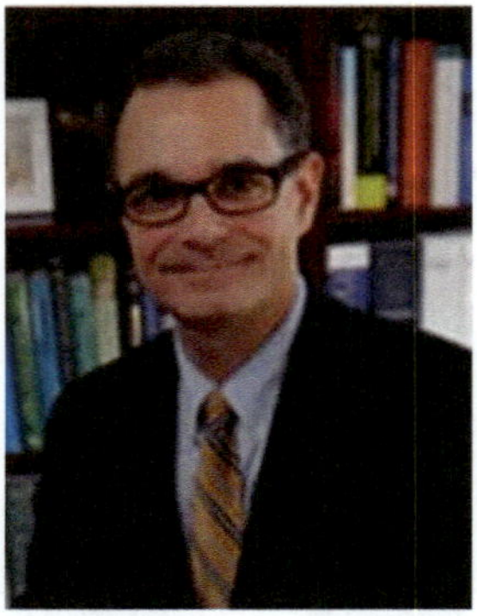

Daniel J. Scott, MD
2016–2017

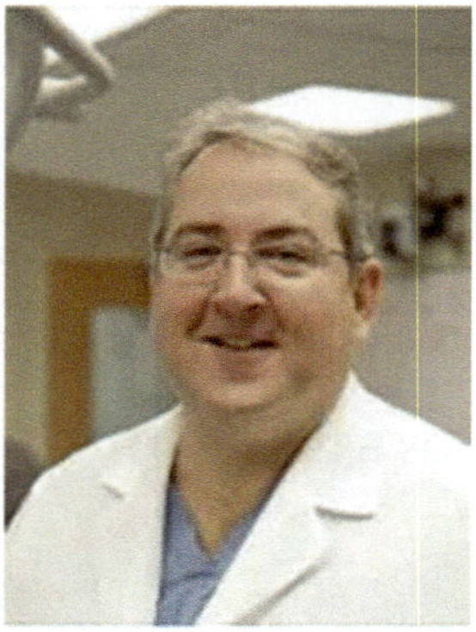

Daniel B. Jones, MD
2017–2018

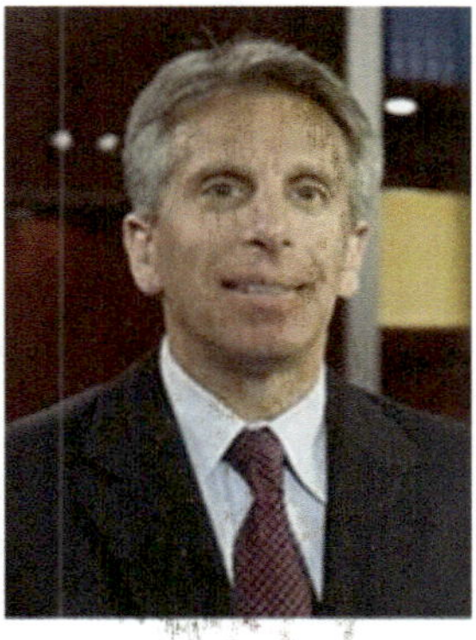

Jeffrey M. Marks, MD
2018–2019

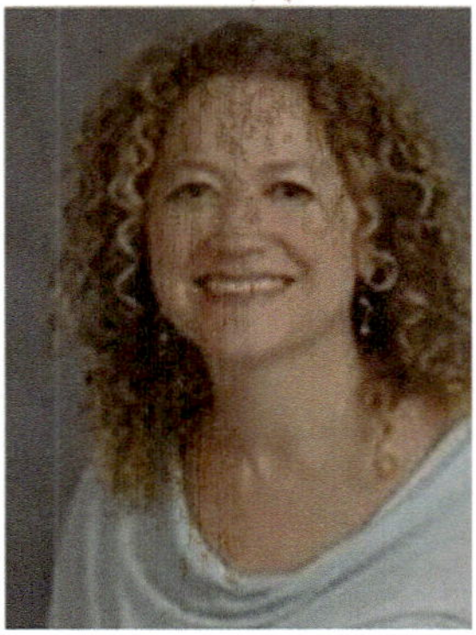

Aurora Pryor, MD
2019–2020

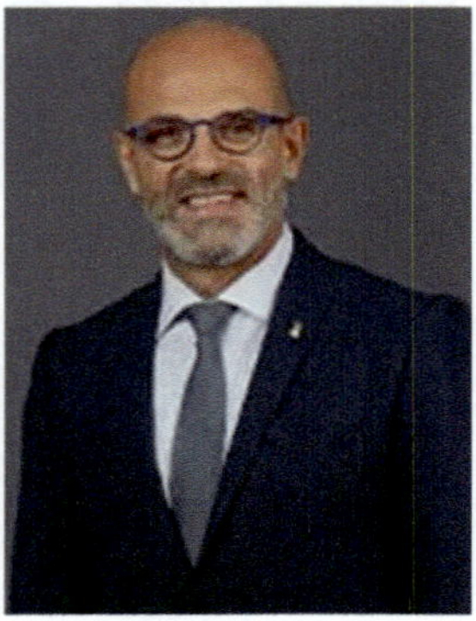

Horacio Asbun, MD
2020–2021

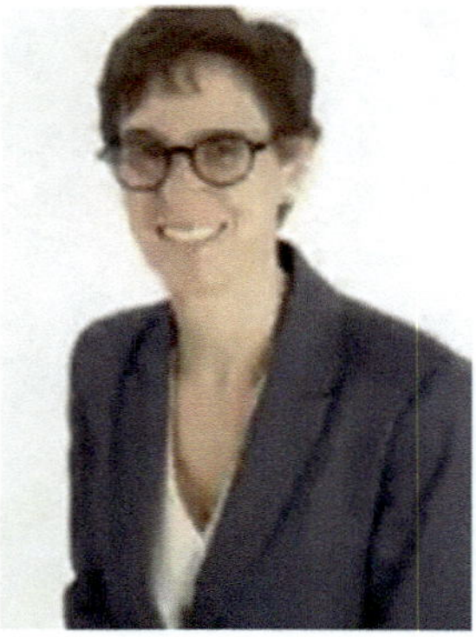

Liane Feldman, MD
2021–2022

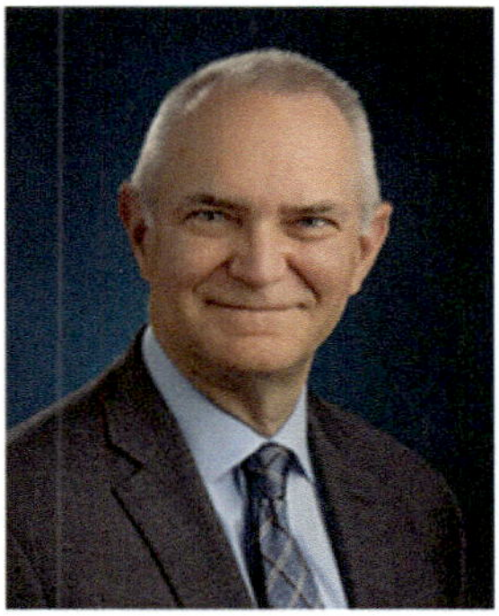

John Mellinger, MD
2022–2023

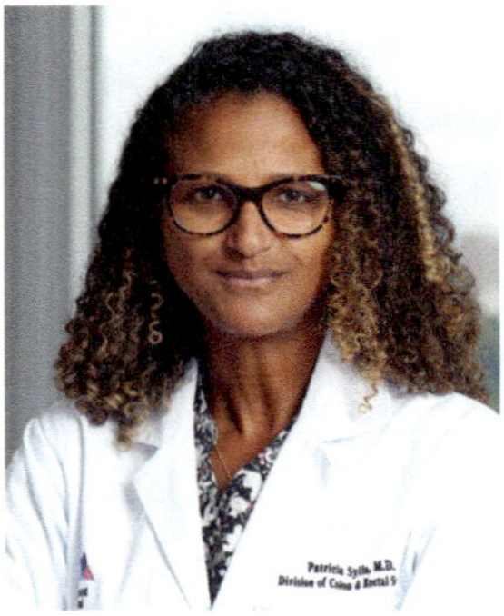

Patricia Sylla MD
2023–2024

Introduction By: Aurora Pryor MD, SAGES Past President (2019–2020)

I am so excited to see this SAGES' manual come to fruition. SAGES is one of the first organizations in surgery to not just embrace techniques and technologies, for our clinical excellence, or research initiatives to build academic strength but also skills to help us build our leadership acumen and excel as surgical leaders. It has been rewarding to see surgeons learn their leadership basics through SAGES and then ascend into leadership roles across the house of surgery. In 2019, we expanded the "We are SAGES" taskforce to include not just diversity, equity, and inclusion, but also the leadership skills to build our future diverse leaders. The newly minted DLPD (Diversity, Leadership, and Professional Development) Committee worked tirelessly to create this manual to help us do just that. The sections in the book start with the basics: Leading Yourself. This section focuses on the foundations of a successful surgical practice. It then expands into Leading Others and, eventually, Leading Systems. This is the typical progression throughout a career as a surgical leader, and I think we have insights for almost every level of surgical leader. Integrating leadership skills from the first stages of your career will set you up for success and immense career satisfaction. I'd personally like to thank all of the authors and the SAGES DLPD Committee for their amazing effort with this manual and share my appreciation for a great tool for building surgical leaders. This manual is the highlights of an MBA—in one easy-to-access location.

Contents

1 **What Is the Mastery Program?** 1
Theofano Zoumpou and Daniel B. Jones

Part I Leading Yourself—Deciding Type of Practice

2 **Understanding Different Practice Types: Private Practice**. 11
Eric Velazquez

3 **Academic Surgical Practice** 23
Ann M. Rogers

4 **Locum Tenens Practice**. 31
Ann M. Rogers and Victoria R. Rendell

5 **Techniques for Negotiating Contracts**. 39
Michael C. Cantrell, Ijeoma A. Ejeh, and Ruchir Puri

6 **Employment Red Flags**. 49
Aaron M. Alford

7 **Financial Considerations When Choosing a Practice** . . . 53
Ruchir Puri and Alia P. Qureshi

8 **Excelling in Training**. 69
Alexandre K. Wang, Dirir H. Abdullahi, Sasha Corbin, and Charis Ripley-Hager

9 **Establishing a Military Surgical Career**. 85
Danielle B. Holt and Andrew T. Schlussel

Part II Leading Yourself—Promotion Across Systems

10 Achieving Promotion Within Different Systems 113
Danny Mou and Scott Davis

11 Strategies to Build a Practice 127
Shawn Tsuda and Jerome Lyn-Sue

12 Practice Adaptation During Crisis 141
Cedrek McFadden, Kenric Murayama, and Shanu Kothari

13 Developing Society Relationships 153
Crystal N. Johnson-Mann

Part III Leading Yourself—Deciding Scope of Practice

14 Determining Scope of Practice and Roles Involved 163
Gregory Leya, Matthew Hutter, and Jahnavi Srinivasan

15 Integrating New Technology and Procedures into Your Practice 171
Benjamin Crisp and Jacquelyn Turner

16 HR, Conflict Resolution, Prioritization, Leveraging New Strengths 189
Angela M. Hanna and Krysta M. Sutyak

17 Utilization of Advancement Opportunities, Expertise, and Marketing to Establish a Practice ... 205
Candice Chipman

Part IV Leading Others—Managing Your Work Environment

18 Evaluating and Assessing Your Team 215
Christopher DuCoin

19 Operationalizing Your Team 233
Vasanth Stalin, Nivedha Muralikrishnan, and Matthew Kroh

20 Effective Team Management 249
Juliet Holder-Haynes and Monique Hassan

21 Establishing an Organizational Culture 265
Eliel Arrey, Shaneeta M. Johnson, and John D. Mellinger

Part V Leading Others—Policy and Administration

22 Policies and Procedures 287
Erica R. H. Sutton

23 Managing Difficult Personalities in the Workplace 297
Mobola Oyefule

24 Dealing Effectively with Challenges 309
Abier A. Abdelnaby and Julie Ann Sosa

Part VI Leading Others—Engagement/Consensus Building

25 Organizational Strategic Planning 329
Danny Mou, Jon C. Gould, Deidra J. Sampson, and Edward Lin

26 Achieving Effective Data Analysis and Research 343
Laura Fischer

27 Leading Surgical Education Teams 379
Clarence E. Clark and Adrian G. Dan

28 Managing Superiors and Your Team 393
Mai Al Khadem and Mujjahid Abbas

29 Goal Implementation 407
Judy Chen

Part VII Leading Systems—Learning Local Context

30 Managing Human Resources and Organizational Talent 417
Joon K. Shim and Ian S. Soriano

31 Leading Systems: Assessment, Innovation, and Sustainability 429
Shukri H. A. Dualeh, Brian T. Fry, and Dana A. Telem

32 Accountability and Effective Communication 441
Juan S. Barajas-Gamboa

33 Educational Opportunities in Strategy and Leadership 459
John R. Romanelli

Part VIII Leading Systems—Building an Efficient System/ Organizational Structure

34 Building an Effective Administration 467
Terrence Fullum and Robert B. Lim

35 Navigating an Academic Career in Surgery 477
Shaneeta M. Johnson, Juan S. Barajas-Gamboa, Aaron M. Alford, and Susan Pories

36 Organizational Change Management in HealthCare 511
Sivamainthan "Siva" Vithiananthan

37 Strategic Thinking and Leadership 535
Shaneeta M. Johnson

38 Good Governance 553
Karenia Landa and Jacob A. Greenberg

39 Creating Opportunities for Tomorrow's Leaders in Surgery 563
S. D. Schwaitzberg and Nargis Hossain

Part IX Leading Systems—Healthcare Delivery

40 Health Policy and Advocacy 581
L. Renee Hilton and Ross Goldberg

41 Ensuring Quality Surgical Care 593
Juliane Bingener-Casey and Haris Khwaja

42 Surgical Quality Considerations in the United Kingdom 611
Michael G. Fadel, Matyas Fehervari, and Haris Khwaja

43 Social Determinants of Health in Surgery 625
Wendy Greene and Michael A. Edwards

44 The Fundamentals of Leadership Development Curriculum 641
Jenny M. Shao and Yewande Alimi

45 Global Leadership and Practice Considerations 655
Linda P. Zhang, Sahle Griffith, and Wesley P. Francis

46 International Medical Graduates: Strategies to Mitigate Challenges in Medical Education 675
Carolina Torres Perez-Iglesias, Fariha Sheikh, and Daniel B. Jones

47 Enhancing the Surgical Value Chain Through Partnership with Industry 685
Sharona B. Ross

48 Diversity, Equity, and Inclusion: Transparency, Measures, and Accountability 701
Shaneeta M. Johnson and Henry Lin

49 Sustainable Surgery 723
Jonathan Vandenberg, Shaneeta M. Johnson, Emmanuel Gabriel, and Patricia Sylla

Index 741

Contributors

Mujjahid Abbas Bariatric Division, Department of Surgery, University Hospitals Cleveland Medical Center, Case Western Reserve University School of Medicine, Cleveland, OH, USA

Abier A. Abdelnaby Department of Surgery, Montefiore Medical Center, The University Hospital for Albert Einstein College of Medicine, Bronx, NY, USA

Dirir H. Abdullahi Department of Surgery, Morehouse School of Medicine, Grady Memorial Hospital, Atlanta, GA, USA

Aaron M. Alford Department of Surgery, Morehouse School of Medicine, Atlanta, GA, USA

Yewande Alimi Department of Surgery, Georgetown University School of Medicine, Washington, DC, USA

Eliel Arrey John P. and Katherine G. McGovern Medical School, Health Science Center at Houston, University of Texas, Austin, TX, USA

Juan S. Barajas-Gamboa Department of General Surgery, Cleveland Clinic Abu Dhabi, Abu Dhabi, United Arab Emirates

Juliane Bingener-Casey Department of Surgery, Mayo Clinic College of Medicine and Science, Rochester, MN, USA

Michael C. Cantrell Department of Surgery, University of Florida College of Medicine, Jacksonville, FL, USA

Judy Chen Department of Surgery, University of Washington School of Medicine, Seattle, WA, USA

Candice Chipman Abington Jefferson Health, Abington, PA, USA

Clarence E. Clark General Surgery Residency Program, Dignity Health System, Chandler, AZ, USA

Department of Surgery, Creighton School of Medicine, Phoenix, AZ, USA

Sasha Corbin Department of Surgery, Morehouse School of Medicine, Grady Memorial Hospital, Atlanta, GA, USA

Benjamin Crisp Department of Surgery, Tulane University School of Medicine, New Orleans, LA, USA

Adrian G. Dan Weight Management Institute—Bariatric Care Center, Akron, OH, USA

Akron City Hospital Campus, Akron, OH, USA

Northeast Ohio Medical Universities, Rootstown, OH, USA

Scott Davis Emory University Department of Surgery, Atlanta, GA, USA

Shukri H. A. Dualeh Department of Surgery, University of Michigan, Ann Arbor, MI, USA

Christopher DuCoin Department of Surgery, University of South Florida, Tampa, FL, USA

Michael A. Edwards Division of Advanced GI and Bariatric Surgery, Department of Surgery, Mayo Clinic, Jacksonville, FL, USA

Ijeoma A. Ejeh Ferncreek General Surgery, Cape Fear Health System, Fayetteville, NC, USA

Michael G. Fadel Department of Bariatric and Metabolic Surgery, Chelsea and Westminster Hospital, London, UK

Imperial College London, London, UK

Matyas Fehervari Department of Bariatric and Metabolic Surgery, Chelsea and Westminster Hospital, London, UK

Imperial College London, London, UK

Laura Fischer OU Health Metabolic & Bariatric Surgery Program, University of Oklahoma, Oklahoma City, OK, USA

Department of Surgery, University of Oklahoma, Oklahoma City, OK, USA

Wesley P. Francis Department of Surgery, UWI School of Clinical Medicine and Research, Princess Margaret Hospital, Nassau, Bahamas

Brian T. Fry Department of Surgery, University of Michigan, Ann Arbor, MI, USA

Terrence Fullum Department of Surgery, Howard University College of Medicine, Howard University Hospital, Washington, DC, USA

Emmanuel Gabriel Department of Surgery, Mayo Clinic Florida, Jacksonville, FL, USA

Ross Goldberg Department of Surgery, Jackson Health System, University of Miami, Miami, FL, USA

Jon C. Gould Division of Minimally Invasive and Gastrointestinal Surgery, Department of Surgery, Medical College of Wisconsin, Milwaukee, WI, USA

Jacob A. Greenberg Duke University in the Division of Minimally Invasive Surgery, Durham, NC, USA

Wendy Greene Department of Surgery, Emory University, Atlanta, GA, USA

Sahle Griffith Department of Surgery, Faculty of Medical Sciences, University of the West Indies, Cave Hill Campus, Queen Elizabeth Hospital, Barbados, Bridgetown, Barbados

Angela M. Hanna Department of Surgery, University of Nebraska Medical Center, Omaha, NE, USA

Department of Pediatric Surgery, Childrens' Hospital and Medical Center, Omaha, NE, USA

Monique Hassan Department of Surgery, Baylor College of Medicine, Scott and White Memorial Hospital and Clinic, Temple, TX, USA

L. Renee Hilton Bariatric Surgery, Center for Obesity and Metabolism, Augusta University Medical Center, Augusta, GA, USA

Digestive Health Center, Augusta University Medical Center, Augusta, GA, USA

Department of Surgery, Medical College of Georgia at Augusta University, Augusta, GA, USA

Juliet Holder-Haynes Michael E Debakey Department of Surgery, Baylor College of Medicine, Houston, TX, USA

Danielle B. Holt Uniformed Services University, Bethesda, MD, USA

Nargis Hossain Department of Surgery, University at Buffalo Jacobs School of Medicine and Biomedical Sciences, The State University of New York, Buffalo, NY, USA

Matthew Hutter Department of Surgery, Massachusetts General Hospital, Boston, MA, USA

Shaneeta M. Johnson Department of Surgery, Morehouse School of Medicine, Atlanta, GA, USA

Satcher Health Leadership Institute, Morehouse School of Medicine, Atlanta, GA, USA

Crystal N. Johnson-Mann Department of Surgery, University of Florida College of Medicine, Gainesville, FL, USA

Daniel B. Jones Department of Surgery, Rutgers New Jersey Medical School, Newark, NJ, USA

Department of Surgery, University Hospital, Rutgers New Jersey Medical School, Newark, NJ, USA

Mai Al Khadem Bariatric Division, Department of Surgery, University Hospitals Cleveland Medical Center, Case Western Reserve University School of Medicine, Cleveland, OH, USA

Haris Khwaja Chelsea and Westminster Hospital & Imperial College, London, UK

Department of Bariatric and Metabolic Surgery, Chelsea and Westminster Hospital, London, UK

Imperial College London, London, UK

Shanu Kothari Department of Surgery, Prisma Health, Greenville, SC, USA

Matthew Kroh Cleveland Clinic, Cleveland, OH, USA

Karenia Landa Duke University in the Division of Minimally Invasive Surgery, Durham, NC, USA

Gregory Leya Department of Surgery, Massachusetts General Hospital, Boston, MA, USA

Robert B. Lim Wake Forest University, Atrium Health Carolinas, Department of Surgery, Charlotte, NC, USA

Edward Lin Division of General and GI Surgery, Department of Surgery, Emory University, Atlanta, GA, USA

Henry Lin Medical Corps, US Navy, Canton, CN, USA

Jerome Lin-Sue Penn State University, Hershey, PA, USA

Cedrek McFadden Department of Surgery, Prisma Health, Greenville, SC, USA

University of South Carolina School of Medicine Greenville, Greenville, SC, USA

John D. Mellinger American Board of Surgery, and Department of Surgery Southern Illinois University School of Medicine, Springfield, IL, USA

Danny Mou Emory University Department of Surgery, Atlanta, GA, USA

Minimally Invasive Surgery, Department of Surgery, Emory University, Atlanta, GA, USA

Nivedha Muralikrishnan Melmaruvathur, Tamil Nadu, India

Kenric Murayama Department of Surgery, John A. Burns School of Medicine, University of Hawaii, Honolulu, HI, USA

Mobola Oyefule General and GI Surgery, Emory University School of Medicine, Atlanta, GA, USA

Carolina Torres Perez-Iglesias Department of Surgery, Beth Israel Deaconess Medical Center, Boston, MA, USA

Susan Pories Department of Surgery, Rutgers New Jersey Medical School, Newark, NJ, USA

Ruchir Puri Department of Surgery, University of Florida College of Medicine, Jacksonville, FL, USA

Alia P. Qureshi Division of General and GI Surgery: Foregut Surgery, Oregon Health and Science University, Portland, OR, USA

Victoria R. Rendell Division of Minimally Invasive Surgery, Department of Surgery, University of Wisconsin School of Medicine and Public Health, Madison, WI, USA

Charis Ripley-Hager Department of Surgery, Lewis Katz School of Medicine at Temple University, Philadelphia, PA, USA

Ann M. Rogers, MD Department of Surgery, Penn State Health, Hershey, PA, USA

John R. Romanelli Department of Surgery, University of Massachusetts Chan Medical School—Baystate Medical Center, Springfield, MA, USA

Sharona B. Ross Digestive Health Institute, AdventHealth Tampa, Tampa, FL, USA

Deidra J. Sampson Emory Healthcare, Atlanta, GA, USA

Andrew T. Schlussel HCA Florida Jacksonville Surgical Specialists, Jacksonville, FL, USA

S. D. Schwaitzberg Department of Surgery, University at Buffalo Jacobs School of Medicine and Biomedical Sciences, The State University of New York, Buffalo, NY, USA

Jenny M. Shao Department of Surgery, University of Michigan, Ann Arbor, MI, USA

Fariha Sheikh Department of Surgery, University Hospital, Rutgers New Jersey Medical School, Newark, NJ, USA

Joon K. Shim Bassett Healthcare Network, Cooperstown, NY, USA

Ian S. Soriano Department of Surgery, University of California San Francisco, San Francisco, CA, USA

Julie Ann Sosa Department of Medicine, Philip R. Lee Institute for Health Policy Studies, University of California San Francisco (UCSF), San Francisco, CA, USA

Department of Surgery, Philip R. Lee Institute for Health Policy Studies, University of California San Francisco (UCSF), San Francisco, CA, USA

Jahnavi Srinivasan Department of Surgery, Emory Healthcare, Atlanta, GA, USA

Vasanth Stalin, MD, FACS, FASMBS Ascension St. Mary's Hospital, Saginaw, MI, USA

Erica R. H. Sutton Morehouse School of Medicine, Atlanta, GA, USA

Krysta M. Sutyak Department of Surgery, University of Nebraska Medical Center, Omaha, NE, USA

Patricia Sylla Division of Colorectal Surgery, Mount Sinai, New York, NY, USA

Dana A. Telem Department of Surgery, University of Michigan, Ann Arbor, MI, USA

Shawn Tsuda Valley Health System General Surgery Residency Program, Las Vegas, NV, USA

Jacquelyn Turner Department of Surgery, Tulane University School of Medicine, New Orleans, LA, USA

Jonathan Vandenberg Department of Surgery, Mayo Clinic Florida, Jacksonville, FL, USA

Eric Velazquez, MD, MBA, FACS, FASMBS Longstreet Clinic Center for Weight Management, Gainesville, GA, USA

Medical Director of Metabolic and Bariatric Surgery, Northside Hospital Duluth, Duluth, GA, USA

Sivamainthan "Siva" Vithiananthan Department of Surgery, Cambridge Health Alliance, Harvard Medical School, Cambridge, MA, USA

Alexandre K. Wang Department of Surgery, Morehouse School of Medicine, Grady Memorial Hospital, Atlanta, GA, USA

Linda P. Zhang Department of Surgery, Icahn School of Medicine at Mount Sinai, Mount Sinai Hospital, New York, NY, USA

Theofano Zoumpou Department of Surgery, Rutgers New Jersey Medical School, Newark, NJ, USA

1 What Is the Mastery Program?

Theofano Zoumpou and Daniel B. Jones

Overview

Welcome to this manual on Strategy and Leadership for surgeons, part of the Society of American Gastrointestinal and Endoscopic Surgery (SAGES) Masters Program (Fig. 1.1). At SAGES, we recognize that the medical field is constantly evolving, and it is crucial for surgeons to stay up-to-date with the latest techniques and knowledge. With this in mind, we have designed the SAGES Masters Program as a platform of asynchronous learning that anyone can access at their availability and per their personal interest [1]. Our aim is to foster and facilitate high-quality postgraduate and life-long education among surgeons, and this manual is a significant step toward achieving this goal.

The SAGES Masters program currently has 13 pathways, including acute care, biliary, bariatrics, colon, foregut, hernia, flexible endoscopy, and robotic surgery (Fig. 1.2).

T. Zoumpou (✉) · D. B. Jones
Department of Surgery, Rutgers New Jersey Medical School, Newark, NJ, USA
e-mail: theo.zoumpou@rutgers.edu; Tz275@njms.rutgers.edu; daniel.jones@njms.rutgers.edu; Dj477@njms.rutgers.edu

S. M. Johnson et al. (eds.), *The SAGES Manual of Strategy and Leadership*, https://doi.org/10.1007/978-3-031-62359-2_1

Fig. 1.1 SAGES Masters Program logo

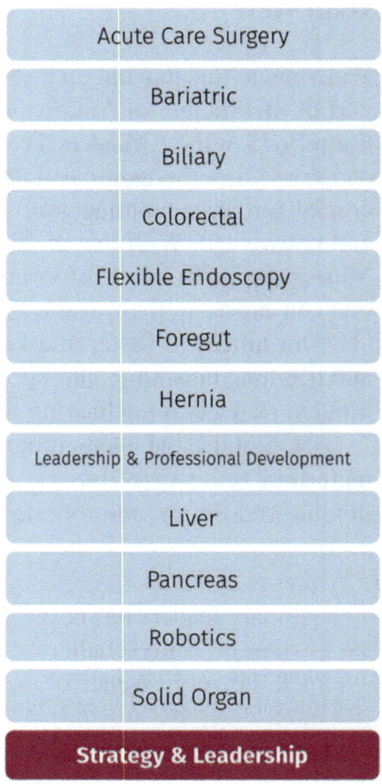

Fig. 1.2 SAGES Masters Program clinical pathways

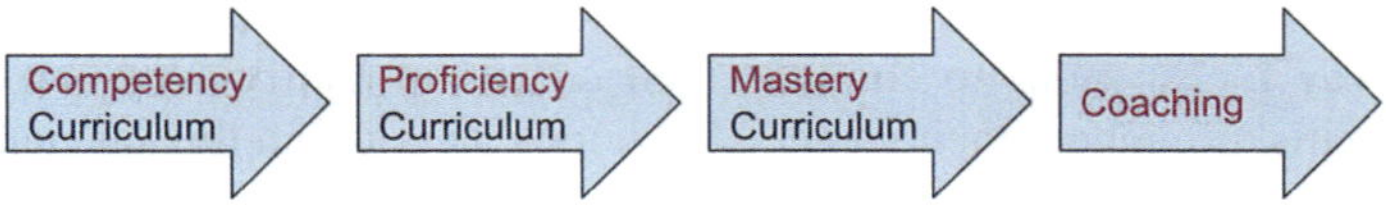

Fig. 1.3 SAGES Masters Program progression

Each pathway is divided into three levels of targeted performance: competency, proficiency, and expertise. The levels originate from the Dreyfus model of skill acquisition, which has five stages: novice, advanced beginner, competency, proficiency, and expertise [2]. The SAGES Masters Program is based on the three more advanced stages of skills acquisition: competency, proficiency, and mastery (Fig. 1.3).

This manual focuses on Strategy and Leadership, which are critical aspects of a surgeon's role. Effective leadership skills are essential for managing complex cases, leading teams, and ultimately improving patient outcomes. This manual covers various topics, including strategic planning, communication, conflict resolution, and team building. We have carefully curated the content of this manual to ensure that it is informative, engaging, and applicable to the challenges that surgeons face in their everyday work. In addition, our team of surgical experts and leaders has drawn from their extensive experience and knowledge to provide practical insights and guidance.

In the ever-evolving healthcare system, leadership has emerged as an indispensable element for achieving excellence, driving innovation, and fostering a culture of inclusivity. Now more than ever, as surgical leadership undergoes a profound transformation propelled by the forces of diversity, the empowerment of women, and other previously marginalized groups, investing in influential and visionary leaders has become paramount [3, 4]. This transformation has not only challenged traditional norms but has also redefined the very essence of surgical leadership. Embracing this newfound diversity, we unlock an immense potential to revolutionize surgical practices, enhance patient care, and shape the future of surgery in an ever more patient-centric, compassionate, and transformative manner.

We believe that the SAGES Masters Program is an excellent way for surgeons to continue their education and develop their skills throughout their careers. We hope that you find this manual to be a valuable resource and an essential step in your journey toward becoming a successful leader in the field of surgery.

Strategy and Leadership Curriculum

This program has been designed to meet the critical and well-described need for surgeons to develop leadership and strategic skills to excel in their roles as clinicians, educators, and healthcare leaders, offering a longitudinal educational opportunity [5, 6].

Surgeons are expected to thrive in a multidisciplinary environment and provide excellent patient care while working with a team of healthcare professionals. Effective leadership and strategic skills are integral to this process, but unfortunately, they are not always part of surgical training programs [7]. This is where the SAGES Masters Program on Strategy and Leadership comes in. Our program provides materials created by faculty with expertise in leadership education, thus providing high-quality content to help you develop the skills needed to excel in your profession.

The SAGES Masters Program and the present SAGES manual on Strategy and Leadership cover various critical topics, including general leadership, managerial skills, business management, communication, teamwork, interpersonal skills, and professionalism [8–11]. They also address self-awareness, personal growth, and wellness, recognizing the importance of physician well-being in achieving optimal outcomes and patient safety [12].

By providing these resources, the SAGES Masters Program aims to effectively promote personal and organizational success. Developing your leadership and strategic skills will improve not only your clinical practice but also your ability to educate others and lead your team effectively. We are proud to offer this resource to surgeons worldwide and are committed to providing the tools to succeed as surgical leaders.

Facebook™ Groups

In addition to the materials provided online and in this manual, the SAGES Masters Program also includes Facebook™ groups. These groups make use of a popular platform to bring together professionals from all over the country and beyond, allowing them to discuss topics, share concerns, and exchange valuable feedback. In addition, participants can connect with like-minded individuals and engage in discussions about various aspects of surgery and leadership. These groups are moderated by experienced leaders in the field and provide a supportive environment where participants can ask questions and interact with their peers.

The SAGES Masters Program Facebook™ groups are a valuable addition to the program, fostering a sense of community and providing the opportunity to learn from others' experiences. We encourage all participants to take advantage of these groups and connect with their colleagues. The community aspect of the program is an essential component of the learning experience, and we are committed to providing a supportive and collaborative environment for all.

Conclusions

This SAGES manual on Strategy and Leadership for surgeons is a critical addition to the field of surgical education. Strategy and leadership are integral aspects of the surgical career, yet they are not typically included in formal curricula. This manual, which was put together by expert surgical leaders and educators, addresses this gap by providing a comprehensive resource on strategy and leadership for surgeons. Furthermore, the manual and SAGES Masters program offers a platform for asynchronous, longitudinal learning and networking, allowing surgeons to learn at their own pace and connect with colleagues worldwide. This manual is part of the SAGES University initiative to foster high-quality life-long surgical education, and we are proud to provide this resource to the surgical community. Thank you for joining us on this journey toward becoming a successful leader in the field of surgery.

SAGES Takeaway

- Continuous Learning Challenge: As healthcare professionals, once trained in a specific subspecialty or after several years in practice, acquiring new procedures, skills, or expanding one's scope of practice can become increasingly challenging.
- SAGES Masters Program: The SAGES Masters Program is designed to offer a structured approach to lifelong learning for surgeons, providing them with the tools and resources needed to stay updated and proficient in their field.
- Strategy Pathway: This manual equips surgeons with essential tools and insights to develop effective and forward-thinking strategies, enabling them to navigate complex healthcare environments and drive meaningful improvements in patient care and surgical practice.
- Leadership Pathway: This manual introduces the Leadership Pathway, which aims to enhance a surgeon's knowledge and skills in leading and driving meaningful change within the medical community and healthcare systems.
- Diverse, Equitable, and Inclusive (DEI) Considerations: In addition to leadership development, the manual also covers essential topics related to the significance of Diversity, Equity, and Inclusion (DEI) within the medical profession, underlining their pivotal role in shaping the future of healthcare.

These key takeaways set the stage for the SAGES manual, emphasizing the importance of lifelong learning, leadership development, and a commitment to DEI in the evolving landscape of surgery and healthcare.

References

1. Jones DB, Stefanidis D, Korndorffer JR Jr, Dimick JB, Jacob BP, Schultz L, et al. SAGES University MASTERS program: a structured curriculum for deliberate, lifelong learning. Surg Endosc. 2017;31:3061–71.
2. Dreyfus SE. The five-stage model of adult skill acquisition. Bull Sci Technol Soc. 2004;24:177–81.

3. Pories SE, Turner PL, Greenberg CC, Babu MA, Parangi S. Leadership in American surgery: women are rising to the top. Ann Surg. 2019;269:199–205.
4. Morris-Wiseman LF, Dent D, Nfonsam VN, Arora TK. Leadership diversity in the Association of Program Directors in surgery: a report of progress. J Surg Educ. 2022;79:e109–15.
5. Sachdeva AK. Acquiring skills in new procedures and technology: the challenge and the opportunity. Arch Surg. 2005;140:387–9.
6. Dimick JB, Scheske J, Lemak CH. Developing leaders in surgery: comment on "training future surgeons for management roles". Arch Surg. 2012;147:944–5.
7. Torres-Landa S, Wairiri L, Cochran A, Brasel KJ. Evaluation of leadership curricula in general surgery residency programs. Am J Surg. 2021;222:916–21.
8. Hanna WC, Mulder DS, Fried GM, Elhilali M, Khwaja KA. Training future surgeons for management roles: the resident-surgeon-manager conference. Arch Surg. 2012;147:940–4.
9. Hill DA M, Jimenez J-C, Cohn SM, Price MR. How to be a leader: a course for residents. Cureus. 2018;10:e3067.
10. Saad AR, Baisden CE, Dent DL, Khoury L, Panzo M, Cohn SM. Evolution of a novel business leadership course for general surgery chief residents. Cureus. 2018;10:e3559.
11. Bearman M, O'Brien R, Anthony A, Civil I, Flanagan B, Jolly B, et al. Learning surgical communication, leadership and teamwork through simulation. J Surg Educ. 2012;69:201–7.
12. Mahmoud NN, Rothenberger D. From burnout to well-being: a focus on resilience. Clin Colon Rectal Surg. 2019;32:415–23.

Part I

Leading Yourself—Deciding Type of Practice

Understanding Different Practice Types: Private Practice

2

Eric Velazquez

Definition and Types of Private Practices

Private practice in the field of medicine is a distinctive model where the physician takes on the role of a self-employed practitioner. This can take the form of a solo practice or a group practice, each offering its own set of advantages and challenges. In this extended discussion, we will delve deeper into the nuances of private practice, exploring the key characteristics of both solo and group practices, the responsibilities they entail, and the factors that influence their success.

Solo Practice

Solo practice, as the name suggests, involves a single physician who operates independently. This setup offers the physician a high degree of autonomy and control over the direction and

E. Velazquez (✉)
Longstreet Clinic Center for Weight Management,
Gainesville, GA, USA

Medical Director of Metabolic and Bariatric Surgery,
Northside Hospital Duluth, Duluth, GA, USA

S. M. Johnson et al. (eds.), *The SAGES Manual of Strategy and Leadership*, https://doi.org/10.1007/978-3-031-62359-2_2

growth of their practice. In essence, they are the captain of their own ship, making decisions related to patient care, practice development, and more.

However, with great autonomy comes great responsibility. In a solo practice, the physician bears the full weight of running the operation. This encompasses not only the clinical aspects of patient care but also administrative tasks and human resource management. From appointment scheduling to medical record keeping, and from hiring staff to managing finances, the solo practitioner wears many hats.

One significant challenge of solo practice is the financial risk it carries. Despite its relatively small scale compared with larger healthcare organizations, solo practitioners must contend with substantial financial burdens. This includes investments in technology such as electronic health record (EHR) systems, medical equipment, and compliance with ever-evolving healthcare regulations. The solo practitioner must navigate these financial challenges with prudence to ensure the sustainability of their practice.

Group Practice

In contrast, group practice involves two or more physicians collaborating to provide medical care within the same facility. This collaborative approach can take various forms, such as an association or a partnership. In group practices, physicians share the overhead expenses, which can help distribute the financial burden more evenly among the members.

Partnerships within group practices extend beyond the sharing of costs. Incomes are also shared, as are personal and medical liabilities. This not only spreads the financial risk but also fosters a sense of camaraderie and collective responsibility among the practitioners.

However, as a group practice expands and more physicians join, some of the autonomy and decision-making authority that solo practitioners enjoy may diminish. Larger group practices often necessitate more structured governance and administrative processes. Yet, they offer advantages such as economies of scale and access to a broader pool of expertise.

The Allure of Private Practice

Private practice is an attractive option for physicians with an entrepreneurial spirit. It allows them to engage not only in the clinical aspects of their profession but also in the strategic design and management of their practice. For those who relish the challenge of building and growing a medical practice from the ground up, private practice can be deeply rewarding.

However, it is crucial to note that private practitioners must possess a certain degree of risk tolerance. The success of a private practice can be influenced by a multitude of factors, including fluctuations in productivity, shifts in patient demographics, and changing healthcare regulations. These variables directly impact the practice's financial stability and, by extension, the physician's income.

One of the significant attractions of private practice is the potential for higher income when compared with salaried or employed positions. With the autonomy to make decisions about billing, fees, and practice growth, private practitioners have the opportunity to maximize their earnings. However, this potential for higher income comes with the caveat of managing the associated financial risks and responsibilities.

Advantages of Private Practice for Physicians

Private practice offers numerous advantages for physicians that make it an attractive career path. These advantages include the following:

1. **Autonomy and Flexibility:** Private practice grants physicians a high degree of autonomy and flexibility. They have the freedom to make decisions about the type of services they offer,

the patient population they serve, and the hours they work. This level of control allows physicians to tailor their practice to align with their professional and personal preferences. For those who value independence and want to take a more personalized approach to patient care, private practice is an ideal choice.

2. **Financial Benefits:** Private practice can be financially rewarding for physicians. They have the ability to set their own prices for medical services, which can result in higher earnings compared with their hospital-employed counterparts. Additionally, private practice physicians often benefit from tax deductions and financial incentives that are not available to physicians working within hospital or healthcare organization settings. This financial independence can be particularly appealing for those looking to maximize their income potential.
3. **Closer Relationships with Patients:** Private practice allows physicians to foster closer relationships with their patients. Unlike hospital-employed physicians who may have limited time for each patient due to heavy caseloads, private practice physicians often have the luxury of spending more time with their patients. This additional time enables deeper patient–physician connections, better communication, and a more comprehensive understanding of each patient's healthcare needs. Consequently, this can lead to improved patient outcomes and higher levels of patient satisfaction.
4. **Greater Professional Satisfaction:** Owning and operating a private practice can provide physicians with a profound sense of professional satisfaction. The ability to take ownership of their practice and make critical decisions about patient care and practice management can be deeply fulfilling. Physicians in private practice often take pride in building and growing their own healthcare businesses, resulting in a heightened sense of accomplishment and job satisfaction.
5. **Practice Customization:** Private practitioners have the flexibility to customize their practice to align with their areas of expertise and personal interests. This allows them to focus on specific medical specialties or niche patient populations, pro-

viding specialized care that can be personally rewarding. Moreover, they can implement innovative approaches and treatment modalities that align with their values and vision for healthcare.

6. **Control Over Practice Environment:** Private practice physicians have control over the physical and operational aspects of their practice. They can design their office space, choose their medical equipment, and create a welcoming environment that reflects their approach to patient care. This control extends to the selection and management of their support staff, fostering a practice culture that aligns with their professional goals and values.

Disadvantages of Private Practice for Physicians

As anticipated, even with its myriad advantages, private practice for physicians does come with its fair share of drawbacks. In the following sections, we will delve deeper into these disadvantages and provide actionable recommendations on how physicians can effectively address or mitigate these challenges in their pursuit of a successful private practice.

1. **Financial Risk:** Starting a private practice can indeed be financially demanding. Physicians often need to secure funding through loans, personal savings, or other means to cover the initial setup costs. To mitigate this risk, consider the following steps:
   - **Create a Detailed Business Plan:** Develop a comprehensive business plan that outlines your practice's financial needs, revenue projections, and strategies for sustainable growth. Seek assistance from financial advisors or consultants to ensure that your plan is sound.
   - **Secure Adequate Financing:** Explore various financing options, including small business loans, grants, or partnerships with investors. Research local and national healthcare funding programs that may offer support to new practices.

- **Budget Wisely:** Maintain strict financial discipline by budgeting effectively. Monitor expenses, prioritize essential investments, and consider cost-saving measures without compromising the quality of patient care.

2. **Administrative Responsibilities:** Managing the administrative aspects of a private practice can be time-consuming and complex. To handle these responsibilities more efficiently:
   - **Hire Administrative Staff:** Consider hiring experienced administrative professionals to handle tasks such as billing, insurance claims, and patient record management. Outsourcing certain administrative functions can also reduce the workload.
   - **Implement Practice Management Software:** Invest in modern practice management software to streamline administrative tasks. These tools can help with appointment scheduling, billing, and EHRs, saving time and reducing errors.
   - **Continuing Education:** Stay updated on healthcare regulations and administrative best practices through continuing education courses and workshops. This knowledge will enable you to navigate administrative challenges effectively.
3. **Limited Resources:** Private practice physicians may face limitations in terms of resources and access to advanced medical technology. To address this issue:
   - **Collaborate with Medical Facilities:** Build partnerships or collaborative agreements with local hospitals or medical centers. This can provide access to specialized equipment and resources when needed for patient care.
   - **Leverage Group Purchasing:** Explore group purchasing options with neighboring practices or medical associations. This can help you access medical equipment, supplies, and technology at more competitive rates.
   - **Invest in Key Resources:** Prioritize essential resources that align with your practice's focus. Assess your patient population's needs and invest in equipment or technology that directly benefits your specialty.

4. **Increased Liability:** Private practice physicians face a heightened risk of liability, including malpractice claims. To mitigate this risk:
   - **Maintain Thorough Documentation:** Accurate and detailed patient records can be invaluable in defending against malpractice claims. Implement a robust EHR system and ensure consistent documentation practices.
   - **Invest in Malpractice Insurance:** Consult with an experienced insurance agent to determine the appropriate level of malpractice insurance for your practice. Adequate coverage is essential to protect your assets and reputation.
   - **Implement Risk Management Strategies:** Develop and implement risk management protocols within your practice. Regularly review clinical processes, engage in peer reviews, and identify areas for improvement to minimize the risk of errors or negligence.
   - **Continuing Medical Education:** Stay current with medical best practices and guidelines through ongoing education. This not only enhances patient care but also reduces the likelihood of medical errors leading to liability issues.

Challenges of Starting a Private Practice

Certainly, Let us expand on the challenges of starting a private practice for physicians and provide more detailed insights, along with actionable recommendations for addressing these challenges:

1. **Financing the Practice:** Launching a private practice can be financially demanding. Physicians often need to secure funding through loans or personal savings, which can create a substantial financial burden, especially if the practice does not generate sufficient revenue initially.

   Actionable Recommendations:
   - **Comprehensive Financial Plan:** Create a detailed financial plan that outlines all startup costs, including equipment, licensing fees, and staff salaries. This plan should

also project revenue and expenses for the first few years of operation.

- **Explore Funding Options:** Research various funding sources, including small business loans, grants, and partnerships with investors. Carefully evaluate the terms and interest rates associated with loans to ensure they align with your practice's financial goals.
- **Budget Management:** Implement a strict budgeting strategy to control costs and allocate resources efficiently. Regularly review financial statements to identify areas where cost-saving measures can be applied.

2. **Finding Office Space: Challenge:** Securing suitable office space is crucial for a private practice's success. Physicians must locate a space that is easily accessible to patients, offers ample parking, and meets specific layout and amenity requirements.

   Actionable Recommendations:

   - **Location Analysis:** Conduct a thorough analysis of potential office locations, considering factors such as proximity to target patient demographics, accessibility via public transportation, and parking availability.
   - **Lease Negotiation:** Engage in careful lease negotiations to secure favorable terms and conditions. Seek out commercial real estate agents with expertise in healthcare property leasing to assist in finding the ideal space.
   - **Customization:** Invest in office layout and design that optimizes patient flow, provides a welcoming environment, and accommodates the medical equipment and technology required for your specialty.

3. **Hiring Staff: Challenge:** Building a competent support staff, including nurses, receptionists, and billing specialists, can be challenging, particularly in regions with a shortage of healthcare professionals.

   Actionable Recommendations:

   - **Network and Collaborate:** Build professional networks and collaborate with local medical schools, nursing programs, and healthcare staffing agencies to identify qualified candidates.

- **Competitive Compensation:** Offer competitive compensation packages and benefits to attract and retain top talent. Consider ongoing training and development programs to enhance staff skills.
- **Culture and Team Building:** Create a positive workplace culture that fosters teamwork, communication, and job satisfaction. Engaged and satisfied staff are more likely to provide excellent patient care and contribute to the practice's success.

4. **Building a Patient Base: Challenge:** Establishing a patient base can be a daunting task, especially in areas with intense competition from other healthcare providers. Physicians may need to invest in marketing and advertising efforts to attract new patients.

   Actionable Recommendations:

   - **Strategic Marketing:** Develop a comprehensive marketing plan that includes online and offline strategies. Consider building a professional website, engaging in social media marketing, and collaborating with local community organizations to increase visibility.
   - **Patient Referral Networks:** Establish referral relationships with other healthcare professionals, such as primary care physicians, to gain access to a consistent stream of patients.
   - **Patient-Centered Care:** Prioritize patient satisfaction and quality of care to encourage word-of-mouth referrals. Delighted patients are more likely to recommend your practice to friends and family.

Tips for Running a Successful Private Practice

Starting and running a successful private medical practice can be a rewarding career choice for physicians. To further explore the tips for achieving success in private practice, let us provide a more comprehensive guide with actionable recommendations:

1. Develop a business plan
   - **Set Clear Goals:** Define your practice's mission, vision, and long-term objectives. Specify your target patient population and the medical services you intend to provide.
   - **Financial Projections:** Create detailed financial projections, including revenue forecasts, expenses, and cash flow analysis for the first few years of operation. This will help you secure funding and navigate potential financial challenges.
   - **Contingency Plans:** Identify potential challenges and develop contingency plans for addressing them. Consider scenarios such as unexpected drops in patient volume or regulatory changes, and outline strategies for adapting to these situations.
2. Seek professional help
   - **Legal Guidance:** Consult with an experienced healthcare attorney to assist with practice setup, including choosing the appropriate legal structure (e.g., sole proprietorship, partnership, and LLC) and ensuring compliance with healthcare regulations.
   - **Financial Advisor:** Work with a financial advisor to manage practice finances effectively. They can help with budgeting, tax planning, and investment strategies.
   - **Marketing Expertise:** Collaborate with marketing professionals to develop a comprehensive marketing strategy. This should encompass both online and offline marketing tactics to increase your practice's visibility and attract patients.
3. Focus on patient care
   - **Patient-Centered Approach:** Prioritize patient satisfaction by adopting a patient-centered care model. Spend ample time with patients, actively listen to their concerns, and involve them in shared decision-making regarding their treatment.
   - **Continuing Education:** Stay updated on the latest medical advancements and evidence-based practices to provide the

highest quality of care. Consider pursuing certifications or attending medical conferences relevant to your specialty.

4. Manage finances carefully
   - **Competitive Pricing:** Research and benchmark your pricing against other providers in your area. Ensure that your pricing is competitive while reflecting the value of your services.
   - **Expense Management:** Implement rigorous expense management practices. Regularly review your practice's expenses and identify areas where cost-saving measures can be applied without compromising patient care.
   - **Invest in Technology:** Strategically invest in the latest medical technology and equipment when it enhances patient care or streamlines operations. Ensure that these investments align with your practice's goals and patient needs.

Summary

Private practice in medicine offers a unique blend of autonomy and entrepreneurship. Whether as a solo practitioner or part of a group, physicians in private practice have the chance to shape their careers, provide patient care on their terms, and, in many cases, enjoy the financial rewards of their hard work. However, it is a path that requires careful planning, a willingness to adapt to changing circumstances, and a strategic approach to managing the associated challenges.

Private practice offers physicians a unique opportunity to exercise autonomy, achieve financial success, build meaningful patient relationships, experience professional satisfaction, customize their practice, and control their practice environment. While it comes with its own set of challenges and responsibilities, many physicians find that the advantages of private practice align with their career aspirations and personal values, making it a fulfilling and rewarding choice in the field of medicine. Although private practice offers many advantages, it also presents significant challenges that require careful planning and strategic management. By taking proactive steps to address financial risks, streamline administrative tasks, optimize resource utilization, and mitigate liability, physicians can navigate the disadvantages of private practice effectively while providing high-quality patient care.

The challenges of starting a private medical practice are significant but can be managed effectively with careful planning, budgeting, and strategic decision-making. By addressing these challenges proactively, physicians can enhance their practice's chances of long-term success and provide high-quality care to their patients.

Private practice offers physicians the autonomy and financial rewards they desire but comes with substantial responsibilities. By following the actionable recommendations discussed in this chapter, physicians can navigate the challenges effectively, ensuring the long-term viability and success of their private medical practice while delivering high-quality patient care and fulfilling their career aspirations.

SAGES Takeaway

- Develop a comprehensive business plan with clear goals, financial projections, and contingency plans.
- Seek professional guidance, including legal, financial, and marketing expertise, to ensure proper setup and management.
- Prioritize patient care with a patient-centered approach and ongoing education to provide high-quality care.
- Manage finances carefully, set competitive prices, monitor expenses, and invest strategically in technology.
- Maintain a focus on both financial viability and delivering exceptional patient care for a fulfilling and successful practice.

3 Academic Surgical Practice

Ann M. Rogers

Nearly half of all active surgeons in the United States are currently in an academic surgical practice [1]. Classically, an academic physician is the Oslerian "triple threat," a master clinician, a research scientist, and a teacher [2]. An additional fourth area of expertise is coming to be recognized, that of administration. This and recent demands for increased clinical productivity make the triple threat aspiration harder for many to meet [3]. Nonetheless, academic surgical departments still aim to fulfill the missions of clinical care, teaching, and research by maximizing clinical full-time employee (FTE) percentage, while allowing for a proportion of protected time for research pursuits, and sometimes even having separate tracks for academics who will seek promotion versus those who will not [4].

A cross-sectional survey was sent to over 25,000 fellows of the American College of Surgeons in 2018. Of the nearly 4000 respondents, about 46% were in the academic practice of surgery, 38% were in private practice, and the remainder reported being in neither [1]. These latter were presumably in an employed/community, military, or locums practice model. This chapter found

A. M. Rogers (✉)
Department of Surgery, Penn State Health, Hershey, PA, USA
e-mail: arogers@pennstatehealth.psu.edu

S. M. Johnson et al. (eds.), *The SAGES Manual of Strategy and Leadership*, https://doi.org/10.1007/978-3-031-62359-2_3

that while academic surgeons reported more weekly hours spent performing nonclinical work than did other surgeons, they were significantly more likely to be satisfied with their career. In addition, and surprisingly, academic surgeons were significantly more satisfied than their non-academic counterparts with their financial compensation. Academic surgeons were also less concerned that competition with other surgeons was a financial threat. Finally, academic surgeons were significantly less likely to find that their experience with malpractice had decreased their job satisfaction.

Academic surgery, while a key component of surgical education and provision of clinical care to a large part of the US healthcare system, is threatened by significant barriers to entry, resource shortages, and high rates of burnout [5]. Formal mentorship programs have been shown to improve scholarly output and professional outlook and thereby satisfaction in academic careers [6]. Such mentorship programs should optimally be provided prior to entry into an academic surgical career, for example, during medical school or residency, although time constraints make this less and less feasible. One of this chapter's aims, therefore, is to accurately describe a potential career in academic surgery, in order to better prepare candidates for such a life. Key themes in academic medicine include not only the clinical aspect of a given career but also various types of research and scholarship, networking and professional recognition, educational opportunities, and teaching activities.

Securing a position in academic surgery can be daunting. An article on obtaining a first job in general cardiothoracic surgery by Sterbling et al. lists the most common resources used by trainees during such a job search, with the top three including (1) information from one's residency program director, (2) knowing about a position already through word of mouth during their residency, and (3) cold calling [7]. Learning about employment opportunities through job boards is often unrewarding. Shubeck et al. expose the well-known practice of posting positions on job boards, despite the job already being earmarked for or having actually been offered to a specific candidate [8]. Finding academic surgical positions through recruitment agencies and other contacts is also relatively unusual at the entry level. One survey of academic chairs showed that there was a strong tendency either to hire "internal candidates," meaning directly recruiting from among their own residents or forging agreements to have them return after fellowship training, or relying on trusted sources, such as division chiefs who know of good faculty who will soon be available for hire. The chapter describes the inherent biases found in such tactics, and how they are less likely to provide for a diverse faculty. Underrepresented minorities not only remain underrepresented in academic surgical departments but may actually be losing ground despite significant pushes to improve diversity, equity, and inclusion [9].

Unsurprisingly, there are also higher barriers to academic surgical entry for women compared with men, with associated ongoing barriers to progression. Abelson et al. project that parity for women versus men at the professor level in surgery may not be reached until the year 2136 [10]. Cochran et al. conducted interviews with 15 mid-career or senior women academic surgeons, seeking information on potential barriers to advancement. In decreasing order of importance, the surgeons listed the following issues: ineffective mentorship, lack of belonging (exclusion), inadequate resources, unclear expectations for advancement, professional role conflict (generally between clinical and scholarly activities), as well as social barriers, such as work-life balance [11]. These appear to be similar barriers to acceptance and advancement experienced by minority groups.

While many academic medical centers are found in larger urban areas, they can be located in suburban or rural areas as well. Promotion and tenure processes, salary, and benefits are all quite variable and depend upon a variety of factors including not only geography but also an area's culture and an institution's history. Identifying the right job for a given applicant takes these and many other topics into account. However, the three stated core goals of excellence in patient care, research, and teaching are fairly standard across academic surgery departments. One problematic issue for academic faculty remains the apparent incongruity between stated criteria for promotion, such as research productivity, versus the significant time requirements for teaching and service that are expected from faculty members [12].

An applicant should understand a given institution's promotion and tenure process prior to signing a contract. Faculty members in general should be evaluated by one of their superiors at least annually, and during these reviews, areas of weakness and strength and ways to successfully approach the goal of academic promotion should be reviewed, with processes set in place for improvement if needed [13]. On an annual basis, the dean of a medical school or the chair of an academic surgery department requests or receives nominations of faculty under consideration for promotion. Nominations are generally made by a department chair, in consultation with a division or section chief and the individual faculty member. Because promotion dossiers can be quite detailed, it is essential for academic faculty to maintain organized vitae and records of accomplishment. In addition to the three central areas of patient care, research, and teaching, most academic medical centers also request information on a faculty member's service to the department, the institution, the profession, and the world at large. Maintaining records of all such activities is vital.

One paper by Cheng et al. described the factors that best predicted promotion in the subspecialty of vascular surgery. The absolute number of publications was the factor most likely to influence promotion from the assistant to the associate professor level, while the number of senior-author publications was the factor most likely to influence promotion from the associate to the full professor level. The "H-index" was also evaluated; this is a function of the number of publications multiplied by the number of citations; this criterion was found to be the one most likely to influence whether a candidate would be promoted to division chief [14].

This leads to the interesting question of subtypes of academic surgical careers and the various pathways to leadership. While it is perfectly acceptable to focus on one's own practice and research, many in academia will seek out opportunities for leadership. This may be within their own department, within an institution, within a medical school, or in surgical societies. All such forms of leadership require the strategic establishment of goals and learning the importance of the art of self-promotion to some extent [15]. Pathways to leadership rely on multiple tools, not the least of which are feedback and mentorship [5]. Exposure to a variety of leaders is helpful in determining strategies for success. There are many competencies involved in being a surgical leader, and these competencies may not fit all personality types [16].

Surgical departments must also be strategic in order to retain good faculty. Recruitment of new faculty to replace those that have left can be extremely expensive [17]. A survey of full-time academic medical faculty by the AAMC found that surgeons' satisfaction with their departments was similar to that of all academic faculty, but that general surgeons reported lower satisfaction with their department than did their counterparts in subspecialties [18]. Overall, the top three drivers of surgical faculty satisfaction with their departments using this survey were departmental leadership, collegiality and collaboration, and a positive direct relationship with a supervisor. The lowest drivers of satisfaction were growth opportunities, medical school leadership, and promotion equality. Armed with this information, academic surgery departments could take meaningful steps to help retain excellent surgical staff.

An academic surgical career can be extremely rewarding in terms of clinical practice, growth, and propagation of knowledge, fellowship within a field of specialization, and the opportunity to teach future physicians and surgeons. In fact, one study found that, despite similar overall ratings of job satisfaction, academic surgeons were much more likely to recommend a career in surgery to medical students than were their non-academic surgeon counterparts [19]. Academic practice will remain a significant driver of entry into the field of surgery, allowing for the future care of all people.

SAGES Takeaway

- The academic track is one of several pathways to a surgical career.
- Finding an academic position and examining its suitability to an applicant can be a lengthy and sometimes complex process.
- While academic surgeons may have less control over their salary and other practice parameters than those in private practice, they are more likely to express satisfaction with their careers and recommend such a career to others.

References

1. Mahoney ST, Irish W, Strassle PD, et al. Practice characteristics and job satisfaction of private practice and academic surgeons. JAMA Surg. 2021;156(3):247–54.
2. Periyakoil V. What would Osler do? J Palliat Med. 2013;6(2):118–9.
3. Zheng EW, Hu J, Levine JS, et al. The catch-22 of promotion: is becoming department chair of surgery a threat to the triple threat? Surgery. 2022;172(5):1422–8.
4. Mullangi S, Blutt MJ, Ibrahim S. Is it time to reimagine academic promotion and tenure? JAMA Health Forum. 2020;1(2):2200164. https://doi.org/10.1001/jamahealthforum.2020.0164.
5. Selvakumar S, Ang D, Elkbuli A. Twelve-step approach for academic development planning in academic surgery: climbing the academic uphill with strong and steady steps. Ann Surg Open. 2022;3(1):1–5.
6. Santiesteban L, McKenney M, Elkbuli A. Mentorship: a millenia-old remedy for learner success amidst the COVID-19 pandemic. J Surg Res. 2021;267:593–7.
7. Sterbling HM, Molena D, Rao SR, et al. Initial report on young cardiothoracic surgeons' first job: from searching to securing and the gaps in between. J Thorac Cardiovasc Surg. 2019;158(2):632–41.
8. Shubeck SP, Newman EK, Vitous A, et al. Hiring practices of US academic surgery departments; challenges and opportunities for more inclusive hiring. J Surg Res. 2020;254:23–30.
9. Abelson JS, Symer MM, Yeo HL. Surgical time out: our counts are still short on racial diversity in academic surgery. Am J Surg. 2018;215:542–8.
10. Abelson JS, Chartrand G, Moo T-A, et al. The climb to break the glass ceiling in surgery: trends in women progressing from medical school to surgical training and academic leadership from 1994 to 2015. Am J Surg. 2016;212(4):566–72.
11. Cochran A, Neumayer LA, Elder WB. Barriers to careers identified by women in academic surgery: a grounded theory model. Am J Surg. 2019;218:780–5.
12. Schimanski LA, Alperin JP. The evaluation of scholarship in academic promotion and tenure processes: past, present and future. F1000Research. 2018;7:1–20.
13. Papaconstantinou HT, Lairmore TC. Academic appointment and the process of promotion and tenure. Clin Colon Rectal Surg. 2006;19:143–7.
14. Cheng TW, Farber A, Rajani RR, et al. National criteria for academic appointment in vascular surgery. J Vasc Surg. 2019;69(5):1559–65.
15. Bleier JI, Kann B. Academic goals in surgery. Clin Colon Rectal Surg. 2013;26(4):212–7.
16. Peters W, Picchioni A, Fleshman JW. Surgical leadership. Clin Colon Rectal Surg. 2020;33(4):233–7.

17. Schloss EP, Flanagan DM, Culler CL. Some hidden costs of faculty turnover in clinical departments in one academic medical center. Acad Med. 2009;84(1):32–6.
18. Wai PY, Dandar V, Radosevich DM, et al. Engagement, workplace satisfaction, and retention of surgical specialists in academic medicine in the United States. J Am Coll Surg. 2014;219(1):31–42.
19. Goudreau BJ, Hassinger TE, Hedrick TL. Academic or community practice? What is driving decision-making and career choices. Surgery. 2018;164(3):571–6.

Locum Tenens Practice

4

Ann M. Rogers and Victoria R. Rendell

Overview

The practice of locum tenens (LT), a Latin phrase that means "to hold the place of," originated in the 1970s as a way to address the need for temporary coverage of physicians in rural areas who needed to be away from their practices [1, 2]. While the benefits of this temporary coverage were easy to understand for the rural physician recipients of coverage, it became clear that these temporary assignments were popular options for many physicians for a variety of reasons, including gaps between permanent positions, a desire for more flexibility in practice, and as a way to "try out" different practice settings.

The usage of temporary physicians by healthcare organizations has increased since the 1970s. Staff Care, which is the largest healthcare staffing organization in the United States, releases a survey of healthcare administrators every few years, and the 2020 survey with data from 204 healthcare facility administrators/exec-

A. M. Rogers
Department of Surgery, Penn State Health, Hershey, PA, USA

V. R. Rendell (✉)
Division of Minimally Invasive Surgery, Department of Surgery, University of Wisconsin School of Medicine and Public Health, Madison, WI, USA
e-mail: rendell@surgery.wisc.edu

S. M. Johnson et al. (eds.), *The SAGES Manual of Strategy and Leadership*, https://doi.org/10.1007/978-3-031-62359-2_4

utives found that 85% use LT physicians to supplement their existing staff [3]. With the increase in LT coverage, concerns have arisen about the impact of temporary staffing on quality of patient care. While there have not been comparative studies in every field, there is no indication in the existing literature that quality suffers. A large retrospective cohort study of Medicare patients found no difference in 30-day mortality between patients treated by LT physicians versus permanently staffed physicians [4]. Similarly, a study of patients treated by LT versus non-LT neurosurgeons found no difference in mortality, complication rates, or length of stay [5]. Despite this, some negative perceptions of the care quality of LT providers by other providers persist. In a survey of pediatric surgeon members of the American Pediatric Surgery Association (APSA), 65% disagreed that LT surgeons provide the same level of care as a full-time community-based surgeon. Most supported LT surgeons only in the context of a short-term coverage plan [6].

Over the years, the utilization of LT surgeons in particular has increased. In 2012, 12% of responding facilities used LT surgeons, which increased to 21% in 2019 [3]. Of the 75% of administrators who were actively looking for LT physicians, 25% were looking for surgeons. In a survey focused on surgeon hiring in rural and critical access hospitals, 20% reported using an LT surgeon in the past 12 months [7].

Key Aspects of LT Positions for Surgeons

For surgeons considering a temporary position, understanding the LT practice and steps to identify and secure a position is helpful.

Identifying Positions

In 2001, the North American Locum Tenens Organization (NALTO), a professional association of temporary physician staffing firms, was established to create and maintain standards and a code of ethics for the industry [1]. Their website lists member agencies that adhere to these established principles and are a resource for physicians seeking these roles. These and many other LT agencies handle hiring for available positions. While healthcare facilities can hire on an individual basis through these agencies, with the increasing use of temporary staffing, more healthcare facilities are outsourcing all management of LT physicians to a Managed Services Provider (MSP) who will take over the recruiting, placement, scheduling, logistics, and billing. Reasonable first steps in the process of evaluating whether an LT position is a good decision for an individual surgeon include talking with surgeons who have served in these positions and browsing the resources available for physicians on the NALTO website, including the LT education center [1].

Basic Features of an LT Position

For a surgeon, most LT positions involve placement for a period of time with varying coverage needs. In a survey of rural hospitals, the median length of time LT surgeons covered was 4 weeks for short-term absences and 26 weeks for long-term positions [7]. These positions are reimbursed at a higher rate compared to what a surgeon would earn for a similar workload with a long-term position. The specific rate is negotiable. LT agencies help to a variable extent with licensing, and in general arrange for travel, lodging, and transportation. Working with a well-established group that provides multi-state positions is recommended in the available literature. When evaluating an agency, working with one that has a larger network can make it easier to find a position that fits individual needs. Using an agency recommended by a colleague who has worked with them before is helpful.

Considerations for an LT Position

There are many factors to consider as a surgeon for an LT agency/ position (Table 4.1) [2, 8].

Table 4.1 Considerations in surgeon locum tenens position selection

Do I have the correct licensing?	– State versus multi-state licensing – Urgent/emergent need licensing
How will I be compensated?	– Base rate – Over-time rate
What is the malpractice coverage?	– Personal versus agency-provided – Claims-based versus occurrence – Tail coverage?
How are travel, lodging, and transportation arranged and reimbursed?	– Reimbursement – Agency-provided
What does the call include?	– General surgery – Specialty surgery – Endoscopy
Do I have clinic obligations?	– How often? – Support staff – Ability to schedule out if planning on returning in the future
Who takes care of follow-up/continuity of care?	– Midlevel providers – Primary care providers
Do I have the equipment I need?	– Vendors and representative access – Critical platforms/tools for individual practice

Licensing

Many agencies will assist with expedited licensing, and some positions are limited to surgeons who already have a medical license in the state to be staffed. The Interstate Medical Licensing Compact (Compact) is a streamlined process, in existence since 2017, that allows physicians to practice in multiple states. To date, 37 states as well as the District of Columbia and the Territory of Guam have chosen to participate in the Compact, which allows physicians to fill out one application for licensure in all participating states. The individual states still issue the licenses, but the process becomes more straightforward. Physicians can apply through the Compact once they obtain a Letter of Qualification issued from a State of Principal License [9]. Some physicians have found the Federation Credentials Verification Service of the

Federation of State Medical Boards to also be helpful [10]. Through this, physicians create a permanent lifetime portfolio of primary-source verified credentials for a base fee, currently $395 for physicians. Most state medical boards accept FCVS, which helps streamline subsequent applications for state licenses but does not replace individual state applications. There are scenarios in which temporary emergency licenses may be issued, usually linked to specific public health emergencies, but this should not be relied upon. LT agencies generally assist with these processes or can provide guidance regarding licensing. Costs can vary but should be understood upfront.

Compensation

When selecting a position, the compensation is negotiated. Understanding the expected work hours for a given base rate is important for negotiation. If there is overtime or extended call coverage, the rate of pay for this should also be addressed. If there is additional compensation for coming into the hospital for operations or for seeing consults, this should be outlined. It is important to understand that LT physicians function as independent contractors who are responsible for federal self-employment taxes. There is an option to be taxed as a corporation or sole proprietorship, which offers some financial advantages. Consultation with an accountant and/or financial advisor can be helpful in determining how to proceed with this strategy. At minimum, recognizing the need for estimated quarterly tax payments to avoid penalties is important.

Malpractice Coverage

LT agencies generally provide malpractice coverage, but there is always an option to carry an individual LT malpractice insurance policy. The policies cover from 6 months to 1 year, and the limits are set per claim and on an annual aggregate basis. Standard terms would include up to one million dollars per claim with a maximum annual aggregate of three million dollars. The types of medical malpractice insurance include occurrence and claims-based insurance. For occurrence insurance, any incident during the policy's activation is covered regardless of when the claim is made.

For claims-based insurance, coverage is for incidents that occur when the policy is active and the claim is filed. This is relevant for LT physicians, who should inquire about "tail" coverage with a claims-based policy. Once the policy is terminated, this can provide additional coverage for claims filed for incidents during the claim-based policy coverage time. There are many online resources explaining the details of the coverage types, and these details should be clarified for each position an LT surgeon considers [11, 12]. Copies of all relevant documentation should be kept even after the position's term is completed.

Details of the Position

Before accepting a position, all the details about the location and logistics should be understood. It is helpful to discuss with the staffing agency, the site managers/contacts, and, if possible, any surgeon who has been placed at the site in the same or a similar position at the healthcare facility. These details include the arrangement of travel, lodging, and daily transportation for sites away from where the surgeon lives. The details of what is expected for call coverage at each healthcare facility should be discussed. There are specific details regarding a general surgery position that are important to cover. What types of cases are performed while on call? Are there expectations for specialty surgery coverage (e.g., pediatric cases)? If the surgeon looking for the position is specialty trained, is this position-specific for that training? What is the case mix for the elective practice? When there is clinic coverage that is needed, the frequency of clinic coverage and the presence of support staff are important to know upfront. If the position is recurring, is it possible to schedule a case from the clinic for the planned future coverage time? In the case of a short-term assignment, who would handle the follow-up for patients on whom you operate? When it comes to operating, what equipment is available at the facility? Do they have a robot, endoscopy towers, laparoscopic equipment, and so on? What vendors and contracts exist for the materials you typically use in practice? What is the training of the scrub staff? How are OR preference lists managed? What is the electronic health record in use, and if a surgeon is unfamiliar, what type of onboarding process is used? Understanding the level of acuity of the facility, the availability of blood products, and the presence of critical care is also important. If there is expectation for coverage of intensive care-level patients, that should be understood. Making sure to ask questions that may seem trivial minimizes surprises and helps the surgeon deliver quality care. The American College of Surgeons released a policy statement intended for LT surgeons, with guidelines and standards for the appointment and assessment of such surgeons [13]. This provides a helpful framework for surgeons looking to ensure they have the resources and arrangements in place to provide high-quality temporary surgery coverage.

Summary

A temporary surgery practice can be attractive to surgeons for a variety of reasons: income supplementation, flexibility of schedule, transitions between permanent positions, and the ability to evaluate many practice locations and styles. Surgeons should evaluate positions using well-respected LT agencies and ensure they ask key questions about prospective positions to ensure a good fit and to assure the availability of infrastructure to provide high-quality care.

SAGES Takeaway

- Utilization of LT (i.e., temporary clinical practice assignments) coverage for surgeons has increased over the past 10 years.
- LT practices offer key advantages for surgeons: schedule flexibility, ability to evaluate practice locations and styles without long-term commitments, and income supplementations.
- When evaluating a potential LT practice, understanding all details of the position, such as clinical expectations, reimbursement, malpractice coverage, and licensing support, is important prior to committing.

References

1. The National Association of Locum Tenens Organizations. https://www.nalto.org. Accessed 1 Jun 2023.
2. Maniscalco MM. A physician's guide to working as a locum tenens. J Am Board Fam Med. 2003;16:242–5. https://doi.org/10.3122/jabfm.16.3.242.
3. Staff Care. 2020 Survey of temporary physician staffing trends based on 2019 data. 2020.
4. Blumenthal DM, Olenski AR, Tsugawa Y, Jena AB. Association between treatment by locum tenens internal medicine physicians and 30-day mortality among hospitalized Medicare beneficiaries. JAMA. 2017;318:2119–29. https://doi.org/10.1001/jama.2017.17925.
5. Chiu RG, Nunna RS, Siddiqui N, Khalid SI, Behbahani M, Mehta AI. Locum tenens neurosurgery in the United States: a Medicare claims analysis of outcomes, complications, and cost of care. World Neurosurg. 2020;142:e210–4. https://doi.org/10.1016/j.wneu.2020.06.169.
6. Nolan TL, Kandel JJ, Nakayama DK. Quality and extent of *locum tenens* coverage in pediatric surgical practices. Am Surg. 2015;81:377–80. https://doi.org/10.1177/000313481508100428.
7. Doty B, Andres M, Zuckerman R, Borgstrom D. Use of locum tenens surgeons to provide surgical care in small rural hospitals. World J Surg. 2009;33:228–32. https://doi.org/10.1007/s00268-008-9820-5.
8. Hauff SJ, Fortune DS. Finding the right job. Otolaryngol Clin N Am. 2022;55:23–31. https://doi.org/10.1016/j.otc.2021.07.007.
9. Interstate Medical Licensure Compact. https://www.imlcc.org. Accessed 20 May 2023.
10. Federation of State Medical Boards. In: Federation of State Medical Boards-Federation Credentials Verification Service. https://www.fsmb.org/fcvs.
11. The White Coat Investor Claims-Made vs. Occurrence Malpractice Insurance. https://www.whitecoatinvestor.com/claims-made-vs-occurrence-malpractice/. Accessed 1 Jun 2023.
12. Staff Care Locum Tenens Malpractice Insurance: Types of Policies. https://www.staffcare.com/locum-tenens-blog/news/guide-to-locum-tenens-malpractice-insurance/.
13. Gantt NL, Davis KA, Sinanan MN. Locum tenens surgery: an opportunity to improve access to quality surgical care. Bulletin of the American College of Surgeons; 2018.

Techniques for Negotiating Contracts

5

Michael C. Cantrell, Ijeoma A. Ejeh, and Ruchir Puri

Introduction

For the past decade, you have sacrificed time with family and friends, holidays, and missed milestones as your child grew too fast; all to get that first, real contract that fairly compensates your expert skills and knowledge. Physicians are delayed gratification connoisseurs, providing indentured servitude for years as residents and fellows, all while patiently waiting to finally make the "big bucks." The letter of intent is in hand, and you see a yearly salary that is 4–5 times what you have been making for the past 5–6 years. You have student loans, a young family, and a mortgage. The easy response is to sign the contract. This chapter will highlight key points to consider when negotiating contracts and create pause. Fight the urge to sign that document as fast as you can! Surgeons have a unique, highly desirable, and lucrative skill set and we carry a tremendous amount of leverage into employ-

M. C. Cantrell · R. Puri (✉)
Department of Surgery, University of Florida College of Medicine, Jacksonville, FL, USA
e-mail: Ruchir.Puri@jax.ufl.edu

I. A. Ejeh
Ferncreek General Surgery, Cape Fear Health System, Fayetteville, NC, USA

S. M. Johnson et al. (eds.), *The SAGES Manual of Strategy and Leadership*, https://doi.org/10.1007/978-3-031-62359-2_5

ment negotiations. Just like most things in life, contract negotiations require that we take the time to educate ourselves and hire an expert in the field of contract review and negotiation to be in your corner [1–4]. This is not always possible when you are hired for your first job and about half of physicians change jobs in their first 5 years post-training [3]. Your next job can avoid all the common contractual pitfalls and prove to be mutually beneficial to all parties, leading to a long and prosperous surgical career. The intent of this chapter is to provide an overview of some important terms as well as highlight items that may be overlooked in surgical contracts.

The Nuts and Bolts of a Contract

If you have ever seen an employment contract, they usually start with compensation and benefits. The contract wants to dangle the carrot of a six-figure salary after a decade of training to entice you to eagerly sign on the dotted line. Buried in the contract are all the responsibilities and services you are expected to provide to the employer. After all, this new relationship is a two-way street. Arguably, the latter portion of the contract is what impacts your quality of life and work-life balance the greatest [3]. So, let us delve into the various responsibilities assigned by the physician contract.

The contract needs to clearly state what is expected of you during the weekdays along with weekends and night calls. Some various iterations of this might include vague terms like "full-time" or a 40-h work week. However, the details are important. For example, full-time should be defined as patient contact hours [3]. If an employer is expecting 40 h of patient contact, the doctor should expect to work significantly longer, considering charting and administrative duties. Expectations for call should also be clearly defined. This should include the amount as well as additional pay for taking extra call. In general, the call should be distributed equally among partners, but it is not uncommon that senior partners who are phasing out, take less call and younger partners building a practice are willing to assume more call responsibility [1–3, 5]. As with most things in life, flexibility is important. However, the language of the contract needs to protect you from the possibility of abuse, making you miserable. There are national benchmarks that provide a good starting point for negotiating call requirements and pay [3, 6]. Having a contract lawyer who is aware of these benchmarks will result in fair expectations.

Another thing to consider is your start date. Not just the day on which you begin employment but everything that is required prior to starting. This could span from credentialing to privileges within a system to the ability to prescribe certain medicines. You will need a state medical and DEA license to name a couple. You also need to be on specific payors' panels so that your services can be reimbursed. Often, doctors will get all this into the hands of someone who handles credentialing in a timely manner. However, despite your best efforts, there may inevitably be delays that are out of your control. The contract should address these situations. At the same time, you cannot ask an employer to pay you for sitting at home while waiting for the process to finish. So, as with most things, there needs to be compromise. One example, if you are partially credentialed, then schedule patients in such a way that you can get reimbursed but recognize that you may have to take reduced hours/reduced compensation while this is resolved. However, certainly, there should not be automatic termination if this is not complete [3].

Hopefully, this start date is followed by a long, fulfilling, and lucrative career. However, at some point, it becomes time to terminate the contract. Termination can be grouped into two major scenarios: with cause and without cause. With cause, termination goes both ways (employer or employee initiated). It is implemented in scenarios when a breach of contract has occurred. For the doctor, claiming a breach in the contract is easy enough to begin this process. It is often for something egregious like not paying compensation that was promised, providing enough block time to operate, or impeding safe and efficient patient care. On the contrary, the employer will likely have a long list of reasons for cause termination. Most of them are not negotiable, and if breached, then there is no arguing with termination. This includes imprisonment, committing a felony crime, witnessing abuse of a patient or coworker, and so on. The important scenario to negotiate is without cause termination. As the name implies, it can come out of nowhere and the one thing in your control is the amount of time to find another job. This should be the same amount of time for both sides and something between 90 and 120 days is often agreed upon [1–4].

Finally, there are miscellaneous items that you need to think about when reviewing a contract. The contract should state the location of where you are going to provide a service and any additional locations. If the contract states you will see patients at an office 45 min away, but you do not address this, then you could be stuck with a very long commute; wasting your precious time. This type of minutiae is something contract review lawyers consider every day. Therefore, having someone with experience with contract negotiations can help mitigate the risk of signing something that commits you to an unpleasant experience.

Compensation and Benefits

Early on in your career, it is advisable to seek employment that offers a base salary. Base salaries will vary widely based on geographic location and practice type whether private, group, or hospital-employed practice. You should be wary of contracts based solely on productivity. The first couple years of your career will be spent building a practice, so productivity will grow but this will take time. There are two types of productivity formulas to be aware of during contract review [3].

First is a formula based on billings or collections. This is a percentage of the amount of revenue your service generates. Often, this percentage will increase after a certain amount of revenue to encourage working harder, paid in the form of a bonus. This formula puts you at the mercy of the payor mix and the amount the billing office can reimburse [3].

The second form of productivity calculations is based on relative value units (RVUs). This formula is often implemented in hospital settings, especially nonprofit institutions. The RVU is standard between different patients with different insurances, so it is easier for large institutions to bill for services and for physicians to know what each service is worth. However, on the contrary, this gives up control, and if someone decides to lower the RVUs for a certain operation, then there is not much you can do about it as a physician. An email survey of physicians in 2017 found that the average annual RVUs generated by US surgeons was 6736. As per the 2021 MGMA report for hospital-based general surgeons, the annual RVUs are 6000. Multiplying the annual RVUs generated by the conversion factor arrives at the annual compensation. The conversion factor varies from $20 to $80 based on the specialty and is $33.0607 per CMS for the year 2023 [3, 6–8].

With respect to bonuses, a productivity formula is often implemented and usually fair. And while bonuses are great, do not settle for a mediocre base salary with the promise that a bonus structure will compensate for any shortcomings. Compensation and RVUs will vary based on geography and competition, so having someone familiar with fair compensation is crucial to negotiating this number. Although less popular, another option is to discuss with colleagues what they are being compensated and use this as a basis of negotiations.

Cold hard cash in the pocket is essential, but there are other aspects of the contract that should be rigorously reviewed. This includes other benefits such as disability pay, retirement benefits, health insurance, and so on. Often, these are icing on the cake and not negotiable. However, knowing what is being offered is essential to comparing various contracts. There are two aspects of group disability that need to be analyzed. This includes the employer's definition of disability and how they will determine if you are disabled, and it needs plain language stating how long the employer will pay if you become disabled [1–4]. This is somewhat negotiable and very important, but it cannot be emphasized enough that every physician, especially surgeons, needs to have a portable, personal disability insurance policy brokered through one of the big six companies that has a legitimate own-occupation, specialty-specific definition of disability.

Retirement benefits are an important aspect to understand, but it is important to know that the employer usually retains the right to change these benefits on a yearly basis without any requirement for employee input. Often, it comes down to the competitive pricing that different brokerages can offer at different times [3].

Finally, there should be no less than 2–3 weeks of paid vacation, often more, paid CME, and additional miscellaneous items such as a private office, block time in the operating room, and ancillary staff to improve your day-to-day workflow to name a few additional benefits [3].

Restrictive Covenants

These are commonly referred to as non-compete clauses. There are many physicians who will argue that restrictive covenants should not exist in a medical employment contract. When there is a physician shortage and a plethora of underserved areas within our country, there should be no limitation on when or where a medical provider can practice. This stance is reasonable at first glance, but it takes putting yourself into the employer's shoes to understand why this covenant may be deemed necessary by employers, at least at first. When first starting a career in a new community, the employer must invest a significant amount of money into growing and promoting your name and services so that you can produce revenue. This covenant protects the employer from providing these services to then have the physician leave and take their skills (and patients) across the street [3]. Clearly, it is an integral protection of their investment, which in this case is you, the surgeon.

So, if restrictive covenants are not going away, the next best option is to educate yourself on how these are written and how to find a reasonable middle ground. There are two key aspects that boil down to place and time. The contract should clearly state the area that the covenant enforces, usually in the form of a radius, in miles, from your main base of operation. It is usually difficult to convince an employer to go any less than 5 miles, so this should be your goal. And the second part states how long this covenant will be enforced after the termination of the contract. The lowest most employers are willing to go is 1 year, so again, this may be considered a reasonable goal [1, 3, 4]. Realistic expectations will vary based on your (sub)specialty, area of practice, and surrounding competition, but these are good general guidelines.

This portion of the contract needs close review from a contract lawyer because the language (legal jargon) is very important. One definition that should be clear includes what exactly you are prohibited from doing. Sometimes, if it does not impact your previous employer's bottom line, then they will waive the covenant and let you practice medicine. However, if this type of stipulation is not stated, then you have no ground to stand on. In addition, there needs to be specific scenarios in which the restriction is waived. For example, being terminated without cause should waive the right to restrict where you go next. And as with most things, money can usually let you out of a restriction [3]. There is usually an expensive buy-out option. However, if your prospective employer has another candidate without this extra baggage, it can be difficult to convince them to hire you instead of them.

Malpractice Insurance

Malpractice insurance is important to all physicians, but especially surgeons. There are two major types of insurance coverages that exist: these are claims made and occurrence-based policies. The most important difference between these is how claims are handled after employment has been terminated. Claims made policies cover any claim that happened during employment (when the policy is covering you). Occurrence policies would cover a particular event if it happened while employed at that location and covered by a policy. So clearly, occurrence policies continue to protect you afterward. But far too often, surgeons find themselves with claims made policies who are ready to move on to another job, only to realize that tail insurance is not covered, exceedingly expensive, and financially prohibitive to leaving. Tail insurance is something either the employee or employer must purchase to cover malpractice after leaving a practice. Thus, having plain language and a solid plan for tail insurance is paramount when negotiating the original contract. This is not something you want to be trying to navigate after the fact. Lastly, keep in mind that this is a moving target, and any employer could change the type of insurance they provide based on competitive pricing at the time [1, 3, 4]. So, if circumstances change, the contract needs to address this new scenario and how tail insurance will be provided.

Negotiations

Negotiation starts from the first recruiting call to signing the dotted line. The best way to prepare for negotiations is to educate yourself and know why you are being recruited. Is it to replace a retiring surgeon and an associate who left with little advance notice or to allow the partners to take more time off or less call? The answers to these questions may give one an idea of their bargaining power. Physicians encourage patients to be involved in their own medical care to improve outcomes and satisfaction. We should do the same and educate ourselves about one of the most important events that impact our lives; employment. There are books dedicated to educating physicians about employment contracts and endless blogs, articles, and podcasts dissecting contracts and the important terms that should be addressed. There is an entire field within the practice of law dedicated to contract review and specifically physician contracts. There is a level of complexity and understanding that is beyond what a physician can be expected to internalize and regurgitate during negotiations [3, 5]. Therefore, in our opinion, it is wise to hire a contract review lawyer who will review every aspect of the contract and even negotiate on your behalf. After all, the people you are negotiating with will soon be your colleagues, ideally. It takes away the pressure of painting a poor portrayal of your character early in your career if negotiations turn ugly. Also, this job is very important, and your employer should think the same. This process should be meticulously scrutinized and negotiated to mutually benefit both parties. You want someone on your team who specializes in physician contracts and gets win–win results on a regular basis.

Conclusion

Physician employment contracts are complex documents packed with complex, legal language. Our aim as surgeons should be to develop a basic understanding of the major sections within the document so that we can intelligently make informed decisions when negotiating terms, and also know what is reasonable and fair. While the compensation and dollar amounts are important, there are several other items within the contract that need meticulous attention. Having a professional on your team is paramount to set your career trajectory on the correct path. As negotiation expert, Chester Karrass, once said, "In business [medicine is a business], you don't get what you deserve, you get what you negotiate" [9].

SAGES Takeaway
- Educate yourself on all aspects of the contract not just the compensation.
- Understand that you do have the leverage to negotiate a mutually beneficial contract.
- Hire a contract review team and/or attorney, especially for the first contract.

References

1. Curtis M. What to negotiate for in a physician contract. The White Coat Investor. 2021. https://www.whitecoatinvestor.com/things-to-negotiate-for-in-a-physician-contract.
2. Dahle J. What physicians need to know about contract negotiation. The White Coat Investor. 2019. https://www.whitecoatinvestor.com/what-physicians-need-to-know-about-contract-negotiation-podcast-133.
3. Hursh D, ESQ. The final hurdle: a physician's guide to negotiating a fair employment agreement. Anesthesiology. 2019;127:403–4.
4. Miller D. Things to ask for in a physician contract. The White Coat Investor. 2022. https://www.whitecoatinvestor.com/things-to-ask-for-in-a-physician-contract.
5. Felberg R. Anatomy of a complex physician contract negotiation. The White Coat Investor. 2017. https://www.whitecoatinvestor.com/anatomy-of-a-complex-physician-contract-negotiation.

6. MGMA. Provider pay and the pandemic. 2021. https://mgma.com/getmedia/c2b0ec3f-a7a9-45d3-b8ec-b02c26abcc4c/DD-ProviderComp-DataReport-May2021.pdf.aspx?ext=.pdf.
7. Michas F. Work relative value units (RVUs) of U.S. physicians as of 2016, by specialty. 2019. https://www.statista.com/statistics/293869/rvus-of-us-physicians-by-specialty/.
8. Foe LM. How will the 2023 MPFS affect your practice? 2023. https://www.facs.org/for-medical-professionals/news-publications/news-and-articles/bulletin/2023/january-2023-volume-108-issue-1/how-will-the-2023-mpfs-affect-your-practice/.
9. Karrass CL. In business as in life—You Don't Get what You Deserve, You Get what You Negotiate. Stanford Street Press; 2013.

Employment Red Flags 6

Aaron M. Alford

Employment Red Flags

While deliberating employment, several factors should be considered prior to signing a binding agreement. Contemplation of several elements by both parties is essential for a symbiotic working relationship to thrive. Considerations should include a focus on the alignment of goals between employer and employee, attention to references and reputation, opportunities for advancement, and attention to "red flags" or signs of concern. The importance of the due diligence process by both parties cannot be overstated. These red flags discovered by either the employer or employee can lead to prolonged negotiations and breed resentment during the hiring process if not handled appropriately. When red flags are discovered and reconciliation cannot be established, then the budding relationship may terminate abruptly. Therefore, it is imperative for conversations around red flags to be bidirectional between employer and employee. Furthermore, these conversations should take place in a fair and non-judgmental manner.

A. M. Alford (✉)
Department of Surgery, Morehouse School of Medicine, Atlanta, GA, USA
e-mail: aalford@msm.edu

S. M. Johnson et al. (eds.), *The SAGES Manual of Strategy and Leadership*, https://doi.org/10.1007/978-3-031-62359-2_6

Successful contract negotiations are frequently predicated upon well-established discovery processes which set the expectations up front and foster transparency. Candidates for employment who are seeking a long-term, productive relationship should also develop self-strategies to delve into the mission, reputation, and existing faculty of the institution. Since the stakes are high in a professional contract, both the employer and employee should have a thorough understanding of the contractual language, the expectations outlined in the agreement, and the protection of both parties embedded within the language.

When areas of concerns are encountered, strategies should be implemented to reconcile the discovered information. Probing further into red flags can foster open communication when approached in a responsible manner. Accusatory or judgmental behavior will likely be detrimental to both parties involved and should be avoided. Having discussions around red flags can be a learned skill through strengthening emotional intelligence and learning how to have crucial conversations. When employers or employees discover red flags, the deliberation process for employment may become more in depth or altogether cease. In some situations, red flags can present as stumbling blocks that are unable to be overcome. In other circumstances, the red flags may be reconciled through productive conversation. Developing skills to hold crucial conversations around difficult topics is essential for both individuals and institutions. Two keys to managing crucial conversations are self-awareness and preparation. Explicit self-awareness can save one from engaging in a conversation in a way that panders to feelings rather than needs [1]. Self-rehearsing or practicing difficult conversations with a colleague are ways to gain experience [2]. Furthermore, remaining objective and open-minded are essential for advancing the conversation in a positive manner. Therefore, when red flags are discovered, efforts should be attempted to proceed with transparent communication which ultimately may provide further clarification of the discovered concerns.

Historically, faculty with pre-employment red flags are significantly more likely to experience subsequent performance deficiencies [3]. As a substantial investment is made in recruiting and hiring new faculty, efforts to identify and assist faculty members at risk can provide academic departments opportunities to offer the best environment for the success of all faculty members. From a faculty point of view, overly complicated or duplicitous contractual verbiage may promote lower satisfaction scores among employed faculty. Thoroughly researching an institution or candidate prior to accepting or extending an offer of employment may help determine if a synergist relationship can prevail.

Interpretation of red flags varies from institution to institution and from person to person. However, there is a general shared understanding of examples of red flags. Red flags that may be noticed by the employer can include behavior deemed unprofessional, delayed response to queries, delayed submission of required documentation, multiple job departures after short periods of time, and extended lapses in between periods of employment. Another red flag is bad-mouthing former colleagues [4]. Red flags that may be noticed by the employee can include disparaging comments regarding former employees, overreaching restrictive covenants, excessively complicated compensation offers, and specific language and terms that are difficult to understand. While hiring legal counsel to go over an employment contract may seem too serious, it should not be omitted. Medical contracts have specific language and terms that are difficult to understand. Working with legal counsel can assist with reviewing the contract, pointing out any red flags and can help figure out negotiation points [5].

Under certain conditions, red flags can go unrecognized. An example is when a candidate is seeking employment in a strongly desired institution or an employer is considering hiring a highly desirable faculty candidate. In these scenarios, the judgment of the employee or employer may be clouded due to the highly sought after employment opportunity. Therefore, it is imperative to remain vigilant for red flags.

Although the perfect job or perfect candidate may empirically exist in the mind's eye, due diligence should be performed to avoid difficult employment relationships that may bring disharmony within an organization. Therefore, before contracts are finalized, modifications may be considered to protect the interests of both parties. Realistic negotiations can help build relationships that lead to productive, long-lasting relationships for the hiring entity and employee.

SAGES Takeaway

- When considering employment, learn how to recognize red flags.
- When red flags are encountered, communication is the key to resolution.
- When transparent communication is prioritized, productive relationships can ensue.

References

1. Weeks H. Taking the stress out of stressful conversations. Harv Bus Rev. 2001;79(7):112.
2. Priftanji D, Hill JD, Ashby DM. Managing difficult conversations. Am J Health Syst Pharm. 2020;77(21):1723–6. https://doi.org/10.1093/ajhp/zxaa149.
3. Cooper WO, Simmons JH, Moore PE, Rush MG, Domenico HJ, Foster JE, Rice TD, Bolina S, Lowe K, Webber SA. Early predictors of performance deficiencies in academic faculty: pre-employment red flags. Acad Pediatr. 2021;21(4):716–22. https://doi.org/10.1016/j.acap.2020.06.144.
4. Emergency Department Management. Avoid hiring the wrong clinicians: ask in-depth interview questions, spot red flags. ED Manag. 1998;10(7):73–6.
5. Bajwa A. Common pitfalls to avoid when signing a contract. Newstex Blogs TechBullion. 2023. https://advance.lexis.com/api/document?collection=news&id=urn:contentItem:680G-NRG1-F03R-N3RJ-00000-00&context=1516831.

7 Financial Considerations When Choosing a Practice

Ruchir Puri and Alia P. Qureshi

> *I have never regretted going into medicine. I'd do it again tomorrow, and I tell that to any youngster who is considering it. Medicine is a calling. It is more than a business. One can make money doing other things. But I chose medicine–surgery–because it combined a quest for knowledge with a way to serve, to save lives, and to alleviate suffering.*
>
> *—C. Everett Koop, MD, FACS, Pediatric Surgeon and former U.S. Surgeon General*

The surgical journey is long and arduous. There is probably a minority of surgeons who "knew from the beginning they would 1 day wield the scalpel," but most surgeons will state that they found their path to medical school after a variable period of explo-

R. Puri
Department of General Surgery, University of Florida COM, Jacksonville, FL, USA
e-mail: ruchir.puri@jax.ufl.edu

A. P. Qureshi (✉)
Division of General and GI Surgery: Foregut Surgery, Oregon Health and Science University, Portland, OR, USA
e-mail: qureshia@ohsu.edu

S. M. Johnson et al. (eds.), *The SAGES Manual of Strategy and Leadership*, https://doi.org/10.1007/978-3-031-62359-2_7

ration and soul-searching during their undergraduate years in college. Many surgeons would also attest to being drawn to surgery during medical school as it allows an opportunity to bring instant, meaningful change into a person's life, as well as immediate gratification for the surgeon. It is only after the ebb and flow of a prolonged surgical residency and fellowship; the surgeon is faced with the realization that they need to find employment. The joy of completing the competitive surgical journey is short-lived and is quickly replaced by anxiety to find the right job and the financial implications thereof. This chapter intends to discuss the financial consideration of the various types of surgical practices and highlight some unique aspects of private practice.

Pertinent to the discussion is to understand that a variety of practice types exist at the end of a surgeon's training. The various practice types are discussed in greater detail in the first chapter. Less than half a century ago, the options available were limited to academic or private practice, which included joining a large group practice. The options available to surgeons now are more diverse than ever and apart from the traditional options include working in large integrated delivery systems, hospital-based practice, group practice, HMO-based model, and finally locum tenens. With so many options, choosing a specific practice type in many regards has gotten more challenging. Apart from a geographic location and setting urban, suburban, or rural, there are several factors a surgeon needs to consider when choosing a practice type. These include but are not limited to the financial debt owed, the amount of independence desired, the family support that needs to be provided, and whether one wants to work in an environment with trainees. With this segue, we will now discuss the financial implications of each practice type.

Part 1: Financial Consideration of Various Practice Types

There has been a dramatic shift in surgeon employment over the last three to four decades. In the early twentieth century, surgeons mostly owned and managed their own practices. In the late 1980s and early 1990s, the advent of managed care organizations and the increasing administrative complexity of owning practices led to a shift toward a hospital-employed practice [1]. By 2008, a slight majority of physicians in the United States (56%) were either full or part owners of their practices, whereas 44% were employed or independent contractors [2]. A recent survey of the American College of Surgeons revealed that 29% of respondents were in a University/Academic practice, 27% in a not-for-profit hospital, and 25% in a group practice [3]. This trend toward hospital employment is not just limited to surgeons and American Medical Association's (AMA's) Physician Practice Benchmark Surveys data of 3500 physicians shows that in 2020, 50.2% of physicians were employees, up from 41.8% in 2012 [4]. With that background, let us discuss the various practice types [5].

(A) **Private Practice**—highest risk/reward ratio
(B) **Group Practice**—less risk/reasonable reward
(C) **HMOs**—least risk/most predictable
(D) **Hospital-Based Practice**—less risk/less reward
(E) **Locum Tenens**—shift work, predictable

Private Practice

The healthcare landscape has changed dramatically over the last few decades and perhaps more so over the last 3 years due to the pandemic. These changes include increasing cost of healthcare in the United States, reduction in payments for services, healthcare reform, increased regulation by the federal government, hospital aggregation and formation of larger healthcare systems, and finally an imbalance between the availability of surgeons in high-demand areas. These changes have had a significant impact on the practice of surgery in general and private practice in particular. In the United States, the number of physicians in private practice has dropped to 26% in 2021, but 46% of practices are still owned by physicians [6].

Solo Practice

As the same implies in a private practice model, the surgeon usually practices alone. They have complete control over the practice and make all the decisions. The surgeon has to determine how they will charge for the service offered. The surgeon may hire companies that specialize in processing claims or train their office staff for billing and coding. The surgeon will have to negotiate the annual payor contract, but solo practitioners may be at a disadvantage due to low patient volumes. The surgeon has to decide if they want to participate in Medicare/Medicaid or stay out of the network. They are also responsible for their own malpractice insurance, management of their finances, regulatory compliance, and all paperwork. In addition, they may need to hire a small office staff and be responsible for their benefits. Financial burdens are usually higher with a higher overhead cost of running the practice and supporting office staff. The practice itself can be unincorporated or incorporated as a limited liability company (LLC) or a professional limited liability company (PLCC) based on local laws. Due to these reasons, the practice may be more affected by economic and market fluctuations.

Depending upon the income desired, the surgeon can tailor the practice to suit their lifestyle. They can also supplement their income by taking more calls, locum tenens work, consulting, or ownership of an ambulatory surgery center (ASC). This model can be quite lucrative and ideal for someone who wants complete autonomy over their schedule and understands that it requires more paperwork than other models. This model is ill-suited for people who desire less paperwork and like to work with a group of people or with trainees. Finally, working solo without help can at times be demanding and can affect wellbeing. The model has not only the highest reward but also the highest risk.

Group Practice

Small Group Practice

As the name suggests, this refers to a few surgeons working in a small group. The surgeons can work together collaboratively, create a specific niche that can lead to improved patient satisfaction, and increase revenue. Apart from helping each other clinically, the surgeons can distribute administrative tasks and share the overhead costs.

Large Group Practice

In this setting, a large group of surgeons share clinical work and office space. Larger groups will require a bigger financial investment as well as a more complex management structure. A larger practice may be less risk-prone and still offer a controlled lifestyle at the cost of having less autonomy and distribution of revenue and may involve some discussion related to succession. A larger group practice will generally lead to lower financial compensation compared with a small group practice.

In general, there is a trend away from solo practice to large practice types and from private to employed practice. Data from ACS show that, of the 25% of respondents in surgical group practice, 12% were in a multispecialty group, while 13% were in solo practice. The same study showed that 36% of surgeons who have changed their practice have moved from private practice to hospital-based employment [7].

HMOs

In this model, the physicians work as salaried employees for an HMO and care for a selected group of individuals referred to as a "panel of patients." The physician-specific management protocols are determined by the HMO. This model is the least risky and most predictable, salaries are standardized, and some incentive bonuses may be offered. A slight variation of this model is the group HMO model where the physicians are contractors and not employees. The HMO contracts with a group of physicians and ensures patient flow to the practice. The physicians get compensated on capitated (per-member-per-month payment) or defined fee-schedule.

Hospital-Based Practice

In this practice type, the physician works in a hospital or department that is owned and operated by the hospital. The physicians have a more predictable lifestyle including work hours, but usually lower income compared with the private practice models. Also, the compensation and benefits are dependent on the well-being and financial success of the institution.

University/Academic Practice

Academic practice has evolved over many years but is still appealing to many individuals. This practice type is ideally suited to those who have either an interest in training other individuals or have a research mindset and want to move science forward. This practice type may also be appealing to individuals who cherish the "camaraderie" and like the challenging patients and operations. Broadly speaking, the compensation is lower than in private or group practice. Administrative burden may be higher if involved with leadership and the politics in larger programs may not be appealing to many.

Not-for-Profit Hospital/Healthcare System

In pure hospital-employed practice, similar to academic practice, trainees may be present in certain situations. Depending on the practice model mid-level providers may be employed to assist the surgeon with patient care. As mentioned earlier, the general trend is toward more hospital-based employment.

Locum Tenens

This type of practice allows the maximum predictability and flexibility. This is usually a temporary employment but in rare cases can be permanent. Generally, special agencies hire physicians, pay them competitive salaries, and provide malpractice insurance but no other benefits such as healthcare insurance and retirement. The surgeon has the ability to select the practice and how much they want to work but work may or may not be available consistently.

Part 2: Financial Considerations When Acquiring a Practice [6]

Private practice is appealing to many surgeons for the reasons mentioned above. In this next section, we will focus on some specific financial considerations related to acquiring a practice. Acquiring a new practice is in many regards similar to buying a new house with certain special caveats and includes paying close attention to the current patient population and financial well-being of the current practice apart from the geographic location. Typically, information about potential practices to buy will come from colleagues, mentors, websites, and journals. The search should start 6–12 months prior to the proposed start.

Before looking into financial aspects, several prerequisites have to be considered.

1. Leadership within the practice

   This is perhaps one of the most important factors to consider when joining a new practice. In the ideal situation, you want a mix of senior/seasoned, mid-career, and young surgeons. The senior surgeons bring their wealth of experience to the practice and can mentor the new surgeon. The mid-career surgeons are more likely to be in tune with the new innovations and the younger surgeons bring the drive and energy for the practice to thrive and grow.
2. Call, holiday, vacation schedules, and work-life balance in the practice

   It is typical in any practice type to provide call coverage. The number of patients, number of hospitals covered, and call days will vary by practice. Unless a completely outpatient type of a practice in most solo practices, the surgeons round on their own patients but may provide coverage to other surgeons on weekends to be able to get weekends off themselves. Similarly, in a group practice, it is typical for the surgeon to round on all the patients covered by the surgeons in a hospital. Depending upon the structure, this may involve taking an acute care surgery (ACS) call as well. The ACS coverage is usually reimbursed by the hospital at a mutually agreeable, contracted rate.

In larger group practices, the number of call days will be lower if all the surgeons are taking call.

Holidays and vacations apart from the national holidays vary with practices. It is not uncommon to have less vacation time in private, especially solo practices, and more in hospital-based practices. Academic practices may afford more time for meetings and conferences than private and group practices.

3. Work culture within the practice

   This is another important factor that may not be as easily evident as some others. A friendly, respectful, collaborative, and non-punitive work culture is the best to ensure the success of a team and ultimately is best for the patients.

4. Prestige in the community being served

   Generally, older practices with reputable surgeons will have a good standing in the community.

5. Quality and strength of the office/support staff

   Running a solo or large practice requires a competent and diligent support staff. The revenue cycle detailed below describes the process of getting paid for surgical services provided. The whole cycle is dependent on capable office staff.

6. Quality and access to the electronic medical record (EMR)

   EMR has revolutionized patient care, but it does require a significant upfront cost and maintenance along with ongoing training.

7. Financial structure, benefits

   Financial structure and benefits will vary significantly with practice types. Solo practitioners are their own bosses and theoretically can earn unlimited amounts after paying the office staff and taking care of overheads. Many group practices offer a base salary and bonuses based on relative value units (RVUs) and productivity. In many practices, there is a pathway to a partnership after a variable number of years which can add to the income. Hospital-based or academic practices are usually more rigid in their compensation. Many academic practices base their compensation on the Association of American Medical Colleges (AAMC) salary data.

Benefits including health insurance, pension, money for meetings, and bonuses are variable across the different practice types.

Once all these factors have been considered and a decision is made to proceed with acquiring the practice, the subsequent steps in the process are as follows. We will now discuss some of these terms in detail.

(A) Determine the fair market value (FMV) and negotiate the purchase price. FMV refers to the value of the practice in an open market if certain conditions are met and is different from the market value and appraised value. These conditions include the parties that are free of any pressure to buy or sell, are acting in their own interest, have all the facts available to them, and have sufficient time to come to a decision. Market value is the price of the practice in the marketplace, and the appraised value is what any expert or assessor assesses the value to be.

The most common method used to assess FMV is the EBITDA (earnings before interest, taxes, depreciation and amortization) method. Professional business evaluators then use of one three approaches to assess value.

(a) Income-based approach—using multiples of EBITDA.
(b) Assets-based approach—calculating all tangible and intangible assets.
(c) Market-based approach—checking what comparable businesses are sold for.

(B) Purchase/self-agreement—a legal document generally prepared by an attorney to acquire a business.
(C) Warranty and representations (statement of facts and indemnity clauses)—these outline the current state of finances and potential for future growth of the practice being acquired. Indemnity or indemnification clause requires one party to reimburse the other from third-party claims.
(D) Transition structure—asset acquisition/stock acquisition/merger.

(E) Valuation—One more method utilized is the discounted cash flow (DCF) method. This is aimed at determining how much money the practice is expected to make in the future compared with other investments. This includes calculating future revenue and discounting it back to estimate the current value of the practice.
(F) Tax issues.
(G) Listing of assets and liabilities.
(H) Non-compete—this refers to a clause within the contract that prevents a physician from operating a practice within a fixed geographic distance or for a certain time frame e.g. A non-compete clause may prevent a surgeon from joining another practice within 25 miles of his past employment for a period of a year.
(I) Terms related to patients [EMRs, Health Insurance Portability and Accountability Act (HIPAA), Stark, Anti-Kick Back (AKB)].
(J) Referring to physician reports.
(K) Transition plan.
(L) Post-closing items—patient/staffing, liability carrier, marketing, and advance notification of federal agencies.

Valuation

Ideally, FMV is the price that both parties settle at when the buyer and seller have knowledge of all the facts and are not under any compulsion. An appraiser collects a number of data points to formulate a report. The cost of the appraisal depends on the complexity of the deal and the litigation involved. Buyers should ensure a strong revenue stream confirmed by data and potential for future growth. Three ways to assess valuation were mentioned above.

Due Diligence

This refers to evaluating all aspects of the practice that is intended to be acquired including its valuation and risk associated. These can be divided into six subheadings:

(a) Corporate due diligence—an investigation into the practice's financial conditions and suitability of the acquisition.
(b) Compliance due diligence—an assessment of the practice's regulatory compliance with federal and non-federal entities.
(c) Tax due diligence—a thorough review of all the tax returns/ audits of the practice.
(d) Financial due diligence—an audit of the financial records and accounts of the practice.
(e) Human resources due diligence—is an assessment of the human resource processes of the practice to include hiring practices, retention, support, and most importantly the culture within the practice.
(f) Information Technology and Intellectual Property due diligence—this includes details of any current and planned IT initiatives/key projects as well as the quantity and quality of any IP owned by the practice.

Figure 7.1 represents a typical transaction cycle when acquiring a new practice.

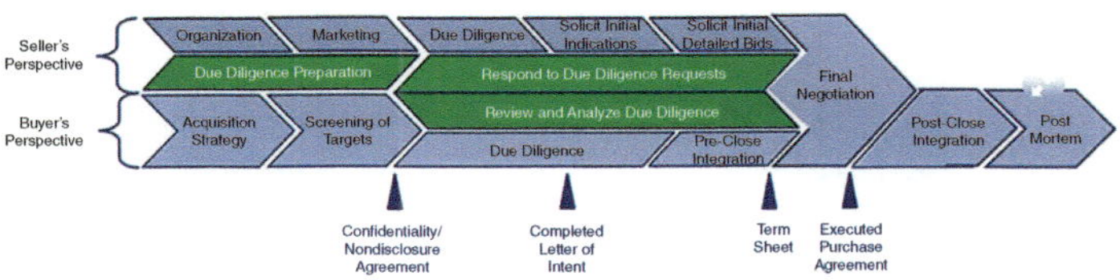

Fig. 7.1 Transaction cycle. (Courtesy: American College of Surgeons: The Surgeon's Guide to Buying a Practice)

The Revenue Cycle [3]

An important concept to master for people who are in or intend to be in private practice is the concept of the revenue cycle (Fig. 7.2). Simply put revenue cycle refers to all the steps required to get paid. In the past, the insurance companies were billed for the service and the patient did not have to make any upfront payment. Today, many practices will collect payment money prior to the service being rendered.

Successful management of the revenue cycle is dependent on 11 key steps.

1. Preregister patients—entering patients' demographic and insurance information prior to arrival.
2. Verify eligibility and benefits—ensure that the patients have insurance coverage.

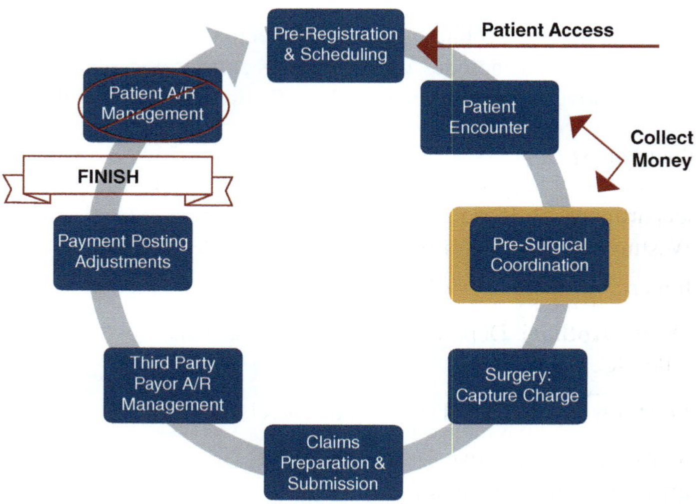

Fig. 7.2 The revenue cycle. (Courtesy: Resources for the Private Practice Surgeon: The Private Practice Surgeon. American College of Surgeons. Vol 2. Oct 2019)

3. Verify patient identity, information, and insurance at check-in—front desk confirms all information.
4. Collect patient financial responsibility amounts at the time of service—ascertain and collect the entire amount at the time of the visit.
5. Collect deposits before a surgical procedure is scheduled—staff sends a cost estimate and collects the amount prior to the surgery.
6. Post charge/submit claim within 48 h—electronically submit the claims.
7. Implement electronic remittance advice for all payors who offer it—automate to avoid manual posting.
8. File explanation of benefits (EOBs) forms in a batch, by posting date—scan EOBs by date and put them in a batch.
9. Use automated work queues in the practice management system (PMS)—as mentioned above to streamline the collections.
10. Check the status of unpaid claims online—correct denials and resubmit on payor websites.
11. Use the PMS collections module to manage patient A/R follow-up.

In addition to the revenue cycle to maintain financial health and run a profitable practice, the surgeons have to review seven financial steps each month. The American College of Surgeons—Resources for the Private Practice Surgeons published in October 2019—provides comprehensive information about many elements related to private practice for surgeons [3].

1. Charges, payments, and adjustments—this report comes from the PMS. The PMS software can streamline the practice of billing and payments, identify trends, and so on.
2. Profit and loss (P&L)—this report is generated from an accounting software and identifies the total revenue and expenses. In essence, this outlines how well the practice is financially managed.

3. Aged A/R, by date of service—is a management tool that generates a report by date of service and can separate patient balances from insurance balances. The reports are typically broken down into 30 days and can help identify patients that may be chronic late payers.
4. Credit balances—this is the amount the practice owes the payors and patients on a monthly basis; ideally, this should be zero or as close to zero as possible.
5. Noncontractual adjustments—this is a part of the bill that is not charged or billed to the patient due to a billing agreement with the insurance companies or any other reason. Assessing these can help identify issues with workflow and collections.
6. Unapplied payments—to ensure accuracy, it is imperative that all collections be posted to a specific category in the PMS. Monitoring the unapplied payments can reveal large sum of money that can be moved to the correct account.
7. Rejection report—this report identifies claims that were rejected by payors; assessing and addressing these rejections can help reduce denials and improve the financial wellness of the practice.

Apart from the topics discussed, success of a practice depends on numerous other factors including the knowledge of coding, billing, and office workflow which are beyond the scope of this chapter. In addition, there is a litany of healthcare regulations and laws that all surgeons should be familiar with including the HIPAA of 1996, the Occupational Safety and Health Act, the Fair Labor Standards Act, and the Family and Medical Leave Act, to name just a few.

Conclusion

In summary, each practice type offers unique opportunities and challenges related to finances, work-life integration, and satisfaction. Ultimately choosing the practice is a very personal decision that requires consideration of numerous factors as mentioned above. While the financial aspects are important, they should not be the only criteria when choosing the right practice. When done thoughtfully, the right practice can lead to years of fulfillment and add to the joy of being a surgeon. Acquisition and success of a private practice requires a thorough knowledge of associated medicolegal and financial aspects.

SAGES Takeaway

- Each practice type offers unique advantages that have to be considered carefully when deciding on which practice type is the "best fit" for an individual.
- Acquiring a new practice requires a thorough investigation into the practice being considered along with a clear understanding of the medicolegal and financial aspects of the acquisition with the help of professionals.
- It is essential for solo and private practice surgeons to understand the revenue cycle which is key to running a successful and a financially viable practice.

Acknowledgments The American College of Surgeons has a variety of resources for practicing surgeons. Two of those were utilized in preparation of parts of this chapter related to practice acquisition and the revenue cycle.

References

1. Charles AG, Ortiz-Pujols S, Ricketts T, et al. The employed surgeon: a changing professional paradigm. JAMA Surg. 2013;148(4):323–8.
2. Boukus E, Cassil A, O'Malley AS. A snapshot of U.S. physicians: key findings from the 2008 Health Tracking Physician Survey. Data Bull (Cent Stud Health Syst Change). 2009;35:1–11.
3. Resources for the private practice surgeon: the private practice surgeon. American College of Surgeon. 2019.
4. Kane CK. Recent changes in physician practice arrangements: private practice dropped to less than 50% of physicians in 2020. American Medical Association; 2021.
5. Darves B. Differentiating among medical practice settings. NEJM. 2011.
6. Satiani B, Bailey-Wheaton JL. The surgeons guide to buying a practice. American College of Surgeon.
7. American College of Surgeons Quantitative Survey Report March 2019. Conducted by Association Laboratory, Inc. of the membership for the ACS.

Excelling in Training 8

Alexandre K. Wang, Dirir H. Abdullahi,
Sasha Corbin, and Charis Ripley-Hager

Introduction

Surgical training is a challenging but rewarding time in your surgical career. It provides the basis of both skills and knowledge upon which you will build for a lifetime. Many of our closest personal and professional relationships are formed during this time, and these relationships often last throughout our careers. Many of us call our faculty from training throughout our careers for professional (and sometimes personal) advice. It is certainly a time of great change, great stress, and great reward. Making the most of surgical training requires hard work, a positive attitude, and the ability to make the most out of the opportunities you are given. The skills required at each level share many similarities but progress alongside your skills, knowledge, and responsibilities. For some, these abilities will come naturally, but for most of us, the environment is new and unlike any other we have experienced. Therefore, learning from others' experiences is vital to success in training.

A. K. Wang (✉) · D. H. Abdullahi · S. Corbin
Department of Surgery, Morehouse School of Medicine, Grady Memorial Hospital, Atlanta, GA, USA

C. Ripley-Hager
Department of Surgery, Lewis Katz School of Medicine at Temple University, Philadelphia, PA, USA

S. M. Johnson et al. (eds.), *The SAGES Manual of Strategy and Leadership*, https://doi.org/10.1007/978-3-031-62359-2_8

How to Be Successful as an Intern

Intern year can be a very nerve-wracking time in your medical career. Research has shown that among General Surgery Residents, the highest rates of attrition occur during internship [1]. However, taking a confident and strategic approach to your intern year will aid in your success. When starting a new service, communicate with your senior. Determine their preferences in how to run the service. Ensure you understand what is expected of you.

Be organized. You will transition between high- and low-volume services. It is very important that you are familiar with each patient on the service. Take notes and make a to-do list for each patient. As you go through your list, focus on one task at a time, one patient at a time. Check off each task when completed. Once all to do's are completed, run the list a second time to ensure nothing was missed. Follow up on any outstanding tasks. Update your seniors on any new pertinent results or changes in patients' clinical status.

Be punctual. Show up early, ready, and eager to complete the day's tasks. Volunteer to assist in any way possible. A team approach will make the load easier.

Know your limitations. There will be times when you are unsure of what to do in a particular scenario. Whenever there is a doubt, ask your senior! It will always be better to seek assistance than to do the wrong thing. Your seniors are available to guide you. General Surgery is a team; you are not expected to make decisions entirely on your own. Patient safety and the quality of patient care are improved when doctors work effectively as a team [2]. When you are called about a patient, go see the patient. The information gained from an in-person assessment will provide vital details that cannot be relayed by a third party over the phone.

As the Intern, you are responsible for teaching the medical students. In this role, remember what teaching styles worked best for you; try to reciprocate those. Take every opportunity to teach around the current patients. This will allow your students to make the connections between the textbook and real-life clinical cases.

This helps them to consolidate the learning points. Take the initiative to teach the students how to be a good intern, as that will be their role soon.

Finally, communication is key. You can never over-communicate. When in doubt, ask for clarification. When there is a change in the clinical status of a patient, alert your seniors as early as possible. Follow up on all outstanding tasks and results, at every given opportunity. Relay any updates to your seniors in a timely manner. You will realize throughout your medical career that communication is essential to success in any position held.

How to Be Successful as a Junior Resident

As a junior resident, the transition can sometimes be abrupt and can feel overwhelming. This is normal, especially for those that start July first on a service in which they are expected to take a primary or independent role seeing consults or leading a team. Your intern year prepared you to gather data, often on complex patients. Your junior resident years ask you to synthesize this data and develop plans independently. As an intern, you likely had a junior or senior resident that you admired for their dedication to patient care and their role as leaders on the service. Now as a junior resident, you have the opportunity to emulate these skills. Questions you must ask yourself are as follows: How can I best be helpful to my interns so they are not overwhelmed? How can I best support my chief to lead the team and take the best possible care of our patients? The role of a junior resident as a leader on the service is constantly in flux, from taking the role of an intern 1 day to taking the role of a senior in another. As such, your role truly can be the most difficult. Knowing when to ask for help and relaying critical information to your seniors and attendings are crucial to one's success. By being a role model for the interns on the service showing them it is ok to ask questions and for help, it will give them the courage to do the same.

Extensive research has been conducted over the past centuries on what qualities a good teacher has. Though most of the research was not focused on general surgery residency, the recurring theme was approachability, compatibility, ability to listen, and interest in one's learning [3]. This directly applies to surgery residency as a junior resident because your actions are observed and seen by all who interact with you from attendings, co-residents, social workers, patients and their families, consultant staff, and many more on a day-to-day basis.

As a junior resident, you may have the opportunity to guide an intern through a procedure or operation for the first time. Ask them how they plan to approach the case, and if they are correct, allow them to proceed with you in the role of teacher. If they are incorrect, use the case as a learning opportunity by allowing them to assist you and instructing them throughout your decision-making. This way, your intern feels seen, and outside of all the floor work and clinic, they can manifest their skills as a surgeon.

Mistakes are bound to happen; it is part of surgical education. However, how one handles a mistake truly makes a difference in their future. If an intern makes a mistake and does not approach a junior, senior, or attending about it as soon as it occurs, it is important to approach them in a respectful manner in privacy. For example, if an intern removed a chest tube from a patient in the morning, ordered a post-pull chest X-ray which showed a large pneumothorax and the intern knew but did not relay the information. In this instance, a patient's life may have been at risk. As a junior resident, as soon as you find out, inform your senior resident and proceed to correct the action by taking care of the patient first. Next, sit down with your intern to discuss what happened. You must first understand what happened that day, understand their workflow, and ask them what they were feeling. After understanding the situation, let them know the consequences if this was not found out earlier, the patient could have died from tension pneumothorax. Let it settle, then ask what they will do differently next time, and hold them to it. The goal is not to reprimand the intern or destroy their confidence, but to address mistakes imminently for patient safety, then have a detailed conversation about what led to the event, what was learned, and how to never repeat it.

Every attending will have variations in how they perform a procedure—even something as simple as a lipoma excision will have variations in their technique and pre- and post-operative management. The best way to learn your attendings' specifics is to ask your senior residents, read previous operative reports on the case you're performing, and ask the surgical tech and nursing team about the tray set the attending uses. Importantly, after you have performed or observed a procedure, take notes about how it was done.

How to Receive Operative Feedback

There is no one way to receive operative feedback, each attending and senior resident provides it differently. Your role as a junior resident is to seek it in any convenient moment you can. Some attendings and senior residents will give you operative feedback during the surgery, guiding you, while some will stay quiet and just intervene when you are not moving forward or close to a danger zone. Regardless, the best time for operative feedback is immediately after the critical portions of the case are complete or at the end of your operative day. Be proactive when asking for operative feedback. Volunteer what you think you did well and what you think you need to improve on and then ask the attending for their feedback as well. Try not to wait until the end of a rotation to ask for feedback, the earlier it is given, the more meaningful and actionable it will be. If you are going to be doing several of the same cases with an attending in a given day or week, asking for feedback between cases will give you actionable items to improve on in the next case and you will see dramatic improvement in your skills in a short period of time. We are now moving toward entrustable professional activities as general surgery residency, which will significantly motivate faculty to provide real-time feedback via an app that is visible immediately to the resident. This will be a requirement based on the American Board of Surgery (ABS) to start with the incoming intern class of 07/1/2028 [4]. This new type of feedback has been studied and verified in multiple other specialties including orthopedics surgery and in PA school [5, 6].

Practice Laparoscopic/Robotic Skills on the Box Trainer/Simulator

There is no one way to practice these skills on a simulator, however, having an accountability partner in your program who also is in need of practice is a useful tool. As a resident, you are busy with service and exhausted after with family and obligations, so setting a certain time and day a week with a co-resident is helpful. Learn each other's schedules, and figure out which 1 or 2 days of the week are best so that you can practice laparoscopic and robotic skills. Individually, practice the day/night before for a specific skill you will need for the next day's case (e.g., laparoscopic knot tying prior to hiatal hernia repair and robotic suturing prior to robotic hernia repair).

Participate in Clinic

Participation in clinic is an often overlooked but critical part of your surgical training. When seeing a patient, perform the physical exam whenever appropriate. This is your best opportunity to develop your skills for evaluating hernias and other physical exam-based diagnoses. After seeing the patient, develop your own plan and present it. You will learn at least as much from the times your plan is wrong as from the times your plan is right. Pay attention to the way your attending manages post-operative questions and complications. Pay attention to the way they discuss procedures with patients. These are skills you will not learn anywhere else in residency and will be critical to your success as a surgeon.

How to Be Successful as a Senior Resident

Leading a Team

As the senior resident of the team, your leadership for junior residents sets the tone for daily rounds and overall patient care. You will know attending preferences the best by now and will serve as an intermediary between attendings and the rest of the team. Organizational and prioritization skills you have built during intern and junior resident years become important to balancing running a team efficiently and being timely to first start cases or clinic. Being able to recognize each resident's role as well as strengths and weaknesses will allow you to assign tasks for each team member to get work done effectively while allowing each resident to grow. However, keep your ears on the ground and communicate often with your team; whether it's after rounds or at the end of the day. Recognizing your team's interpersonal work relationship and recognizing major or minor conflicts early allows time for them to resolve and will improve overall working conditions for everyone. Recognize small wins every day such as improvement in a patient's clinical status, a resident's operative success, or a good catch on the floors by your intern. Positive compliments boost morale and motivation for the team to continue to work hard. Last of all, PM rounding can be a powerful tool to incorporate to ensure that morning plans are properly executed and to evaluate if they are effective. This also allows additional patient care plans to be made for the night, improving overall patient care.

Developing Operative Independence

Becoming a successful senior resident in the OR requires proper planning and preparation before cases. Your operative autonomy grows, and to best utilize each opportunity, it is important to prepare specific skills on the laparoscopic training or robotic simulator. Develop a plan for every case to decide how you want to do the case and what equipment you need or have available. Use every operative opportunity as practice for what you would do if you were in practice on your own. Ask questions about everything from why an attending has a certain preference such as how to enter an abdomen for a particular case to what type of mesh they use in different scenarios. Senior residency is a daily opportunity to figure out what works best for you to incorporate into your future practice.

How to Excel in Clinical Duties

When carrying out clinical duties, have a clear understanding of your role and what is expected of you. Each day, list what needs to be done. Tackle one task at a time, prioritizing the time-sensitive tasks: checking in patients for the OR, discharges, and consulting other services. After rounding, ensure that all orders are placed. Try your best to complete all hands-on tasks on the floors prior to turning your attention to other tasks such as notes. Learning how to triage the work will be the ultimate key to success. This will come over time, with more experience.

When taking consults over the phone, ask the pertinent questions to clearly understand exactly what the consult is for. Get the patient's name, medical record number, location, and a good call-back number. Write everything down. See the consult within 10 min if possible. Once you have seen the consult, compile the information into a precise and comprehensive presentation with all relevant labs, imaging, and your plan, prior to calling to discuss with your seniors. This not only allows for organized communication but also displays your ability to think critically about the disease pathology and display your knowledge and understanding of that topic.

Finally, never hesitate to carry things up the ladder to your seniors. Listen to your patients, and trust yourself and your intuition. If something does not seem right, discuss it with a senior.

How to Gain Operative Experience

Building operative experience throughout residency begins outside of the operating room. It starts at home or in the resident lounge with various knot-tying techniques or your suturing kit for different suturing methods. Repetition outside of the OR is key to maximizing time spent executing and performing skills in the OR. As you progress through residency and your expected level of contribution to complete the case grows, so will the skills you practice.

It is important to understand the indications for why a particular surgery is being performed over another as well as which situations this surgery would be contraindicated. Always read up on the patient prior to the case to give yourself a better understanding of the patient's clinical status and past medical and surgical history. Each of these components may affect which pre-operative antibiotics you give, how you choose to start the case depending on their surgical history, or even what post-operative pain medications you will prescribe to the patient.

Utilize an operative techniques textbook or society video library to learn the key steps and critical mistakes for the operation you are going to perform. Write down the major steps for each case and set goals for yourself on what you want to accomplish for the case. Prior to the case, discuss which steps you are comfortable with and which steps you would like to improve on with attending supervision. Communication is key with your attending and even junior residents in the case so that everyone can learn while ensuring patient safety.

Scrub every case when able, even if it requires double or triple scrubbing for larger cases. There is always an operative technique or skill that can be learned or repeated to mastery. As an intern or junior resident, double scrubbing allows you to watch and learn how instruments are being set up and used for every case so that you will be more familiar with how to operate them in the future. It also allows you to learn from what your senior resident may struggle with and give you an insight into how they overcome them in the OR.

How to Do Well on Tests

Questions, questions, questions. They can be from SCORE or other sources, as long as you are being consistent. Reading is also critical, whether it is from SCORE chapters, an ABSITE review book, or a general surgery textbook. Stick to one or two resources to not get overwhelmed. During your didactics time see if your program will allow 30 min a session for a resident to teach an ABSITE topic. Research has shown that teaching improves memory, cognition, and patient communication with improved bedside manners, as such will help with ABSITE review and with patient care [7, 8]. Set aside time each day (even if it is only 15 min) with a goal of at least 10 questions a day. This will change as you get closer to the exam date. Listen to podcasts on your journey to and from work or while working out. There are many podcasts available; ask your senior residents for recommendations. When you see a disease process clinically, read about it right away. You will remember it better.

Delivering Good Presentations/Lectures

Throughout our education experience from high school to medical school, we learned the importance of being concise yet informative with the point made. Surgeons and many health care professionals will present on several topics throughout training to peer residents and larger audiences including attendings. This includes but not limited to surgical intensive care unit presentations presenting research at a conference with a PowerPoint versus poster presentation. The key is recognizing your audience, conducting extensive research on said topic, limiting the number of words on each slide, and saving enough time for questions.

Applying for Practice

Applying for practice begins with preparing your CV. It can be helpful to include an "About Me" section to give potential recruiters or employers an insight into who you are, specific skills or training that you have to offer, and what you are looking for in a practice. Ask your current attendings about the benefits of an academic or community position. Your level of training may also dictate the environment you choose to practice in. For example, fellowship-trained graduates may grow a practice easier with an academic affiliation and referral for specialized cases. Send emails to department chairs for academic programs of your specific interest. Many email addresses can be found on society pages. On the contrary, general surgery graduates in a community setting may be better able to maintain a broader practice due to the lack of specialist coverage in that area. Have an idea of what you would like to include in your practice and ask jobs in the community about the types of cases being covered. This may range from endoscopies to vascular procedures. While private practice models still exist in general surgery (42.7%), there has been an increase in hospital-employed models. Research and ask recruiters or employers which model they employ [9]. As a hospital-employed surgeon, you are hired directly by the hospital or the company that owns the hospital. Whereas in private practice, the group employs you and at times with the option for a partnership track after a required number of years working for the practice. Ultimately, create a list of the most important factors in choosing a job such as location (city size, suburban, or rural), call schedule, colleague/group collegiality, base income with or without call pay, and robotics availability.

Choosing a Fellowship

Deciding which fellowship to pursue is much like deciding residency specialty in medical school. The major difference is now you have truly done the work. You have been the surgeon. Think back to each of your rotations to this point. Which rotations did you look forward to? Which rotations did you enjoy with the patients? Enjoy the operations? Reflect on yourself and your personality. Do you need a subspecialty with good outcomes or do you want to do the most challenging, last chance cases? Are you okay with getting called into the hospital every night you are on call or do you want a more relaxed lifestyle? Most importantly, which field do you think can sustain you for the next 20–30 years. Remember that this is the first time in your medical training that you will be doing the same thing for more than a few months at a time. Pick something that truly brings you joy and that will sustain you through tough days or weeks. Speak with a trusted advisor about your honest competitiveness in the field of your choice. Are you willing to do an extra research year to improve your competitiveness for your chosen field or is there a similar field that can offer the same joy but is perhaps a little less competitive? Finally, if you have a spouse or other family member who supports you, speak with them about the sacrifices they will be asked to make for your chosen specialty.

A Good Residency/Fellowship Application

The first step in preparing your residency or fellowship application is preparing your CV. This is a good time to build the habit of updating your CV every 6 months with additional research or activities that you have performed or participated in. Ask your medical school or residency for their CV template. Remember to proofread! Ideally ask someone else to proofread for you as well—it is easy to miss our own typos. As you fill out your research activities, no activity is too small. Little things count in your application, just be prepared to talk about everything you list.

Letters of Recommendation

The ideal number of letters of recommendation is typically at least three. These should be balanced between individuals who will write strong letters for you. One who "adores" and highly supports you where the quality of this letter is more important than their national recognition. One who you have worked well with clinically and/or have worked on a project together. Last of all, one who is senior or nationally well-known in the department. Your residency program coordinator or manager is a great resource as they often know who are great letter writers to ask from. If the letters are being acquired for a fellowship application, it can be helpful to include letter writers who are specialists in the field you are applying to.

Preparing for Boards

Qualifying Exam

Preparing for the qualifying exam is much like preparing for your ABSITE. This is a knowledge-based exam and you are expected to know all of general surgery, much like your ABSITE. There has been a shift in focus over recent years with the ABS change to continuous certification for the exams to test current treatment guidelines rather than historical dogma. This is the primary difference between the qualifying exam and ABSITE, you will be asked what the most current guidelines recommend. There are many resources out there—make sure you are using an up-to-date resource as the answers from 2 to 3 years ago may not be accurate today in some fields.

Certifying Exam

The most important thing you can do to prepare for the certifying exam is practice, practice, practice. Ask your residency and fellowship faculty to do mock orals for you. When they do, prepare for these like they are the real thing. This is less a knowledge-based exam than it is a test of your ability to use the knowledge you have safely. The ABS has links to the curriculum and content of the exam on their website. Finally, this is the one exam that is really worth spending money on a preparation course. Many residencies will reimburse you for the cost once you pass.

How to Take Care of Yourself During Training

Even with the 80-h work rule in place by the ACGME in 2003 to help residents with a better work-life balance, surgical residency is still widely accepted as long, demanding, and arduous training [10]. Even so, taking care of yourself should remain the top priority to avoid burnout. Find or keep hobbies outside of medicine that you can enjoy on your scheduled days off. Whether it is spending time with friends, family, or significant other, recognize what keeps you grounded after a long stretch of work days and plan ahead. Balance operative opportunities or clinical duties with time for yourself to rest for the night after work. Know when you are overextending yourself, whether physically or mentally, and learn when to respectfully decline certain responsibilities or projects if your health needs prioritizing instead. Struggling is a normal part of learning during training. Be aware of any resources available to you such as therapy or counseling that may help you overcome difficult periods of your life. Ask for help during these times from your program, attendings, or colleagues. Ultimately, taking care of yourself during training will allow you to optimize your health and mind to learn and gain the most out of surgical residency.

SAGES Takeaway

- Surgical training is a challenging but rewarding time in your surgical career. Learning from others' experiences is vital to success in training.
- At each stage of your training, know your limitations, communicate well and ask for help often.
- Prepare thoroughly for each opportunity and task you are given – from ordering IV fluids to performing a splenectomy, success comes from the preparation before you place the order or walk into the operating room.
- Be an advocate for your own learning, stay humble and seek out constructive feedback.
- Read about the disease processes you see throughout your day – combining reading with clinical experience enhances learning and retention of information.

References

1. Yeo H, Bucholz E, Sosa JA, et al. A national study of attrition in general surgery training: which residents leave and where do they go? Ann Surg. 2010;252(3):529–34.

2. Weaver SJ, Dy SM, Rosen MA. Team-training in healthcare: a narrative synthesis of the literature. BMJ Qual Saf. 2014;23:359–72.
3. Kumari KL, Rao PL, Sekhar RC, Elena GK. Qualities of best medical teacher: a student perceptive study. Int J Res Med Sci. 2016;4(12):5436–9. https://doi.org/10.18203/2320-6012.ijrms20164224.
4. "Entrustable Professional Activities". The American Board of Surgery. 2003–2023. https://www.absurgery.org/default.jsp?epahome.
5. Dwyer T, Wadey V, Archibald D, Kraemer W, Shantz JS, Townley J, Ogilvie-Harris D, Petrera M, Ferguson P, Nousiainen M. Cognitive and psychomotor entrustable professional activities: can simulators help assess competency in trainees? Clin Orthop Relat Res. 2016;474(4):926–34.
6. Mulder H, Ten Cate O, Daalder R, Berkvens J. Building a competency-based workplace curriculum around entrustable professional activities: the case of physician assistant training. Med Teach. 2010;32(10):e453–9.
7. Snell L. The resident-as-teacher: it's more than just about student learning. J Grad Med Educ. 2011;3(3):440–1. https://doi.org/10.4300/JGME-D-11-00148.1. PMID: 22942984; PMCID: PMC3179240.
8. Seely AJ, Pelletier MP, Snell LS, Trudel JL. Do surgical residents rated as better teachers perform better on in-training examinations? Am J Surg. 1999;177(1):33–7. https://doi.org/10.1016/s0002-9610(98)00306-7.
9. Strazewski L. Practice owner or employee? Physicians' specialty may tell the tale. American Medical Association; 2021.
10. Accreditation Council for Graduate Medical Education. The ACGME's approach to limit resident duty hours 12 months after implementation: a summary of achievements. Accreditation Council for Graduate Medical Education; 2002. http://www.acgme.org.

Establishing a Military Surgical Career

9

Danielle B. Holt and Andrew T. Schlussel

Abbreviations

MHS	Military Health System
DHA	Defense Health Agency
DHHQ	Defense Health Headquarters
USU	Uniformed Services University of the Health Sciences
MTF	Military or Medical Treatment Facility
NDAA	National Defense Authorization Act
JTS	Joint Trauma System
CPG	Clinical Practice Guideline
CoSCCC	Committee on Surgical Combat Casualty Care

Disclaimer: *The opinions and assertions expressed herein are those of the author(s) and do not reflect the official policy or position of the Uniformed Services University of the Health Sciences or the Department of Defense.*
This research was supported (in whole or in part) by HCA Healthcare and/or an HCA Healthcare affiliated entity. The views expressed in this publication represent those of the author(s) and do not necessarily represent the official views of HCA Healthcare or any of its affiliated entities.

D. B. Holt (✉)
Uniformed Services University, Bethesda, MD, USA
e-mail: danielle.holt@usuhs.edu

A. T. Schlussel
HCA Florida Jacksonville Surgical Specialists, Jacksonville, FL, USA

S. M. Johnson et al. (eds.), *The SAGES Manual of Strategy and Leadership*, https://doi.org/10.1007/978-3-031-62359-2_9

ATTD	Army Trauma Training Detachment
FRSD	Forward Resuscitative Surgical Detachment
GST	Ground Surgical Team
AFMS	Air Force Medical Service
MEDCOM	US Army Medical Command
BUMED	US Navy Bureau of Medicine and Surgery
eMSM	Enhanced Multi-service Markets
ERSA	External Resource Sharing Agreements
MEDCEN	Medical Centers
OCONUS	Outside of the Contiguous US
OTSG	Office of the Surgeon General
PCS	Permanent Change of Station
ROFR	Right of First Refusal
SMMAC	Senior Military Medical Action Council
DMMAC	Deputy Military Medical Action Council
OASD[HA]	Office of the Assistant Secretary of Defense for Health Affairs
MHSER	MHS Executive Review Board
WRNMMC	Walter Reed National Military Medical Center
SAMMC	San Antonio Military Medical Center
MCC	Murtha Cancer Center
USAISR	Institute for Surgical Research
CCCRP	Combat Casualty Care Research Program
KSA	Knowledge, Skills, and Abilities
C-STARS	Center for Sustainment of Trauma and Readiness Skills
AMCT3	Army Military–Civilian Trauma Team Training
ODE	Off Duty Employment
CRADA	Cooperative Research and Development Agreements
DoDTR	Department of Defense Trauma Registry
GHE	Global Health Engagement
PME	Professional Military Education
MHSSPACS	Military Health System Partnership with the American College of Surgeons

Introduction

A career as a military surgeon can be a highly fulfilling and rewarding path for those with a passion for medicine and a desire to serve their country. As a military surgeon, one is tasked with providing crucial medical care to service members and their families, often in challenging and dynamic environments. Beyond combat situations, military surgeons also play a critical role in the overall health and well-being of service members, from routine procedures to specialized treatments for injuries and illnesses. The sense of purpose and fulfillment that comes from serving one's country and making a tangible difference in the lives of others is a unique and compelling aspect of a military surgeon's career. Additionally, military surgeons can work alongside highly skilled and dedicated medical professionals, receive advanced education and training both clinically and professionally, as well as develop leadership skills that can benefit them both in their military careers and beyond.

To effectively shape your career and achieve success, it is essential to have a comprehensive understanding of both the mission and leadership structure of the military health system (MHS). Military medicine encompasses three primary missions: to provide combat casualty care and ensure that service members are healthy to deploy, to ensure that military medical personnel are ready to provide care worldwide, and to provide medical services at military treatment facilities (MTF) to service members, retirees, and their families. Awareness of the organization and structure of the MHS provides a foundation of knowledge to transition and advance through milestones in one's career.

The Office of the Assistant Secretary of Defense for Health Affairs (OASD[HA]) serves as the chief medical adviser to the Secretary of Defense and oversees the leadership of the MHS which includes the Defense Health Agency (DHA), the Joint Staff Surgeon, the service Surgeon Generals (TSG), and the Uniformed Services University of the Health Sciences (USU).[1] Figure 9.1

[1]https://www.health.mil/About-MHS (accessed May 5, 2023).

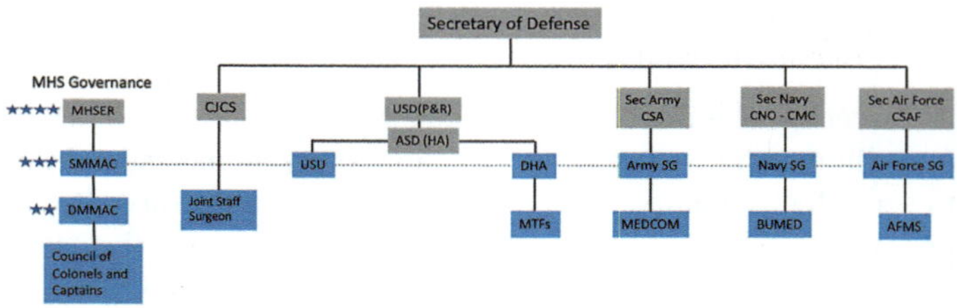

Fig. 9.1 Military health system governance. *MHS* Military Health System, *SMMAC* Senior Military Medical Action Council, *DMMAC* Deputy Military Medical Action Council, *CJCS* Chairman, Joint Chiefs of Staff, *USD[P&R]* Undersecretary of Defense for Personnel and Readiness, *ASD[HA]* Assistant Secretary of Defense for Health Affairs, *USU* Uniformed Services University, *DHA* Defense Health Agency, *MTF* Military Treatment Facility, *CSA* Chief of Staff of the Army, *SG* Surgeon General, *MEDCOM* Medical Command, *CNO—CMC* Chief of Naval Operations—Commandant of the Marine Corps, *BUMED* Navy Bureau of Medicine and Surgery, *CSAF* Chief of Staff of the Air Force, *AFMS* Air Force Medical Service

details the joint structure of MHS governance. Working in partnership, TSGs lead the medical forces while DHA manages healthcare markets and provides support to the combatant commands.[2] Following the 2017 National Defense Authorization Act (NDAA), the MTFs fall under the direction of DHA. Comprehension of your local MTF's mission within DHA, the structure and priorities of your service branch, as well as the relationships within the Department of Defense (DoD) can provide context for establishing and growing your surgical career.

There are three general career pathways to pursue as a military surgeon: clinical and administrative, academic and research, as well as operational and command. Different positions can intersect multiple pathways which makes it important to weigh assignments relative to personal and family considerations, time you plan to spend in the military, and long-term career goals. Many of these options are synergistic; however, there are certain job opportunities, especially in the leadership and command pathways that

[2] https://www.health.mil/About-MHS/OASDHA/Defense-Health-Agency (accessed May 5, 2023).

require a well-designed plan early in one's career. As seniority and administrative responsibilities increase, direct patient care may decrease, posing unique professional challenges. Maintenance of clinical skills requires deliberate planning which may need supplementation if not located at a robust medical center or civilian partnership site. In this chapter, we will explore considerations for your first job and each of these pathways in more detail. We hope that this chapter helps provide a road map with resources to further your career in the military while allowing you to develop a meaningful practice as a surgeon.

Your First Job

The initial job and location assignment will vary based on a variety of factors including branch of service, seniority, fellowship training, Graduate Medical Education (GME) needs, and timing. Special consideration is afforded to surgeons married to other service members or with family members who have specific health needs. Each branch of service has a representative (usually not a surgeon) in the human resources and personnel management areas as well as a consultant to the Surgeon General or specialty leader (who is a surgeon) who will assist in position allocation. Anticipate that your initial position may not be at your first-choice location. If you have a specific assignment in mind or are interested in working with residents, engaging in a proactive discussion with the local chief of surgery and/or program director (PD) will inform local needs and may assist in an assignment at that location. Following graduation from residency, most surgeons will be stabilized for the first year to complete boards and codify skills. Some surgeons may go straight into fellowship after residency, depending on the service and available positions. Military–civilian partnerships which will be discussed in more detail later are possible with some partnerships reserved for fellowship-trained surgeons.

MTFs with surgical capabilities range from small outpatient surgery centers to tertiary academic medical centers. The Army is composed of seven medical centers (MEDCEN) that support surgical GME including Walter Reed National Military Medical Center (WRNMMC), San Antonio Military Medical Center (SAMMC), Madigan, Tripler, William Beaumont, Eisenhower, and Womack Army Medical Centers. SAMMC is integrated with the US Army Institute of Surgical Research Burn Center and WRNMMC is co-located with USU. Army community hospitals that support the operational force are referred to as Medical Department Activity (MEDDAC). As a general surgeon in the Air Force, your first job is typically at an MTF with a utilization code that assigns you to a Ground Surgical Team (GST). There are five GME surgical training programs in the Air Force at SAMMC, Wright Patterson, Nellis, Travis, and Keesler Air Force Bases. The Air Force has more opportunities for overseas assignments, and it is recommended to speak with the consultant regarding these positions. In the Navy, many surgeons will be assigned to operational units such as an aircraft carrier and marine expeditionary force for their first job. The Navy has three GME teaching hospitals in San Diego, Portsmouth, and WRNMMC. The hospital organizational structure usually separates clinical leadership with military administrative and legal functions by assigning surgeons to a local military commander.

Your first year in practice is a great opportunity to determine what drives you as a surgeon. When you find a position or a job you enjoy, cultivate it. Ultimately, the location you are placed is up to the needs of the military; however, if you want to stay in a location, you want to find ways to make yourself valuable. The services review assignments every 3 years and based on military needs, surgeon preferences, fellowship training, GME needs, and seniority will determine whether you will move to another position referred to as a Permanent Change of Station (PCS). Fellowship-trained surgeons typically stay located with GME programs. Ultimately, it is up to you to be proactive in your career, but if you stay humble, be respectful, and work well with your team, you will have ample opportunities to further your development.

Fellowship training is available in the military for those interested in advancing their surgical skills. Available slots and specialties are based on the needs of your branch of service but generally include surgical oncology, colorectal, pediatric surgery, cardiothoracic, vascular, trauma and critical care, plastic surgery, and minimally invasive surgery (MIS). Most fellowships are performed at civilian institutions, with vascular surgery at WRNMMC, trauma and critical care at SAMMC, and the burn fellowship at the US Army Institute of Surgical Research (USAISR). Brigham and Women's Hospital has a dedicated military position in a two-year thoracic focused cardiothoracic fellowship [1]. Both WRNMMC and San Diego have established American College of Surgeons (ACS) Accredited Education Institutes fellowships in surgical education and simulation.[3] These training opportunities will incur active-duty service obligations but can provide a path to a clinically focused career.

Clinical Practice

MTFs provide opportunities to practice a wide breadth of surgery depending on your comfort level, hospital infrastructure, and staffing. The community hospitals typically have general surgeons but often do not have subspecialists allowing you to diversify your practice. If your facility does not have gastroenterology, you may be doing more advanced endoscopy. If you do not have endoscopic retrograde cholangiopancreatography capability, you can consider obtaining a surgical proctor or taking a short course in laparoscopic transcystic common bile duct exploration which can be accomplished with additional equipment. Without interventional radiology, you may have to laparoscopically place drains as in the case of perforated appendicitis which is not suitable for appendectomy or antibiotics. If your hospital lacks nuclear medicine or plastic surgery, consider getting credentials at a local hospital with those capabilities to perform sentinel lymph node biopsies or breast reconstruction with a local plastic surgeon. At places with minimal otolaryngology support, you can

[3] https://www.facs.org/for-medical-professionals/education/programs/accredited-education-institutes/fellowship-accreditation-standards-and-criteria/open-positions/ (accessed May 16, 2023).

develop an endocrine practice but will likely have to learn how to perform your own ultrasound-guided fine needle aspirations and need to ensure you have cytotechnician and cytopathology support. You can incorporate pediatric hernias and appendectomies assuming you have appropriate pediatric anesthesia. Similarly, you can perform video-assisted thoracic surgery if anesthesia can provide single-lung ventilation. For advanced or complex procedures, a request can be made for an inter-facility credentials transfer brief (ICTB) which allows military subspecialists to obtain temporary credentials at your facility to proctor or assist you with specific procedures assuming your hospital can provide appropriate postoperative care.

Expanding your clinical practice will largely depend on the surgical needs of your local market, called a Defense Health Network (DHN). There are nine regionally aligned DHNs lead by a director typically in the rank of general or admiral. Some MTFs may not have enough surgical volume to maintain specialized skill sets. Surgical capabilities will change in response to competing MHS priorities allowing opportunities for augmenting your practice. For example, metabolic and bariatric surgery is one of the most common and consistent referrals to surgeons in the DoD; however, not all MTFs can be staffed with fellowship-trained minimally invasive surgeons, allowing general surgeons to perform these operations. Establish appropriate quality and safety multi-disciplinary care and conferences for more complex surgical patients such as bariatrics. Collaborating within the network forms a valuable partnership that ultimately results in the recapture or providing care for service members and their beneficiaries at the MTF. Most institutions have a managed care department that can assist with this process through the right of first refusal (ROFR). This allows the surgery service at the MTF to care for patients if the capability permits, rather than sending to the network, however, requires careful attention to updating available capabilities in a timely fashion such as when specialists deploy and return. Following the 2023 deputy secretary of defense stabilization memo, efforts should first be directed towards re-attracting patients to the MTF where possible. An additional resource for understanding the surgical care being provided at the MTF and in the network is the Knowledge, Skills, and Abilities (KSA) dashboard which is part of a comprehensive Clinical Readiness Program to maintain the surgical skills and knowledge needed to deploy [2]. The CAC-enabled KSA clinician readiness dashboard depicts the complexity and volume of surgical procedures by domain performed by each surgeon at every MTF in the DoD as well as the types of procedures being performed by practices in the network.[4]

Agreements, Memorandums, Military–Civilian Partnerships, and Other Employment

DHA has multiple support agreements to foster partnerships with outside institutions to expand a surgical practice. Like any contract negotiation, these will take time to create and are executed centrally by the DHA Lead Agreement Manager, DHA Office of General Council, MTF and market directors, as well as the corresponding parties at the civilian institution. The American College of Surgeons *The Blue Book: Military-Civilian Partnerships for Trauma Training, Sustainment, and Readiness* provides best practices for maintaining civilian partnerships. Below is a list of types of agreements that can be made:

1. External Resources Sharing Agreement (ERSA): ERSAs involve a TRICARE contractor whereby the MTF sends MHS providers to a local hospital to provide healthcare services not available at the MTF. This avoids a referral to a network provider and examples include endoscopy, robotics, critical care, and nuclear medicine.
2. Veteran Affairs (VA) Sharing Agreement: This allows you to evaluate and treat patients at the VA with full privileges under a without compensation status. This partnership can significantly help foster relationships between your VA and MTF,

[4]https://carepoint.health.mil (accessed May 11, 2023).

especially if there is a shortage of surgeons at the VA facility or a shortage of operating room, endoscopy, or other clinical space at your facility. Additional funding can be obtained by applying for Joint Incentive Funds (JIF) to encourage innovation and programs that support both the VA and DoD.
3. Support Agreements: These alternative agreements include a Memorandum of Agreement (MOA) which involves resources and a Memorandum of Understanding (MOU) which has no resources involved. MOUs and MOAs are written contracts between two or more parties that outline the terms and understanding of their collaboration, particularly in the delivery of healthcare services. MOUs and MOAs may be used to establish agreements between military medical treatment facilities and civilian medical facilities, or between military treatment facilities and other government agencies. MOAs are typically more formal and legally binding than MOUs because they may be used to allocate resources, define roles and responsibilities, and establish performance standards and metrics.

Following the 2017 NDAA, the services increased opportunities for military–civilian partnerships with the largest number in the Air Force [3]. Surgeons can be embedded full or part-time (including rotational assignments) with most of the full-time partnerships designated for trauma surgeons. The Air Force has both full-time and part-time programs as part of the Center for Sustainment of Trauma and Readiness Skills (C-STARS) at the University of Maryland R Adams Cowley Shock Trauma Center, Saint Louis University, and University of Cincinnati Medical Center as well as Sustained Medical and Readiness Trained (SMART) programs at University Medical Center of Southern Nevada, and UC Davis Medical Center. The Army Military–Civilian Trauma Team Training (AMCT3) is a full-time, embedded program designed to provide bi-directional trauma and emergency preparedness with sites at Cooper University Health Care, Oregon Health and Sciences University, Harborview Medical Center, Vanderbilt University Medical Center, Grady Memorial Hospital, University of North Carolina at Chapel Hill Health, University of Chicago Medicine, and Medical College of

Wisconsin. The Navy has full-time embedded programs at LA County University of Southern California, University of Pennsylvania, and Cook County Hospital. An international military–civilian partnership also exists in Abu Dhabi at Sheikh Shakhbout Medical City.[5]

An additional consideration for building your clinical experience includes participation in off-duty employment (ODE). This program allows military surgeons to perform civilian work outside of their regular duty hours such as locum tenens positions. In the Air Force, ODE can only be performed after successful board certification. ODE cannot interfere with military duties or create any conflicts of interest. This requires military personnel to obtain approval and generally has time limitations and other restrictions. You must ensure that you have medical malpractice insurance as you will not be covered under the Federal Tort Claim Act and must ensure you are not receiving reimbursement for care provided to Tricare patients.

In addition to your surgical practice, licensure and maintenance of board certification also depend on continuing medical education (CME). Military funding for CME varies and depends on your local MTF budget unless the event is centrally funded by the service branches. Although a significant amount of CME can be web-based, there are many opportunities for attending national meetings. The Society of Gastrointestinal and Endoscopic Surgeons (SAGES) continues to waive conference fees for active-duty military personnel. SAGES provides a platform to host the Military Surgical Symposium which allows for a forum to present research, provide expert sessions, bridge the gap between military and civilian surgeons, and provide networking for military surgeons. The Military Health System Strategic Partnership with the American College of Surgeons (MHSSPACS) supports the Excelsior Surgical Society which also provides a yearly military

[5] https://www.facs.org/for-medical-professionals/membership-community/military-health-system-strategic-partnership/ess/about/newsletters/2022/three-new-military-civilian-partnerships-combatting-the-peacetime-effect/ (accessed May 16, 2023).

symposium for education, networking, and collaboration with civilian partners.

Administrative Leadership

Military surgery affords leadership opportunities often much earlier in one's career than civilian surgeons. Be proactive, and volunteer for hospital committees such as risk management, credentials, quality and process improvement (QI/PI), executive committees of the medical staff, pharmacy and therapeutics, patient safety, blood utilization, critical care, simulation, infection control, and multi-disciplinary trauma meetings to name a few. Depending on the size of your facility, you may have the opportunity to serve as the clinic, service, and department chief with more senior leadership roles being available at smaller facilities. The chief is directly responsible for credentialing, peer review, management of service operations, budget, referrals, schedules, policies, certifications, operating room utilization, awards, and military evaluations. The chief will work with the surgical consultants for assignments and will be involved in human resource actions for civilian employees, gaining valuable experience in interviewing and performance assessments. These skills allow you to shape and improve your surgical team. To succeed in a leadership role, one should first develop a solid clinical foundation. This will enhance your ability to effectively lead an interprofessional team of surgeons, advanced practitioners, nurses, technicians, enlisted, and administrative staff. You should not do it all—find opportunities for multiple members of the team to lead as subject matter experts. Treat the team with respect, take suggestions, and try to implement their ideas in an impactful way.

Look for opportunities to lead both in formal and informal roles. Depending on your institution and your specialty, some MTFs hold professional society certifications such as the Metabolic and Bariatric Surgery Quality Improvement Program, ACS Commission on Cancer, and National Accreditation Program for Breast Centers, and trauma verification which you could initiate or re-verify at your hospital. If you do not have a tumor board at your facility, you can likely join one at a local hospital or have civilian specialists come to a tumor board you host. Each MTF has a surgeon champion as part of the ACS National Surgical Quality Improvement Program (NSQIP) which leads multidisciplinary teams and participates in the national DoD NSQIP consortium to improve surgical outcomes. Even if you are not in a GME program, many MTFs have a wide variety of medical learners. You can become a site director or an instructor for the Army Interservice Physician Assistant Program, special forces medics, or corpsmen.

Professional Development and Education

Multiple opportunities exist for military surgeons to further their professional education in management, healthcare administration, and leadership. You can request a nomination to attend developmental courses such as the Army Junior Leader and Iron Major courses, USU's MEDXELLENCE course, the MHS Female Physician Leadership course, the Leadership, Education, Analysis, Development, Sustainment Joint Medical Executive Skills Institute Intermediate Executive Skills Course and Capstone Course.[6,7] Getting involved with professional societies such as SAGES and the ACS also provides opportunities for leadership development through committees, chair, and executive roles and courses (Table 9.1). You can request funding to attend professional society conferences and developmental courses. SAGES offers the Fundamentals of Leadership and Development course for surgeons just starting in a leadership role. ACS offers the Surgeons as Leaders: From Operating Room to Boardroom course for surgeons already in a leadership role.[8] The American College of Healthcare Executives provides fellowship and board certifica-

[6] https://www.health.mil/Training-Center/LEADS (accessed May 8, 2023).

[7] https://medschool.usuhs.edu/pmb/education/medxellence (accessed May 16, 2023).

[8] https://www.facs.org/for-medical-professionals/education/programs/acs-surgeons-as-leaders/ (accessed May 11, 2023).

Table 9.1 Military medical professional societies or surgical societies with military committees and chapters

AAS	https://www.aasurg.org/leadership/committee-objectives/
AAST	https://www.aast.org/committees/military-liaison-committee
AMSUS	https://www.amsus.org/membership/#who-are-our-members
ASMBS	https://asmbs.org/committees/military-committee
Excelsior Surgical Society	https://www.facs.org/for-medical-professionals/membership-community/military-health-system-strategic-partnership/ess/
MHSRS	https://mhsrs.health.mil/SitePages/Home.aspx
SAGES	https://www.militarysurgeons.org/
SOMA	https://specialoperationsmedicine.org/

AAS Association for Academic Surgery, *AAST* American Association for the Surgery of Trauma, *ASMBS* American Society for Metabolic and Bariatric Surgery, *MHSRS* Military Health System Research Symposium, *SAGES* Society of American Gastrointestinal and Endoscopic Surgeons, *SOMA* Special Operations Medical Association

tion in healthcare management.[9] The American Association for Physician Leadership provides both certificate programs and a pathway to become a Certified Physician Executive.[10] Engaging with organizations outside the hospital provides a perspective from other leaders in your specialty that may be influential at your institution. If you would like to pursue formal graduate education, USU offers a full-time in residence Masters in Healthcare Administration and Policy.[11] Army surgeons specifically interested in executive leadership can apply for the Baylor program for a Masters in Health Care Administration (MHA) or combined MHA/Masters in Business Administration (MBA) program which includes 1 year of didactics and 1 year residency which incurs an active duty service obligation.[12] The Naval Postgraduate School in

[9] https://www.ache.org/fache (accessed May 16, 2023).

[10] https://www.physicianleaders.org/credentials/cpe (accessed May 11, 2023).

[11] https://medschool.usuhs.edu/pmb/master-of-health-administration-and--policy (accessed May 14, 2023).

[12] https://hankamer.baylor.edu/army-baylor (accessed May 16, 2023).

Monterrey, CA, offers both in residence and distance Masters and PhD programs such as an MBA.[13]

Academic Medicine and Research

Military undergraduate medical education and GME generate and contribute to the retention of many physicians, influencing the long-term success of the MHS. If you are assigned to one of the GME training platforms, there are multiple options for leadership in education and teaching including the PD, assistant PD, and faculty roles. Generally, GME locations will consist of faculty from surgical subspecialties required to meet ACGME requirements. Even if you are assigned at a smaller hospital without surgery GME, you may work with other specialties such as family and internal medicine residents. USU medical students attend their clerkship rotations as well as Health Professions Scholarship Program medical students for post-clerkship and interview rotations for residency. Each GME program consists of core faculty determined by the PD who participate in curriculum development and clinical teaching. Faculty can lead in research and resident education, serve as the coordinator for medical students, grand rounds, board preparation, and QI/PI, and become the director for simulation.

USU provides in-person and virtual faculty development courses and certificates in teaching, academic leadership, scholarship, and research.[14] Professional societies also provide additional educational content for faculty including the Association for Surgical Education and the Association for Academic Surgery which has a military chapter (Table 9.1).[15] You can also pursue formal graduate programs at USU in health professions via distance learning through the Center for Health Professions Education, including a Master of Health Professions Education and a Master of Education in HPE, as well as a PhD.[16] The

[13] https://nps.edu/degree-programs#masters (accessed May 11, 2023).

[14] http://fac-dev.usuhs.edu/ (accessed May 8, 2023).

[15] https://www.aasurg.org/leadership/committee-objectives/ (accessed May 16, 2023).

[16] https://chpe.usuhs.edu/graduate-programs (accessed May 8, 2023).

Department of Family Medicine at Madigan Army Medical Center offers a 2-year faculty development fellowship where fellows can obtain an MPH or MBA.[17]

USU affords military surgeons the ability to participate in an academic health system with opportunities for academic promotion. It is important both to catalog your educational activities in your curriculum vitae and to create an educator portfolio which is required for promotion.[18] You can apply for an assistant professor as a chief resident or immediately upon graduating residency to expedite time in grade requirements for promotion, which is typically 5–6 years to associate and full professor. Promotion qualifications include scholarship of discovery, teaching, integration, and application as well as institutional citizenship which are defined in the USU Policies for Academic Administration of the Faculty, Instruction 1100A.[19] Contact SUR-Faculty@usuhs.edu in the Department of Surgery to request academic promotion.

Unique opportunities exist for conducting research and investigational protocols within military medicine. If research is one of your top priorities as a surgeon, then you may want to consider spending time at either USAISR in San Antonio or USU and WRNMMC which include multiple research centers such as programs located at the Murtha Cancer Center (MCC) and partnerships with the National Institutes of Health.[20] The U.S. Army Medical Research and Development Command at Fort Detrick serves as the command agency for the USAISR as well as manages the Combat Casualty Care Research Program (CCCRP) which also offers opportunities for collaboration.[21] The Henry Jackson Foundation is an additional resource that can assist with

[17] https://madigan.tricare.mil/About-Us/Graduate-Medical-Education/Faculty-Development (accessed May 16, 2023).

[18] https://sites.google.com/usuhs.edu/sur/faculty/faculty-promotion (accessed May 5, 2023).

[19] https://www.usuhs.edu/sites/default/files/media/documents/usui_1100._signed_pdf.pdf (accessed May 16, 2023).

[20] https://www.usuhs.edu/research/centers (accessed May 16, 2023).

[21] https://mrdc.health.mil/index.cfm/program_areas/medical_research_and_development/ccc_overview (accessed May 5, 2023).

funding opportunities, proposal support, and administrative and research staff to begin a new program of research.[22] In addition, most MTFs have a military department of clinical investigation (DCI) that falls under the Clinical Investigation Program (CIP) at DHA.[23] The CIP is accountable for supervising and conducting clinical investigations, along with providing support for clinical trials, epidemiological studies, and other research projects. Its main objective is to facilitate graduate health sciences education and enhance the health and readiness of military personnel. Furthermore, if available at your facility, you can participate in the Institutional Review Board and Animal Care and Use Committee within DCI.

Identifying a research mentor early will help generate investigational ideas and develop protocols that will benefit the surgical community and be completed in a reasonable amount of time given the requirements and resources within the MHS. When your research goals exceed the resources your local institution can provide, multi-institutional protocols can be designed through collaboration with military colleagues at other MTFs, partnering with civilian academic institutions through Cooperative Research & Development Agreements (CRADA) which allows for data Sharing or remaining in the MHS working with the Joint Trauma System (JTS) to analyze the Department of Defense Trauma Registry (DoDTR). The Military Health System Research Symposium (MHSRS) is the DoD's primary scientific meeting to present your research related to combat casualty care, military operational medicine, and simulation.[24] If you are proactive, understand institutional requirements, and look for opportunities for collaboration, research can be a significant component of your career.

---

[22]https://www.hjf.org/funding-opportunities (accessed May 16, 2023).

[23]https://www.health.mil/Military-Health-Topics/Research-and-Innovation/DHA-Research-and-Engineering/Research-Support-Division/Clinical-Investigations-Program-Branch (accessed May 8, 2023).

[24]https://mhsrs.health.mil/SitePages/Home.aspx (accessed May 5, 2023).

Deployment, Global Health, and Operational Assignments

One distinct and often rewarding aspect of military medicine is participation in an operational mission or deployment. The presence of a surgeon on the battlefield gives service members the will to fight knowing they will be provided exceptional medical care if injured. Deployments allow you to hone your leadership skills and develop the capability to provide surgical support while in an austere environment, giving military surgeons adaptability and resilience that is highly valuable for your career after the military. With the end of the conflict in Afghanistan, the operational or deployment tempo has significantly decreased; however, the US maintains a military presence around the globe. General surgeons will typically be assigned to a NATO Role 2 forward resuscitative surgical detachment or GST with the mission to provide far-forward surgical care on the battlefield.[25] Additional opportunities can be found at Role 3 field hospitals or with special operations teams.

Surgeons interested in assignment to special operations teams can apply through a competitive selection process. Those with a particular interest in special operations can also join the Special Operations Medical Association for tactical, austere, and deployed medicine.[26] Maintain an open line of communication with your military consultant to let them know if there is a certain location or deployed position you would be interested in performing. If you volunteer for a position, it could allow a more predictable timeline and you may feel more purposeful and fulfilled by completing a mission you elected to take. If possible, communicate early with the surgeon you are replacing or colleagues who have been to similar locations to know of any special considerations or equipment needed.

[25] https://www.nato.int/docu/logi-en/1997/lo-1610.htm (accessed May 16, 2023).

[26] https://specialoperationsmedicine.org/ (accessed May 11, 2023).

The KSA platform will aid in the assessment of surgical readiness for an operational mission as an expeditionary or austere surgeon. Although many surgeons do not perform trauma care daily, military surgeons regardless of their specialty must maintain trauma competency for combat casualty care. DHA's Sustaining Expeditionary Medical Skills strategic initiative outlined in the fiscal year 2022–2026 campaign plan utilizes the Clinical Readiness Program and KSA metric to identify opportunities for skills maintenance.[27] Military surgeons have access to multiple courses to maintain the knowledge and surgical skills for deployment such as Advanced Trauma Life Support certification. Under the Defense Medical Education and Training Institute, the Emergency War Surgery Course consists of the Advanced Surgical Skills for Exposure in Trauma and Combat Orthopedic Trauma Surgery courses that utilize perfused cadavers to perform surgical exposures for trauma.[28] The JTS Combat Casualty Care Curriculum Conference provides subject matter expertise to maintain readiness and provides CME.[29] The JTS Clinical Practice Guidelines (CPGs) should be downloaded prior to deployment and provide evidence-based clinical care pathways for the care of injured patients.[30] The JTS Committee on Surgical Combat Casualty Care (CoSCCC) holds yearly meetings to promote evidence-based care for combat casualties.[31] You may participate in team-based readiness training such as the Army Trauma Training Detachment (ATTD) at the University of Miami/Ryder Trauma Center, the Navy Trauma Training Center at Los Angeles County

[27] https://www.health.mil/About-MHS/OASDHA/Defense-Health-Agency/DHA-Campaign-Plan (accessed May 5, 2023).

[28] https://health.mil/Military-Health-Topics/Education-and-Training/DMRTI/Course-Information/Emergency-War Surgery-Course (accessed May 16, 2023).

[29] https://jts.health.mil/index.cfm/education/overview (accessed May 16, 2023).

[30] https://jts.health.mil/index.cfm/PI_CPGs/cpgs (accessed May 16, 2023).

[31] https://jts.health.mil/index.cfm/committees/cosccc (accessed May 16, 2023).

+ University of Southern California Medical Center, or the Air Force C-STARS programs.[32]

Global health engagement (GHE) encompasses a variety of foreign service activities that military surgeons can participate in to include global surgery and humanitarian assistance. The Air Force has a specialized International Health Specialist program, and the Navy has a GHE identifier that can be obtained through education and training. USU offers a global health distance learning certificate.[33] The Center for Global Health Engagement also offers short courses such as the Global Health Strategies for Security.[34] Under US Southern Command (SOUTHCOM), Joint Task Force-Bravo based out of Honduras has an enduring GHE mission where you may be asked to participate in a Medical Readiness Training Exercise.[35] Shipboard GHE includes the United States Naval Ship (USNS) Comfort in SOUTHCOM and the USNS Mercy which conducts the Pacific Partnership, the largest multinational humanitarian assistance and disaster relief preparedness mission conducted in the Indo-Pacific. The Indo-Pacific Military Health Exchange is co-sponsored by the US Indo-Pacific Command (USINDOPACOM) to facilitate military health interoperability.[36]

Military surgeons can also select an assignment with an operational unit. Operational military assignments typically rotate every 3 years for career progression. Advantages for relocating include gaining knowledge and insight from multiple organizations, understanding the role of military medicine in the operational force, as well as the ability in some instances to travel

---

[32] https://www.med.navy.mil/Navy-Medicine-Operational-Training-Command/Naval-Expeditionary-Medical-Training-Institute/NEMTI-Courses/ (accessed May 11, 2023).

[33] https://medschool.usuhs.edu/pmb/education/global-health-distance-learning-program (accessed May 8, 2023).

[34] https://cghe.usuhs.edu/training-and-education/global-health-strategies-for-security (accessed May 8, 2023).

[35] https://www.jtfb.southcom.mil/ (accessed May 16, 2023).

[36] https://www.ipmhe2023.org/about/ (accessed May 16, 2023).

OCONUS with locations in Europe and Asia. You should be deliberate about your plan for skills maintenance if selecting an operational assignment such as operating at your nearest MTF, establishing an ERSA or MOU, or performing ODE. Multiple leadership opportunities exist typically in the role of a medical advisor as the command surgeon or commander of a surgical team such as an FRSD. In the Air Force, junior surgeons interested in operational medicine may request a position as team leads for a GST, and senior surgeons could be selected as Expeditionary Medical Support System (Field Hospital) commanders. Navy general surgeons will often perform operational assignments immediately following completion of residency on an aircraft carrier or part of a fleet surgical team on an amphibious assault ship. Consider engaging in AMSUS, the Society of Federal Health Professionals, which publishes the journal *Military Medicine* and provides collaboration for federal, public, and global health.[37]

Military Career and Command

The role of a military surgeon provides a distinct experience by managing the professional requirements of a career in surgery but also as a military officer. Successfully navigating the intricacies of assignments, evaluations, professional military education, and promotions necessitates a commitment to personal development, as well as building strong networks, seeking out mentorship, and cultivating relationships, especially if you aspire to a command position. The tri-service surgical community is small, estimated at around 500 personnel, emphasizing the importance of maintaining a solid reputation and working with surgical colleagues to complete military requirements.

Officer performance evaluations form the basis for merit-based selection for military schools and promotions. All the services utilize a forced distribution to identify the highest-performing indi-

[37] https://www.amsus.org/ (accessed May 11, 2023).

viduals. Generally, you want to see an upward trend in your evaluations with the highest assessments possible before a promotion board. You need to understand favorable language in evaluations as many are written in an exaggerated style. Positions with larger scopes of responsibility can help in favorable evaluations with strong performance. Best practices include ensuring that your rater is aware of your accomplishments by providing them with formal written communication.

Professional military education (PME) is required for certain leadership and command positions and selection for promotion to higher ranks. Each service requires a minimum level of PME even for surgeons in clinical and academic roles which can be challenging to schedule as it often coincides with the completion of surgical residency. Attending PME in person at more senior ranks such as the command and general staff officers' course (intermediate level education) and senior service college (war college) requires a board process for selection. The length and availability of virtual options for these courses often change, so you want to be proactive in scheduling the best times that can be supported by personal and professional obligations. Furthermore, pursuing additional training such as airborne school, air assault school, or the flight surgeon course, allows for unique skillsets and experiences only possible while in the military.

Command is determined through a centralized selection board that largely uses evaluations to determine the order of merit and requires completion of PME. Surgeons need to opt-in for consideration and should anticipate a reduction or stopping of surgical practice in these roles. You can command both operational medical units and healthcare delivery platforms. Those who continue in these roles will often transition into executive medicine at the enterprise level and can positively impact healthcare administration from a surgeon's perspective. If you desire to return to clinical practice after a command assignment, there are opportunities to be assigned to positions where your primary focus is surgical practice. In such positions, you can receive guidance and mentorship from other surgeons to help safely integrate back to direct patient care.

Selection rates for military promotion vary by service but are generally increasingly competitive with more senior ranks. Leadership positions in any of the career pathways are generally favorable for promotion with nominative and command select positions being most influential. It is important to generally understand the promotion board process which consists of both non-medical and medical officer board members. Medical corps officer board files often look significantly different from those of combat arms (line) officers. Ideally, job titles should communicate your scope of responsibility to a non-medical officer using terms such as officer in charge, department chief, or director where appropriate. Senior leaders will host officer professional development lectures; you can attend to understand promotions and board processes. Selection for flag/general officer is extremely limited and requires at a minimum completion of the senior service college with strong performance in joint, multiple command select, and strategic billet positions.

Conclusion

Establishing your military surgical career presents numerous opportunities across clinical medicine, medical education and training, research, and operational health service support. Leadership opportunities are afforded early, making skills maintenance planning a deliberate process throughout your military career. Building clinical competence lays the groundwork for your career as a surgeon, and at an early stage, you should prioritize opportunities to broaden your surgical practice. Take responsibility for your growth and development, and when you encounter boundaries or limitations, seek out additional mentorship as well as education and training either through military or professional services in your areas of interest. Strive to understand the priorities of your service, DHA, and your organization to advocate for improved surgical care. Do not wait for senior leaders to provide your clinical practice, take the initiative, and shape your clinical practice by becoming a leader in your chosen field. By establishing strong relationships and seeking out new experiences, this will not only benefit you but will also have a positive impact on those in your practice and most importantly for your patients.

In addition to the leadership experience you will gain, your personal and professional relationships can be some of the most rewarding aspects of military medicine. A crucial component of leadership is the transition from self-development to the development of others. Seek out positive ways to engage in your MTF, solve problems with limited resources, find opportunities in challenging situations, and support your teammates. Whether fulfilling your service obligation for only a few years or staying until retirement, a military surgeon can develop a meaningful practice through service to the broader mission of caring for those in harm's way.

SAGES Takeaway

- Military surgeons play a vital role in providing essential medical care in challenging environments, serving both service members and their families, and contributing significantly to their well-being.
- Military surgeons work alongside skilled professionals, receive advanced training, and develop leadership skills, enhancing their professional and technical expertise while serving their country.
- Understanding the structure of the Military Health System and aligning career pathways with personal goals are essential for success.

Acknowledgments MAJ (P) Sean McFarling; Human Resources Command, US Army; COL (Ret) Robert Rush, US Army; Maj Katherine Cameron, US Air Force; LCDR Matt Nealeigh, US Navy; COL John Horton, US Army; LTC Timothy Plackett, US Army.

References

1. DeBarros M, Jaklitsch M, Bueno R, Mase VJ Jr. Formal military civilian affiliations are a template for low military cardiothoracic surgery volume. Ann Thorac Surg. 2022;114(3):621–4.
2. Holt DB, Hueman MT, Jaffin J, Sanchez M, Hamilton MA, Mabry CD, Bailey JA, Elster EA. Clinical readiness program: refocusing the military health system. Mil Med. 2021;186(Suppl 1):32–9.
3. Gurney JM, John SK, Whitt EH, et al. Data driven readiness: a preliminary report on cataloguing best practices in military civilian partnerships. J Trauma Acute Care Surg. 2022;93(2S):S155–9.

Part II

Leading Yourself—Promotion Across Systems

Achieving Promotion Within Different Systems

10

Danny Mou and Scott Davis

Understanding the Institution's Promotion Tracks

Understanding an institution's various promotion tracks equips physicians with a blueprint of how to progress in their careers. Importantly, the promotion tracks of an institution often reveal its priorities and values. For those who are seeking new employment positions, the promotion tracks should serve as a guide to whether that institution is suitable for them. A clinician who prioritizes high-volume clinical output may not be as suitable for an institution that prioritizes academic achievement. Likewise, an aspiring academic clinician may not be the best fit for an institution that promotes mostly based on clinical volume. That said, many institutions have different promotion tracks that cater to different career trajectories and thus may be suitable for clinicians with different professional goals.

Though there are variations across institutions, there are generally four categories of physician promotion tracks in health care

D. Mou (✉)
Department of Surgery, Emory University, Atlanta, GA, USA
e-mail: danny.mou@emory.edu

S. Davis
School of Medicine, Emory University, Atlanta, GA, USA
e-mail: sdavisj@emory.edu

S. M. Johnson et al. (eds.), *The SAGES Manual of Strategy and Leadership*, https://doi.org/10.1007/978-3-031-62359-2_10

institutions: **research, clinical, education, and service/administration**. These promotion tracks may be under different names across different institutions (i.e., investigator track vs. research track), so the most accurate way of comparing them will be to review the promotion track criteria. It should be noted that the promotion tracks usually do not measure outputs that are mutually exclusive from each other; certain skills such as excellence in teaching may contribute to both clinical and teaching promotion tracks. Additionally, promotion is often predicated on achievement in different categories. For example, an assistant professor may need to demonstrate excellence in both academic output and education for consideration for promotion to associate professor.

The research track focuses on academic output as measured by peer-reviewed manuscripts, intramural and external grants, editorship or editorial boards of academic journals, and membership of academic committees. It is important to be aware of the variations across institutions. For example, some institutions allow for physicians to be promoted to the most senior rank of professor in the research track without sustained extramural funding, while others require sustained extramural funding to be even considered for promotion to associate professors. Thus, if a clinician is interested in research but does not wish to write grants as a major part of his/her career, he/she should consider employment at the former type of institution. Next, there is the clinical track, on which advancement is typically based on clinical excellence, teaching, and often service. Some institutions may also require publications that advance clinical practice. Another promotion track focuses on educational activities such as consistent clinical teaching of resident physicians and medical students on rotations, publishing manuscripts in the field of education, and holding formal educational positions such as the program director, fellowship director, surgery simulation laboratory director, advisor roles, dean of education, or membership of local, regional, or national education committees. Depending on the institution, promotion may require publications and grants to advance the field of education. Once again, it is important for the clinician to be familiar with these details so that he/she will not be surprised by his/her career progression over time. Continually keeping education-related documentation such as mentee testimonials, e-mails, formal evaluations of the physician as a mentor, letters, and so on is a strongly encouraged practice in preparation of the promotion package. Finally, there is the service/administration track, which promotes physicians based on administrative contributions that support the healthcare system. Examples include leadership or managerial roles (e.g., bariatric surgery division chief), hospital operations roles (e.g., operating room (OR) logistics committee member), and other relevant positions (e.g., positions in quality improvement, hospital marketing, electronic health record management, faculty development, etc.). This promotion track has considerable variability and may not exist at certain institutions or is incorporated into another track such as the education track. Unlike the more classical research, clinical, and education promotion tracks, the administrative/service is newer, and its milestones may be more subjective. Measuring grant funding, number of publications, and impact of impact of publications may often be more straightforward than measuring a physician's impact as a member on the quality improvement team.

Within each promotion track, there are faculty ranks that are relatively standardized across institutions. Most academic institutions have instructor or assistant professor as the starting title for their clinicians. The instructor role below the assistant professor is often designed to allow for more time for the clinician to build up a sufficient work portfolio to be considered for promotion to the next level, which is often time-bound. Institutions often have a window of time before a clinician is expected to be evaluated either for promotion or for reappointment for that same position. For example, an institution can require evaluation for promotion/reappointment every 3 years for assistant professors and every 5 years for associate professors. Other institutions may have policies that have a time limit for a specific rank. For example, assistant professors may be required to be promoted within 7 years. It is advisable for the physician to understand the intent of these rules. More aggressive institutions may have a culture of "promote or out," where it is expected that clinicians advance through the promotion ladder at a specified pace. Discussing with peers and mentors at that institution is critical to understand if such a time pressure is present, as this may influence the clinician's choice of employment. On the flip side, institutions may have minimum years required to be at a rank. For example, an institution may require clinicians to be an assistant professor for at least 4 years before being considered for promotion. Beyond assistant professor, the associate professor rank is typically granted to clinicians who have attained a regional and national presence in their fields. The most senior position is typically the full professor, and these are usually granted to clinicians who are considered national or international authorities in their fields. The tenure position is a title given to clinicians who have demonstrated sustained extramural funding often from multiple sources (e.g., National Institute of Health, Department of Defense, industry funding, foundation funding, etc.). Consideration for tenure usually begins at the associate professor level. Some institutions only confer tenure to certain tracks such as research.

Beyond the name and prestige, promotion to the next faculty rank is often associated with increased compensation, voting power for institution-related matters, and eligibility for leadership positions. Clinicians may often be surprised (pleasantly or not so pleasantly) by the increase in compensation for each faculty rank promotion. The compensation differential may correlate with the difficulty of promotion. Some institutions only allow assistant, associate, and full professors to vote on committees that oversee faculty searches, promotions, leadership nominations, university-level committees, and so on. Finally, there are often leadership positions that have minimum faculty rank requirements such as department chairs (often full professor), division chiefs (often associate professor), program directors, and so on.

Criteria for Promotion

Having a good grasp of an institution's promotion criteria will empower a physician to both choose the appropriate promotion track and to tailor his/her work portfolio to satisfy the milestones for promotion. For example, an institution may have three primary areas of assessment: scholarship, teaching, and service.

Each of these areas may be assessed and graded on four achievement levels: involvement, achievement, reputation, and leadership both at the institutional/regional level and at the national/international level (Fig. 10.1). Consider the following example for the service/administration track. For assessment at the institutional/regional level, "involvement" may describe clinical excellence, participation in hospital committees, and advising patient advocacy groups (Table 10.1). "Achievement" may include leading quality improvement (QI) teams, serving a substantial division role such as division chief, and serving on the organizing committee of a regional meeting. "Reputation" may include serving departmental leadership roles such as department vice chair, serving in advisory roles for local or regional governmental agencies, and leading a core program/service with regional impact. Finally, "leadership" may include serving as department chair or executive vice president of the hospital, serving as president of a major regional chapter of a national organization, and achieving national recognition for his/her leadership roles. At the national/international level for service assessment, "involvement" may include holding senior membership at a national professional society, serving as ad hoc reviewer for mid-level impact journals, and serving as moderator at major society conferences. "Achievement" may include serving as a member of the major committee of professional societies, serving as an ad hoc reviewer of leading journals, and serving as a protocol leader of major collaborative network initiatives. "Reputation" may include leading a major

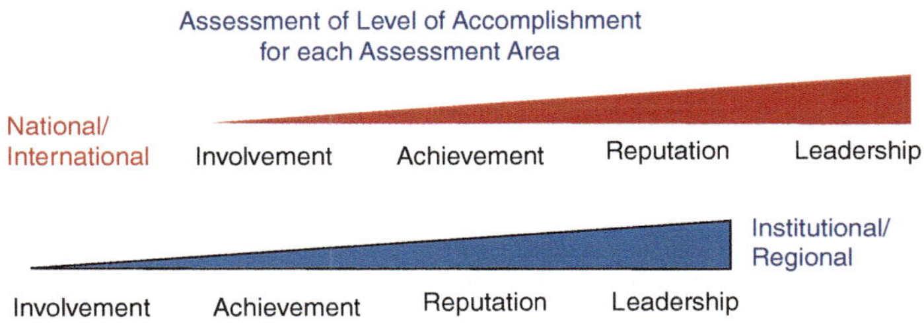

Fig. 10.1 Graphical display of how the achievement levels align between institutional/regional and national/international achievement scales

committee at professional societies, holding membership on editorial boards of leading journals, and implementing national/international clinical or research programs. Finally, "leadership" may include leading professional societies (e.g., board of directors, officer, president, etc.), holding key editorial roles at leading journals, and serving as program committee chair for national meetings.

For this service/administration example, a level of achievement can be assigned to each "area of distinction" achieved by a

Table 10.1 Example of an institution's definitions of different achievement levels on the institutional/regional scale

Institutional/regional professional service benchmarks	
Involvement	• Providing high-quality patient care • Participating in quality improvement activities • Participating in divisional or departmental service activities • Participating in a hospital committee • Organizing recurring departmental meetings (e.g., grand rounds and M&M conferences) • Advising community or patient advocacy groups
Achievement	• Providing clinical service above and beyond peers in quantity and quality • Leading quality improvement teams • Developing a clinical program that attracts patients from the state or region • Chairing a divisional, departmental, or hospital committee or serving on multiple committees • Serving as a member of major university or school committees • Receiving division/department service award • Serving in a substantial division role (e.g., section chief, etc.) • Serving in a leadership role of small, accredited training or graduate programs • Serving in a supportive leadership role of large, accredited training or graduate programs • Serving as director of a core facility/service center • Serving on the organizing committee of a regional meeting • Participating as a committee member for a state/regional society

Table 10.1 (continued)

Institutional/regional professional service benchmarks	
Reputation	• Leading a core program/service that has a regional impact • Chairing major university, school, or health system committees or serving on multiple institution-wide committees • Receiving major institutional service awards • Serving in a leadership role of accredited allied health, training or graduate medical programs • Serving in a departmental leadership role (e.g., department vice chair, division chief, section chief, etc.) • Holding a titled leadership position within the school, university, or healthcare partner (e.g., chief quality officer, chief medical officer, hospital service chief, etc.) • Leading/developing a center that involves multiple departments, school, or other components of the institution • Serving as committee chair or elected officer for state or regional organizations • Serving as chair of the program organizing committee for local or regional CME meetings • Serving in advisory roles for local or regional governmental agencies • Earning service awards from state or regional professional societies or medical organizations
Leadership[a]	• Serving as department chair, executive associate dean, dean, executive vice president for health affairs, president, or the equivalent • Serving as president of a major regional chapter of a national organization

[a]The candidate should be recognized nationally for their institutional/regional leadership role

physician and summarized in a table, which then can be compared with an institution's requirements for promotion (Table 10.2). This assessment applies to the other promotion tracks, with different output measures. For example, the research promotion track may focus more on the number and quality of manuscripts, reviews, book chapters, abstracts, invited presentations, and grants. Institutions rarely have a predetermined number of manuscripts or grants that are required for promotion. Rather, it is usu-

Table 10.2 Example of an institution's criteria for promotion to associate professor (A) and full professor (B). The institution has three mission areas: scholarship, teaching, and service

Area of Distinction	Mission Area		
	Scholarship	Teaching	Service
A (Associate Professor Candidate)			
Scholarship	≥ Emerging[a] national/ international **reputation**	≥ Regional, institutional, national or international **involvement**	≥ National/International **involvement**
Teaching A	≥ **Involvement**	≥ Institutional/regional **reputation**	≥ Institutional/regional **achievement**
Teaching B	≥ **Achievement**	≥ Institutional/regional **reputation**	≥ Institutional/regional **involvement**
Professional Service A	≥ **Involvement**	≥ Institutional/regional **achievement**	≥ Institutional/regional **reputation**
Professional Service B	≥ **Achievement**	≥ Institutional/regional **involvement**	≥ Institutional/regional **reputation**
B (Full Professor Candidate)			
Scholarship A	≥ National/ international **reputation**	≥ National/ international **achievement**	≥ National/International **achievement**
Scholarship B	≥ National/ international **reputation**	≥ Institutional/regional **achievement**	≥ Institutional/regional **reputation**
Teaching	≥ Substantial[b] **involvement**	≥ National/ international **reputation** OR ≥ Institutional/regional **leadership**	≥ Institutional/regional **achievement**
Professional Service	≥ Substantial[b] **involvement**	≥ Institutional/regional **achievement**	≥ National/ international **reputation** OR ≥ Institutional/regional **leadership**

[a]Emerging reputation: Blend of items in achievement and reputation categories
[b]Substantial involvement: Blend of items in involvement and achievement categories

ally a composite of the number and impact of the work that is evaluated. Finally, the threshold to promote may differ across institutions. A productive researcher may qualify for a full professor position at one institution and only an associate professor position at another. Typically, the more academically prolific institutions have higher thresholds for promotion.

Preparing the Promotion Package

Once a physician familiarizes himself/herself with the promotion tracks and the associated promotion criteria, he/she can then begin to prepare the promotion package. This typically includes a curriculum vitae (CV), personal statement, service portfolio, teaching portfolio, letter from the department chair, letters of evaluation, and representative publications. Before compiling the promotion package, the physician should seek out institutional resources for guidance and advice. Most institutions have a faculty development committee that specializes in its staff's professional development. This resource can advise physicians regarding the appropriate timing of promotion, assist with promotion package preparation, and provide references to relevant advisors. Beyond formal institutional resources, a physician should certainly reach out to his/her network of peers and mentors. Peers who have recently been successfully promoted can be especially valuable given their immediate experiences and willingness to share. More senior and established peers or mentors may be able to provide perspective from the evaluation side, as they may serve on relevant promotion committees.

The CV, literally translated as "course of life," is a summary of a person's academic and professional progress. It is one of the most important components of the promotion package, as it should capture all the relevant career accomplishments. Though there are variations of CV formats, institutions often require or recommend a specific format. It should be emphasized that abiding by these formats is important as it facilitates the evaluation of the contents by the promotions committee. This will not only make the promotion committee's job easier but will also ensure that relevant details for promotion are accurately and systematically captured. Ideally, the framework for the CV should be created and updated regularly as a physician accumulates achievements and accolades. This practice will minimize the amount of work when the time of promotion evaluation comes and will also provide an updated CV for any other purposes such as grant applications, job interviews, and so on. Importantly, if there are sections of the CV template that one currently does not have any accomplishments to populate, do not delete this section heading. This heading will serve as a reminder in subsequent drafts and may be populated in the future. Despite the CV format variations, there are some best practices. The physician's full name and the date should be included on the first page. Pages should be numbered to facilitate referencing. A single font should be used throughout the document, and acronyms should be avoided. All sections should be arranged in chronological order. The document should be thoroughly reviewed for any typos or grammar mistakes. When citing bibliography, a standardized citation format should be used. Furthermore, it is helpful to bold or underline one's name in the line of authorship to facilitate assessing the degree of contribution. Accomplishments should never be duplicated in different sections of the CV; it is obvious when someone is attempting to "pad the CV." The final product should be up-to-date, comprehensive, and succinct. The formatting should make the CV easy and pleasant to read.

Next, the personal statement is typically a two- to five-page document that conveys one's background, area of expertise, and future career plans. Unlike the CV, which is a list of accomplishments and accolades, this document provides a linear narrative of one's professional career. It should begin with what one has done, what one is currently doing, and what one aspires to do in the next 5 years. It should tell a cohesive story that highlights how a promotion candidate has contributed to the institution's missions. A compelling personal statement convinces the promotions committee that a candidate has the track record, experience, potential, and motivation to advance the institution's priorities. This document allows the writer to highlight areas of achievement and craft how achievements may be viewed. For example, being a Committee Chair on Educational Resources can be considered an achievement in either education or services. Depending on what the physician needs for promotion, there is flexibility in adapting this achievement to optimize his/her promotion portfolio.

Oftentimes, institutions may allow promotion candidates to submit teaching and service portfolios, which complement the personal statement with more detailed activities. For example, the teaching portfolio may include a collection of teaching-related achievements and activities that match the CV. However, unlike the CV, this is an opportunity to expound on specific positions and convey the relevance and impact of one's contributions. For example, the CV may indicate that a clinician has been the residency program director for the past 5 years while the teaching portfolio may describe how he/she doubled the size of the residency, reduced the residency program attrition rate, and increased research output per resident. Additionally, the teaching portfolio may include a list of the promotion candidate's former trainees and their current positions. Supporting documentation such as letters of support, trainee evaluations, lecture evaluations, and even e-mails conveying gratitude from former trainees can be included. A representative sample of formal trainee evaluations of the clinician can also be included. Finally, if the clinician has developed curriculum, given lectures, or moderated talks, representative examples of these can be included. Teaching portfolios may be limited to around 50 pages.

Similar to the teaching portfolio, the service portfolio is typically a templated document that elaborates on one's unique or exceptional roles in the various service areas. If a clinician implemented a new patient-reported outcome measures (PROMs) platform that has been used across multiple clinical divisions, he/she can describe the impact of this work, such as clinical workflow optimization, research output, and patient care improvement. Quantifying the impact with the number of PROMs collected, the number of divisions impacted, the number of manuscripts published, and so on will help the promotion committee assess the impact. Letters of support from collaborators may be included. The service portfolio is typically limited to around ten pages.

Beyond the CV and work portfolios, a promotion candidate will need to obtain letters of support to highlight accomplishments across the four domains. Aside from the CV, this is arguably the second most important component of the promotion package. Institutions often specify the number and type of letters required for each promotion rank. For example, consideration for associate professor may require at least three letters of support, of which at least two are from external institutions. In contrast, consideration for full professor may require at least eight letters of support, of which six are from external institutions and two from full professors within the institution. Oftentimes, institutions may ask the promotion candidate to identify these individuals so that the promotion committee will reach out to them directly. The selection of letter writers requires some thoughtful reflection. Ideal evaluators should be leaders in the field, genuinely supportive of the promotion, and free of conflict of interest (i.e., not a former mentor or direct collaborator). If the institution requests that the candidate reach out to the letter writers, it is always good practice to provide them with significant advance notice. Additionally, it may be helpful for the promotion candidate to send the letter writer his/her CV to facilitate the writing process. Typically, evaluators are required to be at or above the promotion candidate's aspired rank.

The Promotion Process

Understanding an institution's promotion process and timeline is critical to a successful promotion. The process can be involved and protracted as the promotion package will be reviewed by multiple committees. Most institutions review promotions annually on a regular timeline. The following is a representative example of a promotion timeline at an academic institution. There is an annual review of faculty members who are eligible for promotion.

Input from division chiefs is solicited during this review. The accomplishments of the promotion candidates are then de-identified for a "blinded review," where the faculty development committee assesses whether the promotion process should proceed. If not, the promotion process ends. If so, the promotion package undergoes a full review, where the candidate's promotion package is comprehensively reviewed by the promotions committee. Should the committee favor promoting the candidate, this message is conveyed to the division chief and department chair, who will then write a letter of support. This letter, along with the promotions package, will be sent to the Dean's office for review and approval. For promotions associated with tenure, the promotion package may also need to be approved by the university provost's office. It should be evident that given the required review and approval of multiple committees, this process can take many months. Early preparation and a good understanding of the promotion process will ensure an efficient progression through the promotion process.

Conclusion

Though the promotion process can appear daunting at first, it should be seen as an opportunity to appropriately recognize and award a physician's contribution to his/her organization. Understanding the promotion tracks, criteria for promotion, the components of the promotion package, and the promotion process will maximize the chances of a successful promotion. The promotion process should generally reflect an institution's priorities and values. Thus, it can be used to assess whether a physician would be a good fit. Seeking advice from recently promoted peers and mentors is invaluable to optimizing a promotion outcome. Finally, the responsibility of appropriate promotions should not only fall on the employee but also on the employer. Leaders such as division chiefs and department chairs should regularly assess their faculty for appropriateness for promotion. Doing so will improve talent retention and physician well-being.

SAGES Takeaway

- Career promotions should be seen as an opportunity to be recognized for professional achievements as opposed to a comparison to one's peers.
- Different institutions may have different promotion tracks and criteria. Understanding them will confer a significant advantage in advancing one's career.
- Mentors and peers who recently underwent the promotion process can provide invaluable advice that can optimize a candidate's chances for a successful outcome.

11 Strategies to Build a Practice

Shawn Tsuda and Jerome Lyn-Sue

Practice Types

Surgical practice types can be determined by size, employment structure, affiliations, and revenue structure. Practice models can include a solo practice, partnership, or group. Models of direct employment by a hospital, medical school, healthcare group, or integrated system are becoming more commonplace. Finally, direct pay, concierge, and contractor structures such as locum tenens round out the models [1]. Solo practice offers the advantage of autonomy for the general surgeon practitioner and the disadvantage of financial risk, lack of collegial partners, and potential issues regarding on-call coverage. There are data suggesting that solo or partnership general surgery practices have been declining in the past decade. Between 2012 and 2020, the percentage of surgeons in practices of 1 or 2 declined from 19% to 12%, while surgeons in groups of 500 or more grew from 20% to 31% [2].

S. Tsuda (✉)
Valley Health System General Surgery Residency Program, Las Vegas, NV, USA
e-mail: drshawntsuda@vipsurg.com

J. Lyn-Sue
Penn State University, Hershey, PA, USA
e-mail: jlynsue@pennstatehealth.psu.edu

S. M. Johnson et al. (eds.), *The SAGES Manual of Strategy and Leadership*, https://doi.org/10.1007/978-3-031-62359-2_11

Group practices can be single-specialty and multispecialty practices, ranging in size from 2 to 1000 or more practitioners. In contrast to solo practices, group practices may help mitigate overall financial risk, provide more employee/owner benefits, and allow greater flexibility in shift scheduling.

Increasingly, physicians are being employed within one of several practice models, with over 24,000 new openings projected per year over the next decade through 2033 [3]. Hospitals, healthcare organizations, physician-run groups, and academic institutions serve as employers, with the advantages of baseline or guaranteed compensation, productivity-based bonuses, employee benefits, and potentially improved lifestyle through shared clinical responsibilities. Autonomy in employment, however, is diminished compared with the above practice models and surgeons may have limited bargaining power within their group structure.

Alternative practice models have emerged in recent years, classified by the non-traditional payment systems. These include concierge or cash-only practices that can be solo or group-based in structure. These practices either function without the use of insurance payments for services or with a retainer for direct concierge care in addition to insurance coverage for services. Although more common in primary care practices, the concierge medicine model was sized at USD 6.1 billion in 2022 and is expected to grow at a compound annual growth rate of 10.32% from 2023 to 2030 [4]. There is some concern that the rise of concierge and cash-pay models may impact access to care for underserved populations [5].

The decision on what type of surgery practice to enter remains salient throughout the lifecycle of a surgeon's career, from graduation until retirement. Healthcare and economic trends, geographic availability, as well as evolving personal goals affect this decision. This chapter will focus on the issues and strategies for forming a successful practice primarily from the standpoint of a solo practitioner, or a group practice owner. However, because the issues regarding building a successful business model in medicine are agnostic to practice type, some content may be relevant to administrators, directors, or officers of employed groups either just starting or seeking to optimize aspects of their practice. The dynamics of practice-building may have vastly different circumstances depending on the country of practice, but this chapter will focus primarily on the U.S. system.

Licensure, Credentialing, and Insurance

State, territory, or other government licensure is a requirement for surgical practice in most regions and can often be a limiting factor for starting a practice in a new location or after graduation from residency or fellowship. In the United States, unique challenges can affect foreign medical graduates transferring for work as surgeons. The average time to medical licensure is state-dependent and ranges from 6 to 12 weeks, with the average being 60 days [6]. Factors that can affect the timeliness of licensure include existing full state licensures, practice experience, graduation from an ACGME or AOA-accredited medical school or one in the International Medical Education Directory, passing of each component of the USMLE, COMLEX-USA, or equivalent exam in less than three attempts, specialty board certification, disciplinary actions, criminal history, substance abuse history, malpractice history, and any current investigations. Application for state licensure should be the first step following a decision or acceptance to practice in any U.S. state as any of these factors may impede or lengthen the licensure process. In other areas such as Canada, licensure occurs through a central organization (The Medical Council of Canada) but may carry similar challenges.

Following state licensure, facility credentialing at hospitals or ambulatory surgery centers is a second hurdle. Similar barriers to state licensure can impede this process, but the delineation of privileges will be a tertiary hurdle for some practitioners who do not have the volume of cases to support immediate credentials (e.g., flexible endoscopy, advanced laparoscopy, esophageal surgery, robotic surgery, bariatric surgery, etc.). A period of proctorship may be required in these cases, along with postgraduate courses, or in rare situations, additional formal training.

Insurance underwriting often has to occur simultaneously or even precede state licensure and facility credentialing. Malpractice insurance in the United States will be universally mandatory, sometimes with set minimums for coverage. Employers may pay for malpractice insurance for employed surgeons, but transferring from another practice may require negotiation over tail coverage. In private practices, additional general liability insurance for office locations, cybersecurity insurance, disability insurance, and employee health insurance are all other types of liability coverage that need to be considered.

The Importance of Payor Contracts

Once licensure and credentialing is secured, one of the most important building blocks of a successful practice is insurance payor contracts. Third-party payor contracts in the United States determine the reimbursement, access, delivery, and market competitiveness of a surgeon or practice. Understanding the landscape of insurance payors is essential to identifying, engaging, and prioritizing contractual agreements (Table 11.1).

Regardless of the practice type one is establishing, a contracted medical credentialer can be a valuable resource. Credentialing specialists will often have pre-existing clients with contracts, insider knowledge, and a wide network of contacts to begin an insurance credentialing process. While credentialers can expedite licensing and hospital credentialing, the processes for insurance contracting can have complexities that are often outside of the

Table 11.1 Types of insurance payors

Commercial insurance • Health maintenance organization (HMO) • Preferred provider organization (PPO) • Exclusive provider organization (EPO) • Point-of-service (POS)
Self-funded employee plans
Third-party administrators
Government providers (Medicare, Medicaid, and VA)
Accountable care organizations (ACO)
Integrated healthcare delivery organization

armamentarium of the typical general surgery graduate. In addition to a credentialing specialist, a contract lawyer with specific experience in insurance contracts may be essential for establishing payor rates that are competitive.

The terms of insurance contracts determines the compensation, risk-sharing, exclusivity, and longevity of the relationship. Most insurers have structured relationships with providers in some version of "value-based payment," although the exact meaning of this methodology can vary [7]. The terms of payor contracts include the fee-for-service reimbursement schedule. These may be set by statute or rules which are the case for government payor programs, or on the other spectrum, may be completely negotiable as with some self-funded payors. Reimbursement may also be subject to the payor's chargemaster (standard charges for given services to patients) or subject to their usual, customary, and reasonable (UCR) rates, or their maximum allowed payments. For commercial payors where contracted reimbursement can be negotiable, solo or newer entrants into a market may lack the bargaining power to achieve competitive rates on their repertoire of services. An experienced contract attorney can be valuable in these cases. Self-funded employer programs will often have the most leeway and agency in determining their rates to providers and can create a competitive coup for surgeons or practices that have unique services, or carve-outs. An example of this would be providing surgeries in a market where they are not readily available, such as complex minimally invasive surgery, hepatobiliary surgery, advanced endoscopy, or bariatric surgery.

Self-funded providers sometimes work through third-party brokers to provide bundled payment models that include facility, anesthesia, and surgeon provider fees at a capitated fee. These fee schedules will require coordinated negotiation between facilities (hospitals or ASCs) and an anesthesia provider but can often include exclusivity and favorable reimbursement. However, careful consideration has to be given to shared risk based on risk stratification of the patient population and considerations of insurance against complications. On the contrary, the risks of shared culpability can be offset by shared savings, quality incentives for superior outcomes, and higher-than-average reimbursement and exclusivity.

The relationship with payors is contiguous with the entire lifecycle of a surgery practice and has to be re-assessed at least annually. The use of expertise in both credentialing and contract negotiation, as well as the surgeon's own understanding of the third-party insurance market, can be critical components of gaining financial feasibility as an entrant into the healthcare market.

Practice Management

While licensing, credentialing, and insurance contracting establish the regulatory foundation for practice, practice management sets the functional and competitive groundwork for the surgeon. Sound practice management for a starting practice requires initial capital, requiring at minimal a $100,000 USD line of credit [8]. Funding can be obtained through a traditional bank loan, term loan, short-term loan, or business loan. Some loan servicers specifically underwrite physicians starting a new practice or expanding upon one, often providing favorable terms and liberal underwriting requirements. The following practice management components will focus on specific strategies to create a solid foundation for a practice as well as strategic competitiveness.

Office Space and Equipment

The surgeon's patient care office is public and customer-facing. A professional and attractive office setting, as with any business, can influence the retention and referral of patients. Ample waiting room space with comfortable chairs and a restroom available to waiting patients can be essential. Conveniences such as water, coffee, tea, or refreshments can affect impressions. Even in practices not treating bariatric patients, the prevalence of obesity would benefit from having adequate-sized and weight-rated chairs, doorways, exam tables, and toilets ([9]) (Table 11.2).

Patient exam rooms are ideally well-lit, ventilated, spacious, and comfortable. Patient pamphlets have been well-established to enhance patient health knowledge, although data suggests that

Table 11.2 Facility requirements to accommodate patients with obesity

Chairs	Weight-rated or supported toilets
Beds	• Weight-rated floor mounted
Doorways	• Weight-rated wall mounted
Showers	• Supported floor mounted
	• Supported wall mounted

Metabolic and Bariatric Accreditation and Quality Improvement Program [9] Optimal Resources for Metabolic and Bariatric Surgeons

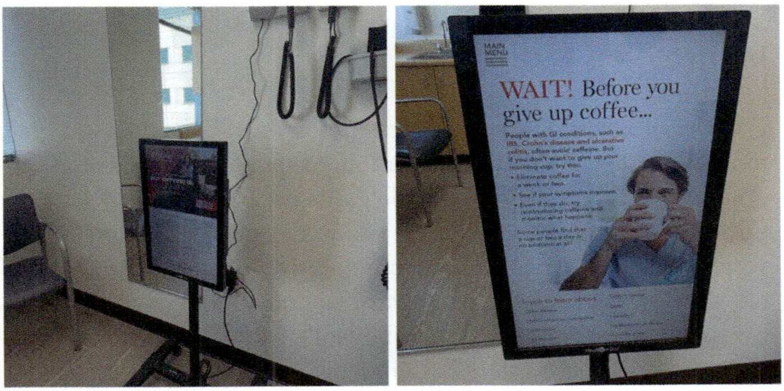

Fig. 11.1 In-office digital patient pamphlet

video versions of patient educational material can have a higher yield in health literacy [10]. An exam room with an interactive digital tablet with information and videos can shorten the subjective wait times of patients while providing guided information for your patient population's health issues (Fig. 11.1).

Office Staff

Having the right and correct number of staff affects your office's efficiency as well as the patient experience. Although the calculated number of required full-time employees (FTEs) can be as low as 0.75 per physician in a practice, that number is affected by the amount of in-house services provided [11]. Lab draws, billing, and ancillary health education like dietary and psychosocial services can increase the number of required FTEs. Physician extenders such as advanced practice registered nurses or physician assistants may impact practices in both tangible financial gain as well as workflow safety [12]. They also serve as additional points of contact for patients that can relieve on-call demands on the surgeon, although the supervision requirements for physician extenders vary by state and should be confirmed prior to employment.

Information Technology

The use of health information technology (HIT) is almost a given in today's larger health organization, as the drive to be compliant, efficient, and competitive mandates its use. Solo or smaller practices may have more resistance or inertia in the adoption of HIT, which provides a substantial competitive disadvantage as such technology has been shown in various domains to have unequivocal financial and patient safety advantages [13]. Various areas of HIT should be considered a vital investment for the successful practice (Table 11.3).

With telehealth, the regulatory and reimbursement policies governing its use in the post-COVID pandemic era are still in flux, but the cost-benefit and outcome improvements over a wide variety of fields and disease states have been well-established [14]. However, with many of the other digital technologies such as electronic payment, analytics, patient flow, appointment-making, and electronic health record systems—the barrier is simply pro-

Table 11.3 Health Information Technologies (HIT) that augment practice efficiency and safety

• Electronic health records • Patient portals • Automatic check-in, reminders, and patient scheduling • Telehealth	• Electronic patient pamphlets • Digital payment • Data analytics • Patient flow trackers • Health monitoring devices

vider resistance or initial capital investment. The benefits of these technologies are essentially non-negotiable, and the absence of them in a surgery practice will equate to a competitive disadvantage. However, HIT should not be adopted without careful research, training, attention to compatibility with existing systems, and with a structured pro forma dependent on the current growth and needs of the practice.

Marketing and Web Presence

The adage that "marketing is everything and everything is marketing" applies to a patient-focused business as it does any customer-facing one [15]. Marketing in today's digital world goes beyond the outreach lunches brought to referring physician offices, print ads, or billboards. While these traditional modalities still have value, the importance of web and social media marketing cannot be understated. These include search engine optimization (SEO), online forums, social network posts, online patient reviews, blogging, and email lists (Fig. 11.2). Even if a physician has experience in social media, online blogging, or website creation—the time and effort for maintaining an ongoing digital presence precludes a practitioner from taking on their own marketing campaign without the use of a third-party professional or company. Of all the modalities available, SEO is likely the most important as it is the primary way—outside of referrals and word-of-mouth—that patients become aware of your practice. Unless the practice is in an area or specialty without significant competitors, SEO usually has to be paid for through a "pay-per-click" model. In heavily saturated territories, a virtual online battle for maintaining visibility at the top of search engines can often drive prices up for competing practices. However, choosing to disengage from the SEO campaign can quickly lead to a significant loss of online referrals. Whether a practitioner is starting off on their own, or joining an existing practice or employment contract, assuring that a strategic plan for the digital (and traditional) marketing of themselves is an important aspect of the overall business roadmap.

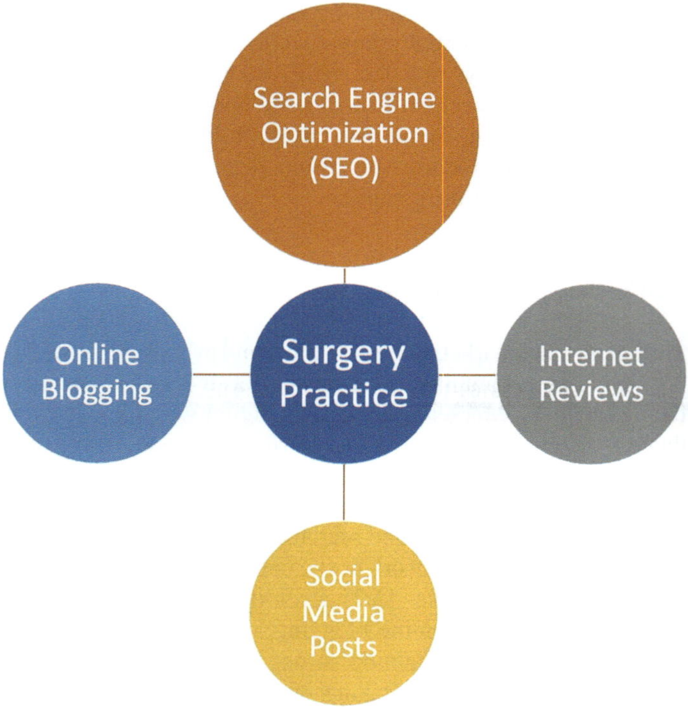
Search Engine Optimization (SEO)
Online Blogging
Surgery Practice
Internet Reviews
Social Media Posts

Fig. 11.2 Example of online marketing campaign for a surgery practice

Miscellaneous Strategies

Preventing Burnout

The Society of American Gastrointestinal and Endoscopic Surgeons Re-Imagining the Practice of Surgery Task Force identified several stressors that affect the well-being of surgeons-in-practice: Work-life Integration, Administration-related Concerns, Time and Productivity Pressures, Operating Room Factors, and Lack of Respect [16]. Guarding surgeons within a practice against burn-out is an investment in the quality and longevity of patient care. Work-life balance with adequate time off, the use of mid-level providers, or mentorship from within and without the practice are all ways to help ensure a satisfying work environment. For a group leader, open communication and an ombudsman program may help to keep channels open with physicians within a practice. For solo practitioners, engaging in a surgeon mentoring or coaching program—several of which are available through national societies or private entities—can be useful for the first few years of practice. Validation and autonomy are key drivers of many surgeons' sense of purpose. Being proactive by seeking committee or leadership positions within provider facilities can often create a sense of collegiality with hospital or ASC administration, give back some agency in policy-making, and create a sense of accomplishment without an excessive time commitment.

Trend-Watching and Diversification

One of the most common pitfalls of a surgical practice is missing a trend or technological disruption. The advent of minimally invasive surgery or even robotic surgery are examples of disruptions that have become prevalent enough to leave those who did not adopt at a significant disadvantage. Maintaining an eye on innovations, technological advances, medical trends (e.g., new weight loss medications in the bariatric field), and even cultural shifts can keep a practice on the cutting edge rather than left behind. Besides staying up-to-date on literature and guidelines, partnering with your marketing or social media company, or staying active on discussion forums or blog-writing can keep a surgeon current and relevant. Attending local chapter meetings for national societies and teaching within a residency program or medical school are also ways to stay abreast of the latest trends if attending national meetings or taking part in heavy research and reading are not feasible with a busy surgery schedule. There is also the possibility that a major locoregional or national disruption can severely affect a specific practice—such as a change in reimbursement to a commonly performed procedure or a large, corporate group entering the same market. For this reason, having some diversification of practice services can hedge against external threats to the practice. These can include performing minor office procedures, prescribing medical treatments for surgery-adjacent diseases, and taking courses or mini-fellowships to become certified in specialized areas. Examples of these would be a bariatric surgeon using FDA-approved weight-loss medications to augment the treatment of their patients or treat those who do not qualify for surgery or becoming facile at advanced endoscopic techniques to supplement laparoscopic or open approaches to surgery.

Summary

The healthcare landscape evolves over time, and the surgeon seeking to build a successful practice must be willing to educate themselves in the fundamental aspects of practice-building, as well as engaging technology or novel trends in their field to stay competitive. By doing so, staying nimble while rooted and committed to quality care, a long-lasting and fulfilling practice can thrive in today's healthcare landscape.

SAGES Takeaway

- After licensing and credentialing, competitive insurance contracts are an essential foundation for a successful practice in the United States.
- Engaging in health information technologies (HIT) will increase competitiveness, while failing to engage in HIT can severely degrade the market positioning of a practice.
- Keeping an eye on trends and technological disruptions is a hedge against major setbacks to a surgeon's practice.

References

1. Online ACP. ACP Online. In: Types of Medical Practice; 2023. https://www.acponline.org/about-acp/about-internal-medicine/career-paths/residency-career-counseling/resident-career-counseling-guidance-and-tips/medical-practice-types. Accessed 13 Sep 2023.
2. Anderson ST, Hammond JB, Hogan JS, et al. Current trends in U.S. general surgery practice consolidation. Am J Surg. 2022;223:477–80. https://doi.org/10.1016/j.amjsurg.2021.12.016.

3. U.S.Bureau of Labor Statistics. Physicians and Surgeons. 2023. https://www.bls.gov/ooh/healthcare/physicians-and-surgeons.htm#:~:text=in%20May%202022.-,Job%20Outlook,on%20average%2C%20over%20the%20decade. Accessed 13 Sep 2023.
4. Grand View Research. U.S. Concierge Medicine Market Size, Share & Trends Analysis Report By Specialty (Primary Care, Pediatrics, Osteopathy, Internal Medicine, Cardiology, Psychiatry), By Ownership (Standalone, Group), And Segment Forecasts, 2023–2030. 2023. https://www.grandviewresearch.com/industry-analysis/us-concierge-medicine-market-report.
5. Doherty R, Medical Practice and Quality Committee of the American College of Physicians. Assessing the patient care implications of "concierge" and other direct patient contracting practices: a policy position paper from the American College of Physicians. Ann Intern Med. 2015;163:949–52. https://doi.org/10.7326/M15-0366.
6. Medium. How Long Does It Take To Get A Physician License In Each State?. 2023. https://medium.com/nomad-health/how-long-does-it-take-to-get-a-physician-license-in-each-state-f83c88d78a06. Accessed 13 Sep 2023.
7. American Medical Association. Payor Contracting. 2023. https://www.ama-assn.org/system/files/payor-contracting-toolkit.pdf. Accessed 8 Oct 2023.
8. Freedman, Max. How to open a private medical practice, step by step. 2023. https://www.businessnewsdaily.com/8910-opening-a-medical-practice.html.
9. Metabolic and Bariatric Accreditation and Quality Improvement Program. Optimal resources for metabolic and bariatric surgeons. 2019.
10. Ludens M. A digital initiative to improve patient health literacy. S D Med. 2022;75:453.
11. Cloud-Moulds PJ. Calculating the right number of staff for your medical practice. Physicans Practice; 2014.
12. Seyidova N, Lin SJ. Impact of physician extenders and Midlevels in plastic surgery. Plast Reconstr Surg. 2023;151:1097–103. https://doi.org/10.1097/PRS.0000000000010048.
13. McClellan SR, Casalino LP, Shortell SM, Rittenhouse DR. When does adoption of health information technology by physician practices lead to use by physicians within the practice? J Am Med Inform Assoc. 2013;20:e26–32. https://doi.org/10.1136/amiajnl-2012-001271.
14. Mahtta D, Daher M, Lee MT, et al. Promise and perils of telehealth in the current era. Curr Cardiol Rep. 2021;23:115. https://doi.org/10.1007/s11886-021-01544-w.
15. McKenna R. Marketing is everything. Harv Bus Rev. 1991;69:65–79.
16. Hughes D, Hanson MN, Alseidi A, et al. Factors influencing surgeon well-being: qualitatively exploring the joy of surgery. Surg Endosc. 2023;37:6464–75. https://doi.org/10.1007/s00464-023-10135-5.

Practice Adaptation During Crisis

12

Cedrek McFadden, Kenric Murayama, and Shanu Kothari

Handling a crisis is an essential aspect of medical training. Residency programs instill in trainees fundamental patient assessment and triage skills, source control, stabilization, and definitive management to keep patients alive when they are often sickest. After training, medical trainees become adept at navigating and flowing through algorithms designed for various clinical scenarios. These algorithms, rightly so, serve as a method to recenter and focus amidst the often-chaotic environment of trauma bays or operating rooms, where patients frequently transition to unstable medical conditions without prior warning. At the end of residen-

C. McFadden (✉)
Department of Surgery, Prisma Health, Greenville, SC, USA

University of South Carolina School of Medicine Greenville, Greenville, SC, USA
e-mail: cmcFadden@prismahealth.org

K. Murayama
Department of Surgery, John A. Burns School of Medicine, University of Hawaii, Honolulu, HI, USA
e-mail: kenricm@hawaii.edu

S. Kothari
Department of Surgery, Prisma Health, Greenville, SC, USA
e-mail: Shanu.kothari@prismahealth.org

S. M. Johnson et al. (eds.), *The SAGES Manual of Strategy and Leadership*, https://doi.org/10.1007/978-3-031-62359-2_12

cies, study materials emphasize a stepwise process to ensure a passing score when preparing for oral certifying examinations. Learning how to master this seemingly unconscious and seamless thought process and effectively translating it into direct patient care is arguably one of the most underappreciated accomplishments in medical education. Interestingly, while surgeons are trained to expect the unexpected in the operating room, there is often a lack of training regarding system-wide practice crises.

Like patient care, effective leadership must withstand moments of crisis. A competent leader maintains control of the team during these challenging situations. If a leader displays ineptitude, the organization or group they are guiding will struggle to focus on their mission. In critical moments within the operating room, the proactive involvement of the attending staff in assuming control is vital to ensure favorable patient outcomes. However, one study conducted by Parker et al. revealed a concerning trend: the presence of unexpected developments in the operating room often leads to a breakdown in positive leadership behavior [1].

In the Academy Award-winning movie, Titanic, the captain vividly exemplifies a more appropriate leadership responsibility. The portrayal of Captain Smith instills a deep appreciation for the ability to steer the team's efforts toward prioritizing the well-being of the passengers, even in the face of a sinking ship. Quite literally! Even before his crew members inform him of the Titanic's collision with an iceberg, Captain Smith demonstrates the empathetic nature of a good leader by rousing from sleep and promptly engaging his team to address the situation. After a brief pause to assess the gravity of the crisis, he delegates responsibilities for safely evacuating the passengers onto lifeboats. Despite foreseeing the grim outcome, he remains resolutely focused on fulfilling his duties within the constraints of the crisis. Here are several valuable lessons we can learn from Captain Smith's leadership:

1. A competent leader remains attuned to the essence of the organization. In addition to understanding and actively working toward its vision and mission, a good leader develops a heightened intuition about the organization. This intuitive sense

serves as a guide, enabling them to make informed decisions and anticipate potential dangers and crises.
2. A skilled leader knows their team members' strengths and weaknesses before a crisis occurs. This awareness allows them to delegate responsibilities appropriately when faced with challenging situations. Moreover, the leader must possess realistic self-awareness of their strengths and weaknesses. A study conducted in Scotland examined how surgeons assessed their leadership style, revealing a significant discrepancy in viewpoints. While most surgeons described their leadership style as collaborative, the rest of the surgical team perceived it as autocratic [2]. This disconnect poses potential challenges not only in communication but also in the execution of workplace operations.
3. A strong leader allows the organization's vision and mission to steer their actions during times of crisis. In Captain Smith's case, his priority was ensuring the safety of the passengers. Likewise, healthcare leaders must prioritize maintaining the highest quality of patient care at the forefront of their work, regardless of the circumstances.

It is worth noting that Captain Smith tragically perished at the helm of the sinking Titanic. The authors do not generally advocate for the literal or metaphorical demise of a leader with an organization. However, it is essential to acknowledge that having a profound passion that guides one's actions enables the leader to remain fully committed and actively engaged even in the most challenging moments of crisis.

Moments of crisis are an unavoidable reality of life. The ability to pivot, assess, and take appropriate action that aligns with the severity of the situation is crucial. An all-too-common mistake is a failure to adapt and modify workflows and operational procedures. In such times, the leader is vital in resetting the team's approach and establishing a new sense of normalcy. In this chapter, the authors draw upon their experiences of navigating crises in their respective practices, offering valuable lessons that shed light on the necessary adaptations required to maintain stability and successfully overcome challenging situations.

Crisis 1: Sudden and Unexpected Departure of a Key Team Member: Navigating the Unforeseen Change

January is an exceptionally demanding time in medical education. The interview season is in full swing as aspiring residents compete for program positions. The role of the residency coordinator is vital during this period, as they handle the crucial tasks of selecting applicants for interviews, scheduling interview dates, coordinating faculty schedules, and evaluating candidates to determine the most desirable ones for the program. This responsibility entails countless phone calls and emails with applicants while managing the existing residents' preparations for in-service exams and their demanding 80-h work weeks. Our program was fortunate to have one of the finest residency coordinators who effortlessly fulfilled these responsibilities year after year. She had a nurturing instinct that endeared her to the residents, yet she could also provide firm guidance to keep them on track.

However, several years ago, amidst this busy season, we were struck by a tremendous loss—our beloved residency coordinator's sudden and unexpected death. Our department was filled with grief, standing in solidarity with her family while grappling with the profound sense of loss. Yet, despite the overwhelming emotions, the work needed to continue. In the wake of this devastating event, we gained valuable insights and resilience.

Here, we share the lessons we learned during this challenging period that reshaped our perspective.

1. *Avoid working in silos.* Our residency coordinator was highly skilled and efficient but often worked alone. Her unexpected passing left many unanswered questions about past, present, and future projects. We struggled to locate the necessary files and passwords unknown to the rest of the team. While she had a well-established protocol for managing residency applicants during the mid-cycle of the application season, this knowledge was not shared with others. In the days following her death, we had to invest significant time sorting through and retrieving

vital information. To prevent such challenges in the future, we learned to consider maintaining a file shared with other key stakeholders, including important passwords and processes, ensuring smooth continuity of work in any situation.

2. *Develop a succession plan for the entire team.* Having a succession plan is crucial for everyone, not just department leaders. It is a wise approach to identify potential sources of incoming talent, document current workflow processes, and plan if someone might need to step into your position at any moment. Coaches also follow this approach. The game does not come to an end when a player gets injured. They always have a backup player in mind and know precisely who is prepared to step in and continue playing. Unlike sports, recruiting new talent for positions in healthcare can be time-consuming, taking months or even years. By proactively preparing for such transitions, we can minimize disruptions and ensure a smooth continuation of work during these transition periods.
3. *Meet with your team.* Take the opportunity to gather with the remaining team members and evaluate the current and future needs while establishing timelines for the necessary tasks. Dedicate time to communicate both as a group and individually with the team. Listen to their concerns and uncertainties about their work, providing support as they step up to maintain productivity. Expressing your appreciation for team members who demonstrate their dedication is crucial. Offer verbal acknowledgments and gestures such as staff lunches, outings after work, or thank you cards to show gratitude. Remember that transitions challenge everyone on the team, not just you as the leader.
4. *Embrace the change for positive growth.* It is essential to constantly and critically examine opportunities for realignment and reset. When a team member departs unexpectedly, it can catalyze a positive period of transformation. View departures as opportunities rather than setbacks. This departure provides a valuable chance to re-evaluate the team's efforts in that particular position and explore areas for improvement. When team members are re-engaged, centered, and taught to enhance

performance in these moments of crisis, there is a remarkable improvement in leadership, cooperation, communication, decision-making, and situational awareness, not just in that particular moment but also in future performance [3]. By embracing this opportunity, the team can identify strengths, weaknesses, and potential areas for growth and allow for fresh perspectives, new ideas, and the chance to reshape strategies and goals to ensure ongoing success.

Crisis 2: Global Crises Requiring Internal Adaptation

Shortly after the COVID outbreak, we held our first Department COVID-19 Command Team Call. This meeting directly responded to the sudden growing global awareness of the coronavirus outbreak. In the following days and months, like all health systems, we faced an unprecedented crisis that demanded swift action. We made difficult decisions, such as postponing non-urgent surgical procedures, restricting patient visits, implementing hospital visitor limitations, and carefully managing our doctors, nurses, and office staff to minimize close contact. Our work landscape underwent a profound transformation within a matter of days.

Here, we outline the lessons learned from the practical adaptations we implemented during this sudden crisis that profoundly impacted our practice and the world around us.

1. *Maintain focus*. We needed to focus on our organization's central vision and mission during the near-global lockdown. Despite challenging circumstances, we kept our doors open, serving as a reminder of our dedication to the health and well-being of our patients. Patient calls and visits to the emergency department continued, keeping our mission right in front of us. However, in cases where the mission and vision may be less apparent, it is essential to proactively and regularly restate them to team members during times of crisis. Doing so can organically reinforce the purpose and ensure alignment in times of uncertainty.

2. *Continue the work.* Before the pandemic, we had recognized the potential of telemedicine to improve efficiency. Initially, our surgeons expressed skepticism, highlighting various reasons it may not be feasible. However, as the pandemic unfolded, those concerns became irrelevant, prompting us to embrace video and telephone visits as viable alternatives. We swiftly adjusted our processes to accommodate these remote consultations, simultaneously reducing the number of in-person office visits. Another example of our adaptive response was shifting from face-to-face to telephone conversations when communicating with patients' families post-surgery. Our dedication to providing quality care to our patients and their families remained steadfast while we modified our methods to ensure effective delivery.

   Amidst these changes, an unexpected positive emerged. Our work adjustments inadvertently revealed inefficiencies in our existing processes, prompting valuable insights and improvement opportunities. One notable enhancement was the optimization of patient communication pathways through the implementation of hospital-based patient portals. This development further solidified our commitment to efficient and effective care delivery.
3. *Communicate openly and often.* From the outset of the first Command Team Calls, we established a proactive plan for regular and frequent meetings. Initially, we convened weekly, but as the situation escalated, we increased the frequency, sometimes multiple times, even over the weekends. These crucial meetings consistently took place after standard work hours in the early evening to ensure broad participation. We actively sought input from key stakeholders, including division chiefs, resident representatives, and practice operation managers, recognizing the importance of their perspectives. Throughout these discussions, we strongly emphasized fostering an open environment that encouraged the contribution of opinions and ideas from all team members. This approach was particularly vital as our adaptations directly impacted their work, and their insights played a crucial role in shaping our strategies.

4. *Collaborate with others.* Our department is privileged to enjoy strong working relationships with other hospital departments within our health system. We actively shared the best practices we uncovered and seized the opportunity to learn from their experiences. Additionally, we fostered connections with hospital systems in our region and city, collaborating closely to explore innovative approaches to patient care. By working together, we aimed to minimize the necessity for patient transfers and ensure optimal care within our reach. By opening dedicated COVID care centers, our surgeons stepped up and provided essential surgical expertise for tracheostomies and obtaining central venous access while working with our medical intensivists. Their collaborative efforts with our medical intensivist further ensured comprehensive patient care during these challenging times. In times of crisis, our collective strength and collaboration became even more vital, reaffirming that we are stronger when united.
5. *Embrace discomfort and step outside your comfort zone.* Moments of crisis have a way of pushing teams beyond their usual routines. Work processes undergo changes, roles and responsibilities shift, and expectations expand. Team members should expect to encounter frustration, uncertainty, and feelings of unease, and they must be prepared not to be caught off guard or unsettled by these emotions. In times of crisis, a competent leader offers the team a sense of psychological safety, creating an emotional safety net that fosters learning and facilitates growth [4]. In response to the pandemic, our team experienced significant changes. Several members took on additional and different responsibilities, such as prioritizing the need for central venous access. Recognizing that our residents possessed the necessary expertise in this procedure, we had to rely on them in our dedicated COVID care centers. We temporarily redefined their roles and modified the conventional aspects of their education for the greater good.

Crisis 3: Crises from Cybersecurity Breaches

We prioritize the trust of our patients and their families, which entails safeguarding their privacy throughout their care journey, whether in our offices or the hospital setting. Maintaining their trust includes protecting the personal, financial, and health information they share. Unfortunately, healthcare data breaches have increased, creating a crisis affecting patients and health systems. Disturbingly, the Department of Health and Human Services' Office for Civil Rights has reported over 5000 healthcare data breaches involving 500 or more records over the past two decades [5]. These breaches have resulted in the exposure of nearly 400 million healthcare records, surpassing the population of the United States by more than 1.2 times. In 2022 alone, an average of three healthcare data breaches involving 500 or more records were reported daily [6].

Our health system and practices have not been immune to data breaches impacting patient and employee health and personal information. When these breaches occurred and affected patient information, our system leadership immediately acted and maintained open communication with the affected parties, offering complimentary protective services for their credit records as a proactive measure. In response to high threats of cybersecurity, our health system implemented several layers of security measures to protect employee information. However, a considerable responsibility was empowering and educating team members about potential areas of weakness, reminding them they are vital to protecting sensitive information and were "the last line of defense."

Our information technology department led us through these moments and implemented crucial adjustments to prevent future breaches and crises. They consistently kept their software up to date and strengthened the encryption of protected health information to ensure its security during ransomware attacks. Additionally, we implemented two-factor authentication for hospital records to enhance overall data protection. We foster a culture of transparency and provide team members with up-to-date information about present and future risks. We actively encourage them to contact our information technology service centers with areas if they receive a strange email, telephone call, or text message. Initiatives, such as the weekly sharing of "cybersecurity tips," effectively convey practical information that reinforces the importance of protecting the personal and health information of both team members and patients, regardless of whether they are in crisis.

To conclude, this chapter explored the importance of practice adaptation during crises in healthcare. From handling unexpected departures of key team members to global problems such as the COVID-19 pandemic, and cybersecurity breaches, we recognize valuable lessons on navigating and overcoming these challenges. The ability to adapt and modify practices during times of crisis is absolutely necessary for maintaining stability and successfully overcoming challenges. By embracing change, and implementing proactive measures, healthcare leaders and teams can survive and thrive while staring down the barrel of adversity. Through these adaptive practices, healthcare organizations can continue to provide high-quality care while observing their vision, maintaining their mission, and ensuring the well-being of their patients and their families.

SAGES Takeaway

- During a crisis, effective, competent leadership is key.
- A competent leader remains attuned to the essence of the organization. This leader understands the essence of the organization and actively works toward its vision and mission.
- Knowledge of team members' strengths and weaknesses before a crisis is essential for good leadership and adaptation if/when a crisis occurs.
- Prioritization of the highest quality patient care must be at the forefront for any organization, especially during a crisis.

References

1. Parker SH, Flin R, McKinley A, et al. Factors influencing surgeons' intra-operative leadership: video analysis of unanticipated events in the operating room. World J Surg. 2014;38:4–10.
2. Flin R, Yule S, McKenzie L, et al. Attitudes to teamwork and safety in the operating theatre. Surgeon. 2006;4:145–51.
3. Roberts NK, Williams RG, Schwind CJ, et al. The impact of brief team communication, leadership and team behavior training on ad hoc team performance in trauma care settings. Am J Surg. 2014;207:170–8.
4. Edmonson A. Speaking up in the operating room: how team leaders promote learning in interdisciplinary teams. J Manage Stud. 2003;40:1419–52.
5. Dorsey & Whitney. HHS OCR settles HIPAA investigation with business associate for $350,000. 2023. Available via JD Supra. https://www.jdsupra.com/legalnews/hhs-ocr-settles-hipaa-investigation-1194053/. Accessed 05 May 2023.
6. Healthcare Data Breach Statistics. https://www.hipaajournal.com/healthcare-data-breach-statistics/. Accessed 05 May 2023.

Developing Society Relationships

13

Crystal N. Johnson-Mann

Introduction

At our core, humans are social beings. In this regard, we are not unlike many in the animal kingdom. Success, or failure, with social interactions can have several helpful or harmful downstream effects. The ability to form meaningful social relationships can also play a significant role in the ability to achieve professional success.

Socialization among our peers and developing or maintaining social relationships are key to the human experience. It is our social networks that led to protection and provided a survival advantage to our ancestors. Both negative and positive social experiences result in not only physiologic effects but also psychological ones [1]. This is vital in medicine, where social support among our peers is a needed part of coping mechanisms for physicians' unique experiences with medical trauma, patient deaths, complications, and general work-related stressors. Social isolation is a risk factor for experiencing burnout, a fact made more apparent during the recent COVID-19 global pandemic [2, 3].

C. N. Johnson-Mann (✉)
Department of Surgery, University of Florida College of Medicine, Gainesville, FL, USA
e-mail: Crystal.johnson-mann@surgery.ufl.edu

S. M. Johnson et al. (eds.), *The SAGES Manual of Strategy and Leadership*, https://doi.org/10.1007/978-3-031-62359-2_13

Belonging is a necessary part of the human experience and, ultimately, a factor in career satisfaction and progression. This chapter will discuss the essential aspects of developing society relationships and achieving professional success.

Getting Involved and Networking

Opportunities to become engaged in medical/surgical societies are numerous, but the exact process varies by each individual organization and professional level. Even medical student-level individuals can often get involved as student members of multiple societies and become active on medical student committees, which is a fantastic way to start involvement early and begin the networking process. At the resident level, the same opportunities exist in multiple societies for residents/fellows to become actively engaged. One well-established example is the Resident and Associate Society of the American College of Surgeons (RAS-ACS). Becoming involved can lead to elected leadership positions on committees, with the potential to become elected as an officer to the executive committee, and subsequent opportunities to further engage with the faculty leadership of the ACS and set oneself up for future opportunities once transitioned as a Fellow Member of ACS.

Societal engagement through committee involvement is just the tip of the iceberg. Individuals who actively engage in committee work and volunteer/lead committee projects with good results are often rewarded with additional opportunities, including appointments as committee chairs and/or invitations to serve as invited session directors, moderators, and speakers of corresponding surgical society meetings.

Saying "Yes"

> Our lives are defined by opportunities. Even the ones we miss—
> F. Scott Fitzgerald

The adage passed down along the generations in medicine is to say "yes" when an opportunity presents itself – be it for a talk, book chapter, joining a committee, assuming a leadership role, and so on. This is generally true, as these opportunities may not represent themselves in the same manner again in the future. There are several benefits of saying "yes," as highlighted by Amy Blaschka in a 2019 *Forbes* article: [4].

1. It creates new opportunities and challenges.
2. It invites collaboration.
3. It empowers and affirms others.
4. It creates an environment where it is safe to try, fail, learn, and innovate.
5. It makes life more fun.

Opportunity does not always come around more than once, depending on the specific opportunity. Personal and professional growth often means stepping outside of one's comfort zone. By doing so, growth occurs, and additional opportunities may arise if an individual has demonstrated a solid work ethic and the ability to produce good results in a timely fashion.

In medicine, especially surgery, collaboration is a vital part of the research mission, leading teams, teaching, providing excellent patient care, and implementing initiatives that benefit the diverse members of medical societies. A willingness to collaborate also opens the door to diverse voices, allowing people to sit at the table and share their opinions, a continued need in society and medicine [5].

Empowering and affirming others is part of leadership. Saying "yes" allows an individual to wholly lean in and support the viewpoints and needs of others, contributing to the building of trust necessary for team dynamics. It is the action point of demonstrating that they are seen and heard.

Creating an environment where it is safe to try, fail, learn, and innovate is essential across many sectors. However, this is especially true in healthcare, where we are also focused on educating and training the next generation of physicians and allied health professionals. A supportive culture is also necessary for innovation, which is the cornerstone of advancements in medicine.

Finally, saying "yes" invites some degree of fun into one's life through new professional and personal adventures. New relationships formed through collaborations and new opportunities can lead to long-lasting professional benefits and create new friendships that can last a lifetime.

However, an additional consideration to saying "yes" *carte blanche* is to contemplate, by saying "yes," what that would mean for the other items on one's plate. Surgeons, by virtue of our chosen profession, are primed to take on anything that may come our way. As a result, we are not infrequently overextended. Part of saying "yes" is ensuring that there is enough gas in the tank to cross the finish line, whatever the task may be. In other words, make sure enough bandwidth and **time** exists before committing. If not, here is when knowing when and how to say "no" in a manner that does not derail future opportunities is an advantage. Saying "no" is a learned yet equally as important skill as saying "yes." As pointed out by Amanda Imber in a 2021 *Ascend* article for *Harvard Business Review*, saying "yes" is much easier than saying "no" because it does not require an explanation and takes less time [6]. Ultimately, when contemplating a response to opportunities that arise, your time and existing commitments (professional and personal) should be considered. If saying "yes" to something will derail prior commitments to other projects or responsibilities, perhaps saying "no" in that setting is the best option. Another consideration should be adopting hard rules that govern how you deliberate over decisions. For example, Imber covers an example regarding networking that can easily be extrapolated into medicine and large networking events [6]. If attending large networking events is anxiety-producing, but you recognize that it is a necessary part of forming relationships for the advancement of your career, then reframe how you approach networking by reaching out to individuals on a one-on-one basis to spark conversations that will allow you to build networks, but in a less anxiety-producing manner.

Knowing when to take advantage of opportunities and when to defer based on time and prior commitments is an art but a necessary skill set in developing networking and societal relationships for career advancement.

Mentorship and Sponsorship

In addition to connecting with colleagues in your specialty who may become lifelong friends, the same individuals can also provide meaningful mentorship and/or sponsorship relationships vital to your professional success, whether in training, private practice, or academic medicine.

The value of mentorship cannot be understated. It is a vital factor associated with improved career satisfaction, academic promotion, research productivity, and overall wellness [7, 8]. Effective mentorship is essential for the career development of women and underrepresented minorities, and the lack thereof has been described as a barrier to career progression, especially in academic medicine [8, 9]. Mentoring relationships are designed to be longitudinal, with mentees often having more than one mentor to best serve their spectrum of needs. However, effective mentorship as a stand-alone entity is insufficient for career development [10].

Sponsorship is necessary to create new opportunities that can change the course or direction of an individual's career. Mentors can also serve as sponsors, as sponsorship is episodic in nature and involves putting forth an individual's name for a committee, speaking opportunity, nomination for a leadership position, and so on. One part of being set up by sponsors for opportunities is having a *niche* – having an area of focus, and valuable expertise is critical when being considered for speaking engagements and leadership positions, along with a track record of successfully delivering when called upon for prior opportunities [11].

The overlap of solid mentorship and sponsorship is a critical factor in professional relationships [10]. Other integral factors include benefits for both involved parties, multiple relationships, and a baseline of trust, loyalty, and respect. The presence and outcomes of effective mentorship and sponsorship throughout one's career are necessary for career advancement.

Summary

Socialization and a sense of belonging are critical aspects of well-being, preventing isolation and decreasing the risk of burnout. Networking, involvement in surgical societies, knowing when to say "yes" to opportunities, and effective mentorship and sponsorship relationships are the foundation of promoting oneself and developing society relationships to achieve desired career advancement and satisfaction.

SAGES Takeaway

- Getting involved in surgical societies is an integral aspect of professional networking.
- Learning how to accept/decline opportunities is a skill.
- Mentorship/sponsorship relationships are critical for professional success.

References

1. Eisenberger NI. An empirical review of the neural underpinnings of receiving and giving social support: implications for health. Psychosom Med. 2013;75(6):545–56. https://doi.org/10.1097/PSY.0b013e31829de2e7.
2. Southwick SM, Southwick FS. The loss of social connectedness as a major contributor to physician burnout: applying organizational and teamwork principles for prevention and recovery. JAMA Psychiatry. 2020;77(5):449–50. https://doi.org/10.1001/jamapsychiatry.2019.4800.
3. Shanafelt TD, West CP, Dyrbye LN, et al. Changes in burnout and satisfaction with work-life integration in physicians during the first 2 years of the COVID-19 pandemic. Mayo Clin Proc. 2022;97(12):2248–58. https://doi.org/10.1016/j.mayocp.2022.09.002.
4. Blaschka A. Five reasons why saying 'yes' is the best decision for your career. Forbes, Forbes Magazine; 2019. https://www.forbes.com/sites/amyblaschka/2019/11/21/five-reasons-why-saying-yes-is-the-best-decision-for-your-career/. Accessed 4 Jul 2023.

5. Riner AN, Herremans KM, Neal DW, et al. Diversification of academic surgery, its leadership, and the importance of intersectionality. JAMA Surg. 2021;156(8):748–56. https://doi.org/10.1001/jamasurg.2021.1546.
6. Imber A. When (and how) to say 'no' to opportunities. Ascend, Harvard Business Review; 2021. https://hbr.org/2021/08/when-and-how-to-say-no-to-opportunities. Accessed 4 Jul 2023.
7. Walensky RP, Kim Y, Chang Y, et al. The impact of active mentorship: results from a survey of faculty in the Department of Medicine at Massachusetts General Hospital. BMC Med Educ. 2018;18(1):108. https://doi.org/10.1186/s12909-018-1191-5.
8. DeCastro R, Griffith KA, Ubel PA, et al. Mentoring and the career satisfaction of male and female academic medical faculty. Acad Med. 2014;89(2):301–11. https://doi.org/10.1097/ACM.0000000000000109.
9. Crown A, Berry C, Khabele D, et al. The role of race and gender in the career experiences of black/African American academic surgeons: a survey of the Society of Black Academic Surgeons and a call to action. Ann Surg. 2021;273(5):827–31. https://doi.org/10.1097/SLA.0000000000004502.
10. Ayyala MS, Skarupski K, Bodurtha JN, et al. Mentorship is not enough: exploring sponsorship and its role in career advancement in academic medicine. Acad Med. 2019;94(1):94–100. https://doi.org/10.1097/ACM.0000000000002398.
11. Stain S. Setting yourself up for leadership roles. In: The surgical section presents our 2023 webinar series. Surgical Section National Medical Association; 2023. https://surgical-nma.org/. Accessed 24 August 2023.

Part III

Leading Yourself—Deciding Scope of Practice

Determining Scope of Practice and Roles Involved

14

Gregory Leya, Matthew Hutter, and Jahnavi Srinivasan

Introduction

There are a limitless number of surgical practice types when it comes to the scope of practice and roles involved, and determining the most appropriate arrangement for yourself requires a nuanced, honest understanding of yourself and the broader, macro-environmental context within which you work. While our clinical training equips us with the tools necessary for clinical excellence, it is often devoid of the practical logistical, managerial, and leadership tools necessary to transform those clinical insights into a successful practice structure. By using basic principles and concepts taught at every business school and learned from our own clinical experience, we herein hope to provide a guiding road map to help you determine your own best scope of practice. While we do not provide clear answers on the best scope

G. Leya · M. Hutter (✉)
Department of Surgery, Massachusetts General Hospital, Boston, MA, USA
e-mail: mhutter@mgh.harvard.edu

J. Srinivasan
Department of Surgery, Emory Healthcare, Atlanta, GA, USA
e-mail: Jsrini2@emory.edu

S. M. Johnson et al. (eds.), *The SAGES Manual of Strategy and Leadership*, https://doi.org/10.1007/978-3-031-62359-2_14

and roles for your individual situation, we hope to provide you with the questions you should be asking yourself and some frameworks by which to answer those questions. We cite managerial and business literature references throughout for a deeper dive into the concepts discussed.

To better understand yourself and your macro-environmental context, you first need to consider your own personal and career goals, as well are your forecasted career trajectory. Doing so requires a balanced consideration of personal factors unique to yourself—micro factors—and broader contextual and environmental factors common to everyone in your field—macro factors [1]. Micro factors focus on knowing and leading yourself and include, but are not limited to:

1. Personal career goals;
2. Opportunities that are available to you now and in the future—e.g., clinical, administrative, managerial, research, innovation, education, and family opportunities;
3. An honest appraisal of your talents and shortcomings with regard to how you relate to others and manage yourself;
4. Understanding what brings you joy;
5. The personal revenue stream of your activities.

Complementing these micro factors are the macro-contextual factors that you should consider, including, but not limited to:

1. The competitive market environment for your clinical services and other services;
2. The private, academic, or “priva-demic” nature of your practice (a detailed discussion of which is outside the scope of this chapter);
3. Growth opportunities within your clinical field, founded on basic supply and demand principles;
4. Volume–outcome relationships in your field, and any pressures for increased sub-specialization within your field;
5. A needs assessment of your community and institution;
6. The institutional revenue stream of your activities.

In reviewing the above schema, it is easy to draw comparisons to basic management and leadership principles taught in business schools all over the world. The same principles that apply to the effective management and rollout of a startup company also apply to the management of yourself early in your career. You are your own startup company, and, similarly, you need to consider your competitive advantage, marketing strategy, resources at your disposal, financing, overarching strategy, cultural reputation, and partnerships [2, 3]. Furthermore, you should use the same principles that companies use to understand and analyze an industry in order to better understand the macro-contextual factors at play in your own specialty. One such commonly used framework is the SWOT analysis—strengths, weaknesses, opportunities, and threats within your macro-environment [4] (Fig. 14.1). If, in planning your own scope of practice and roles involved, you use the principles used to guide successful start-up companies and the

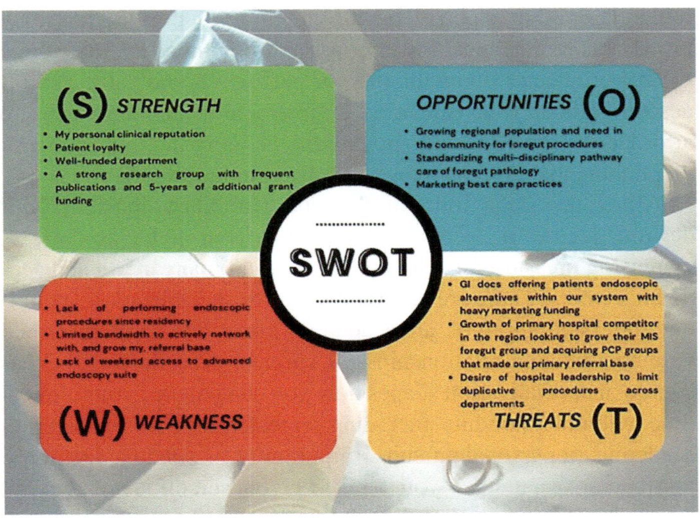

Fig. 14.1 Abbreviated SWOT analysis of MIS foregut surgeon in privademic practice

tools used by all successful companies to analyze their competitive market environment, you undoubtedly are more likely to be successful in your own pursuits.

Micro Factors: Leading Yourself and Personal Context

Determining your best scope of practice begins with self-awareness and an authentic assessment of your personal context and goals [1, 5, 6]. Importantly, your roles and responsibilities change dynamically throughout your career. These changes require you to constantly reassess your own scope, roles, and macro-context. Early on in your career, as a junior attending, your focus should be on establishing a strong clinical reputation and brand through effective self-marketing of your unique value proposition [7]. Just like Apple, Google, or Patagonia, you are your own brand. Your success depends not only on your clinical, research, or other expertise but also on how you present that value to patients, colleagues, institutions, and communities [8]. While the importance of maintaining your personal brand value continues throughout your career, as a more senior attending you are afforded the opportunity to potentially be more flexible and work on pursuits that do not have externally visible rewards.

Along the same train of thought, you must consider your desired degree of specialization within your field, as there is increasing pressure for sub-specialization in many urban and academic centers. There are several benefits to specialization, including the facilitation of an academic focus and well-described volume–outcome relationships for surgical procedures [9]. Your degree of specialization shapes how you can balance your clinical time with other pursuits, including protected time for managerial, academic, or personal pursuits. Importantly, as you consider these non-operative pursuits, you need to be conscientious of the fact that being an active surgeon informs and adds context to your other pursuits, and operating garners the respect of your colleagues if you hope to lead others.

In considering specialization, you need to understand your personal competitive advantage—what unique features you bring to the table that enhance your value relative to other surgeons. Just as businesses are taught to understand their competitive advantage and funnel resources, shape their business strategy, and focus marketing toward the competitive advantage, so too should you focus your energy on strengthening your competitive advantage rather than being distracted by areas where your value proposition is less. Creating a strategy focused on your competitive advantage allows you to position yourself around clinical, research, innovation, and other tasks that are difficult for other surgeons to match. Finding your competitive advantage takes genuine, frank introspection.

While surgeons have traditionally been known to neglect personal life for work, there has been a favorable shift toward recognizing the importance of work-life balance, just as there has been a shift in recognizing the importance of culture and workforce well-being in other industries. In determining your scope and role, you should evaluate how much protected time off clinical work you will have to pursue other interests, which is determined by your clinical partners available for coverage and your collaborators in extra-clinical pursuits [10]. Related to work-life balance is the value of learning to say "no." Surgeons are often naturally inclined to take on more work than they can handle or deliver at a high quality, and learning to say "no" maintains your integrity, work ethic, and value of your word [11].

Additionally, your financial goals will play a significant role in shaping your scope of practice. At every corner, you need to consider the costs and benefits of receiving a payout now versus a payout later. As anyone who has completed medical school, residency, and fellowship can attest, fixed-cost investments early on in your career can lead to payouts in the future. Examples of such fixed investments include subspecialized surgical training, additional graduate school degrees, or advanced training once you are an attending surgeon in robotics or endoscopy. Are both your clinical and extra-clinical pursuits financially viable, or do you plan to use one to subsidize the other? Are your roles and responsibilities scalable and sustainable financially? The reality of our careers is that money talks, and the clinical and non-clinical decisions you make will impact your salary and future leadership positions—your ability to provide revenue to your institution, through clinical work, innovation, or grants, will impact your ability to get a seat at the leadership and decision-making table. A notable exception is society leadership, which, while often providing non-monetary rewards, does afford you the opportunity to promote yourself and your brand while earning a seat at the table.

Finally, non-monetary rewards are likely to provide as much, if not more, personal reward that any monetary goals can. Pursuing personal goals that allow you to positively impact your patients and communities, that allow you to advance public health, or that allow you to shape the policy, art, and science of your field can provide priceless fulfillment. At the end of your career, it is incumbent on you alone to consider how you will assess your life and the success of your career, and financial rewards are seldom the most fulfilling accomplishment of any retiring surgeons.

Macro Factors That Shape Your Scope and Roles

Whereas previously we focused on important personal considerations that should shape your scope of practice and other roles, we now pivot to a framework to understand how the broader context within which you practice should affect your scope and roles. You always need to keep a finger on the pulse of your local and national contexts, including, but not limited to, the funding environment, changes in your professional societies, and business and political pressures shaping the healthcare landscape. SWOT analysis is a tool ubiquitous in the business and finance world to understand the opportunities and threats that should shape a company's ongoing strategy. A SWOT analysis involves listing the strengths, weaknesses, opportunities, and threats that your firm faces, with the first two focusing on your firm's internal characteristics and the second two focusing on external contextual factors. You can apply a similar analysis to your own surgical career with the broader socioeconomic context to drive your strategy and positioning going forward [4]. For instance, how does the increasing nationwide pressure toward hospital consolidation and centralization of care affect your own clinical practice? What are the growth opportunities in your field (e.g., robotic or endoscopic)? Who are your main competitors (e.g., MIS surgeons or GI endoscopists)? What pressures are there for you to sub-specialize or not? [12].

Macro-context is not only limited to national socioeconomic and political forces but also includes a focus on your team and institution. Applying the intentional and strategic analysis to understand the needs of your team, partners, and institution can make you an indispensable key player.

Conclusions

Determining your appropriate scope of practice and roles involves is a personalized and nuance decision that depends on your own personal goals, competitive advantage, resources at your disposal, timeline, and context. The underlying principles that guide the effective management of organizations and startups should similarly guide your own career and brand as you set off to create a successful, individualized surgical business model.

SAGES Takeaway

- Understand your personal and career goals, talents, and what brings you joy to determine your best scope of practice.
- Consider personal factors like career goals and talents (micro) and broader factors like market environment and institutional needs (macro).
- Apply business frameworks, such as SWOT analysis, to manage your surgical career effectively.
- Balance work and personal life while considering the benefits of specialization in your field.
- Financial goals are important, but non-monetary rewards, such as personal fulfillment and impacting your community, are also valuable.

References

1. Kaplan R. What to ask the person in the Mirror. Harvard Business Review; 2007. https://hbr.org/2007/01/what-to-ask-the-person-in-the-mirror.
2. Eisenmann T. Why start-ups fail. Harvard Business Review; 2021. https://hbr.org/2021/05/why-start-ups-fail.
3. Gulati R, DeSantola A. Start-ups that last. Harvard Business Review; 2016. https://hbr.org/2016/03/start-ups-that-last.
4. Minsky L, Aron D. Are you doing the SWOT analysis backwards? Harvard Business Review; 2021. https://hbr.org/2021/02/are-you-doing-the-swot-analysis-backwards.
5. George, et al. Discovering your authentic leadership. Harvard Business Review; 2007. https://hbr.org/2007/02/discovering-your-authentic-leadership.
6. Ibarra H. The authenticity paradox. Harvard Business Review; 2015. https://hbr.org/2015/01/the-authenticity-paradox.
7. Avery J. A new approach to building your personal brand. Harvard Business Review; 2023. https://hbr.org/2023/05/a-new-approach-to-building-your-personal-brand.
8. Dawar N. When marketing is strategy. Harvard Business Review; 2013. https://hbr.org/2013/12/when-marketing-is-strategy.
9. Birkmeyer, et al. Surgeon volume and operative morality in the US. NEJM. 2003;349(22):2117–27.
10. Groysberg B, Abrahams R. Manage your work, manage your life. Harvard Business Review; 2014. https://hbr.org/2014/03/manage-your-work-manage-your-life.
11. Tulgan B. Learn when to say no. Harvard Business Review; 2020. https://hbr.org/2020/09/learn-when-to-say-no.
12. Decker, et al. Specialization and the current practices of general surgeons. J Am Coll Surg. 2014;218(1):8–15.

Integrating New Technology and Procedures into Your Practice

15

Benjamin Crisp and Jacquelyn Turner

Throughout history, technological innovation has allowed for an enhanced operative experience for both the patient and the surgeon. This review will discuss how to go from encountering new technology in the market to integrating technology into practice and sustaining the skills to use the technology for patient care. One common theme of this review is that consistency and standardization are key principles in the integration process necessary to deliver high-quality outcomes, maintain procedural safety, and manage costs.

Overview of New Technologies

A Look Back at the Growth of Surgical Technology

Surgical technology has evolved over centuries of innovation. In modern-day history, minimally invasive surgical techniques, for example, have skyrocketed with innovation. The use of robotics is a great example of technological growth in surgery. Since NASA's first exploration into telesurgery in the 1970s, the development of

B. Crisp · J. Turner (✉)
Department of Surgery, Tulane University School of Medicine, New Orleans, LA, USA

S. M. Johnson et al. (eds.), *The SAGES Manual of Strategy and Leadership*, https://doi.org/10.1007/978-3-031-62359-2_15

robotics in surgery has been at the forefront of technological advancement, pushing the evolution of surgery forward. In 1983, orthopedic surgeons began using robots to assist with limb positioning. Two years later, the benefit of reduced hand tremors was recognized, and robots were used to reduce errors in brain biopsy. The first laparoscopic cholecystectomy was also performed in 1985, which served as an integral step forward in minimally invasive surgeries [1]. By the 1990s, laparoscopic surgery was more common, new procedures were being performed, and novel systems were invented to facilitate this surgical technique. By the year 2000, Intuitive Surgical Operations, Inc.™ received FDA approval for its da Vinci® robotic platform [1]. Over the ensuing decades, additional robotic platforms have been developed, enhanced, and expanded to become more user-friendly and with advanced features to assist the surgeon.

Areas of Technologic Advances in General Surgery

A tremendous amount of growth has taken place with robotic surgery over the last decade. However, while robotic surgery serves as a single example of emerging technology in surgery, there are a growing number of technological advancements currently being developed that will be integrated into daily surgical practice. In fact, the evolution of robotic and minimally invasive surgery has driven forward the markets for staplers and energy devices.

Staplers and energy devices carry added advantages in surgery including improvements in operative time and efficiency as well as improvements in tissue handling. As fast as research and development improves the technology in this market, vendors are promoting such new devices. This leads to surgeons taking advantage of the many improvements. Ultimately, the growing use of these devices and new procedures leads to improvements in the surgical industry standards. For example, in June 2022, Johnson & Johnson's Ethicon™ introduced its next-generation Echelon 300 stapler. The device provides greater articulation and a wider jaw aperture to give surgeons enhanced control over stapling [2].

Medtronic offers Tri-Staple™ technology, which includes three rows of varied-height staples to generate less stress on tissue during compression and clamping [3]. Both of these products are available as battery-powered devices. Intuitive's da Vinci® System also continues to develop and enhance its SureForm staplers which uses SmartFire technology to gauge the tissue. This technology uses more than 1000 measurements per second to make automatic adjustments to ensure a consistent staple line is created and prevent tissue damage [4]. Furthermore, there are currently several different types of energy devices used in surgery. Covidien™ (Medtronic), Ethicon™ (Johnson & Johnson), and Gyrus™ (Olympus) dominate the laparoscopic space [5]. However, compared with other technologies, development of novel energy devices has stagnated.

Future Advances in Surgical Technology

To further push the envelope and deliver improved clinical outcomes, there may be a shift from robotic-assisted surgery to performance-guided surgery. A major factor in accepting augmented intelligence (AI) as an emerging technology is recognizing it as an enhancement to human (surgeon) intelligence, rather than a replacement. AI and machine learning (ML) will become integral parts of surgery from the planning in the preoperative preparation phase through the postoperative analysis of results and outcomes. Intraoperatively, AI could help guide decision-making and perhaps assist or perform portions of the procedure. Tasks may include measuring defects and recommending mesh type/size, measuring bowel length, and gauging tissue thickness to facilitate with the procedure [6]. Limitations in technology and principles surrounding patient care prevent robotic surgery from being totally autonomous currently. For now, early AI should be used as a "navigation system" rather than perceived as an autonomously driven vehicle, though that may become reality in the not-to-distant future.

Integrating New Technologies into Your Practice

Encountering New Technology

Interactions with representatives from the medical device industry can be useful when discovering and implementing new technology into practice. Vendors and company representatives can facilitate the process of simulation/learning, device acquisition (sourcing, pricing, contracting), and intraoperative use (performance evaluations, troubleshooting). Continuing medical education (CME) is vital to the growth, development, and maintenance of surgical skills. However, it is important to distinguish between CME sessions that are educational versus those that are simply marketing opportunities for device companies [7].

Once an encounter with device representatives has occurred at conferences or CME courses, it is acceptable to further explore opportunities to implement the use of new products. Nevertheless, it is imperative to avoid creating a conflict of interest. If a physician chooses to pursue interactions with industry representatives, it is critical to clear vendor credentialing with higher-level administration to ensure compliance and the ability to follow supply chain protocols. It is equally important for hospitals to have an official vendor management policy.

Systematic Process of Acquiring and Integrating New Technology into Practice

To begin the process of integrating a new desired product into practice, the surgeon should first contact the Director of Supply Chain Operations of the institution they desire to incorporate the product. The Director of Supply Chain Operations oversees the supply chain management which is "the coordination of production, inventory, location, and transportation among the participants in a supply chain to achieve the best mix of responsiveness and efficiency for the market being served" [8]. The healthcare supply chain consists of managing medical and surgical supplies as well as pharmaceutical products [9].

Specifically, the Director of Supply Chain Operations is responsible for the daily operations of all supply chain functions conducted in the hospital facility including the operating room. This person oversees the inventory management and supply expenses. This person will also have a working relationship with the various product vendors. Furthermore, integrating each of the service lines in the hospital and making sure that the service lines are functioning within the hospital's primary purposes are also key functions of the Director of Supply Chain Operations. It is important for the director to develop and implement policies and procedures that guide or support services and perform assessments to improve department performance [10]. The Director of Supply Chain Operations should be involved in every step of the integration process.

Vendors should also be involved early in the process of integrating the device into the practice. The lifecycle of the typical vendor process often begins with "Identification of Need." The physician and/or vendor identify a need that can be met by the proposed device [11]. After identifying the need for a product, there are several steps to get the new product in stock and available for use. These steps include product review, trial period, approval of product, and purchasing (Fig. 15.1). During the product review, the product of interest is initially assessed for its benefits of use and potential risks by the Director of Supply Chain Operations. The director can pull information from reporting systems about the product. For example, an ECRI report is a reporting system that checks for product recall, equipment malfunction, and areas of potential harm. Such a reporting system improves the effective management of specialized requests such as capital equipment, which accounts for 15% of all new product requests evaluated. Health systems should use such reporting systems, especially when considering investing in costly decisions to incor-

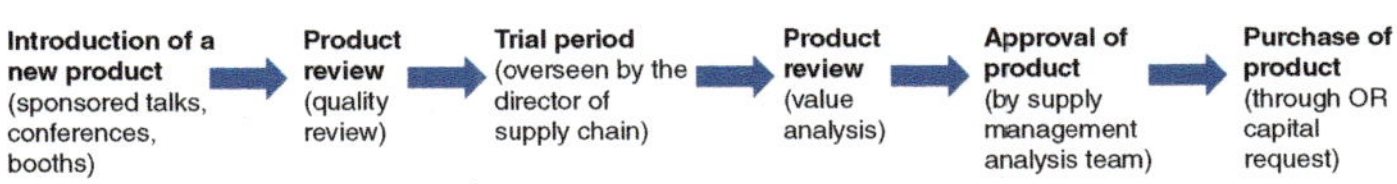

Fig. 15.1 Steps for integrating new products and technology into practice

porate requested items by physicians, med-surg supplies, and/or capital equipment [12].

Usually, all new medical equipment and devices must be trialed before purchasing. With the approval of the Director of Supply Chain Operations, the product can then be approved for use for a trial period. There may be contracts provided by the vendor to trial the equipment. The trial period is a set period of time where the vendor brings the product into the patient care facility to allow surgeons to use the product on patients during their practice. The Director of Supply Chain Operations should oversee the trial period and ensure that a safety system is in place during the trial period to protect the patient. Furthermore, when applicable, the equipment/device must be processed by the hospital policies. The vendor should also work with the director and central processing to comply with any special processing needs of the trial device [13]. At this point, it is important to monitor the performance of the device and compliance with planned protocols and contracts. Throughout the time of the trial period, the surgeon is assessing the benefits and downfalls of the equipment. The surgeon can compare the new product with existing products and consider replacing current alternatives if alternatives exist. This part of the process comes to an end when the contract ends or when the project closes [11]. Surgeons participating in the trial period should determine if they would like to move forward with acquiring the product.

Many hospitals have committees that may fall under a variety of names such as a "Value Analysis Committee" or "New Technology Committee" to determine if the product should be considered for acquisition and/or purchase at their institution. This committee will review the feedback from the surgeons during the trial period. They will also determine if the product is more cost-effective or provides more benefits than the current alternative(s). The supply management team along with the Director of Supply Chain Operations may also assess all data and determine if the product is approved for use at the institution. This process is often known as the "Go-to-Market/Sourcing Process." During this step, other options are explored evaluating the value and quality of the product in comparison with its alternatives. This allows for an informed decision that best fits the needs of the institution. Various vendors can be evaluated prior to selecting the most-qualified vendor(s) based on agreed criteria.

Once the appropriate teams and committees have approved the product to be safe and to be more beneficial than the existing product, then the product must go through the operating room capital request process. Of all the services in the hospital, operating rooms have the most inventory. Operating room cost centers are responsible for about 60% of total hospital costs [14]. Therefore, a process must be in place that balances out the push for low inventory costs and the request from surgeons to purchase new products that should enhance their operative techniques and improve outcomes [15]. Once a legal contract is signed, the vendor is set up within the institution and purchase orders can be written to execute the contract. Legal contracts can include nondisclosure agreements, purchase terms, rental terms, product repairs and replacement, and product upgrades. Finally, devices are delivered, and use is implemented [11].

After the new product has been approved and purchased by the operating facility, the focus must be turned to maintaining the safety of use among the proceduralists and assistants. In some cases, the entire operative team including operating room nurses and operating room technicians may need to have an in-service on the product, the procedure it is used for, and the involved equipment. Surgeons who desire to use the product and are not familiar with the product may need to demonstrate appropriate training before use.

Ongoing Quality Improvement

Once a product is in use at a hospital, it is best to continue an ongoing review process to achieve and sustain high-level performance, deliver quality care, and maintain efficiency. To accomplish this, it is beneficial to have a Quality Improvement Committee in place. The committee should comprise members of the supply chain operations including the director, proceduralists, and assistants who have used the new devices, and others involved in the use and maintenance of devices such as representatives from central processing. According to SAGES guidelines for the introduction of new technology and techniques [16], the following parameters should be monitored after the introduction of new technology:

1. Safety profile.
2. Cost.
3. Patient outcomes (specific to technology and technique).

Monitoring of the following should also be considered and can be useful in guiding ongoing use of new technologies:

1. Effectiveness compared with alternatives.
2. Required resources (e.g., training of individual and/or team).
3. Benefits to the patient (e.g., patient satisfaction, quality of life).
4. Benefits to surgeon.
5. Benefits to hospital.
6. Existing or anticipated volume of use.
7. Barriers to adoption (before introduction).
8. Existing resources (before introduction).
9. Whether the anticipated benefits prove real after introduction.

Committee members should review product usage and outcomes to ensure that primary endpoints and goals are being met, and if not, recognize faults in the system and processes that can bring outcomes back to the desired level [17].

Integrating New Procedures into Your Practice

New technology and devices are often paired with new procedural practices. Most often than not, patient care facilities require documentation proving that the procedure is safe and that the proceduralist is competent to perform the procedure. Surgeons seeking privileges to perform new procedures may be required to complete training courses, participate in case observation, and/or operate under supervision with a proctor for their cases. The remainder of this section will focus on the credentialing, privileging, and monitoring safety of the proceduralist.

Defining Credentialing and Privileging

According to He et al., credentialing is the process of appointing a surgeon to medical staff at a healthcare facility and involves reviewing medical staff licensure, insurance, education, training, skills, and experience. Privileging is the process of allowing surgeons to undertake specific procedures at certain facilities [18]. Credentialing and privileging are safety mechanisms used by hospitals and patient care facilities to maintain safe patient care among providers. Providers must prove that they are proficient in the technical skills needed to use the technology and that their proficiency has been maintained. The joint commission requires institutions to have specific policies related to credentialing [19]. However, the credentialing process is controlled by individual patient care facilities and/or larger healthcare systems. This lack of standardization of credentialing processes causes large variability among institutions. Yet some technologies, such as laparoscopic surgery, are robustly integrated into training programs and are a requirement by specialty board entities upon completion of training [20, 21]. However, credentialing and privileging for the use of newer technologies and procedures widely varies.

Achieving Competency

Residency and fellowship training programs, competency-based training pathways, and curricula are an essential part of the discussion of integrating procedures and new technology into practice. Trainees must show proficiency in the skills needed for the procedures to carry on with them when they begin their individual practices. When new technology and procedures are introduced, modifying existing curricula and creating new curricula to teach these practices will help reduce the risk of preventable complications, mitigate instrument or system malfunction, and affect hospital credentialing. Furthermore, providing a sound curriculum may play an important factor in medical-legal issues that may arise [18, 22]. Many surgical training programs, for example, are still in the process of updating their existing curriculum and/or creating new curricula to integrate robotic surgery into their education and practice. With robotic surgery through da Vinci® by Intuitive, trainees are eligible for a certificate of training for robotic surgery. To obtain the certificate, residents and fellows must complete online, video-based structure didactics. The trainee will then participate in a dry lab that includes an overview of the equipment, simulated docking, port placement, console overview, and system management. Once this portion of the training has been completed, the trainee will complete an online assessment and obtain an online training certificate. The trainee is then eligible to begin an operative experience which includes the primary role of bedside assistant and the primary role of console surgeon (Fig. 15.2). A letter from the training program is solicited to verify the trainee's participation in the process. After submitting a copy of the online training certificate, case logs, and letter of verification, the trainee will then be eligible to receive a certificate of system training that might be used at some hospitals for credentialing [23].

While most training programs have structured curricula, informal training of advanced skills is also often done. For instance, the apprenticeship model is sometimes used where the volume of cases is a marker for competence. Through this model, trainees learn through observation and perform procedures under supervision. This model is commonly used in non-accredited programs and transitional years. One drawback of this model is the elusiveness of defining the minimal number of recommended volume of cases to achieve competency. Competency-based curriculums are favored as they tend to address the degree of involvement during

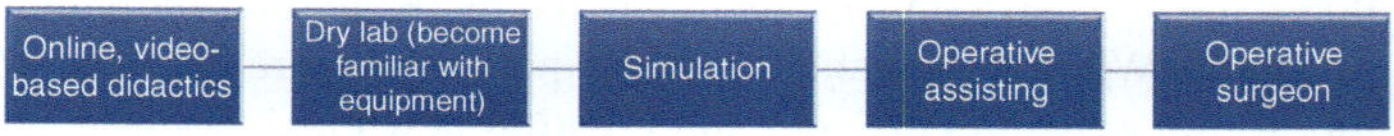
Online, video-based didactics
Dry lab (become familiar with equipment)
Simulation
Operative assisting
Operative surgeon

Fig. 15.2 A graduated competency model for trainees

training, diversity of case exposure, and level of difficulty. By achieving competency, it is implied that the trainee can independently perform the procedure upon completion of training [24]. According to the American Society of Gastrointestinal Endoscopy (ASGE), competency of a major skill or a skill that involves a new technology or procedure comprises a high level of complexity and/or interpretive ability should include the following:

1. Understanding of the indications, benefits, risks, and alternatives to the procedure.
2. Having the ability to perform the procedure proficiently and safely.
3. Identifying and managing adverse events that may arise.
4. Interpreting findings accurately.
5. Incorporating these into the overall clinical evaluation of the patient.
6. Providing a comprehensive pre- and post-procedural plan [25, 26].

When incorporating this framework for a competency-based paradigm, it should be procedure-specific. Furthermore, the training and action plan required for that provider may vary depending on the level of skill of the trainee. A couple of limitations of competency-based curricula include the lack of consensus of target achievements to obtain competency and the subjectivity of competency-based evaluations which could lead to bias [24–26].

There is also a need to provide access to skills and training resources outside of structured curriculums, especially for practicing surgeons. For example, some new procedures may be performed by few experts which may limit trainers who would be able to teach the necessary skills. Also, proceduralists in clinical practice may be limited by time and restrictions of their practicing institution. For these instances, live and hands-on courses may be available at national and international conferences, at sponsoring institutions, and through professional societies. A limitation of national and international courses is that they do not assess and/or affirm the competence of their participants [24].

Institution-Specific Credentialing and Privileging

Once a proceduralist has achieved the appropriate level of competency, that provider can apply for privileges at their institution and begin the credentialing process. Credentialing and privileging vary greatly among patient care institutions. Huffman et al. examine institutional credentialing requirements for robotic surgery. The authors were able to review credentialing policy from 42 institutions including 18 universities in 24 community-based hospitals from 24 different states across the United States. According to their review, most hospitals (83%) require surgeons to have privileges for the equivalent open or minimally invasive procedure for which they are applying for robotic privileges. Most hospitals (60%) required the credentialing surgeon to be board-certified or board-eligible. Less common, 38% of hospital credentials required surgeons applying for robotic privileges to have completed an ACGME/AOA accredited residency program and 14% of the hospital defined the maximum amount of time allowed after completion of robotic training to first proctored case (4.32 months) [19].

Credentialing and privileging can also vary based on the surgeon's experience. More experienced surgeons may need less requirements for obtaining privileges. For example, surgeons with a case volume of more than 50 robotic cases in a 12-month period may not require proctoring. Practicing surgeons who are learning a new skill or integrating a new technology in their practice may at their existing institution need to show documentation of an industry-sponsored training course, completion of online modules, provide a minimum number of training hours, document completion of a skills lab or simulation component, require case observation, and/or require proctored cases. A recent trainee from a residency or fellowship program (defined as one who completed a training program less than 3 years before applying for privileges) may be required to provide a letter from their residency or fellowship program director detailing the graduate's experience. Further requirements might be required of the recent trainee based on the number of cases submitted such as a defined number of proctored cases. Interestingly, 55% of hospitals require surgeons to provide a robotic case log. Of those hospitals, 26% specified a minimum number of total robotic cases to be completed [19]. Transferring surgeons may be required to provide a letter from the chair of the department from their previous institution to verify the surgeons' ability. Moreover, some institutions require transferring surgeons to provide documentation of privileges held at their previous institution and/or submission of case logs. Many hospitals require a specific number of cases per unit of time (e.g., 20 robotic colectomies over 12 months) to obtain privileges for that procedure.

After reviewing the credentialing documentation, new trainees or practicing surgeons performing new procedures may be granted provisional status. Provisional status suggests that surgeons can perform the new procedure under the direct supervision of a proctor. At most institutions, to obtain provisional status, surgeons must have board certification, hold clinical privileges, and perform an appropriate annual volume of indicated procedures. Surgeons who have provisional status should complete their initial cases within a defined period of time, usually within the first 2 months, after training to ensure that they have maintained the skills for the procedure [27]. The number of cases a surgeon must complete under provisional status may vary by procedure. Once the criteria of the provisional status have been met, the surgeon can then proceed to independent practice without a proctor. Some hospitals require surgeons to complete a certain amount of basic cases before attempting to have privileges for complex and advanced cases. An operative steering committee should monitor their surgeons' cases and work in conjunction with quality improvement and/or credentialing steering committees for the annual renewal of surgeon privileging. For example, a robotic steering committee should monitor the case complexity and outcome of each individual surgeon performing robotic cases and provide recommendations to the appropriate credentialing committee concerning surgeon credentialing on the robot [28].

Maintenance of Skills

Maintenance of skills will largely be dependent on the volume of cases the proceduralist performs. Plans to incorporate a new procedure should include predictions of future case volume to ensure that the proceduralists can maintain their skill and justify the need to continue to perform the new procedure. Knowledge-based exams and scheduled reporting of the practicing providers' case log may be required by specialty boards to qualify and maintain board certification [24, 29]. The American Board of Surgery, for example, requires a knowledge base exam every 3 years post initial board certification [30].

From the healthcare institution perspective, recredentialing with institutional-specific requirements may occur every 12–24 months. Failure to meet these requirements may subject the surgeon to losing privileges and/or to being placed on a focused professional practice evaluation plan. Furthermore, large gaps of time between surgeries should also be monitored. Large gaps should be addressed with that surgeon possibly triggering additional training and proctoring. When looking at robotic privileges among institutions, for example, the average maximum allowable gap in robotic cases on average is 5 months [19].

Finally, many new procedures may not have Current Procedural Terminology (CPT) codes. The lack of CPT codes for some of the new procedures can make both reimbursement and tracking of these procedures difficult. Furthermore, the lack of a CPT code and the associated reimbursement may deter surgeons who are contemplating performing the new procedure. CPT codes are updated annually by the CPT Editorial Panel authorized by the American Medical Association (AMA). Medical specialty societies, physicians, hospitals, and even third-party payers may submit applications for additions and changes to CPT codes to the AMA CPT Editorial Panel and for possible further review by the AMA CPT Advisory Committee [31]. Until the CPT code is updated or added, surgeons who are trying to bring a new procedure without an updated CPT code to their institution should be diligent in working with their institution/practice regarding the tracking and billing of the new procedure.

Summary

Undoubtedly, every surgeon will likely experience integrating new technology and procedures into practice at some point in their career. Vendors and industry representatives can be vital resources in this process. Likewise, surgeons should be prepared to work with hospital administration (Director of Supply Chain Operations, New Technology Committee, Quality Improvement Committee, etc.) to ensure the safe and effective implementation of new technology. On an individual level, surgeons and healthcare institutions should ensure that adequate credentialing and privileging are completed. Moving forward, it is vital to maintain skills and continue medical education to familiarize oneself with emerging technologies with the ultimate goal of driving change to improve patient care. Implementation of new technology is a collaborative effort. If proper steps are taken, it can be completed safely, efficiently, and effectively to benefit all involved.

SAGES Takeaway

- Evolution of Surgical Technology: The field of surgical technology has undergone significant evolution, particularly in the realm of minimally invasive techniques and the integration of robotics. This progress has revolutionized surgical procedures, making them more precise and less invasive. For example, robotics and advancements in stapling and energy devices have played a pivotal role in advancing surgical techniques.
- Integration of New Technologies Requires a Systematic Approach: Integrating new surgical technologies and procedures into practice involves a systematic process. This includes interactions with industry representatives, supply chain management, product reviews, trial periods, and ongoing quality improvement. Collaboration between surgeons, industry representatives, and hospital administration is crucial for successful implementation.
- Importance of Credentialing and Privileging: Credentialing and privileging are critical safety mechanisms used by healthcare facilities to ensure that surgeons are qualified to perform

specific procedures. The process involves reviewing a surgeon's qualifications, experience, and skills and granting them privileges accordingly.

- Ongoing Skill Maintenance and Quality Improvement: Surgeons must actively maintain their skills through regular practice. Quality Improvement Committees, monitoring, and evaluation are essential for ensuring that surgeons continue to provide high-level performance and quality care.

References

1. Gaines J. The past, present and future of robotic surgery: after decades of merely assisting doctors, are sophisticated machines ready to take charge? Knowable Magazine; 2023. https://knowablemagazine.org/article/technology/2022/handing-surgeon-scalpel-to-robot. Accessed 28 May 2023.
2. Newmarker C. Ethicon launches next-gen surgical stapler. MassDevice; 2022. https://www.massdevice.com/ethicon-launches-next-gen-surgical-stapler/. Accessed 10 May 2023.
3. Medtronic. Tri-Staple™ Technology. https://www.medtronic.com/covidien/en-us/products/surgical-stapling/tri-staple-technology.html. Accessed 28 May 2023.
4. DaVinci Stapling SureForm with SmartFire technology. https://www.intuitive.com/en-us/-/media/ISI/Intuitive/Pdf/sureform-staplers-brochure-1045912.pdf. Accessed 28 May 2023.
5. Malik S, Khairi F, Wijerathne S. Electrosurgery and energy devices. In: Lomanto D, WTL C, Fuentes MD, editors. Mastering Endo-laparoscopic and Thoracoscopic surgery. Singapore: Springer; 2023.
6. Fernando, A. The Evolution of Robotic Technology: From Robotic Assistance to Augmented Intelligence to Elevate All Surgery. Medical Device and Diagnostic Industry. 2021. https://www.mddionline.com/robotics/evolution-robotic-technology-robotic-assistance-augmented-intelligence-elevate-all-surgery. Accessed 10 May 2023.
7. HHS-OIG. Physician relationships with vendors. https://oig.hhs.gov/compliance/physician-education/iii-physician-relationships-with-vendors/. Accessed May 28, 2023.
8. Hugos M. Essentials of supply chain management. 3rd ed. New Jersey: John Wiley and Sons, Inc; 2011.
9. Landry S, Beaulieu M. The challenges of hospital supply chain management, from central stores to nursing units. Handbook of healthcare operations management. New York: Springer; 2013.

10. HCA Houston Healthcare. Director Hospital Supply Chain Operatons. https://careers.hcahealthcare.com/jobs/12253123-director-hospital-supply-chain-operations. Accessed 28 May 2023.
11. Senters K. Your Guide to Vendor Management Best Practices. Symplr; 2020. https://www.symplr.com/blog/your-guide-to-vendor-management-best-practices-symplr. Accessed 12 May 2023.
12. ECRI. Value Analysis Workflow. https://www.ecri.org/solutions/value-analysis-workflow#:~:text=ECRI%27s%20transparent%20value%20analysis%20management,requests%20often%20can%20be%20complex. Accessed May 28, 2023.
13. NHS University Hospital Sussex. Medical equipment and product trials. NHS Foundation Trust; 2020. p. 1–22.
14. Weiss A, Hollandsworth HM, Alseidi A, et al. Environmentalism in surgical practice. Curr Probl Surg. 2016;53(4):165–205.
15. Ehsan A, Masel DT, Metcalf AY, Schuller K. Inventory management of surgical supplies and sterile instruments in hospitals: a literature review. Health Syst. 2019;8(2):134–51.
16. Stefanidis D, Fanelli RD, Price R, et al. SAGES guidelines for the introduction of new technology and techniques. Surg Endosc. 2014;28:2257–71. https://doi.org/10.1007/s00464-014-3587-6.
17. Varkey P, Peller K, Resar RK. Basics of quality improvement in health care. Mayo Clin Proc. 2007;82(6):735–9.
18. He B, de Smet MD, Sodhi M, et al. A review of robotic surgical training: establishing a curriculum and credentialing products as an ophthalmology. Eye. 2021;35:3192–201.
19. Huffman EM, Rosen SA, Levy JS, et al. Are current credentialing requirements for robotic surgery adequate to ensure surgeon proficiency? Surg Endosc. 2021;35:2104–9.
20. The American Board of Surgery. Becoming certified. https://www.absurgery.org/default.jsp?examoffered. Accessed 25 Apr 2023.
21. Accreditation Council for Graduate Medical Education. Case log system. https://www.acgme.org/archived-web-pages/data-collection-systems/case-log-system/. Accessed 25 Apr 2023.
22. Schreuder H, Wolswijk R, Zweemer RP, et al. Training and learning robotic surgery, time for a more structured approach: a systematic review. BJOG: Int. J Obstet Gynaecol. 2012;119:137–49.
23. DaVinci by Intuitive. Certificate of da Vinci® System training for residents and fellows. https://www.intuitive.com/en-us/-/media/ISI/Intuitive/Pdf/equivalency-certificate-requirement-210352-.pdf. Accessed 25 Apr 2023.
24. Yang D, Mihir SW, Draganov PV. The status of training in new technologies in advanced endoscopy: from defining competence to credentialling and privileging. Gastrointest Endosc. 2020;95(5):1016–25.

25. ASGE Standard of Practice Committee, Faulx AL, Lightdale JR, Acosta RD, et al. Guidelines for privileging, credentialing, and proctoring to perform GI endoscopy. Gastrointest Endosc. 2017;85:273–81.
26. ASGE standard for clinical application. Methods of privileging for new technology in gastrointestinal endoscopy, vol. 50. American Society for Gastrointestinal Endoscopy Gastrointestinal Endosc; 1999. p. 899–900.
27. AAGL Advancing Minimally Invasive Gynecology Worldwide. Guidelines for privileging for robotic-assisted gynecologic laparoscopy. J Minim Invasive Gynecol. 2014;21:157–67.
28. Green C, Levy J, Martino M, Porterfield J Jr. The current state of surgeon credentialing in the robotic era. Ann Laparosc Endosc Surg. 2020;5 https://doi.org/10.21037/ales.2019.11.06.
29. The American Board of Surgery. Booklet of Information Surgery 2022–2023. https://www.absurgery.org/xfer/BookletofInfo-Surgery.pdf. Accessed 28 May 2023.
30. The American Board of Surgery. Program requirements—continuous certification. https://www.absurgery.org/default.jsp?exam-mocreqs. Accessed 28 May 2023.
31. CPT Editorial Panel. The CPT code process. https://www.ama-assn.org/about/cpt-editorial-panel/cpt-code-process. Accessed 28 May 2023.

HR, Conflict Resolution, Prioritization, Leveraging New Strengths

16

Angela M. Hanna and Krysta M. Sutyak

Introduction

Current leadership models have shifted from previous pathways. In decades past, leaders were promoted through personal accomplishment and pedigree and there was a large element of "learning as you go." [1, 2] In comparison, now we are seeing individuals selected for leadership positions who have awareness, training, and education, as well as skills in team building and emotional intelligence in the workplace [1, 3]. Many of these characteristics were traditionally seen as soft or not tough enough but are now seen as essential components of effective leadership [1]. Traditionally, many leaders did not have any formal training or resources available, and leadership ability was about innate skill with the right personality. This too has shifted: leadership training and preparation today includes not only numerous resource books

A. M. Hanna
Department of Surgery, University of Nebraska Medical Center, Omaha, NE, USA

Department of Pediatric Surgery, Childrens' Hospital and Medical Center, Omaha, NE, USA

K. M. Sutyak (✉)
Department of Surgery, University of Nebraska Medical Center, Omaha, NE, USA
e-mail: krysta.sutyak@unmc.edu

S. M. Johnson et al. (eds.), *The SAGES Manual of Strategy and Leadership*, https://doi.org/10.1007/978-3-031-62359-2_16

and papers but also courses, both university and association or societal-based courses, seminars, as well as advanced degrees [2]. Current-day practice involves hiring leadership, mentorship, and professional coaches to strengthen these exact skills and take the guesswork out of ability [1, 3]. This demonstrates a shift in not only outlook but also vision to put effort into learning to lead and strengthening human relationship skills to reach successful leadership.

The first step to leading a team is leading yourself. To lead yourself, you have to identify your own core values, mission, and goals to then set the stage for how these intersect in the environment in which you work and with the individuals you are tasked to lead. Understanding this first will help maintain strong skills essential for personal effectiveness and productivity that will set you up to be successful in leading others. Learning how to lead yourself will help you develop a career path to then build a legacy, and in turn, help build overall job satisfaction and fulfillment, while increasing resilience and decreasing burnout.

Conflict resolution is a necessary skill to learn as a leader. Peters et al. suggest that conflict is not only inevitable but necessary [4]. They explore the viewpoint that if you are not experiencing conflict, there is likely a lack of ideas, improvement, or growth [4]. However, what is the best way to manage conflict when it arises? There are tools and skills you can develop to learn how to successfully navigate through conflict, both individual and team conflict.

After developing a set of core values, a mission statement, and goals, prioritizing should follow. Without laying the framework, it is impossible to understand how to prioritize. Prioritizing involves delegating and handing over control at times, which can be difficult, but can be learned and will help build trust and provide opportunities for mentorship.

Learning how to leverage our strengths and recognizing our weaknesses requires self-awareness and input. A component of this may involve learning how to "manage up" and ask for what we want. Finding the opportunity to show our strengths can lead to increased leadership roles and responsibilities, and ultimately, contribute to our pathway to a satisfying career.

Building on this new paradigm, we will discuss how to lead yourself to address these specific leadership needs: successfully navigate human relationships, engage in conflict resolution, learn prioritization, and finally, leverage strengths, to prepare to lead in a manner that moves to build your career on a path that is sustainable, builds resiliency, minimizes burnout, and adds to your own personal legacy.

Human Relations

Cited as the number one most influential business book of the twentieth century, Steven R. Covey changed the landscape of leadership with his groundbreaking book, The 7 Habits of Highly Effective People [5]. He studied effective leaders and found common traits leaders possessed and delineated them clearly: being proactive, being with the end in mind, putting first things first, thinking win/win, seeking first to understand then to be understood, synergizing, and sharpening the saw [5]. Each of these tenets leads to how to optimize your interactions with others, but what Covey really submits is that it all begins with you and your paradigm. He suggests that we all have a personal paradigm that affects how we interpret the world [5]. This paradigm affects our actions and responses, and we may be unaware of what that even is. Successful interactions are a result of honing in on your own character traits through paradigm shift or change.

A good place to start in leading yourself is "begin with the end in mind." [5] What does it mean when Covey says this? It goes beyond thinking about what you want out of a simple conversation or interaction. As a leader, before you can begin, you must know where you are coming from. It is common for teams to draw up a team charter or a mission statement, so why are not we doing this as individuals? Thinking about and clearly defining what your core values are as a person will help lay the foundation for you to then create an individual mission statement and goals which will serve as your guide and roadmap. This is the first crucial step in leading yourself, the first step to "begin with the end in mind." [5] Once you have these "roadmaps" as a foundation, then you can lead a team. The first place to start with the team is by delineating these same team core values and then mission statement and goals.

Successful interactions are indeed the core to team dynamics. However, learning how to manage relationships well is not solely about personality or likeability. Emotional intelligence is a key ingredient to successfully navigating both individual and team dynamics and relationships. Emotional intelligence refers specifically to the tenants of self-awareness, self-regulation, motivation, empathy, and social skills [1]. These are skills we may all possess at different levels, but they can also be learned and taught through practice and feedback [1]. Emotional intelligence is not a new scientific study or field of research. Daniel Goleman wrote *Emotional Intelligence* in 1995, it was featured in a Harvard Business Review article in 1998, and by 2021, there were 6819 PubMed-indexed publications that cite emotional intelligence in the year alone. As emotional intelligence has gained more visibility, it is being recognized as a critical component of the qualities a leader possesses and, in some cases, is more important to the role than specific job qualifiers [1, 3]. For example, Boyatzis found that in a study of 2000 supervisors, 14/16 of the traits identified in their high performance were emotionally based [6]. Goleman found that when looking at the ratio of technical skills, IQ, and emotional intelligence of individuals who were categorized as excellent performers, emotional intelligence was twice as important as the other categories examined [1]. Even more interesting, as leadership increases, the difference in these variables increases and the difference in technical skill decreases [1].

There are courses that teach emotional intelligence, but research shows these are not necessarily skills to learn from listening to a lecture or reading a book [1]. As a function of the limbic system, neurocognitive research shows that emotional intelligence is better learned by application, reinforcement, and feedback [1].

A key tenet of emotional intelligence, self-awareness, is an all-inclusive term that includes being aware of your emotions, how they cause you to act, and how that affects the people around you [1]. It also includes your perception of others, their perception of you, and knowing your own strengths and weaknesses, your drives and values, and recognizing how this impacts the choices you make. This directly circles back to Covey's theory of the individual paradigm. Self-awareness develops self-regulation, and eventually, prioritization. Self-awareness is the acknowledgment of the emotions or reactions you are experiencing, and self-regulation is the way you choose to respond [1]. An example of this, Goleman suggests, is when working on a deadline causes extra stress and brings out negative behavior, thus you plan effectively and adhere to a strict schedule so as to complete work in a timely fashion and not be rushed. The groundwork here is prioritizing through self-regulation, how you act and respond to the stressful deadline.

It is important to note that self-awareness can be misleading. Approximately 10–15% of individuals are self-aware; however, some individuals may think or feel they are self-aware, but their perception is unrealistic, not honest, or exaggerated [7]. How do you evaluate if you are self-aware? There are ways to increase your skill: reflection is the key part of this. Start by asking those around you about their perception of your interactions and assessing your perception. Do they match? Look back on your interactions throughout the day and reflect on responses you felt were successful and ones that were not. Assess your tone and choice of words. How are you presenting yourself and how do you think you sound?

Think about the leaders who mentored you to this point—how did they respond to you when you missed a deadline, performed something wrong, or were involved in a conflict? How did they respond when you received awards and recognition or were successful on projects? Then, think about the leaders from your past and present who you do not feel share your values and do not represent the kind of leader you wish to be. When you ask yourself the same questions about how they responded to your successes and failures, this can help you identify what you should avoid doing in your own leadership interactions and responses. Again, this circles back to Covey's concept of identifying our personal paradigm and then working on changing it as needed for successful interactions.

A professional coach can help with this reflective process in an even more neutral objective way. Coaches can record meetings, interactions, and conversations you have and then play it back to you for an "observer's" secondhand perspective [1]. The coach can then walk you through the process of evaluating and reflecting on the results. Reflection, feedback, and practice are all steps to improve your self-awareness [1]. Once you are self-aware, then the next step is to work on self-regulation. Self-regulation involves consciously making decisions about your responses and actions, even planning your response in some situations. Being able to slow yourself down, think about what you want to accomplish out of the interaction, and how best to obtain that with your response will help you avoid reacting in the moment [8]. Once even partially mastered, self-regulation will improve the overall team environment and in leading by example can have a top-down effect [1].

Social skill is another key principle of emotional intelligence that is critical for leaders to develop. Social skill is the ability to build and foster mutually beneficial relationships, such as networking and building up a support system that can serve as guidance, support, and mentors when needed [1]. Social skill also includes building yourself to authentic leadership and providing mentorship from the top down. Mentorship is repeatedly cited as a majority contributor to the success of leaders. Developing mentorship abilities is an important skill and takes work. Primal leadership written by Daniel Goleman describes six distinct styles of leadership: visionary, coaching, affiliative, democratic, pacesetting, and commanding [9]. A visionary leader guides others through inspiration and motivation. They lead by connecting with their team and using positive energy to unite the team toward a common shared dream or goal [9]. Coaching style implements guiding the team through the task while pushing and supporting them to achieve on their own. At the core of Coaching is helping others focus on their strengths and improve their weaknesses [9]. Affiliative style promotes emotional intelligence and excels by human connection [9]. At the core of the democractic style are team decisions and promoting decisions as a group and combining individuals' inputs to the group decision [9]. Pacesetter leadership style hones in on setting and meeting goals. This leadership style is based on achievement, high-level performance, and task-oriented work ethic [9]. Finally, the commanding style works to guide the team as the true leader, at the "helm of the ship." In this style, the person in charge makes the decisions for the group [9]. Any one of us may gravitate toward one particular style that is either innate to us and our personality, or that we are inherently good at. As a result, we may utilize this style in the majority of our interactions [9]. However, different circumstances may require a variety of leadership styles. Developing the skill to show flexibility and the capacity to change leadership styles as needed will not only enhance social skills overall but also lead to more authenticity in leadership as well as open the door to providing mentorship. Different team members may respond better to different styles of leadership. Having the ability to flex into what the team member will best respond to will open the opportunity to then provide mentorship as well.

Continuing to part from previous models of leadership, the leader who is feared or not available is no longer seen as being successful or realistic [2]. Society has shifted from leaders who command and control to those who cultivate and coordinate [10]. Being authentic, accessible, and approachable are key characteristics to the success of the overall team. With an open-door policy where team members know they can always come and speak freely, as leaders, we will be in the know of both positives and negatives that are occurring [2]. The term "positional leader" is the idea that people will follow your lead within the purview of your hired position [11]. However, you can grow beyond this: strive for authenticity in yourself and what you display to the people whom you lead. One strategy is constant self-checks or reality checks [11]. This circles back to both self-awareness and holding to your own personal core values and mission statement. By being a leader people learn they can come to honestly, this will lead to respect, trust, and admiration, and result in their support of you, not because they must but because you earned it [11]. Their trust in you as the leader will then foster team trust and loyalty to the team values, goals, and mission statement. This can all be part of you building your career and ultimately your legacy as a leader.

Conflict Resolution

Conflict resolution deals with not only how to resolve conflict but also how to minimize it. As a leader, you will undoubtedly encounter conflict either directly involving you or among team members. As we are pushing boundaries, asking for change, and encouraging others to do the same, we will inherently find turmoil along this path [4]. The conflict itself can be stressful, but also the response to the conflict can be stressful, so finding ways to deal with it in mutually respectful and beneficial ways can deescalate the stress of the situation. Working on healthy and appropriate resolution strategies is vital as ignoring the conflict or handling it inappropriately can be devastating to the relationship, the team, and the overall goal [1, 4].

Multiple conflict resolution theories exist, and almost all are based on very similar tenants. Principles of respect, transparency, and communication are the foundation for most techniques for conflict resolution. As leaders, we are pushing our teams and asking for their opinions, ideas, thoughts, and contributions In order to grow and be safe in this space when conflict arises, we have to be transparent on how we address it. We also have to be self-aware and honest about our role and what we can and cannot do in the situation. As a leader, never be above apologizing if you owe an apology. This will establish trust with the people you are leading if they can see that you can admit when you are wrong.

In any interaction between two people or two groups, each side has its own story and at the center of the interaction is what crucial conversation authors Grenny et al. refer to as the "pool of shared meaning." [8] This "pool of shared meaning" is what each story contributes to the shared goal of the interaction. In any conflict, the first place to start is to look at the other side and to take the approach of: what is their story and how does it contribute to the pool of shared meaning? This is where the fourth tenant of emotional intelligence, empathy, comes into play.

Empathy is cited as a key quality in leaders, regardless of their field [1, 3]. In any conflict, the first step is to look for self-regulation and apply empathy. Try to look at the situation from the other person's perspective. If we maintain the premise that everyone is acting with good intent, how does this change how we view their story? When we start looking at the conflict first with this approach, it helps us to understand their story and to stay focused on what the mutual purpose of the interaction is. Maintaining the mutual purpose can help redirect the goals and deescalate the conflict. This can also lead to a win–win situation when we stay focused on mutual purpose and goals when finding a solution to the conflict [8]. Taking less direct approaches, such as trying to deescalate by agreeing to agree, or staying neutral, even when you disagree, is common but is also ineffective in truly resolving the conflict and ultimately limits advancement and productivity [3].

Communication theory also plays a role in conflict resolution. The LARSQ theory is used by mediators to assist with difficult discussions and finding common ground. This involves listening, awareness of emotions, reframing, summarizing, and questions [4]. There is no set way to proceed through these techniques but rather moving from one to another when appropriate. Utilize pauses and echoing statements to express interest in understanding what the other side is saying and let them finish explaining or answering a question without interrupting [4]. An additional approach to communication in conflict resolution is: inquiring, advocating, and connecting. Inquiry involves asking and non-judgmental listening. Ask questions until you fully comprehend the points they are making. As Covey suggests with Habit #5, seek first to understand and then to be understood [5]. Then the next step is to implement advocating. Explain why you as the leader are or are not able to do what they are asking or why the department has chosen to do something else and try to maintain mutual purpose despite not being able to give them what they want. Acknowledge how this affects the viewpoint they have already shared with you and stay away from aggressive or defensive language, tone, statements, and behavior [10]. Finally, while conflict is sure to be plentiful, you must wisely choose your battles. In this regard, flexibility as a leader means thinking, reviewing, and considering where you can budge and where must you hold firm.

Prioritization

Prioritization comes at the intersection of self-awareness and self-regulation. However, the other piece involved comes back to your core values and mission statement as an individual. As Covey has as Habit #3: first things first—you have to know what your priorities are before you can prioritize them [5]. This will be the driving force behind your goals and how you will prioritize them.

A key component of prioritization is knowing what your limits are and how to delegate. Many leaders mistakenly think if they cannot do it all, they are failing. Many leaders also have a hard time giving up "control" by handing off tasks or assignments. This is a common error we hold ourselves to [10]. Successful leaders know how to prioritize which items need their specific attention and management as opposed to those they can delegate. Delegation has other inherent benefits as well. This should not be viewed as giving up control, but rather allowing opportunities for other people to rise to the occasion and to shine in their abilities as well [2, 10]. Delegation establishes trust among team members, builds them up, and provides an avenue for mentorship. Through delegation, you are sending the message that you are investing in your team. This leads to strengthening the team dynamics, the team goals, and mission.

Finally, part of prioritization is understanding which tasks may not get done or which tasks need to be deescalated or put on the back table. Through this process, you may realize that there are some tasks that no longer fit into the values or mission for you as the leader or no longer fit for the team. This can help "declutter" agenda items that are no longer relevant so everyone can focus on what truly does take priority.

Leveraging New Strengths

An important aspect of building yourself up and truly leading yourself is leveraging your strengths. This takes self-awareness and often input from other peers, mentors, and leaders, to be able to identify what truly are your strengths. With this, it is important to also identify your weaknesses.

Ancona et al. in their Harvard Business Review article, "Praise for the Incomplete Leader," discuss the idea that no leader by themselves can excel at everything [10]. Instead, they highlight their strengths and then fill in the gaps of their limitations with their team members. We must be able to shift our paradigm to accept that as leaders, we cannot do everything on our own and that we will have to lean on others. If we are aware of what our strengths and limits are as leaders, then we can build teams where team members have strengths that fill in those holes. While this may be the idea that we are an incomplete leader, incomplete does not equal incompetent [10]. The difference is that, if we recognize our weaknesses as qualities to be worked on and highlight others' strengths to help make up for that, then we are still being an effective leader. Incompetency would be instead, out of fear or insecurity, hiding our weaknesses, or worse, acting out based on feeling threatened that someone will overshadow us. Ultimately, building up others' strengths will help mentor them and help them excel on their own pathway. This strategy also shows your strength as a leader. Again, this will not only bring trust to you as a leader but also help establish your legacy.

Leveraging your own strengths sometimes means knowing how to "manage up." Sometimes you have to be proactive and ask for what you want. Your own leaders may not know what some of your strengths are or may not have had the opportunity to see them yet. Do not be afraid to ask for opportunities to use these strengths and show them where you can be successful. Seek out opportunities to use these strengths and put them on display, such as serving on committees or offering to take on tasks from your leaders. If there is a strength you want to leverage, look for ways you can enhance that skill to provide more evidence for why you want the opportunity. For example, if you want to use your minimally invasive skills to start doing a new operation at your hospital that has not been done before, find a course that you can attend to hone that skill and lend support for your qualifications when you ask to bring the procedure to your facility. Once you have shown these new strengths and your reliability, it opens the door for new and growing leadership opportunities for you. It shows trust and accountability. Leaders who carry out their accomplishments successfully tend to get more assignments and more leadership opportunities. Also, by truly seeking out what we are interested in, we remain engaged and participatory in our jobs and building our careers. This can decrease burnout.

With building up strengths and looking at weaknesses, it is important to address the topic of burnout. Burnout is the syndrome characterized by exhaustion, cynicism, and reduced effectiveness. It affects physicians more than any other field in the US. It can lead to depersonalization of work, decreased patient satisfaction, decreased quality of care, and increased physician turnover, as well as personal problems such as depression and broken relationships [12]. Burnout may be assigned as a character flaw or a lack of resilience, but this is incorrect. Burnout is a systems problem and addressing it requires understanding where the system is failing rather than blaming individuals.

There are ways to combat burnout. Creating avenues for appropriate work-life balance, finding meaning in your work, flexibility, engagement in your job, and having intersecting values between you and your job are all ways to counter burnout and build resilience. Dr. Julie Freischlag brings together the concepts of leveraging your strengths to build resilience. In her address at the ACS Clinical Congress in 2015, she said, "Giving chances to others and taking our own chances help us all bounce up. Giving chances demonstrates our humanity, and taking chances enhances our resilience and improves our ability to achieve our dreams. Giving and taking chances are essential leadership skills." [13] Having resilience does not mean you will not encounter tough times or even emotional hardships as a leader. However, building on the ability to manage through it and rise above it is what builds and maintains resilience and then lends it to others we lead.

Conclusion

To become successful leaders who can lead others, it is important we first develop and lead ourselves. Key components to leading yourself include first strengthening your management skills, understanding effective conflict resolution, learning how to prioritize, leveraging your strengths, and building on your weaknesses. There are a few resounding principles that keep resurfacing in discussing these topics. First, identify your own core values to build upon. Second, each of these areas of strengthening leadership skills requires self-awareness. Third, practicing emotional intelligence provides a foundation to approach each of these arenas successfully. Fourth, as a leader being honest, authentic, and transparent will build and retain trust and successful relationships. Dr. Julie Freischlag suggests that it is not the strong but the responsive that survive [13]. Sense of belonging, recognition, self-esteem, and the ability to live up to expectations are basic needs for achievement [14]. In the world of leadership, protecting, cultivating, and promoting our people is sacrosanct. Tarnoff et al. suggest that we "embrace a new approach where we care about the opinions and well-being of our teams as much as we care about the opinions and well beings of our patients." [14] All of these successes as a leader, and in building our career, will ultimately help us to build resilience, decrease burnout, and build a lasting legacy that we can be proud of.

SAGES Takeaway

- Current leadership stands on principles of successful human relationships. Start by defining your core values and your mission statement, leading to a roadmap you can follow. Reflect on the way you lead, the way you take and give feedback, and your own strengths and weaknesses. With introspection, look to mentors and even coaches to identify what changes you may need to make to lead successfully.
- Emotional intelligence contains tenets of interaction and understanding that are crucial in successful relationships and leadership. If not innate, these can be learned skills through practice and coaching. In today's workplace, emotional intelligence skills are often viewed as having significant—and even greater—value than technical ability or performance.
- Conflict is always a part of human interactions. Prepare to navigate these challenges with resolution strategies grounded in respect, transparency, and clear communication. Establishing trust, employing empathy and flexibility, and maintaining

mutual purpose in conflict resolution can help deescalate situations and lead to shared wins.

- Through self-awareness, you can begin to prioritize. Prioritization can help you delegate tasks to team members, in turn, building trust, strengthening team dynamics, and demonstrating to your team that you are investing in them.
- Work with mentors and peers to highlight your strengths. Acknowledge the limits of your own weaknesses and turn them into a strength by building a team with members who highlight and fill in the gaps. Leverage your strengths to build resilience, combat burnout, and lead to a legacy that you are proud of.

References

1. Goleman D. What makes a leader? Harv Bus Rev. 2004; https://hbr.org/2004/01/what-makes-a-leader.
2. Rikkers L. Presidential address: surgical leadership-lessons learned. Surgery. 2004;136:717–24.
3. Gewertz B. Emotional intelligence: impact on leadership capabilities. Arch Surg. 2006; https://doi.org/10.1001/archsurg.141.8.812.
4. Peters W, Picchioni A, Fleshman JW. Surgical leadership. Clin Colon Rectal Surg. 2020;33(4):233–7. https://doi.org/10.1055/s-0040-1712976.
5. Covey S. The 7 habits of highly effective people. New York, New York; 2004.
6. Boyatzis R. The financial impact of competencies in leadership and Management of Consulting Firms. Department of Organizational Behavior: Case Western Reserve University; 1999.
7. Eurich T. What self-awareness really is (and how to cultivate it). Harv Bus Rev. 2018; https://hbr.org/2018/01/what-self-awareness-really-is-and-how-to-cultivate-it.
8. Grenny J, Patterson K, McMillan R, et al. Crucial conversations. 3rd ed. New York, NY; 2022.
9. Goleman D. Primal leadership: realizing the power of emotional intelligence. Boston: Massachusetts; 2002.
10. Ancona D, Malone T, Orlikowshi W, et al. In praise of the incomplete leader. Harv Bus Rev. 2007; https://hbr.org/2007/02/in-praise-of-the-incomplete-leader.
11. Maxwell J. The 5 levels of leadership: proven steps to maximize your potential. New York, NY; 2013.

12. Freischlag J, Silva M. Bouncing up: resilience and women in academic medicine. J Am Chem Soc. 2016;223(2):215–20.
13. Knight B. How to develop empathy for someone who annoys you. Harv Bus Rev. 2018; https://hbr.org/2018/04/how-to-develop-empathy-for-someone-who-annoys-you
14. Tarnoff M. Dissecting the important difference between good surgeons and good leaders. JAMA Surg. 2020;155(9):801–2.

17 Utilization of Advancement Opportunities, Expertise, and Marketing to Establish a Practice

Candice Chipman

How to Utilize Advancement Opportunities

Utilizing advancement opportunities is highly specific to your practice environment, be it academic, community hospital, or private practice. The goals and definition of success look very different in each one of these settings.

Expertise is the way to advance in our current environment of surgery. Fellowship training, specific certification, or becoming niche specialized equal not only promotion and higher salary but also job security.

In this age of medicine, there has been an increased interest and preference for physicians and surgeons to be specialized or fellowship-trained. The reason for this recent trend is not only due to residents not feeling prepared to step out on day 1 after graduation as an attending surgeon, but also due to credentialing changes and competition in overlapping procedures/specialties. There are still some general surgeons; albeit typically rural general surgeons, who perform vascular procedures, surgical oncologic procedures of the abdomen and breast, urology procedures,

C. Chipman (✉)
Abington Jefferson Health, Abington, PA, USA
e-mail: Candice.chipman@jefferson.edu

S. M. Johnson et al. (eds.), *The SAGES Manual of Strategy and Leadership*, https://doi.org/10.1007/978-3-031-62359-2_17

and, in some cases, gynecological procedures. However, for the most part in urban and suburban hospitals, these are relegated to fellowship-trained surgeons. While it may vary from hospital to hospital, the credentialing at most hospital centers and the conditions of one's contract, also require formalized training and a certain number of procedures, be they done in fellowship or over a period in a proctored setting. Some of these hospitals or private practice groups require board certification in those subspecialties in addition to letters of support from a chairman of that specialty.

Specialized training or even training in a specific procedure or technique modality can set you apart from your counterparts and render you a title, increased pay, and preference for specific patients. This occurs because the organization benefits from being able to offer the additional cutting-edge procedure and the additional revenue of doing something so specialized. This equates to a higher base salary and relative value unit (RVU) generation. Of note, if the RVU has not been assigned or the complexity of the procedure does not match the amount of work or skill required, do not be afraid to negotiate a higher RVU allocation within your private practice, hospital, or even with insurance companies. This is particularly important when it comes to collections. Collections can be renegotiated and can vary even amongst surgeons in the same practice.

If you have been practicing for a few years without fellowship training and would like to add more procedures that require subspecialty training, you may negotiate to step away from your institution to complete a full-time fellowship, or begin training for the procedure under surgeons in your institution who are doing it, or participate in courses outside of your hospital and begin operating with guided proctoring.

It is advantageous to keep up with the advances of surgery as time goes on as it will spell decreased consults/referrals not only from Google and social media-educated patients, but also from primary care physicians who become aware of the advances in surgery and want the best for their patients.

Doing what you like increases satisfaction and adds to overall wellness.

A survey on career addict showed that 82% of respondents would quit their job because of a "lack of career opportunities" and 35% "would consider returning if they were offered a better salary or a higher position" [1]. For a surgeon, the expectation is no different.

When we talk about the career advancement of a surgeon, the setting of which their practice is should be taken into utmost consideration. For example, an academic surgeon will be more focused on research and teaching versus a private practice surgeon may gain seniority based on the volume of cases, RVU generation, and the number of years at the practice.

Promotion and revenue generation go hand in hand in any setting.

Prior to us delving into promotion, I want to make a special note that we will often not only talk about how to be promoted based on titles and remuneration, but we will often go back and forth with tying in how making the hospital money in the academic setting as well as in a private practice also translates to more money for you be it guised as a quality bonus within academics or as an end of year bonus as a partner in a private practice or even as a junior surgeon within the private practice. Paying attention to overall revenue and your or your practice's contribution to that overall number is important when considering roles for chairman and chief of surgery as well as chairman of your respective specialty department at the hospital even within private practice. Within the private practice setting, this can mean better negotiation with the hospital for reimbursement for clinics run at the hospital and reimbursement for surgical procedures done on those patients seen at the hospital clinic.

It would be advisable to take a billing course or get in touch with your department billers to help understand what brings in more revenue. You can ask to have regular meetings with the billers and also to have one or two billers assigned to your group to maximize coding and billing. This should be done when beginning to practice or even if you are several years in practice as you may want to touch base with them to see if you are missing an opportunity for better RVU capture and a means to increase collections. This will also increase collections for your department/

practice. Increased revenue for the department or practice equates to more budget allocated to the department for various hiring needs or hardware needed. In private practice, more collections mean a higher bonus at the end of the year. Higher collections also mean preference when it comes to operating room time.

Even in academic settings, quality bonuses are often linked to cost reduction in the operating room and one's ability to finish notes in the appropriate time. Finishing notes on time and keeping costs down are not just part of patient care, but they translate to revenue because you must bill within a certain time frame and keep profits higher than costs. Understanding which diagnoses net higher collections is beneficial to understanding not only your contribution but also in setting expectations when the hospital sets annual budget expectations.

Promotion in academic settings.

In terms of academic promotion, it is important to understand the levels of advancement and what is needed at each stage as there are specific forms of scholarly or clinical activity that need to be completed within a specific time frame. For example, there are clinical and academic/research levels of professorship and only certain levels of research such as original research that will qualify for advancement within the roles. The research will also need to be completed within specific time periods outlined by the institution. At the time of job acquisition, speak with your chairman of surgery about getting an outlined description of what it would take to advance through each level. It is important to do this when you start the job as many of the advancements must happen within a certain time period of your start, particularly if you want tenure. If you are in an academic setting, the Liaison Committee on Medical Education (LCME) requires that every faculty member teaching a resident has a title and declares a track.

You may also consider picking a niche within education to consider if research is not your interest. This means getting involved with medical students, residents, fellows, or faculty development. The American College of Surgeons as well as The Association of Surgical Education has comprehensive courses that are short or long term in getting you ready for a career in training adult learners. Seeking a master's degree in health education or healthcare management would also be of benefit and can also help with the transition to an administrative role in the future. Often, we think of a Master of Business Administration as the key to advancement within the administration, but there are other tracks to consider as well to add the feather in your cap needed in order to be an invaluable asset to your institution.

Promotion within private practice.

In a private practice setting, career advancement may look very different because the goals are more in alignment with small business practices. Sometimes, this can be difficult to grasp as a new attending out of fellowship or residency as you have been trained to always put the patient first, no matter the cost-literally or figuratively.

Your position in the practice is more time dependent on time with the practice, experience, reputation, ability to bring patients to the practice, niche-related, and your ability to increase the volume of cases. All of this equates to higher collection from insurance companies, which is paramount in the private practice world. When signing a contract with a private practice, never sign on without an indication of how long it would take to become a partner. The timeline for partnership should be within 3–5 years. Without a contract outlining this promise and the parameters to meet in order to accomplish that goal, there can be any number of things the practice may use to thwart your advancement to partnership. There are some who claim that being a partner is only an administrative role and does not increase salary or bonus, this is not true, being a partner will increase money and power within the practice to allocate your time and case volume, which still equates to more money. The main titles to gain within a private practice may be partnership within the practice or a director/chairmanship role in the hospital that the practice may operate at. Similarly, research shows that many employees in various industries of small business point out they usually do not move into a new role every year but do feel as though they have outgrown their position and at times may become bored. The solution for a limited environment for big changes would be to add new responsibilities within the same role as a form of career advancement. Clutch survey showed that 67% of employers expect to receive more responsibility at their job each year, but only 46% of people do [2]. This can also be applied within a private practice where sometimes a specific number of years in the practice or a certain number of RVUs are needed to attain partnership or executive levels within the hospital system the practice operates at.

Of special note, if you are ever considering moving out of private practice to an academic role, it would behoove you to prepare for all possibilities by participating in research. If you are not interested in clinical research, consider quality projects that need to be completed as part of the maintenance of a center of excellence. You can publish these data.

If you are in a position of leadership, it is important to map out various paths for your employees' goals. The map should be detailed in that it delineates exactly what needs to happen for them to achieve that goal and a rough timeline to meet their learning objectives or goal. Additionally, these conversations on career advancement should be kept separate from performance reviews [2]. This way, the employee does not feel that their performance is linked to the goals set for career advancement, and the conversation is not deemed punitive or contingent on a specific performance to gain X advancement.

Marketing in a Surgical Setting

Whether the practice is academic or private practice, marketing needs to be something earmarked for considerable investment, in terms of time and money. A separate budget should be allocated to not only the usual avenues of television and radio but also encompass face-to-face meetings and embrace the new social media platforms of Facebook, Instagram, Twitter, and dare I say, TikTok. A person tasked with only marketing should also be allocated to maintain the relationships in person or online.

Maintaining relationships is key. The electronic medical record allows you to automatically send progress notes or operative notes to primary care physicians. Referring to that physician is also helpful. Keep conversations respectful when you disagree with care, always try to find the middle ground, and dual compromise. Offering to do a lecture when needed for residents or attendings is a sign of good faith. The lecture not only gives the attendings an opportunity to know what it is you surgically are doing in detail but also helps them recognize complications or other means of taking care of the patient as it relates to your surgery. Never underestimate the power of the relationship between a primary care physician and their patient. The patient often has been with this physician for many years, even decades, and will abide only by the opinion of the primary care physician.

Last, but certainly not least, your patient is your best marketing tool that you never spent a dime on. Being affable and available never goes out of style, but the key piece is to ensure that your patients understand what you are doing and why. Make whatever changes they need to make for the surgery preoperatively or postoperatively most amenable to their lifestyle and that means doing the simple thing everyone says, "listen to the patient." Be reasonable with what people have the time for and what they can afford. A surgeon who hits every box is key to gaining high numbers of reviews and high-quality reviews be they online, word of mouth, or through the primary care physician. Ensure that they write reviews for you and stay on top of and track what a simple Google search of your name may bring.

There is so much to unpack what was discussed in this chapter. Getting an executive leadership coach to help you become better organized can be a game-changer. Once in a career, it is important to develop an advisory board of mentors, not just a single mentor. This advisory board becomes your sounding board for any challenges along the way or they inspire you to rethink the same success or look at the issue needing to be solved with a different lens.

In conclusion, ask yourself, what makes me unique within my practice, department, and even in my hospital system? What is my value? Am I replaceable, or is there something I can add to my toolbox that can set me apart? Is there something that I am interested in that my hospital needs that can also increase my value? Value is something that changes over time just as the innovation and evolution of current procedures in our field. Never be afraid to be the gray-haired person in the room learning "that new thing."

SAGES Takeaway

- Assess your skill and need for upgrading.
- What is required for advancement at your organization? Have you hit the ceiling there and is it time to move on? Is your advancement tied to teaching, research, or RVU production? How can you maximize even further what you currently do?
- Diversify your contribution to the field of surgery. Look at your participation in your hospital system, the American College of Surgeons, or your specific specialty society/organization.
- Celebrate your success and ensure that it is known through marketing.

References

1. Career Addict. Why people quit their jobs. 2020. https://www.careeraddict.com/careeraddict-study-quit.pdf.
2. Elliott, J. How to create growth opportunities for employees even if You're a small business. 2021. https://www.uschamber.com/co/run/human-resources/creating-advancement-opportunities-for-employees.

Part IV

Leading Others—Managing Your Work Environment

18 Evaluating and Assessing Your Team

Christopher DuCoin

Introduction

When we think of a team in surgery, we think of the surgical team better known as the operative team. A simple statement to sum up this team would be a highly organized and specialized group of individuals with specific tasks and objectives who collaborate to provide safe, effective, and efficient surgical care to patients. Yet, there is so much more to our teams in surgery. These teams will cross the clinical setting from the operating rooms to clinics, from our offices in the outpatient setting to the offices in the executive suite. The ability to navigate, improve, and lead all of these teams is critical for the modern surgical leader. To understand the team, one must also understand the individual and the organization. This is an extremely complex and layered process. The aim of this chapter is to highlight the theory on team development while also providing concise and specific tools to help you evaluate and assess your teams across the house of surgery.

C. DuCoin (✉)
Department of Surgery, University of South Florida, Tampa, FL, USA
e-mail: cducoin@usf.edu

S. M. Johnson et al. (eds.), *The SAGES Manual of Strategy and Leadership*, https://doi.org/10.1007/978-3-031-62359-2_18

The Difference Between Individual and Team Assessment

Team assessment and individual assessment are two distinct approaches used in evaluating the performance, skills, contributions, and collaboration of individuals within an organization. While there are a litany of tools that can be used for either individual or team assessment, each approach serves a specific purpose and provides insights into different aspects of an individual's or a team's ability. To understand team assessment, we must also understand individual assessment. In most scenarios, there is either a solid understanding of the individual or an assessment of individuals prior to moving toward a team assessment.

Individual Assessment

Individual assessment focuses on evaluating ~~the~~ strengths and weaknesses, current performance within the scope of the position, gaps for improvement, and future potential. This assessment is singular and usually does not focus on this individual's relationship within the team dynamic, but rather their relationship with individuals on the team such as their direct superior, inferior, and close collaborators. Individual assessments rely on how well someone is doing at their specific job responsibilities and contributing to institutional goals in congruence with the institute's mission. Usually, these assessments will be conducted with job-specific evaluation forms, direct observation and feedback, 360-degree tools, and self-assessment. The assessment itself usually has minimal time requirements. The goal of these assessments is to provide direct feedback, set goals, and identify areas of improvement. These data are then used for incentives such as promotion or a financial benefit, possibly to hold individuals accountable for their next evaluation, or identify areas for training. Regardless of the assessment tool or outcome, the entire act of individual assessment is solely concentrated on the individual, so the most likely to benefit will only be that individual. Usually, a leader will perform individual assessments prior to moving on to team assessments.

Team Assessment

Team assessment evaluates a group of individuals who work together as a unit or team. There is no minimum or maximum number of individuals that defines a team; there just needs to be more than one person. Team assessment looks at how a group functions and behaves among themselves, with other teams, and within an organization. Team assessment and evaluation is fluid, multifactorial, layered, and challenging. There is an array of tools, outcomes, interventions, and needs for team assessment. These assessments usually require additional time and possibly third-party involvement. The aim of team assessment is to increase the overall synergy of the team regarding their specific purpose, to ensure individuals are functioning at their peak within their specific roles, and to identify areas of collective improvement while ensuring that the team is aligned with the organization's goals. The ultimate goal is to create a high-performance team that has the ability to adapt itself and change to both internal and external stressors.

Teams in Surgery

Teams in the surgical setting will take on a litany of roles. The classic team we think of is that of the "Operating Room" team. This team has extremely specific roles and responsibilities, has a predetermined hierarchy with a true in-the-moment "leader," and has a very clear goal and outcome. This is the easy team to focus on, but there are so many more teams involved in surgery; understanding them all and being able to assess them is key. The additional clinical teams could include the office or outpatient clinical team, the pre- and post-operative teams, or the ward nursing teams who care for the patients. Again, these teams usually have clear roles and responsibilities. As systems become larger and surgeons become more engaged within these systems, the teams will most likely change from clinical to administrative settings. These teams can include such groups as the University -based Departments, Divisions, and Sections, along with hospital-based committees such as Operating Room Governance, Credentials, or Executive Suite. And in private practice, it would include those vested in the business. These teams cross the expanse of clinical, administrative, and business settings. Having a tool kit to evaluate and assess these teams is critical. In the following, we will review various scenarios and tools that can be used to evaluate the team.

Of note, a team is never static, and you need to understand the "moment" or "emotion" of the team. This is critical for any role within the team, from leader to member. As the leader, you can have a direct effect on the "emotion" of the team. If you bring your outside emotions to the team dynamic, do not be surprised if the team mirrors your behavior or shuts down as a critical response. As a member of the team, always speak up, engage, and participate, but do so in a constructive and productive manner even if this conversation is critical in nature. A good rule of thumb is to talk 20% of the time and listen 80% of the time. The listening model should be active and engaged with purpose.

Team Assessment

Team assessment and evaluation must be a systematic, timely, and organized process with a purpose and goal that are both measurable. Prior to assessment and evaluation metrics and the measurable data points must be established and agreed upon. These goals could include any measurable aspect that could be affected by the team. Examples could include for the operative room team—first case on time start; for the Surgical Division team—surpassing an RVU budget; for an outpatient clinical team—having an elevated patient satisfaction survey score; and for the administrative time—producing a balanced budget. Once the goals and metrics are established, the team can begin to function and move through its life cycle. Key areas to focus on your team include: (1) trust among team members; (2) clear communication (described as equality in talking and purposeful listening); (3) defined roles and responsibilities; (4) engagement; and (5) collective goals [1].

When thinking of evaluation and assessment, we usually focus on evaluating the individual and not the team. The team is large, complex, and hard to get into a single location for assessment. However, evaluating the team is so critical for growth, efficiency, patient care, and creating a culture of trust (and fun). Team evaluation should be both scheduled and well thought out. When assessment and evaluation are utilized, there is a lower rate of the team relapsing to previous behavior, a higher rating of job and personnel satisfaction, and evolution of the team [2]. Ultimately, this has been shown to lead to improved patient safety and quailty [2]. Again, while there is great value in using the tools to follow for your surgical team, consider also using them for your clinical, administrative, and executive teams. Also, these tools should be used for specific scenarios, and it is not a "one tool" fits all toolbox. Leaders at times have a habit of using one tool in a repetitive pattern for differing, and sometimes incorrect, scenarios. This can lead to fatigue and frustration secondary to the repetitive nature of the evaluation and a sense of lack of worth in time spent in the process. Using the incorrect tool can also result in bad data if the assessment tool is being utilized in the wrong scenario.

The preferred method of evaluation is to first fully understand each team member. Once the leader understands the team members, then it is the responsibility of the leader to identify where the team is on their project and growth journey and choose the correct tool for evaluation and assessment. We will now review some of the more common tools for team evaluation and assessment.

Tools for Team Assessment and Evaluation

Team Self-Assessment

Using this method, each team member will assess their own performance and contributions to both the team and the institution as a whole. The goal is for open and honest communication and feedback in a non-punitive manner. This can be done via standard survey data, 1:1 discussion, or the preferred method in a group setting.

In a group setting, it is critical to ensure that all team members have the opportunity to speak, while at the same time ensuring that there is purposeful listening. It is encouraged that during group team assessment, ground rules are established upfront, the goal of the meeting is explained, and the situation in which the team is currently in is discussed. It is not critical that the group create any resolution or plan, reminding everyone this is only an assessment to evaluate the team's current situation. In this setting, a third party can be utilized to mediate the conversation. This tool is frequently used when team morale and trust are high, and the team is already comfortable with one another.

360-Degree Feedback

This is a type of survey data with scripted questions to drive at result-based answers. This is anonymous in nature and given to a large enough sample group to ensure anonymity. Using this method, each team member will be evaluated by leadership, those they manage, and their peers. It provides dense information and highlights blind spots and gaps in the leadership regarding the team's performance. Used in a team setting, the data can identify areas for improvement within the team itself. This scenario could be used when there is a concern or deficit in trust within the team.

Team Dynamic Evaluations

These tools help assess how well team members collaborate, communicate, work together, and highlight specific strengths of the team. These evaluations will also identify conflicts, communication breakdowns, and other issues that can impact the team as a whole.

Prior to utilizing a "Team Dynamic Evaluation," one must first understand the basic tenets of team formation, development, and growth better known as dynamics. This was first described by Tuckman in 1965, who stated that these phases are all necessary and inevitable in order for a team to grow, face up to challenges, tackle problems, find solutions, plan the work, and deliver [3]. Tuckman originally described four phases, but later added a fifth phase in 1977. This phase is called adjourning and describes the team at the completion of the task (Fig. 18.1). Adjourning will not be discussed in this text as it has to do with team dismantling, which is not the focus of this chapter.

- ***Forming:*** The team meets to learn objectives and establish goals. Team members will act independently, are on their best behavior, and focus on their own work. Members will attempt

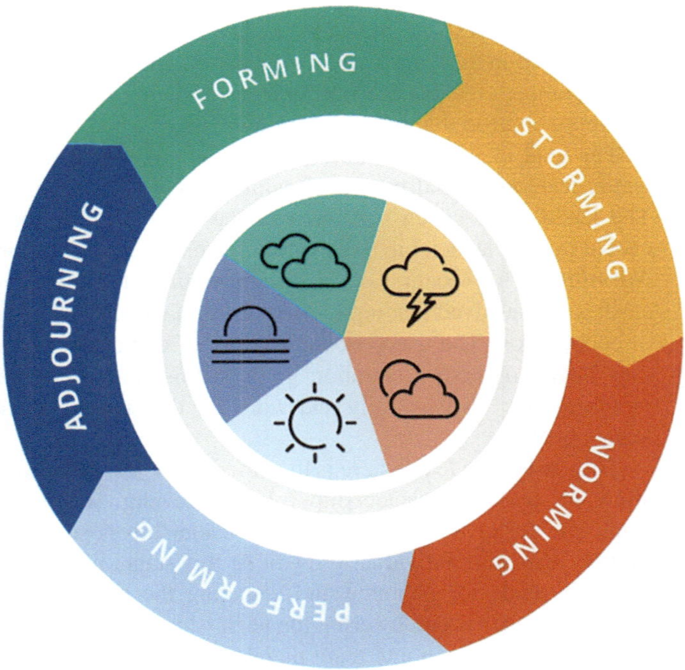

Fig. 18.1 Phases of team dynamic evaluation

to become oriented to the task and to each other. Ground rules are created and toward the end of this phase members start to test boundaries. To move to the next stage, members must risk the possibility of conflict.

The goal of the leader here is to purposefully pick the team, help the team identify goals, and foster team development. The leader is to coordinate behavior, but a mature leader will allow the team to progress to storming. Too many "diplomates" or "peacemakers" in leadership roles could prevent the team from maturing to "storming" and thus prevent the team's full potential.

- ***Storming:*** This is a challenging stage, but if the team endures, group trust will be the final outcome. In this stage, conflict will arise as power is assigned and individuals will voice their opinions. Disagreement and conflict must be resolved before the team can progress to the next stage. Thus, tolerance and patience within the team are critical with the goal of having the team members resolve their differences allowing for stronger and more comfortable relationships to be established.

  The goal of the leader here is to act as a resource for the team, develop mutual trust, and calm the work environment. The leader is to coach behaviors of the team, helping them evolve in their leadership roles within the team and institution.
- ***Norming:*** This occurs once disagreements and personal clashes are resolved leading to greater intimacy and the spirit of cooperation. The team becomes aware of competition, and they begin to share a common goal. In this stage, all team members take responsibility and work for the success of the team's goal.

  The goal of the leader here is to get feedback from the team, allow for additional leadership roles to develop within the team, and foster the transfer of other leadership positions to support team and individual growth. At this stage, time needs to be set aside for planning and engaging the team. In this stage, the leader is empowering the leadership of others.
- ***Performing:*** At this point, team members are now competent, autonomous, and able to handle the decision-making process without supervision. Leaders now become active team members.

Here the goal of the leader is to allow for flexibility in team roles while at the same time assisting in the timing and selection of new team members. Their role is to also create future leadership opportunities for their team members, supporting and encouraging individual growth even at the expense of the team, for example, losing a key team member. In this stage, leaders support the behaviors of others.

The "Tuckman Team Maturity Questionnaire" is composed of 32 questions and can be used to evaluate the team at any one of the above phases. The questionnaire is given to the team to evaluate which of the above categories they fall into. It can also be used to evaluate the individual to see if they are in a discordant relationship with the team. For example, if the team feels they are in the performing stage, while an individual feels the team is in a storming stage. This questionnaire is used to explain where the team is in its current status, while the theory is used to explain to the team what could be its natural progression. This can be used at any point within the team regardless of the current status or level of trust.

SWOT Analysis

Strength, Weakness, Opportunity, Treat (SWOT) analysis is good to help identify not only internal areas of improvement but also external areas that could affect the stability and purpose of the team. The name is an acronym for the four components the technique examines [4]:

- **Strengths**: Characteristics of the business, project, or *team* (internal) that give it an advantage over others.
- **Weaknesses**: Characteristics that place the business, project, or *team* (Internal) at a disadvantage relative to others.
- **Opportunities**: Elements in the *environment* (external) that the business, project, or team could exploit to its advantage.
- **Threats**: Elements in the *environment* (external) that could cause trouble for the business, project, or team.

	Helpful	Harmful
Internal origin	Strengths	Weaknesses
External origin	Opportunities	Threats

Fig. 18.2 SWOT matrix

The results of the assessment are often presented in the form of a matrix (Fig. 18.2). Strengths and weaknesses are usually considered internal, while opportunities and threats are usually considered external [5]. Most authors will advocate assessing external factors before internal factors [6, 7]. To emphasize this point even more, some will suggest that SWOT analysis should be looked at as a "TOWS" strategic plan. TOWS is not just SWOT spelled backward, but rather this is to place the emphasis on your external environment first.

What you end up with are four new categories focusing on external factors over internal ability [7]:

- SO (Strength Opportunities)—Use internal strengths to gain on external opportunities.
- WO (Weakness Opportunities)—Improve internal weakness by gaining on external opportunities.
- ST (Strength Threats)—Use internal strengths to gain on external threats.
- WT (Weaknesses Threats)—Defensive position when poorly positioned. Avoid threats to minimize weakness.

SWOT has been modified to other acronyms such as SOAR (strengths, opportunities, aspirations, and results) and SVOR (strengths, vulnerabilities, opportunities, and risk) [8].

DISC Assessments

Dominance, Influence, Steadiness, and Conscientious (DISC) is a behavioral assessment tool. The evaluation is to aid in predicting job performance and interactions between various types of personalities. The DISC theory uses four types of central behavioral traits [9]:

Dominance—Relating to Control, Power, and Assertiveness
People who score high in the "D" style factors are very active in dealing with problems and challenges, while low "D" scores are people who want to do more research before committing to a decision. High "D" people are described as demanding, forceful, egocentric, strong-willed, driving, determined, ambitious, aggressive, and pioneering. Low "D" scores describe those who are conservative, low-keyed, cooperative, calculating, undemanding, cautious, mild, agreeable, modest, and peaceful.

Influence—Relating to Social Situations and Communication
People with high "I" scores influence others through talking and activity and tend to be emotional. They are described as convincing, magnetic, political, enthusiastic, persuasive, warm, demonstrative, trusting, and optimistic. Those with low "I" scores influence more by data and facts, and not by feelings. They are described as reflective, factual, calculating, skeptical, logical, suspicious, matter of fact, pessimistic, and critical.

Steadiness Relating to Patience, Persistence, and Thoughtfulness
People with high "S" styles want a steady pace and security and do not like sudden change. Low "S" intensity scores are those who like change and variety. High "S" persons are calm, relaxed, patient, possessive, predictable, deliberate, stable, and consistent and tend to be unemotional and poker faced. People with low "S" scores are described as restless, demonstrative, impatient, eager, or even impulsive.

Conscientious—Relating to Structure and Organization
Persons with high "C" styles adhere to rules, regulations, and structure. They like to do quality work and do it right the first time. High "C" people are careful, cautious, exacting, neat, systematic, diplomatic, accurate, and tactful. Those with low

"C" scores challenge the rules and want independence and are described as self-willed, stubborn, opinionated, unsystematic, arbitrary, and careless with details.

No type of DISC assessment is better than another. This tool is used to identify personality types to help gain insight into the individuals on your team. Most would assume correctly that having a multitude of types is preferred over one single type. This becomes key in ensuring that all stakeholders and team members have a choice to speak. For example, on a team heavy with "D"s and "I"s, it would be critical to identify the "S"s and "C"s and ensure them space to be heard.

DISC assessment is a great way for the leaders to get to better know the team members while at the same time allowing the team members to better understand each other. This tool can be used at any point along a team's natural history of growth and can be used at any point regardless of level of trust. However, this tool should not be used in a repetitive format as one would not expect personalities to change drastically over time. This tool is great for improving morale, building culture, and helping the team get to know one another better. It can be used when there has been turnover on a team or expansion with an additional member, but again, it should not be used repetitively with the same team members.

Myers-Briggs Type Indicator (MBTI)

MBTI is a psychometric questionnaire used to measure psychological preferences in how people perceive the world and make decisions. There are fundamentally two dichotomous cognitive functions:

The "Rational" (judging) functions: thinking and feeling
The "Irrational" (perceiving) functions: sensing and intuition

These functions are then expressed primarily in either an introverted or extroverted form [10]. MBTI then sorts these psycho-

Fig. 18.3 Myers-Briggs type indicator with dichotomies, resulting in 16 psychological types

Dichotomies	
Extraversion (E)	Introversion (I)
Sensing (S)	Intuition (N)
Thinking (T)	Feeling (F)
Judging (J)	Perception (P)

logical differences into four opposite pairs, or dichotomies, with a resulting 16 psychological types (Fig. 18.3). Most individuals will naturally prefer one overall combination of type differences [11]. These 16 psychological types are usually reported with four-letter abbreviations, for example, ESTJ: extraversion (E), sensing (S), thinking(T), judgment (J), and so on [11].

To take this one step further, another personality model, the Personality Assessment System (PSA), identifies people's inherited tendencies. In this model, people can either accept and foster them or go on to compensate and modify them as functioning adults. With compensation and modification, the PSA model can classify up to 512 personality types [12].

MBTI is much like the DISC assessment in that it can be used at any point along a team's natural history of growth and can be used at any point regardless of level of trust. Also, like DISC, it should be used infrequently and not in a repetitive manner as personality traits should not change drastically over time.

The Foundation of the Team

Any assessment or evaluation will have little value if there is not a benchmark to compare it to. Thus, having a good foundation with clear communication will set the team up for success. Here are some key tactics to setting ground rules and building your team.

Clear Objectives and Expectations: Establish clear and measurable objectives for each team member. Make sure that they understand their roles, responsibilities, and performance expectations. Clear communication of goals is essential for accurate assessment. This sounds simple and straightforward but is often overlooked as it sometimes is implied within the position. Ensure that the team members *understand* their roles. If this is lacking, the team will be in a state of confusion and members will be unsatisfied.

Regular Feedback: Provide ongoing feedback to your team members. Offer both positive reinforcement for their accomplishments and constructive criticism for areas that need improvement. Regular feedback helps employees stay on track and motivated. A regular cadence should be established, and this communication should be in the format of coaching. The regular cadence will allow the team members to understand that these are creative conversations and not always punitive. These conversations will allow for the development of relationships and trust.

Performance Metrics: Define relevant performance metrics or key performance indicators for each team member's role. These metrics should align with the team's and the organization's objectives. Quantifiable metrics make assessment more objective. This is critical and a must for every position.

Self-Assessment: Encourage team members to conduct self-assessments. This allows them to reflect on their performance, identify strengths and weaknesses, and take ownership of their development. Self-assessment can facilitate open discussions during evaluation meetings.

Recognition and Rewards: Acknowledge and reward exceptional performance. Recognition can boost motivation and morale, contributing to a positive team environment. Provide an opportunity for every team member to be highlighted, but only highlight team members who deserve the recognition.

Goal Alignment: Ensure that each team member's individual goals align with the team's and organization's objectives. This alignment fosters a sense of purpose and teamwork. This is challenging and should be explained to each team member to ensure that they are aware of their purpose within the team and institution.

Performance Improvement Plans: In cases where team members are consistently underperforming, develop performance improvement plans that outline specific actions, timelines, and support mechanisms to help them improve. However, documentation is key if the team member needs to be removed from the work environment. Documentation will empower human resources into action, and without documentation, sometimes little can be done.

Adaptability and Flexibility: Recognize that team dynamics and individual circumstances may change over time. Be flexible in your approach to assessment and be prepared to adjust strategies based on changing needs. Stay updated on best practices in performance assessment and management. Continuously refine your evaluation methods to adapt to changing business needs and employee expectations.

Legal and Ethical Considerations: Ensure that your assessment practices comply with legal and ethical standards, treating all team members fairly and avoiding any form of discrimination or bias.

The above are some of the key components in setting up ground rules and expectations for your team, which will in turn lead to a foundation and culture defining the team. Once this has been established, goals and objectives are created which give your team purpose and drive. At the same time, the leader should understand the roles of each of the team members and learn who they are and what motivates them. At this point, individual assessments and evaluations are excellent tools. Once the team is understood, then team evaluation tools can be used to track the team along its natural course of team development.

Mistakes in Team Building and Evaluation

Prior to evaluating the team, you need to ensure that you have the right team members in place. The idea here is you do not want to strengthen and empower your team when there are members on the team that are not in alignment with the core nature of the team or the institutional goals. The leader must ensure that the right people are maintained on the team, while those who are in misalignment are either let go or moved on. The key here is not implementing key decisions or team building too early, but rather the building of the team takes precedence, and once the team is built, it is then defined. By defining, what is meant is that each member, and the team itself, has clear goals and expectations. Once the expectations have been established, then the plan must be implemented. Here is the critical time to evaluate the team. Look at this as a cyclical process (Fig. 18.4). Once the team is built and actionable, another mistake is to try to manage this alone. Leverage your key team members by providing them with the tools to assist you in whatever the task and the freedom to accomplish it (try to avoid micromanagement). The process is cyclical and ever-changing. The team will constantly bring on new members while letting others go. The goals, objectives, and plan change may change but should always remain in alignment with the institution.

Another mistake of a high-functioning team is to think one member is key or irreplaceable. While there are members on a

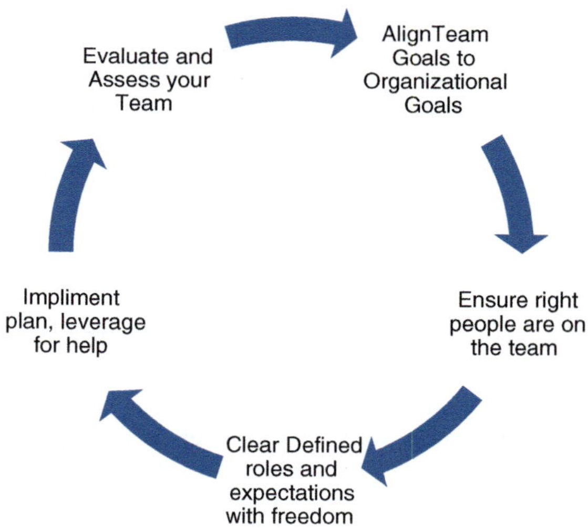
Evaluate and Assess your Team
AlignTeam Goals to Organizational Goals
Ensure right people are on the team
Clear Defined roles and expectations with freedom
Impliment plan, leverage for help

Fig. 18.4 The life cycle of a team

team who will be critical, a highly functioning team will be able to adapt if these members leave the team. A mistake is to try to maintain one of these members when they desire to transition. The team should always support the career of the individual and celebrate their success and career advancement. This single act, in my opinion, is the soul and core of what defines a high-performing team. It is the team that should always support growth and fight against the status quo.

Summary

Team evaluation and assessment are critical in the development of the team. It should come secondary to defining goals and objectives which will in turn make clear the purpose of the team. The purpose of the team needs to be aligned with the intuitional mission. With an aligned purpose in place, the team can be built, and at that point, individual assessment should take place. Once the individuals on the team are understood, then the leader can move on to team evaluation and assessment.

To complete team evaluation and assessment, we have a number of tools to help with the process. They range from survey data and questionaries such as 360 evaluations and Team Dynamic Evaluations to identifying team personal traits using methods such as DISC assessment, MBTI, and SWAT analysis. A key to remember is that there are better tools depending on the scenario, and the right tool could depend on aspects of the team such as level of trust and where the group is according to Tuckman's scale of team development.

SAGES Takeaway

- To understand the difference between individual and team assessment.
- The ability to frame your team for success.
- Review the lifecycle of a team.
- Learn how to evaluate a team in a systematic and objective manner.

References

1. Lencioni P. The five dysfunctions of a team. Jossey-Bass; 2002.
2. Lentz CM, De Lind Van Wijngaarden RAF, Willeboordse F, Hooft L, van der Laan MJ. Dedicated teams to optimize quality and safety of surgery: a systematic review. Int J Qual Health Care. 2022;34(4):mzac078.
3. Tuckman B. Developmental sequence in small groups. Psychol Bull. 1965;63(6):384–99.
4. Ansoff HI. Strategic issue management. Strateg Manag J. 1980;1(2):131–48.
5. Minsky L, Aron D. Are you doing the SWOT analysis backwards?. Harvard Business Review. 2021. Retrieved 7 November 2021. The results of a SWOT analysis can be (and almost always are) presented simply as a 2 × 2 grid, with one dimension representing the internal versus external factors, and the other depicting positive versus negative valence. ... To improve the inventory collection, you should start with the external factors, then turn your attention to the firm's internal ones. See also Sevier 2001.
6. Weihrich H. The TOWS matrix—a tool for situational analysis. Long Range Plan. 1982;15(2):54–66.
7. Watkins MD. From SWOT to TOWS: answering a reader's strategy question. Harvard Business Review. 2007. Retrieved 7 November 2021.
8. McLean GN. Will SOAR really help organization development soar?: an invited reaction to Zarestky and Cole, 2017. New Horiz Adult Educ Hum Resour Dev. 2017;29(1):25–8.
9. Martinussen M, Richardsen AM, Vårum HW. Validation of an ipsative personality measure (DISCUS). Scand J Psychol. 2003;42(5):411–6.
10. Eysenck HJ. Genius: the natural history of creativity, vol. 12. Cambridge University Press; 1995.
11. Myers IB, McCaulley MH, Quenk NL, Hammer AL. MBTI manual (a guide to the development and use of the Myers Briggs type indicator). 3rd ed. Consulting Psychologists Press; 1998.
12. Krauskopf and Saunders. Discusses specific relationship of the MBTI and the PAS. 1994, 66, 69, 127.

Operationalizing Your Team 19

Vasanth Stalin, Nivedha Muralikrishnan,
and Matthew Kroh

Operationalization is **the process of defining abstract concepts through measurable observations and quantifiable data.** What does it mean to operationalize a team? Operationalized outcomes are when every metric or objective within your organization is based on outcomes. This is how you can keep disparate teams invested in a shared definition of success. It is a means **to align each functional team around what is most important. Creating and operationalizing** effective team processes are essential to scaling your team's impact. However, many challenges are associated with creating alignment, balancing overhead, driving adoption, and measuring success.

V. Stalin (✉)
Ascension St. Mary's Hospital, Saginaw, MI, USA

N. Muralikrishnan
Melmaruvathur, Tamil Nadu, India

M. Kroh
Cleveland Clinic, Cleveland, OH, USA
e-mail: Krohm@ccf.org

S. M. Johnson et al. (eds.), *The SAGES Manual of Strategy and Leadership*, https://doi.org/10.1007/978-3-031-62359-2_19

Alignment

Objectives and Key Results (OKRs) create alignment and transparency for how each team and individual impacts the company. When you go through the process of picking simple goals/OKRs that actually matter, you will have tremendous clarity. Communicating a certain "vision" for the organization is distinct from a goal/OKR and helps people understand where they fit. When written proposals (pros and cons lists) are encouraged, conversations move from a potentially charged "my solution is better" environment to a healthier discussion focused on tradeoffs. When there is still no agreement, escalation to a higher management level is the way to go.

Overhead

A leaner overhead can be created in your process by defining "outcomes" first instead of starting with defining a "process." Team initiatives can then be aligned to generate those outcomes. For example, this could be something that looks like shifting the team conversation from "we need to ship 'x' feature" to "how do we move 'y' metric (i.e. customer behavior)."

Adoption

Culture is a potent driver for effective processes. In general, people tend to emulate rewarded behavior. Not hesitating to demonstrate vulnerability reduces the fear of contributing feedback and ideas to improve your team. This has to be modeled in order to be generated and replicated as part of the team culture. Iteration cannot happen without clear feedback and honest input from your team.

Measurement

Leadership needs to be methodical with how the team spends time as it scales. For example, what percentage of the team's time is focused on maintenance activity "keeping the lights on" compared with the proportion of time spent on actions moving the organization forward? Team "health monitors" can provide a fairly accurate idea of how effectively your team works together. They can specifically measure how well teams uphold their commitments and provide a signal of how good they are at upholding trust and reliability.

Key Aspects of Operationalization

Define Behaviors

Take the time to identify some desired behaviors associated with each core value. Involve a select group of employees, possibly your culture committee. Provide clear context around each value. Provide examples of behaviors that are in tune with the intent of the value. Highlight behaviors that would make any employee proud to work for the company. Underscore behaviors that are aligned with the culture you are designing. On the contrary, also identify behaviors that do not align with each value, just to shed light and provide clarity on right and wrong. Defining behaviors, thus, allows employees and executives to translate the values into how they will do business, serve customers, and serve each other.

Define Outcomes

For each value and behavior, the associated desired outcomes should be defined, including outcomes of operationalizing the value versus the alternative if employees do not align with the value. Putting behaviors and outcomes in the limelight provides employees with a clear picture of why each value is vital to the organization. It also allows them to align and, in some cases, maybe not (in which case, they may self-select out).

Effectively Communicate the Values

Communication is one of the most critical steps in growing your desired culture. Values and behaviors cannot just be defined, posted on a wall, and expected to be imbibed. They have to be communicated effectively and socialized. There are many ways of doing this, including:

- Starting with the hiring process—a conversation about core values should be had during employee interviews. A scenario can be outlined, and the interviewee can be asked to provide examples of how they would address the scenario through living the core values. Questions should be asked about their core values and queries to identify if they align with the company's core values should be put forth.
- For candidates that "pass the test,"—candidates should sign a statement detailing your core values, acknowledging that they know and understand what the values are, what they mean, and what the associated behaviors are. This methodology of hiring based on the core values is another way to socialize and operationalize the values.
- During orientation—time should be set aside to discuss the core values and what they mean to the business. Dialogues about the employee experience and the customer experience should also happen, which should already be baked into your core values in some way, shape, or form.
- Orientation should not be the last time you talk to employees about the core values and what they mean to them and the business. Annual refreshers propounding "core value training" could certainly be beneficial. The aspiration should be to make the annual refresher obsolete by doing everything right.

- Focus on a core value each month—dedicate the month to talking about what a particular selected core value means, share stories about employees who have embodied the core value in the past, provide examples to employees, set up rewards, and recognize those people who live and breathe that value, use peer recognition to allow colleagues to call out co-workers who exemplify that core value, have a lunch-n-learn dedicated to all things about that value, bring in a speaker to highlight the importance of the value and to talk about ways that it is impacted their life, ask employees to write what that value means to them and post those notes on a "values wall," and so on.
- Name floors, hallways, conference rooms, break rooms, restrooms, and so on, after the values which keep the values center stage daily.
- Talk about the values in all meetings—share stories about how employees helped each other or interacted with customers that reflect on and represent ways values have been operationalized.

Model the Values

Executives need to lead by example and model the behaviors associated with the core values to get employees to adopt the behaviors. The employees are constantly observing the executives' actions. What is good for the goose is good for the gander too—if executives place themselves "above the law," why should employees be expected to obey the law? Adoption will fail if leadership personnel do not demonstrate commitment to the core values and become an example for employees.

Reinforcement of Values

Reinforcing the values is perhaps the most crucial component of operationalizing them. There are many ways to do this, including incentives, rewards, and recognition. A few other ways to reinforce the values include the following:

- Hiring or Firing for culture fit: X, formerly Twitter, and Amazon are great examples, offering employees who do not believe they fit the culture monetary compensation to leave the organization. Similarly, when employees espouse behaviors not in line with the core values, those must become terminatable offenses.
- Coaching sessions should be built around the ability to clearly display and breathe the company's core values, with performance evaluations being prepared and promotions determined based on this capacity.
- Development of processes and policies and decision-making aligned with the core values.

One key point to keep in mind—if your target is a customer-centric culture, the values, and behaviors must include clear direction and connection to customers and the customer experience.

A case study involving a hypothetical, freshly minted Bariatric Surgeon seeking to Operationalize a Bariatric Surgery team/program, as outlined below, can serve as an effective example to gain a better understanding of the subject or process.

After many years of training, you are finally a fully equipped Bariatric Surgeon ready to practice Medicine. The first decision you must make is whether to join an existing Group practice or to go Solo. This significant decision will affect your financial health and family life and thus must be considered carefully. If you join a group practice, you must be prepared to adhere to the established rules of the group and follow operational policies that are probably already in place. If you decide to open your own Solo practice, you make your own rules, but you will also start from scratch and be responsible for everything from finding office space to buying office equipment to hiring personnel. If you are starting a Bariatric Surgery program for your Healthcare facility, they will coordinate with you on most of these decisions. An equally important decision is selecting an appropriate place to practice. It is imperative that you have enough patients to support your practice. Geographic and demographic assessments are vital in deciding where to locate a practice.

Marketing availability and costs are other considerations. For example, what is the cost of advertising with the local newspaper or television station? To thoroughly evaluate the expenses of opening a practice in a particular area, you must consider the cost of office space (renting vs. buying property), cost of living, salaries for nurse(s) and personnel, office supply costs, and marketing costs. You will want to know the going hourly rate for personnel salaries in that area and the typical benefits offered so that you can be competitive with other practices. These are essential elements to be aware of before you start Operationalizing your Bariatric Surgery team. The more comprehensive your analysis is of a particular area you are considering, the greater the likelihood of success.

Navigating Your Way to Creating a Successful Program

The most critical factor for success in building a Surgery team and Operationalizing a new program is an institutional commitment at the highest level (institutional, medical, and administrative). If you are being interviewed for the position of Program Director to create a program, take note of who specifically (i.e., what level administrator) is conducting the interview. Ideally, you should meet face-to-face with the Chief Medical Officer and/or Chief Executive Officer to ensure that the hospital is fully committed (including requisite resources) to creating your program. Next, create a task force or a "steering committee" that oversees the various aspects of creating a program. For example, for a Bariatric program, this committee should be charged with fulfilling the Metabolic and Bariatric Surgery Accreditation and Quality Improvement Program (MBSAQIP) criteria for "comprehensive center" accreditation. These criteria serve as a valuable blueprint for establishing a Bariatric program. The process of going through the requisite needs to meet each MBSAQIP criterion is invaluable for the multidisciplinary team (MDT) as part of the accreditation process involves satisfying the requirements on a list, which includes evaluating the equipment, meeting the team, and going over the Pathways. Therefore, do a "walk-thru" of the entire hospital. With the appropriate planning and resources (and commitment from the hospital administration), it is possible to establish a surgery program with high-quality outcomes. Patient selection at the outset is important. Building the program based on established criteria is an effective method of ensuring that adequate resources are in place to provide safe and effective care to the surgery patient.

The MDT includes core members central to optimizing the care of patients with obesity. In addition, many other support services are needed. The core members include the bariatric surgeon, bariatric physician, dietician, psychologist, anesthesiologist, and bariatric nurse coordinator. These core members need the support of a cardiologist, pulmonologist, smoking cessation specialist, physiotherapist, interventional radiologist, critical care physicians, gastroenterologist, operating room team, and perioperative nursing staff. The MDT works best when the message delivered to patients, their families, and referring physicians is consistent.

The following key elements must be considered when operationalizing a high-quality surgery program in concordance with the standards for accreditation:

1. Commitment to quality care.
   - Leadership and governance (physician and executive).
   - Credentialing.
   - Designated personnel.
2. Infrastructure.
   - Equipment.
   - Critical care support.
3. Annual procedure volume and patient selection.
4. Clinical pathways outlining the continuum of care.

Metabolic and Bariatric Surgery (MBS) Committee

The control of the program resides in the MBS Committee. At a minimum, it should involve a surgeon director, all surgeons performing MBS at the center, a coordinator, a clinical reviewer, and institutional administration representatives involved in caring for metabolic and bariatric surgical patients. While having a surgeon champion and administrator lead the charge in the MBS quality movement is necessary, it is just as critical to have all surgeons practicing MBS at the center participate on the committee. All committee participants should provide input toward the final decisions in developing the MBS program's structure, process, and improvement plans.

Surgeons as Leaders

Leadership is an essential attribute that surgeons operating a practice in today's healthcare environment must possess. An effective leader supervises with ease and establishes a comfortable, rewarding environment in which staff work together to improve the practice and meet the practice's goals. Goals within the practice should be clearly defined, as should guidance and ideas on how to accomplish them in a manner that gains respect from employees, colleagues, and superiors. Creating a policy manual might be helpful for dealing with routine problems, goals, and employee issues and concerns. The bariatric surgeon, as the team leader, must make sure that everybody has a clear description of their jobs and responsibilities as they relate to the overall workflow and structure so they can effectively perform their functions. Responsibility and accountability for the accomplishment of various tasks must be built into the organizational structure and shared with staff. It is vital to match the correct people to the correct job. This means that you or your office manager must have skills in human resources. Human resources involves more than hiring—it also involves the creation of job descriptions and such policies as salary and bonuses, sick leave, vacation time, and punitive measures if problems occur, such as sexual harassment. In developing and implementing a policy manual for your practice, human resource skills will significantly benefit your team.

The ability to motivate the group is one of the most important characteristics of a good leader. A leader is a person who has the ability to influence others. The main difference between a leader and a supervisor is that a leader can influence others to perform beyond the sphere of his or her authority. A leader is characterized by charisma, a magnetism that creates an atmosphere in which all team members want to reach a common goal, and by the ability to explain his or her vision. Men and women often use different skills in their leadership roles. Women tend to rely on charisma, expertise, and interpersonal skills to influence others. Some men, on the contrary, tend to use positional power to direct and control organizing activity. A good leader resolves conflicts by different methods, depending on the situation. These methods include avoidance, compromise, force, accommodation, and collaboration. Sometimes, you find that the reason other people in the team do not care as much as you do is because they do not have the context—likely they do not know how it applies to them. The nuance is how to motivate people to understand that context and prioritization so that everything being asked of the team can actually be accomplished.

Teaching demonstrates that you care about the individual and the team's growth. It addresses the disparity of experience and the need to provide a deeper understanding of what the team is working to accomplish. Carving out time to teach can be ad hoc and does not need to fit neatly onto the calendar.

Solving problems and making decisions are an integral part of being a Surgeon. Some of the significant steps in the decision-making process include: (1) identifying the problem; (2) collecting relevant information; (3) developing alternatives; (4) exploring each alternative; (5) selecting the best alternative; (6) implementing the decision; and (7) following up and evaluating the decision.

A good leader must have above all else quality communication skills. Communication skills include identifying appropriate words to convey meaning and delivering those words and messages in a manner that invokes attention and is appreciated and understood by the other team members. It is the quality that bridges any gap in understanding, alleviates stress and chaos, and keeps people motivated. You do not have a team if you do not have communication—you have individuals working independently on things that may or may not ladder up to the team's goals. Strong communication goes far beyond being a good talker—it is demonstrated through body language in meetings, the ability to read people and understand when you are or are not connecting with them, being able to make connections between things and draw new conclusions, being open minded to differing opinions, and changing your opinion. By the same token, the quality of being a sound listener is also essential to good leadership, requiring self-control, empathy, and acceptance of others' perspectives. As a lucid communicator, you will also have to serve as a bridge between all staff, who possess differing levels of understanding on many topics. In a group atmosphere, it is essential to develop and maintain the role of an effective communicator to better resolve conflicts, implement discipline, present clear messages, and create an established environment of positive control. When you operationalize your team, it is essential to have the ability to implement change in a positive and motivational manner. The necessity for changes within a practice comes with new developments in your internal organizational needs and evaluations, the general healthcare industry, different types of standards, practice management, and the medical marketplace as a whole. You can build and operationalize your Bariatric Surgery team with good communication skills, staff innovational skills, competent conflict resolution methodology, and the ability to lead the practice with sound direction and decisions.

The center's mission, vision, goals, and objectives of the program are discussed and agreed upon within the MBS Committee. It provides a setting for sharing best practices, reducing practice variation, and responding to adverse events. After identifying opportunities for improvement, committee team members must be willing to enact changes to decrease complication rates and improve the patient's overall experience at the center.

Surgeon Credentialing

Well-trained surgeons are essential in delivering high-quality care to MBS patients in a consistent manner. Credentialing criteria for metabolic and bariatric surgeons should be thoroughly discussed among the MBS committee members and approved before being submitted to the hospital's credentialing committee for official use by the hospital.

Hospital Facilities and Personnel

In healthcare institutions recognized as accomplished in bariatric surgery, there should be a demonstrated commitment to provide adequate facilities and equipment and a properly trained and funded appropriate bariatric surgery support staff. Minimal standards in these areas are set by the institution and maintained under the direction of the Program Director, in charge of a Bariatric surgery management team. This team includes experienced, committed surgeons and physicians, skilled nurses, specialty-educated nutritionists, experienced anesthesiologists, and, as needed, cardiologists, pulmonologists, rehabilitation therapists, and psychiatric staff.

The operating room environment required for the performance of bariatric surgery has special operating room tables and ancillary equipment available to accommodate patients weighing up to 750 lbs. Appropriate bariatric retractors, staplers, and long instruments are available.

Anesthesia for bariatric surgical procedures is performed by individuals specially trained in this area and regularly assigned to bariatric procedures as a member of the bariatric surgery team. Specialized operating room staff familiar with the equipment, instruments, and procedures are identified as members of the bariatric surgery team. The staff of the recovery room and intensive care units are experts in the immediate postoperative care of the morbidly obese patient and their unique needs, particularly for ventilatory and respiratory support. The facilities should conform to standards mandated by the Joint Commission on Accreditation of Health Care Organizations.

The recovery room should be capable of providing critical care to morbidly obese patients. ICUs should have similar capabilities. The preoperative/postoperative assessment of morbidly obese patients may require special radiology equipment. The perioperative care of morbidly obese patients requires special beds, chairs, and commodes. Nursing personnel are trained and skilled in giving respiratory care, managing nasogastric and abdominal wall drainage tubes, assisting with ambulation of the morbidly obese patient, knowledge of common perioperative complications, and recognizing potential intravascular volume, cardiac, diabetic, and vascular problems.

Systematic long-term follow-up after obesity surgery is essential and includes dietary instruction, vitamin and mineral supplementation, exercise therapy, and, where feasible, patient support groups. Long-term follow-up care facilities including rehabilitation facilities, psychiatric care, and nutritional rehabilitation should be available.

Critical Care Support and Training for Patient Safety

All relevant staff must be educated on the care pathway, patient safety, and complication recognition to prevent "failure to rescue situations, in which differences in mortality proposed to result from the failure to recognize, and effectively manage, a postoperative complication timely." Additional training for the surgical teams and the integrated health personnel in postoperative complication recognition and management may improve outcomes.

Annual Procedure Volume, Patient Selection, and Procedure Choice

Deciding what operation to perform or on which patient we should strongly consider not offering a surgical alternative for treatment can often be difficult. Simply put, complex cases should not be performed at a center that only performs a few metabolic and bariatric procedures per month.

Data Review and Identifying Deficiencies and Implementing Quality Improvement

Accurate data collection, feedback, and data review are necessary to develop a high-quality MBS program. Critical analysis and interpretation of data will help identify opportunities for improvement. Once deficiencies are recognized, the center can apply interventions for quality improvement.

Participating MBSAQIP centers can compare their individual center data to all centers entering data into the database; thus, they can determine where they rank among their cohorts. These data can be analyzed between all surgeons, known as the institutional collaborative, and can take place during the MB Committee meetings.

Team Culture

Culture is a powerful lever for effective processes. People emulate rewarded behavior. Vulnerability reduces fear to contribute feedback and ideas to improve your team. This has to be modeled in order to be generated as part of the team culture. You cannot iterate without clear feedback and honest input from your team. One of the most important ways to get team members to adopt the behaviors associated with the core values is for the Surgeon(s) to lead by example and model the behaviors. Other members of the Bariatric team are always watching what the leader is doing: what is good for the goose is good for the gander. If the Surgeon leadership does not demonstrate commitment to the core values and become an example for others, adoption will fail. Reinforcing the values and core management algorithms is probably the most important component of operationalizing them. There are many ways to do this, including using incentives, rewards, and recognition. Spend a bit of time talking about, socializing, and operationalizing your core values to develop the culture you desire from your team. One key point to keep in mind—if your target is a patient-centric culture, the values and behaviors must include clear direction and connection to patients and the patient experience.

Compassion

Strong communication and clear context will get you a long way in motivating your team. However, when you are a manager who has influence without authority, the Surgeon must lead with compassion. If you are but a cog in the Giant Hospital machinery and you are an indirect manager of people, there is no immediate threat to someone for not following your lead—you are not their boss, you are not responsible for their compensation, and you are not the person giving them their promotion (they may or may not understand how much influence you do actually have, but that depends a lot on how feedback works in your system). So, if you want to motivate your team and effectively operationalize your team without making threats or constantly escalating, compassion would be the most substantial quality that leads to immediate action on the team. When you care that the team has to stay late and stay with them, making sure they have had dinner or taken a break, and you tell them you appreciate them for going the extra mile (in the moment, not in an email later)—you will find that people will be more inclined to put in more work. When you create a fun environment and introduce little games or rituals to things that might otherwise feel monotonous, you will find that people enjoy them a little more. When you demonstrate that the work is serious but do not take yourself too seriously, you will have a team that will follow you through the trenches of even the most challenging obstacles. You might be able to get somewhere with brute force or threats or motivate with money or rewards, but without feeling a connection to the Surgeon leader, the people in your team will eventually burn out.

Summing It Up

This is the approach that any leader can take when working in a new environment that would allow them to form quick bonds with their team members and make a lasting impact over a short time. It is how the Team leader would demonstrate to their team that they genuinely care about their success and create the environment they work in a better place. It is about the Captain of the ship putting themselves in the shoes of those they are managing and interacting with, thinking about how they themselves would want to be treated and communicated with, and then practicing those behaviors. It is what keeps the team focused and proactive during the times when you cannot break down all of the work because they know that you are looking out for them. There is no substitute for authenticity and no more significant motivator in a leader.

SAGES Takeaway

- Create alignment, balance overhead, drive adoption, and measure success.
- Define behaviors and outcomes while communicating, modeling, and reinforcing values.
- Commitment to quality, infrastructure, volume, and critical pathways is vital.
- Effective leadership includes problem-solving, communicating, motivating, teaching, and establishing a comfortable work environment.
- Inculcate the desired team culture by modeling behavior.
- Build a team that is bigger than the sum of its individuals.

Effective Team Management 20

Juliet Holder-Haynes
and Monique Hassan

Introduction

Healthcare is a dynamic, shifting, and complicated environment in which leaders must work to develop strong network connections with members of different cultures. Today's teams are complex in that each member works independently, often remotely, and interdependently on their task to contribute to the organization's primary goal. Effective team management is a process that involves supporting, communicating with, and uplifting team members so that they perform to the best of their abilities and continue to grow as professionals.

J. Holder-Haynes
Michael E Debakey Department of Surgery, Baylor College of Medicine, Houston, TX, USA
e-mail: holderha@bcm.edu

M. Hassan (✉)
Department of Surgery, Baylor College of Medicine, Scott and White Memorial Hospital and Clinic, Temple, TX, USA

S. M. Johnson et al. (eds.), *The SAGES Manual of Strategy and Leadership*, https://doi.org/10.1007/978-3-031-62359-2_20

Leadership

"Leadership Is Like the Abominable Snowman Whose Footprints Are Everywhere But Who Is Nowhere to Be Seen" [1]

Leadership has been defined in numerous ways as scholars have attempted to explain this concept. For example, Yukl defines leadership as "the process of influencing others to understand and agree about what needs to be done and how to do it, and the process of facilitating individual and collective efforts to accomplish shared objectives" [2]. Northouse defines leadership as "a process whereby an individual influences a group of individuals to achieve a common goal" [3]. These definitions suggest that leadership is an ongoing process.

Effective leadership builds a competitive edge for organizations and hospitals. The difference between the leader and the leader's development is the concept that defines that leader. The organizational members define the leader. Team effectiveness occurs when positive leadership develops between the leader and team members.

Quality of care is a vital element for achieving high productivity levels within healthcare organizations and is defined as the degree to which the probability of achieving the expected health outcomes is increased and in line with updated professional knowledge and skills within health services [4]. The Institute of Medicine has described the six aims of high-quality care to be: (1) safe, (2) effective, (3) reliable, (4) patient-centered, (5) efficient, and (6) equitable. Measuring health outcomes is a core component of assessing quality of care. Quality measures are structure, process, outcome, and patient satisfaction [4, 5]. According to the National Quality Measures Clearing House (USA), a clinical outcome refers to the health state of a patient resulting from healthcare. Measures on patient outcomes and satisfaction constitute shorter patient length of stay, hospital mortality level, healthcare-associated infections, failure-to-rescue ratio, restraint use, medication errors, inadequate pain management, pressure ulcers rate, patient fall rate, falls with injury, medical errors, and urinary tract infections [6]. Numerous publications recognize leadership style as an essential element for healthcare quality. Effective leadership is among the most critical components that lead an organization to effective and successful outcomes.

Leadership Styles

Transactional Leadership

Transactional leadership is a style that motivates team members through rewards, punishment, recognition, or corrective measures. Team members work independently with minimal commitment to co-workers or the organization [7]. The focus tends to be task-oriented. Transactional leadership effectively promotes incremental improvements in quality and efficiency in the system and hinges on choosing metrics that best reflect the system's goals [8].

Transformational Leadership

Burns initially conceptualized transformational leadership in the 1970s [9]. Transformational leaders tend to use charismatic influence to convey a sense of loyalty through shared goals, motivating others to do more than they originally intended or imagined [7]. In contrast to transactional leadership, where motivation is driven by self-interest, transformational leaders motivate others by focusing on a shared vision for the collective good, building trust, and acting with integrity. Transformational leadership is typically needed when significant organizational change is required [8]. Subthemes of transformational leadership include Idealized Influence, Inspirational Motivation, Intellectual Stimulation, and Individualized Consideration [9, 10]. This leadership style has been identified as one of the most effective in healthcare services, resulting in demonstrated organizational benefits such as a better practice environment, higher work engagement, increased productivity, and superior nurse retention [9, 10].

Autocratic

The autocratic leader has complete control over setting goals and directing all activities and goals with minimal or no input from team members [8]. Under the autocratic model, leadership follows a strict hierarchy. While the servant leader seeks to serve others, the autocratic leader seeks self-interest only. Loyalty by the team members is controlled through a paycheck, and tasks are only performed as assigned. In healthcare settings, autocratic leadership discourages members from providing meaningful work, pursuing personal growth, and speaking up for patient safety [11]. On the contrary, in emergencies and times of crisis, the autocratic model may be necessary to accelerate decision-making and properly manage resources [12], such as during the pandemic [13], but are only effective short-term for the reasons cited above.

Laissez-Faire

The laissez-faire leadership style avoids and abdicates one's responsibilities [14]. The laissez-faire leader is absent from employee-related issues. This leadership style has been consistently found to be the least effective and least satisfying management style and is the most prevalent form of negative leadership [9, 14]. These leaders fail to invest in the leader–employee relationship, and as a result, certain employees may be inclined to reduce their organizational commitment. In addition, laissez-faire leaders fail to provide feedback and recognition to subordinates and act on work-related concerns, harming the organization and subordinates [14, 15]. This form of leadership is distinct from other negative leadership styles as it results from the absence of constructive behaviors rather than the presence of destructive actions [14].

Servant

Servant leadership, based on the work of Greenleaf in the 1970s, focuses on achieving outcomes through interdisciplinary teamwork, shared decision-making, and ethical behavior [7]. These leaders view a position of power as an opportunity to serve others and exemplify humility, integrity, accountability, gratitude, empathy, and a desire to serve a greater purpose beyond themselves [11]. Under a servant leader, team members feel empowered and serve and build the organization through a sense of accountability.

Passive Avoidant

The passive-avoidant leadership style is one of the least effective styles. It is characterized by an aversion to decision-making, avoiding conflict, and an inability to take responsibility. Leaders with this style are likely to outsource decision-making to others out of fear of making the wrong decision or inability to make decisions. Poor employee retention, a lack of trust, and low engagement are often the result of teams defined by this mode of leadership [7].

Leadership Skills

- Integrity.
  - Integrity may be defined by honesty, ethical conduct, and professionalism [16]. We look to our leaders to act with honesty and transparency, even under challenging circumstances. Consistency enhances trust, engenders reliability, and provides an environment where members can focus on being more productive and innovative. Ethical leaders adhere to moral principles, treat others with respect, and are willing to admit errors openly.
- Vision.
  - We rely on our leaders to convey a clear vision to inspire team members toward achieving organizational goals. Under ideal circumstances, the vision provides a rallying point, unites the team, and inspires innovative ideas to reimagine tactical approaches. A clearly communicated vision engenders trust and buy-in from stakeholders, especially when the outlined approach is novel. Charismatic and visionary leaders promote team engagement and encourage others to perform beyond their imagined capabilities.

- Communication.
  - Effective communication's hallmarks include clear, concise, and relatable communication to the target audience. Effective communicators are self-aware and aware of the impact of non-verbal communication on their target audience. Individual team members may differ in their communication styles. In addition to being receptive to feedback, an effective leader understands the need to utilize various modes of communication.
- Developing people.
  - Modern management in healthcare requires leaders who understand the need for teams due to the inability to process the vast amount of information acquired over the last several decades. However, functional teams do not come naturally to physicians, especially surgeons, as our training and culture reward individual performance [17, 18]. Within this framework, the challenge for healthcare leaders is to have the emotional intelligence and self-awareness to put forth the effort to collaborate and develop others. Developing talent relies on providing the following: an environment that encourages learning, regular feedback, practicing active listening, clear communication and goals, and leadership by example.

Management

Management produces order and consistency and is responsible for organizing all elements within the organization to successfully execute the vision of leadership [19]. Managers must appreciate how profoundly the organizational climate can influence financial results. It can account for nearly a third of financial performance. Organizational climate, in turn, is influenced by leadership style—how managers motivate direct reports, gather and use information, make decisions, manage change initiatives, and handle crises. There are six basic leadership styles.

The coercive style. This "Do what I say" approach can be very effective in a turnaround situation, a natural disaster, or when working with problem employees. However, in most situations, coercive leadership inhibits the organization's flexibility and dampens employees' motivation.

The authoritative style. An authoritative leader takes a "Come with me" approach: she states the overall goal but gives people the freedom to choose their means of achieving it. This style works incredibly well when a business is adrift. However, it is less effective when the leader is working with a team of experts who are more experienced than he is.

The affiliative style. The hallmark of the affiliative leader is a "People come first" attitude. This style is beneficial for building team harmony or increasing morale. However, its exclusive focus on praise can allow poor performance to go uncorrected. Also, affiliative leaders rarely offer advice, leaving employees in a quandary.

The democratic style. This style's impact on organizational climate is not very high. By giving workers a voice in decisions, democratic leaders build organizational flexibility and responsibility and help generate fresh ideas. Nevertheless, sometimes, the price is endless meetings and confused employees who feel leaderless.

The pacesetting style. A leader who sets high-performance standards and exemplifies them himself has a very positive impact on employees who are self-motivated and highly competent. However, other employees tend to feel overwhelmed by such a leader's demands for excellence—and resent his tendency to take over a situation.

The coaching style. This style focuses more on personal development than on immediate work-related tasks. It works well when employees know their weaknesses and want to improve, but not when they resist changing their ways.

Management Skills

Plan–Do–Check–Act Cycle

The Deming Cycle of continuous quality improvement is a concept introduced in the 1950s in Japan by W. Edwards Deming. It is also known as the Plan, Do, Check, Act Cycle, or PDCA. It may also be described as PDSA (plan, do, study, act). PDCA is useful when introducing a process, service, or product change and consists of four iterative steps [20]. It produces a systematic approach to problem-solving and encourages organizations to continuously assess their processes and implement changes based on data analysis and alignment with company objectives.

Plan

Planning involves defining problems and finding solutions, organizing processes, identifying pitfalls, and mitigating them. Of all the steps in the PDCA cycle, the planning step often takes the most time and attention. First, the project targets and methods for reaching those targets or goals need to be identified. Next, the manager prioritizes tasks and sets appropriate timelines and metrics to meet deadlines. Securing resources in terms of talent and funding is critical to ensuring the smooth implementation of the plan and identifying and overcoming potential obstacles. Effective communication is essential to gaining buy-in from stakeholders and team members. Planning also involves analyzing data and evaluating stakeholder needs.

The most commonly cited goal-setting methodology uses the SMART framework. SMART goals are Specific, Measurable, Actionable, Relevant, and Time-bound. Alternatives to the SMART framework include CLEAR goals: Collaborative, Limited, Emotionally engaging, Appreciable, and Refinable. CLEAR goals are preferable to SMART goals when prioritizing stakeholder collaboration and engagement. When more audacious goals are preferred, consider BHAG or Big Hairy Audacious Goals as conceptualized in Built to Last [21]. OKRs (Objectives and Key Results) may be implemented in fast-paced, dynamic environments requiring innovation and adaptability [22]. John Doerr adopted this objective-setting framework at Google based on the work of Intel CEO Andy Grove [22].

Do

Once the plan is established, the next step involves providing team members with appropriate education and training to implement the plan on a small scale and collecting data to determine the plan's effectiveness in the next step.

Check

Checking involves evaluating the results of the plan's implementation against the goals and objectives outlined. It helps to answer the question, "Did your implemented plan work?" This can take the form of formal and informal assessments. Failures identified may require a root-cause analysis. Based on the results, gaps and opportunities for further improvement can be identified. A flexible approach allows for the plan to be modified as needed.

Act

Based on the results of the Check stage, the next step is to act. First, if the outlined targets are not met, the reason for failure must be determined. Next, a modification or a new plan to achieve the outlined goals and targets should be considered. The PDCA cycle is then repeated.

Leader Versus Manager

Leadership and management are different skill sets, although they are used interchangeably (see Table 20.1) [23]. Management depends on the formal assignment of power to influence others, whereas leadership relies on a social influence process through a series of interactions. Leaders are identified by their acts and not appointed positions [24]. Leaders drive change, focus on thinking ahead, and capitalize on opportunities [25]. Aligning individuals toward a common goal is among the goals of leadership. Leaders focus on rallying people, while managers focus on deploying people tactically while executing a process [23].

Management tends to focus on the execution of processes that deliver predictable, orderly results [18]. Management is an intrinsic part of leadership, and good leaders tend to be good managers, although the opposite is not necessarily true [8]. Good managers can identify the unique traits of their team members and deploy them in the best way possible in a coordinated plan of attack [26, 23].

Table 20.1 Leadership versus management. Adapted from [19]

Leadership	Management
Establishes direction • Creates a shared vision • Identifies the bigger picture • Sets goals and strategies in place	Plan and budget • Resource allocation • Time management and process steps • Establish agendas
Connecting people • Communication of goals • Team building and networking • Aims for commitment	Employment and organizing • Maintain structure • Staffing placements • Enforce rules and procedures
Motivate and drive • Inspire and motivate • Empower followers • Identify and work toward needs	Control and problem solve • Reward systems • Identifies problems • Solves problems/takes corrective actions

Team Building

Building effective teams takes time and effort as they evolve through different stages of development. Tuckman's model explains that as the team develops maturity and ability, relationships are established, and leadership style changes to more collaborative or shared leadership [27]. During each stage of team development, team members have recognizable feelings and behaviors; therefore, understanding why things are happening in specific ways on a team can be an essential part of the self-evaluation process.

Stage 1—FORMING

During the Forming stage of team development, team members are usually excited to be part of the team and eager about the work ahead. Members are asking, "Why are we here?" Members often have high positive expectations for the team experience. However, there can be feelings of anxiety and confusion, and sometimes less work is accomplished. The principal work for the team during the Forming stage is to create a team with a clear structure, goals, direction, and roles so that members begin to build trust. The team should establish its charter, strategy, roles, tasks, and goals at this early stage. These must be defined as an effective team that will learn how to work together.

Stage 2—STORMING

During the Storming stage, the team members ask, "Can we work together?" Team members are trying to see how the team will respond to differences and how it will handle conflict. Power plays may occur, i.e., who is in charge and what actions must be taken toward goals. Behaviors during the Storming stage may be less polite than during the Forming stage, with frustration or disagreements about goals, expectations, roles, and responsibilities being openly expressed. At this stage, it is vital to encourage transparent and fair communication and affirm that disagreement is healthy and resolvable. The team may also need to develop task-related skills, group processes, and conflict management skills. A redefinition of the team's goals, roles, and tasks can help team members overcome the frustration or confusion they experience during this stage.

Stage 3—NORMING

During the Norming stage of team development, the team asks, "How will we work together?" Team members begin to resolve the discrepancy between their expectations and the reality of the team's experience. Rules get created, and team members learn to work together productively. Team pride develops, and norms are established for how people treat each other, meetings are conducted, who will do what work, and how the goals will be achieved based on the strengths and weaknesses of the team. Team members accept each other, making a conscious effort to resolve problems and achieve group harmony. Team members shift their energy to the team's goals and show increased productivity in individual and collective work. The team may find this an appropriate time to evaluate team processes and productivity.

Stage 4—PERFORMING

In the final stage of team development, the team asks, "How can we work smarter?" The team becomes fully engaged and functional. It is harmonized and achieves results by working seamlessly together as they diagnose, solve problems, and make decisions. Members feel attached to the team as something "greater than the sum of its parts" and feel satisfaction in its effectiveness. Differences among members are appreciated and used to enhance the team's performance. This is the highest stage of creativity and productivity, and the team can handle new tasks by working together or delegating work. Commitment to the team's mission is high, and the competence of team members is also high. Team members should continue to deepen their knowledge and skills, including working to improve team development continuously. Accomplishments in team processes or progress are measured and celebrated.

Typically, the process is linear as the team goes from one stage to the next. However, as new challenges arise, the team can move in and out of stages 2 (STORMING) to 4 (PERFORMING) more quickly because of the trust built over time. Teams that achieve this level are high-performing teams (HPTs).

A high-performance team consists of individuals with a common purpose, often with different skill sets or perspectives yet with high levels of collaboration and innovation, that produce superior results [28]. In healthcare, increased team diversity can improve the team's ability to innovate, communicate with patients, and assess patient risk [29].

Conclusion

Effective communication and teamwork are essential for delivering high-quality, safe patient care, and healthy team dynamics are essential for effective teamwork. Effective healthcare leadership requires a commitment to navigating the complexities of the competitive healthcare landscape, which encompasses promoting healthcare excellence, delivering quality outcomes, building collaborative teams, inspiring innovation, and driving organizational goals. The effective leader must be an inspiring communicator who models the highest moral standards and provides transparency in planning and decision-making. The modern era of healthcare requires effective leaders to listen actively, promote empowerment, and develop new leadership talent, all while considering organizational strategy, risk management, and marketplace trends. With the rapid advancement in technology, changes in reimbursement, and society's demand for increasing quality and transparency, today's leaders are challenged to maintain a commitment to continuous quality improvement and adaptability. Their leadership style should be adaptable to various environments as well. Making data-driven decisions while leveraging innovation and technology must be balanced with a humane approach to providers and patients.

SAGES Takeaway

- The best leaders are also good managers, although it is rare to find the best traits of both in one person.
- Management can be simply defined as the organization of processes and people to achieve a desired result.
- Planning is the most critical skill of managers. Success is difficult at best and impossible at worst without planning.
- An HPT is committed, coordinated, focused, and adaptable and has diverse skills and talents.
- Building effective teams takes time and effort as they evolve through different stages of development.

References

1. Bennis WG, et al. Leaders: strategies for taking charge. Harper & Row; 1985.
2. Yukl GA. Leadership in organizations. 8th ed. Pearson; 2013.
3. Northouse PG. Leadership. 8th ed; 2019. SAGE
4. Leavitt M. Medscape's response to the Institute of Medicine Report: crossing the quality chasm: a new health system for the 21st century. MedGenMed. 2001;3(2):2.
5. Sfantou DF, Laliotis A, Patelarou AE, Sifaki-Pistolla D, Matalliotakis M, Patelarou E. Importance of leadership style towards quality of care measures in healthcare settings: a systematic review. Healthcare. 2017;5(4):73. https://doi.org/10.3390/healthcare5040073.
6. Lang TA, Hodge M, Olson V, Romano PS, Kravitz RL. Nurse-patient ratios: a systematic review on the effects of nurse staffing on patient, nurse employee, and hospital outcomes. J Nurs Adm. 2004;34(7-8):326–37. https://doi.org/10.1097/00005110-200407000-00005.
7. Specchia ML, Cozzolino MR, Carini E, Di Pilla A, Galletti C, Ricciardi W, Damiani G. Leadership styles and nurses' job satisfaction. Results of a systematic review. Int J Environ Res Public Health. 2021;18(4):1552. https://doi.org/10.3390/ijerph18041552. PMID: 33562016; PMCID: PMC7915070
8. Onaca N, Fleshman JW. Types of leadership and how to use them in surgical areas. Clin Colon Rectal Surg. 2020;33(4):228–32. https://doi.org/10.1055/s-0040-1709457. Epub 2020 Jun 3. PMID: 32624720; PMCID: PMC7329368
9. Moon SE, et al. Measuring transformational leadership in establishing nursing care excellence. Healthcare. 2019;7(4):132. https://pubmed.ncbi.nlm.nih.gov/31689901
10. Hayati D, Charkhabi M, Naami A. The relationship between transformational leadership and work engagement in governmental hospitals nurses: a survey study. Springerplus. 2014;3:25. https://doi.org/10.1186/2193-1801-3-25. PMID: 24455469; PMCID: PMC3895439
11. Stahel PF, Ahankoob N, Nguyen C. Servant leadership: an endangered species? Patient Saf Surg. 2022;16:9. https://doi.org/10.1186/s13037-022-00321-0.
12. Rosing F, Boer D, Buengeler C. When timing is key: how autocratic and democratic leadership relate to follower trust in emergency contexts. Front Psychol. 2022;13:904605. https://doi.org/10.3389/fpsyg.2022.904605. PMID: 35992493; PMCID: PMC9382123
13. Sanders J, Balcom C. Clinical leadership during the COVID-19 pandemic: reflections and lessons learned. Healthc Manage Forum. 2021;34(6):316–9. https://doi.org/10.1177/08404704211044587.
14. Robert V, Vandenberghe C. Laissez-faire leadership and affective commitment: the roles of leader-member exchange and subordinate relational

self-concept. J Bus Psychol. 2021;36:533–51. https://doi.org/10.1007/s10869-020-09700-9.
15. Hinkin TR, Schriesheim CA. An examination of “nonleadership”: from laissez-faire leadership to leader reward omission and punishment omission. J Appl Psychol. 2008;93(6):1234–48. https://doi.org/10.1037/a0012875.
16. Devine CA, Chin ED. Integrity in nursing students: a concept analysis. Nurse Educ Today. 2018;60:133–8. https://doi.org/10.1016/j.nedt.2017.10.005.
17. Arroliga AC, Huber C, Myers JD, Dieckert JP, Wesson D. Leadership in health care for the 21st century: challenges and opportunities. Am J Med. 2014;127(3):246–9. https://doi.org/10.1016/j.amjmed.2013.11.004. Epub 2013 Nov 23
18. Stoller JK. Developing physician-leaders: a call to action. J Gen Intern Med. 2009;24(7):876–8. https://doi.org/10.1007/s11606-009-1007-8. Epub 2009 May 20. PMID: 19455370; PMCID: PMC2695517
19. van Diggele C, Burgess A, Roberts C, Mellis C. Leadership in healthcare education. BMC Med Educ. 2020;20(Suppl 2):456. https://doi.org/10.1186/s12909-020-02288-x. PMID: 33272264; PMCID: PMC7712520
20. Deming WE. Out of the crisis, center for advanced engineering study. Cambridge, MA: Massachusetts Institute of Technology; 1982.
21. Collins J, Porras JI. Built to last: successful habits of visionary companies. Harper Business; 2004.
22. Doerr J. Measure what matters: OKRs: the simple idea that drives 10× growth. Penguin Group (SA) Limited; 2018.
23. Leadership vs Management: What’s the difference? Harvard Business School. October 31, 2019. https://online.hbs.edu/blog/post/leadership-vs-management
24. Fennell K. Conceptualizations of leadership and relevance to health and human service workforce development: a scoping review. J Multidiscip Healthc. 2021;14:3035–51. https://doi.org/10.2147/MDH.S329628.
25. Gavin M, Gomez L, Bernet P. Diversity improves performance and outcomes. J Natl Med Assoc. 2019;111:383–92. https://doi.org/10.1016/j.jnma.2019.01.006.
26. Buckingham M. What great managers do. Harv Bus Rev. 2005;83(3):70–9, 148. PMID:15768677
27. Tuckman BW. Developmental sequence in small groups. Psychol Bull. 1965;63(6):384–99. https://doi.org/10.1037/h0022100.
28. Katzenbach J, Smith D. The wisdom of teams: creating the high performance organization. Boston, MA: Harvard Business School Press; 1993.
29. Gomez LE, Bernet P. Diversity improves performance and outcomes. J Natl Med Assoc. 2019;111(4):383–92. https://doi.org/10.1016/j.jnma.2019.01.006. Epub 2019 Feb 11. PMID: 30765101.

Establishing an Organizational Culture

21

Eliel Arrey, Shaneeta M. Johnson, and John D. Mellinger

Introduction

Organizational culture can be defined as the collection of common norms, values, expectations, and beliefs shared by its members [1, 2]. Such culture is foundational in any healthcare context, as it provides the template for acceptable practice in accomplishing the organization's work in delivering or leading healthcare. Some have referred to organizational culture as the organization's DNA, which reflects the mutual outlook, assumptions, and standards of its membership [1]. Nothing plays a more significant role in shaping organizational culture than leadership [3, 4]. Competent leaders are vital to developing, shaping, and maintaining a successful organizational culture [5]. To be effective, a leader must

E. Arrey
John P. and Katherine G. McGovern Medical School, Health Science Center at Houston, University of Texas, Austin, TX, USA
e-mail: earrey@msm.edu

S. M. Johnson
Department of Surgery, Morehouse School of Medicine, Atlanta, GA, USA
e-mail: shajohnson@msm.edu

J. D. Mellinger (✉)
American Board of Surgery, and Department of Surgery, Southern Illinois University School of Medicine, Springfield, IL, USA
e-mail: jmellinger@siumed.edu

S. M. Johnson et al. (eds.), *The SAGES Manual of Strategy and Leadership*, https://doi.org/10.1007/978-3-031-62359-2_21

understand the varying dimensions and related artifacts or expressions of organizational culture and, perhaps most importantly, recognize the values, tribes, and goals that comprise the organization and their interrelationships.

A strong organizational culture within a healthcare system can promote team unity, provide guidance in dealing with complex scenarios, promote job satisfaction and employee commitment, and even serve as a predictor of the success of quality improvement initiatives [1, 5]. Cultural strength can be a competitive advantage to any surgical practice. This chapter aims to impart to the surgeon leader the keys to establishing and maintaining a successful organizational culture in their surgical practice setting.

Defining Organizational Culture

Elements of Organizational Culture

Peter Drucker, a respected leadership consultant and author, is credited for the famous quote, "Culture eats strategy for breakfast" [6]. This statement was not meant to undermine the importance of strategy and execution within any enterprise but highlights an important point: the culture of an organization plays a vital role in determining whether strategic plans will be executed effectively and if organizational goals will be achieved [2, 7]. Culture can both prevent and promote strategic goals from being realized and often does so in ways that are at the subconscious level of organizational behavior.

Thus, the first step in establishing the organizational culture of a surgical practice is recognizing the various artifacts that contribute to it. These artifacts can be divided into two categories: superficial and deep, or tangible and intangible. Superficial artifacts include the physical (or visible) elements of the organization's culture, such as physical structures, language, rituals, ceremonies, stories, and legends. Conversely, shared values and common or underlying assumptions represent the deeper aspects of culture [2, 8, 9].

Tangible Aspects of Organizational Culture

The visible and more tangible aspects of an organization's culture represent some of its most potent elements. They depict the outward face and, in some cases, the longitudinal history of more inwardly held organizational tenets. These could be represented in physical structures, such as how employee workspaces are arranged or located, or whose pictures are displayed on walls for public recognition. Such structures often belie function. Are employee stations set in open spaces to promote collaboration? Are managers and senior leaders embedded with teams or in a separate area to themselves? If this was a surgical practice, are the provider stations organized in a way that promotes accessibility or visibility to the nursing and ancillary staff? [10]. In other words, much of an organization's culture can be observed by simply being in its physical space and considering features such as what it highlights, directs, orders, and prioritizes. Standing habits governing communication, celebration, and behavior as embodied in language, rituals, or ceremonies also showcase much of an organization's culture. Rituals and ceremonies refer to company reward systems or policies that promote or reward the propagation of a specific culture. The presence of pictures from previous company picnics or gatherings, the employee of the month or year awardees, or patterns for how employees dress on certain occasions (for example, casual Fridays) all serve as superficial or openly visible manifestations of the organization's culture.

Intangible Aspects of Organizational Culture

The deeper and less tangible aspects of an organization's culture are shared values and shared assumptions [2]. Shared values refer to conscious beliefs, shared principles, common standards, or goals [2, 8]. These are powerful and assist members of the organization in evaluating what is good, bad, right, or wrong in the organization's eyes and are often stated or enfranchised in credos or codes consciously endorsed by the organization. Conversely, shared assumptions lie at the deepest and often unarticulated levels of organizational culture. These are generally unconscious or unspoken, can be of positive or negative influence, and often involve beliefs about fundamental issues, such as how the organization sees humanity and reality [2, 8]. An example of an assumption could be that employees are easily replaced and interchangeable, leading to human resource policies that prioritize fiscal thrift and downplay the importance of social capital development and talent retention. Shared assumptions create implicit mental models and translate into how more superficial artifacts are presented within the organizational space.

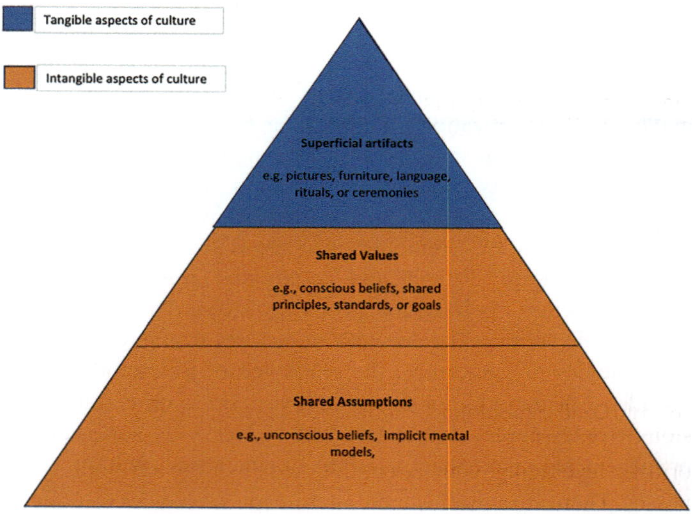

Understanding and recognizing these various elements of organizational culture is imperative to running a successful healthcare system. A culture that recognizes the foundational importance of shared values and assumptions is much more effective in channeling and directing employee behavior than one that focuses only on extensive company rules and policies [8]. The former takes into account shared internal motivations, while the latter may be weakened by potentially only factoring in external behavioral influences. A weak culture that is naïve to assumptions and unspoken mental models can unknowingly undermine organizational performance. In contrast, a strong culture that reflects on and enfranchises shared values and consciously embodies them in more superficial artifacts will offer a competitive advantage [7].

This theme of alignment between deeper, subconscious, and less tangible cultural elements such as shared values and assumptions, and more superficial elements or artifacts that ideally express or mirror those values can be assessed through organizational culture profiling. Each organization has a unique culture profile determined by the various cultural dimensions working individually but synergistically to shape the overall organization.

Organizational Culture Models

Hofstede's Model

Geert Hofstede is credited with defining and establishing that an organization's culture profile comprises several dimensions of practice rather than simply stated values [11]. A culture profile is thus a depiction of organizational behavior rather than intention alone. These dimensions vary among organizations based on the industry of the organization and are vital in identifying, measuring, or managing an organizational culture more effectively. They provide a behavioral framework that can then be compared with intentions for consistency of expression or alignment. These dimensions include the following, as embodied in specific groups of employees who behaviorally manifest them:

- Innovation: Refers to the subgroup of employees who are continuously experimenting, taking risks, and seeking new opportunities. They tend not to follow the rules but rather bend or break them to explore new areas and ideas.
- Stability: Employees within this subgroup are predictable and consistent, promote a sense of security within the organization, and are rule-oriented.
- Respect for people: Employees within this subgroup promote fairness and tolerance of diversity.

- Outcome orientation: Members of this subgroup have high expectations of themselves and their colleagues and are results-oriented.
- Attention to detail: These employees are precise and very analytical.
- Team orientation: These members vigorously promote collaboration and value human resource capacity. They tend to emphasize equality, wellness, dignity, and employee rights.
- Aggressiveness: Members of this dimension are competitive and promote a win-at-all-cost mentality with a low emphasis on social responsibility.

Multiple dimensions are typically found within the same organization across various departments or subgroups. Thus, these categories may be cross-sectional or matrix-like in their organizational presentation. As an example of how these dimensions might interrelate, an innovation-strong but stability-low organization could innovate itself into bankruptcy, but the converse could be so conservative as to fall behind and be eclipsed by competitors. Similarly, an organization that was strong on aggressiveness and low on respect for people might emphasize individual achievement in such a way that corporate citizenship, teamwork, and collective intelligence were undermined. Thus, not only dimensional strengths but the interplay of these dimensions that predict organizational performance and units that are constructively inclusive of multiple dimensions may be most effective.

Organizational Subcultures

Leaders of healthcare organizations should not assume that all members of the organization recognize and embrace the prevailing artifacts of the organizational culture. There are always subcultures within any business entity. The dominant culture is the set of values, norms, and beliefs shared by most of the members of the organization, while a subculture is a set of values shared by a small minority of the organization's members [2].

Subcultures may serve as countercultures that oppose some aspects of the dominant culture. These may arise as a result of conflicts or experiences shared by members of the organization. Leaders must pay extra attention to minimize employee social dislocation and alienation within their organization, including through recognition of and sensitivity to subcultures and countercultures [12]. Some scholars argue that countercultures serve as a source of surveillance and critical review of the organization and a source of emerging values [2]. Countercultures are thus not necessarily destructive in their influences and potential and may manifest in superficial and/or deeper elements of an organization's culture.

Mckinsey 7S Framework

Developed by McKinsey consultants Tom Peters and Robert Waterman, the McKinsey 7S model is a widely adopted model to evaluate and strengthen organizational culture [13]. The model utilizes seven skills stratified into hard and soft skills to determine the organization's effectiveness and culture. All seven skills are connected, meaning that a change in one area will affect change and necessitate change in others. The seven skills are listed in Table 21.1.

Hard Skills:

- Strategy: Refers to the sources of competitive advantage and the organization's strategic priorities.
- Structure: This skill evaluates how tasks, people, and activities are distributed and grouped to accomplish the goals of the organization.
- Systems: Evaluation of the formal processes and procedures to manage the organization, such as performance measurement, reward systems, planning, and resource allocation systems.

Table 21.1 Mckinsey 7S framework

Hard skills	Soft skills
Strategy	Staffing
Structure	Skills
Systems	Style
	Shared values

Soft Skills:

- Staffing: Refers to the team makeup of the culture, such as who are the team members and their backgrounds and competencies. It also evaluates the organization's approach to recruitment, selection, and socialization.
- Skills: This element evaluates the unique competencies within the organization with regard to its people, management practices, systems, and technology.
- Style: Evaluation of the leadership style of the leadership and management team of the organization, as well as the overall operating style. This will impact the customs of the people within the organization, including how they work and interact.
- Shared values: Perhaps the most important of the skills, shared values represent the core values that are accepted and represented in the organization. These values should serve as guiding principles and have a significant meaning to the organization's members.

Use of this framework is important to understand the organization's existing culture and drive culture change or strategy based on shared values and expectations. The organization's culture should be frequently reevaluated to ensure that the team's alignment is in concordance with the interests and values of the leadership and team.

Iceberg Culture Model

The Cultural Iceberg model was developed by Edward Hall in 1976 [14]. The model visualizes organizational culture as comprised of both visible and invisible elements that form the fundamental assumptions of the organization's culture. The tip of the iceberg contains the visible elements of the organization's culture. These elements include the vision, strategy, mission, policies, and external presentation of the organizational culture. The invisible elements include attitudes, feelings, values, norms, unwritten rules, relationships, and personal fundamental needs (e.g., safety, belonging, and acknowledgment). These elements, which lie beneath the surface, often determine the overall vision, strategic direction, culture, and success of the organization. The model stresses that organizational culture can only be shaped by addressing the invisible elements of the organization. The pulse of the organization must be measured, and a deeper dive into the cultural composition of the organization performed to allow for more significant change and growth toward shared goals.

Tribes Within an Organization

In their book, Tribal Leadership: Leveraging Natural Groups to Build a Thriving Organization, Dave Logan et al. describe organizations as a collection of small towns wrapped into a bigger city [15]. These small towns, he called tribes. Tribes are not necessarily teams within an organization, but a collection of mindsets and personalities who "behave as [they] see their world" [15]. Tribes thus represent an embodiment of subcultures and may be passively or aggressively oriented and in alignment or opposition to prevailing or dominant cultural themes. Within this model, as organizations are the sum of the tribes, tribes are ultimately how things get done within an organization. Tribes can be powerful in changing organizations or rejecting a new organizational leader. Some tribes want to change the world, while others are content with multiple coffee breaks. Thus, tribal culture is of significant cultural importance and, if understood and intentionally directed, can become a powerful tool within any organization.

Tribal Culture

Tribal culture determines strength and influence within an organization, and effective tribal leadership can help support and sustain a thriving corporate culture. A healthcare system is a classic example of tribes at work. It is often said that the third-year medical student spends most of their time finding their tribe, which, of course, means their specialty niche or focus within the overall medical system. Tribal culture extends beyond specialty choice and reflects how we decide to practice medicine within specialties or other work units. In this model, every tribe can be categorized as operating at a different stage, reflective of that group's standing within the organization, which in turn can motivate desires to increase the tribe or unit's position and influence. Logan et al. further stratify tribal cultures into five distinct stages and their associated thematic expressions of life within the organization (see Table 21.2). They argue that the majority of employees in most workplaces are between stages 2 and 4 and that an organization's ultimate goal would be to progressively embody a stage 5 tribe. Those in stage 1 tribes demonstrate hostility and despair within the organizational culture. People in stage 2 tribes are passively antagonistic and cross their arms in judgment, and their laughter is quietly sarcastic because "they've seen it all before and watched it all fail" [15]. People in this tribe want to protect other tribal members from the intrusion of management and leadership. Stage 3 is the most heavily populated workforce element in most organizations. This cohort generally represents the lone warriors who are willing to work and feel a need to win, especially if someone else loses. Members of this tribe are too busy, have no time, and often express their disappointment for others who "don't have their ambition of skill" [15]. Tribes with a stage 4 mindset feel united and pulled by the group, ready to face a larger foe. Members of this tribe have little patience for personal agendas or politics. Finally, stage 5 tribes comprise the smallest cohort and represent high-level leadership with a strong sense of inspiration and vision. Members of this tribe speak one language, focused on potential and making history. A strength of this model is its standardization of the multiculture or subculture theme in a way that is typical of many organizations. Another strength is in its ability to succinctly

Table 21.2 Stages of tribal culture according to Dave Logan

Tribal stage	Defining mood	Main theme
1	Hostility and despair	"Life sucks"
2	Passively antagonistic and the apathetic victim	"My life sucks"
3	The lone warrior	"I'm great … and you are not"
4	Tribal pride	"We are great"
5	"Innocent wonderment," pure leadership, vision, and inspiration	"Life is great"

Adapted from Dave Logan et al. [15]

outline a path toward strengthened organizational health and effectiveness based on a vision that moves from critical self-centeredness to an aspirational and collective mindset.

Tribal Leadership

Logan et al. contend that leaders within each tribe have the most meaningful influence on elevating their tribe to the next stage [15]. Individuals with credibility and influence, and not simply titles, can lead in this regard and often do so by example or role modeling as well as through other means of articulated or demonstrated embracement of higher-level mindsets. It is important to note that tribal leadership is a dynamic process, not an outcome. The more tribes an organization has operating at higher levels (i.e., stages 4 and 5), the better the company's performance [2, 15]. The concept of tribal culture and leadership speaks to how employees within an organization see themselves and their roles. Thus, tribal leadership becomes a potentially transformative strategy and a lens through which organizational leaders might view their employees' behavior at a deeper level, enabling them to become more effective motivators and change agents.

Developing a Successful Organizational Culture

Having defined organizational culture and some ways it might be characterized and understood or operationalized, we now turn our attention to some points of further application. These will include defining cultural strengths and predominant qualities of high-performing cultures and briefly outlining strategies for change management and merging cultures.

Cultural Strength

The strength of organizational culture is determined by the degree to which members of the organization personally hold or align with its dominant values and assumptions. The objective of a leader in a healthcare organization should first be to define the elements and dimensions of their culture clearly. When the culture so examined is reflective of the organization's needs, then that culture should be articulated, highlighted, and enfranchised through corporate practices and habits such as those reflected in credos, structures, celebrations, and policies. Suppose the culture is identified as not reflecting the organization's aspirations. In that case, leaders can help address this through new employee selection or leveraging change agents and change management strategies that emphasize the new cultural elements and move the organization in the desired cultural direction [2]. The subject of change agents and change management in an organization could make an entire book by itself. Stated succinctly, one can describe a change agent as a person who acts as a catalyst for the change management process within an organization [16, 17]. These agents can be internal (manager, senior executive, human resource personnel, etc.) or external (e.g., third-party consultants) [16]. Their roles within an organization are generally targeted and involve transforming how an organization operates by inspiring and influencing members of the organization. Change agents are pivotal in helping promote, champion, enable, and support an organization's change implementation agenda or culture. In a key model of leadership developed from research across cultures and disciplines, effective leaders, in general, model desired behavior, inspire collective or shared visions, challenge processes that impede or impair, enable action by group members, and encourage the hearts and motivation of constituents [18]. Notably, the dominant culture must be institutionalized through artifacts, as previously mentioned, such as language, rituals (programmed routines), ceremonies (planned activities for an audience), or physical layouts (office designs, wall hangings, etc.) that convey the cultural meaning.

Finally, cultural strength lasts longer when it originates with organizational founders or top leadership. The Mayo Clinic is typically cited for its culture of excellence which was birthed in its conception with Dr. William and Charles Mayo setting out to develop a surgical mecca of excellence, innovation, professionalism, and care for the sick [2, 19, 20]. A strong culture can function as a robust control system, social glue, and sense-making apparatus for members and guests within the organization.

Qualities of Strong Organizational Culture and Organizational Outcomes

As mentioned, a strong organizational culture can be a source of competitive advantage. A strong culture is much more potent at orienting and directing employee behavior than extensive company rules and policies [7, 8].

Qualities of a healthy organizational culture are those that promote employee well-being and maximize employee performance. Employee engagement, integrity, diversity, collaboration, and teamwork, alongside opportunities for growth, a unified sense of purpose, open communication, and core values, are some of the most commonly cited qualities of a solid and productive organizational culture [2, 21–23].

Changing Organizational Cultures and Dealing With Mergers

With the advent of emerging healthcare systems and practice mergers, one of the most challenging aspects of acquiring healthcare organizations, or organizations seeking to blend on equal terms, is changing or adapting the existing organizational culture(s). This is a delicate process, as merging or changing entrenched cultures is more challenging than creating them. The first step to joining cultures is performing a bicultural audit. A bicultural audit evaluates cultural relations between organizations and estimates the extent to which cultural clashes will occur [2]. This is generally done using focus groups, questionnaires, and identifying existing cultural artifacts to best identify the cultural differences and potential friction points between the merging companies [24, 25]. A successful bicultural audit can be used to orient strategies to minimize conflict during the merger process and allow the creation of an action plan to bridge the identified cultural differences.

Following a successful bicultural audit, the following processes take place (to varying degrees) within the newly formed organization:

- Assimilation: The employees of the acquired healthcare institution embrace the new acquiring culture.
- Deculturation: The acquiring healthcare system imposes its culture and practices on its newly acquired staff.
- Integration: In some cases, composite cultures (a heterogeneous mix of multiple cultures) preserve the best features of a plurality of past cultures.
- Separation: The newly merged organization decides to keep respective corporate cultures and practices that remain distinct.

Recognizing which of these processes are occurring or desired as an outcome of the merger process can help leaders define and respond to the cultural challenges of organizational change entailed in mergers and acquisitions.

Strengthening and Maintaining Organizational Cultures

The final section of this chapter focuses on strengthening and maintaining the culture within a healthcare organization after it has been defined and established. Culture being a dynamic structure, failure to recognize the importance of efforts to intentionally sustain desired features can lead to deviation or deterioration over time despite strong beginnings.

Attraction, Selection, and Attrition

Proper attraction, selection, and socialization are the lifeblood of strengthening any organization's culture. The attraction-selection-attrition theory, first introduced by Benjamin Schneider, refers to the strengthening of an organization's culture by:

1. Attracting applicants that self-select based on compatible values;
2. Allowing the organization to select applicants with compatible values;
3. Letting go (or removing) employees with incompatible values (attrition) [2, 26–28].

Beyond the attraction-selection-attrition theory, healthcare leaders must consistently introduce powerful artifacts such as culturally consistent rewards and recognitions and the continued support provided through workplace stability and reinforcing communication to strengthen their organizational culture continuously/steadily. Workforce stability minimizes turnover which can profoundly weaken organizational culture, and a strong culture is dependent on frequent, open, and transparent communication [2, 15, 25].

Maintaining Organizational Culture by Socialization

Organizational Socialization

Coupled with the strengthening of organizational culture is the concept of organizational socialization, which refers to the continuous learning of values, expected behaviors, and social norms for members of an organization [2]. This learning process provides members of the organization with the necessary knowledge to assume their roles within the organization with coherence and alignment. Organizational socialization allows new members of the organization to understand and make sense of the various elements or dynamics of an organization's culture and eases the adaptation process to new roles or team structures.

Stages of Organizational Socialization

Organizational socialization generally occurs over three stages best explained by the Feldman model: pre-employment (anticipatory) stage, encounter (newcomer or breaking in) stage, and role management [2, 29, 30].

- During the anticipatory stage, a prospective recruit gathers information about the organization from the outside, anticipating the experiences they will encounter, and begins to adapt accordingly. An example might be a fourth-year medical student visiting or discussing with residents at their future training institution before starting an internship.
- During the encounter or accommodating stage, the newcomer undergoes initiation to their tasks and workgroups with the goals of changing and reshaping inaccurate, unrealistic expectations.
- In the role management stage, the recruit is now an insider, practicing new role behaviors and typically striving to resolve two types of conflicts: outside life conflicts and conflicting demands at work.
- The desired outcome of this socialization model is to increase productivity, satisfaction, and loyalty and mitigate stress and turnover which are two factors that can deeply undermine organizational culture.

Organizational socialization can be further improved by providing prospective newcomers with a realistic job preview (a balance of positive and negative information about a potential job) as well as maximizing exposure to supervisors and co-workers who make excellent socialization agents, and themselves role model high function and alignment within the organization [2].

Conclusion

Establishing an effective organizational culture can be challenging but is a necessary aim of the healthcare leader. By embracing cultural tenets and values, the aspiring leader can be better prepared to define, select, and implement changes that produce a productive and successful culture for the organization.

SAGES Takeaway

- Organizational culture can be defined as the collection of norms, values, expectations, and beliefs of individuals shared by members [1, 2].
- To be effective, a leader must understand the different artifacts, dimensions, and tribes of the organizational culture.
- Good cultural strength and cultural qualities have an enormous impact on organizational outcomes and employee well-being.
- Proper attraction, selection, and socialization are the lifeblood of strengthening and maintaining any organization's culture.
- A strong organizational culture can be a source of competitive advantage for a healthcare system.

References

1. Chalmers R, Brannan GD. Organizational culture. In: StatPearls [Internet]. Treasure Island, FL: StatPearls Publishing; 2022.
2. McShane SL, Von Glinow MA. Organizational behavior and theory. McGraw-Hill; 2018.
3. Sfantou D, Laliotis A, et al. Importance of leadership style towards quality of care measures in healthcare settings: a systematic review. Healthcare. 2017;5(4):73–89. https://doi.org/10.3390/healthcare5040073.
4. Dixon-Woods M, Baker R, Charles K, et al. Culture and behaviour in the English National Health Service: overview of lessons from a large multimethod study. BMJ Qual Saf. 2014;23(2):106–15. https://doi.org/10.1136/bmjqs-2013-001947.
5. ALFadhalah T, Elamir H. Organizational culture, quality of care and leadership style in Government General Hospitals in Kuwait: a multimethod study. J Healthc Leadersh. 2021;13:243–54. https://doi.org/10.2147/JHL.S333933. PMID: 34703349; PMCID: PMC8528408
6. Engel J. Why does culture 'eat strategy for breakfast'? Forbes. 2018. https://www.forbes.com/sites/forbescoachescouncil/2018/11/20/why-does-culture-eat-strategy-for-breakfast/?sh=5631065e1e09. Accessed 15 May 2023.
7. Cochrane BS. Leaders go first: creating and sustaining a culture of high performance. Healthc Manage Forum. 2017;30(5):229–32. https://doi.org/10.1177/0840470417718195.

8. University of Minnesota. Organizational behavior. 2017. https://doi.org/10.24926/8668.1501. Accessed 15 May 2023.
9. Schein EH. Organizational culture and leadership. San Francisco, CA: Jossey-Bass; 1992.
10. Stegmeier D. Innovations in office design: the critical influence approach to effective work environments. Hoboken, NJ: John Wiley; 2008.
11. Hofstede G. Dimensionalizing cultures: the Hofstede model in context. Online Read Psychol Cult. 2011;2(1):8. https://doi.org/10.9707/2307-0919.1014.
12. Cutler C. Subcultures and countercultures. Encyclopedia of language and linguistics. 2nd ed. Elsevier; 2006. p. 236–9. ISBN 9780080448541. https://doi.org/10.1016/B0-08-044854-2/01312-2.
13. Bradach J. Organizational alignment: the 7-S model. Harvard Business School; 1996. 9-497-045
14. https://www.spps.org/cms/lib/MN01910242/Centricity/Domain/125/iceberg_model_3.pdf. Accessed 25 Aug 2023.
15. Logan D, King J, Fischer-Wright H. Tribal leadership: leveraging natural groups to build a thriving organization. Harper Business of Harper Collins Publishers. New York, NY; 2011.
16. Malik P. The role of a change agent: characteristics, types, skills. 2022. https://whatfix.com/blog/change-agent/. Accessed 2 Aug 2023.
17. MasterClass. Change agent: characteristics of an effective change agent. 2022. https://www.masterclass.com/articles/change-agent. Accessed 2 Aug 2023.
18. Kouzes JM, Posner BZ. The truth about leadership: the no-fads heart-of-the-matter facts you need to know. 1st ed. Jossey-Bass A Wiley Imprint: San Francisco, CA; 2010.
19. Anaya-Prado R, Rubí MG. William and Charles Mayo: their influence on American medicine. J Invest Surg. 2007;20(6):325–9. https://doi.org/10.1080/08941930701772116.
20. Toledo-Pereyra LH. The Mayo brothers: an American surgical legacy. J Invest Surg. 2010;23(5):244–8. https://doi.org/10.3109/08941939.2010.519969.
21. Rogel C. The 12 attributes of a strong organizational culture. 2014. https://www.tlnt.com/the-12-attributes-of-a-strong-organizational-culture/. Accessed 15 May 2023.
22. Wong. Organizational culture: definition, importance, and development. 2020. https://www.achievers.com/blog/organizational-culture-definition/. Accessed 15 May 2023.
23. Rozen. The seven characteristics of successful company cultures. 2015. https://www.huffpost.com/entry/the-seven-characteristics_b_11339884. Accessed 15 May 2023.
24. Solomon C. Culture audits: supporting organizational success. Alexandria, VA: American Society for Training and Development; 2004.

25. Strathern M. Audit cultures: anthropological studies in accountability, ethics and the academy. Portsmouth, NH: Routledge; 2000.
26. Schneider B. The people make the place. Personnel Psychol. 1987;40(3):437–53.
27. Schneider B, Goldstein HW, Smith DB. The ASA framework: an update. Pers Psychol. 1995;48(4):747–73.
28. Ryan AM, Sacco JM, McFarland LA, Kriska SD. Applicant self-selection: correlates of withdrawal from a multiple hurdle process. J Appl Psychol. 2000;85(2):163–79.
29. Kennedy E, Lawton L. Developments in business simulation and experiential exercises. 1990;17.
30. Feldman D. The multiple socialization of organization members. Acad Manag Rev. 1981;6(2):309–18.

Part V

Leading Others—Policy and Administration

Policies and Procedures 22

Erica R. H. Sutton

Vignette

Your department is making a strategic policy change because it has had a longstanding reputation for a lack of ethnic and gender diversity. The new chairperson has promised leadership that will usher in a more equitable and diverse future, and the department's newly appointed vice chair of Diversity, Equity, and Inclusion (DEI) has assured the dean that if the new DEI policy is implemented (and funded), deliberate recruitment efforts will engage greater numbers of diverse faculty and trainees. In addition, research trials will become more inclusive and worthy of funding, and the institution will become trusted by the communities they serve.

The New DEI Policy States

The Department of Highly Fundable Esoterics is committed to treating all people equally and with respect, regardless of their age, disability, marriage or civil partnership, pregnancy or mater-

E. R. H. Sutton (✉)
Morehouse School of Medicine, Atlanta, GA, USA
e-mail: esutton@msm.edu

S. M. Johnson et al. (eds.), *The SAGES Manual of Strategy and Leadership*, https://doi.org/10.1007/978-3-031-62359-2_22

nity, race, religion or belief, gender or gender reassignment, or sexual orientation.

While the dean is generally supportive, the institution's legal counsel responded to the vice chair and the DEI committee with a lengthy email of a somewhat critical tone, posing serious questions. *What are you trying to accomplish overall? What do you want employees to do as a result of your policy? How does one report a violation of this policy? What are the consequences of violating this policy? How will adherence to the policy be monitored or deemed effective?* Though discouraged, the DEI committee commits to revising the policy but realizes that there is much more to be learned about what a policy is and does, and plainly, how to write a good one. Furthermore, it will need to understand the difference between a policy and a procedure.

Is It a Policy or Is It a Procedure?

It can be easy to confuse the two. Usually, a policy is written first, and then specific procedures to implement the policy are written later. A procedure is a detailed description or instructions of how policy is carried out (when and how). It is specific to a particular workplace and can include a variety of issues including health and safety, dress codes, how to perform remote working, HR practices, and so on.

A policy is "a set of ideas or a plan of what to do in particular situations that has been agreed to officially by a group of people, a business organization, a government, or a political party." This definition by the Cambridge Dictionary highlights two features central to all definitions of policy: it is **a plan of action that is agreed to by a group [1].** In the workplace, a policy states what management expects from employees (what to do, behaviors) and often provides reasoning that aligns with organizational values. In this way, policy is intended to guide decision-making.

Types of Policies

To better understand policymaking, first know that it is divided into two areas: public and organizational. Public policy refers to governments that put policy in place for large groups of people in countries, states, or counties. The American political scientist Theodore J. Lowi [2] proposed four types of public policy: distributive, regulative, constituent, and redistributive. Distributive policy deals with land distribution, subsidies, and tariffs. Regulative policy concerns rules regarding standards for health and safety, advertising, and so on. Constituent policy handles setting up agencies, reapportionment, and so on. Finally, redistributive policy is involved with controls on credit, social security, taxes, and so on [2]. The public interest is the main focus of public policymaking but can be influenced by politics.

John W. Kingdon [3] recognized politics as part of his construct of public policy. It was part of a multiple streams framework that included the problem, the policy, and the politics, which all operated independently of each other. When these streams converge, this creates a policy window that allows for change [4]. The problem stream recognizes a public problem that may require government action. This step can be quite low-key or it can be more dramatic where an organization uses protests or advertising to make the public and policymakers aware of a problem. The policy stream is concerned with brainstorming possible solutions via policies. Kingdon [3] asserts that only problems with proposed solutions will become the focus of policymakers. The politics stream involves a variety of influences from public opinion to lobbying to changes in government that can sway policymakers to draft and enact policy to fix a problem. This generates the policy window when policy is finally written and put into effect.

Organizational policy is similar to public policy in that decisions are made to regulate behavior but of a smaller group of people. The purpose is to protect individuals against incidents that would disrupt workflow within the organization and protect workers [5]. Organizational policies are often categorized based on purpose: employee health and safety, benefits, leave, organizational culture, HR policy, and so on [6]. Policies can also be classified based on how they are expressed, such as oral policies, written policies, and implied policies. Organizational policies simply are expressions of what the organization expects from its employees and what the employees can expect from the organization. Understanding the categorization of a company's policies will aid in creating and introducing new policy.

Procedures

Organizational procedures explain how the policy is to be carried out, often in step-by-step instructions that may include process steps or checklists. Procedures tell who is responsible for each task and who to report to, what steps need to be taken in order to carry out policy, and what must be done when there are violations of policy. In other words, a procedure outlines a specific plan to enact a policy.

Before Writing a Policy and Procedure

In general, writing either a policy or a procedure have similar steps in the beginning. First, a need for a policy or procedure must be identified. The organization or department must decide if the policy or procedure will be written in anticipation of a situation or in response to one. For example, in the vignette above, the Department of Highly Fundable Esoterics realizes that its university (or headquarters of a major organization) has a new leader who strongly is advocating DEI broadly within the entire organization. Because the department has lagged behind in DEI ethics, it has written a policy in anticipation of an organization-wide policy on DEI. In another scenario, the department could have witnessed a DEI injustice within its purview and now realizes it must create a policy to present future injustices. Policies written in anticipation of a situation can also occur when an organization expects a federal or state requirement for which the organization must comply. This provides legal protection for the organization.

Sometimes, policies are written to streamline internal procedures or processes and can help guide employees through unexpected incidents and emergencies.

Once the need is recognized, select someone to take leadership in creating a policy or procedures committee. This team should include representatives not only from your specific department but also from other departments who have knowledge about writing policies and procedures. Those experts will become valuable resources in how to handle the process. The team will then gather information, including legal responsibilities, about the topic of the policy. Consulting appropriate stakeholders would be valuable in order to identify the potential effect of the new policy and to discuss any potential glitches in implementation that may need to be addressed. In addition, look at how other organizations have written policy statements and procedures similar to what your department or organization wants to do.

Writing Good Policy: Language

There are two views on writing policy. One is to be very specific, outlining every contingency. The other is to be more flexible or general in wording. Most policy is written in more general terms when there will be detailed procedures outlining the implementation of the policy. In either case, write in clear language that is easy to read. Make sure that the policy is issue-specific, includes all employees, and is easy to manage or implement. In particular, make sure that the wording is strong enough to be relied upon in a court of law.

Writing Good Policy: Purpose Statement

Write a strong purpose statement that explains why the policy is being implemented and what the desired outcome will be. This statement should reflect the legal authority of the organization to require this policy.

Writing Good Policy: Statement of Policy

The statement of policy should be clear about the behavior surrounding the identified issue for which the policy was written.

Writing Good Policy: Specification Section

This section includes details of who the policy applies to and may include general consequences for noncompliance. Detailed explanations of occurrences where the policy will be applied and what will happen for infractions are usually included in the detailed procedures that follow the policy.

Writing Good Policy: Implementation Section and Effective Date

The implementation section shows who is responsible for implementing the policy and who will enforce it and how. The date when the policy will be in force will be shown on the effective date.

Writing Good Policy: Seek Feedback

It is always wise to seed feedback when writing organizational policy and procedures. Provide copies of the draft of the policy and/or procedures to supervisors, employees, and other stakeholders to see if the policy is written in a clear language that is understandable. Ask those who consulted with the policy/procedures team during the prewriting stage, especially those who had written similar policies before, to see if this meets their standards. Listen to all feedback and make a team decision on changes to the document. If necessary, send the edited document around for another review. Continue to make changes until the document precisely reflects what you want to cover in your new policy.

Writing Good Policy: Send Policy for Approval and Implementation

When the policy is ready, send it out for approval and implementation. In the scenario above, the Department of Highly Fundable Esoterics sent their policy statement to the legal department of their organization. That is probably a good first place to start the approval process. Once the legal aspects are approved, send the document up through the broader organization for approval.

Writing Good Policy: Monitor, Review, Revise

Policies and procedures should change as your organization changes. In general, review them annually and make adjustments and changes as necessary. Always include employees from within the wider organization for policies and procedures that apply to all employees.

Writing a Good Procedure

Writing a good procedure involves similar steps to those for writing policy but with one difference. Make sure that the language of the procedure is very detailed. Include all instances where the policy will be applicable. Be specific in what is permitted and what is not and to whom that applies. For example, if it is a dress code policy that says all employees must dress appropriately, specify that business professional attire is required for all employees at every business event, except on Fridays where they may wear business casual dress. Note where employees may go for instruction about policy if they have questions about its implementation.

Vignette Revisited

The policy that the Department of Highly Fundable Esoterics presented was lacking elements. Its statement of policy really was a preamble to the purpose of the new policy. It said:

> The Department of Highly Fundable Esoterics is committed to treating all people equally and with respect, regardless of their age, disability, marriage or civil partnership, pregnancy or maternity, race, religion or belief, gender or gender reassignment, or sexual orientation.

It lacked more detail about why the new policy was important to implement. It did not also state that the DEI policy would be applicable to other practices and procedures already established on recruitment, new hires, compensation, benefits, promotions, transfers, terminations, professional development, and building the culture of the organization. The policy that the department wrote did not also include how the DEI policy would look in the workplace, regarding respectful cooperation and communication, respectful conduct on and off the workplace at organizational events, representation, work/life balance, and employer/employee contributions to the wider community to promote respect and understanding of DEI. In addition, there was no mention of disciplinary action if an employee was found to have displayed inappropriate behavior nor was mention made of where employees could report discrimination. The legal department asked for more details in the policy which were necessary, but a much lengthier procedure document will provide more specifics on implementation of the policy and how to handle infringements of it.

SAGES Takeaway

A good policy:

- Clearly articulates the desired actions or attitudes and employee should demonstrate.

- Explains the consequences and the methods for reporting violations.
- Is monitored for effectiveness and reviewed regularly.

References

1. The Cambridge Dictionary. 2023. https://dictionary.cambridge.org/dictionary/policy.
2. Lowi TJ. Four Systems of Policy, politics, and choice. Public Adm Rev. 1972;32(4):298–310. http://links.jstor.org/sici?sici=0033-3352%28197207%2F08%2932%3A4%3C298%3AFSOPPA%3E2.0.CO%3B2-X
3. Kingdon JW. In: Kingdon JW, editor. Agendas, alternatives and public policies. Boston, MA: Little, Brown & Co.; 1984.
4. Mackey TK. Opening the policy window to mobilize action against corruption in the health sector comment on "we need to talk about corruption in health systems". Int J Health Policy Manag. 2019;8(11):668–71. https://doi.org/10.15171/ijhpm.2019.65.
5. Francisco EB. Policies and procedures: a guide for workplace professionals. Safety Culture. 2023. https://safetyculture.com/topics/policies-and-procedures/
6. Volunteer Now. How to develop policies and procedures. DIY Committee Guide. https://diversity.iu.edu/doc/anti-racist/resources-articles-lit/How%20to%20Develop%20Policies%20and%20Procedures%20%20DIY%20Committee%20Guide.pdf

Managing Difficult Personalities in the Workplace

23

Mobola Oyefule

Defining the Problem

Defining Difficult Personalities

In the workplace, difficult personalities describe individual traits that are challenging to manage due to their impact on team dynamics and overall morale These traits are subject to amplification or attenuation depending on contextual factors and professional milieu. Just as individuals exhibit multifaceted behaviors across different domains of life, difficult personality traits manifest differently within varying settings It is important to recognize that the term "difficult personality" does not encapsulate the entirety of an individual's being but describes specific personality traits that hinder the cultivation of a healthy workplace environment.

M. Oyefule (✉)
General and GI Surgery, Emory University School of Medicine, Atlanta, GA, USA
e-mail: mobola.oyefule@emory.edu

S. M. Johnson et al. (eds.), *The SAGES Manual of Strategy and Leadership*, https://doi.org/10.1007/978-3-031-62359-2_23

The Impact of Difficult Personalities in the Workplace

Difficult personalities in the healthcare workplace can disrupt team dynamics, erode morale, and hinder productivity. Like the proverbial bad apple, individuals exhibiting negative behaviors have the potential to "infect" others, leading to heightened tension and strife. Research indicates that negative workplace behaviors, including those displayed by difficult personalities, contribute to decreased job satisfaction and increased stress levels among healthcare professionals. These difficult personalities can create an overtly or insidiously toxic work environment that significantly impacts the overall productivity and well-being of employees [1].

Failing to effectively address or manage these individuals can result in escalated conflicts and higher employee turnover/trainee attrition rates as employees are more inclined to seek alternative employment if they perceive the workplace environment as toxic [2]. Particularly within the healthcare context, individuals with difficult personality traits may exhibit uncivil behaviors that compromise safety and the quality of patient care. When healthcare professionals feel intimidated or unfairly treated, they are less likely to speak up or report errors, which ultimately hampers educational and patient care outcomes [3]. It is crucial to recognize and appropriately manage difficult personalities to foster a safe and supportive work environment that promotes optimal patient care [4].

Identifying Difficult Personalities

Difficult personalities come in different forms. Below are seven distinct archetypes of difficult personalities that can be found in the workplace [5].

Domineering Daniel(a): The Assertive and Controlling Personality

This personality tends to consistently dominate team meetings, disregarding others' input in favor of making decisions unilaterally. In an attempt to convey their passions and deeply held beliefs, they frequently interrupt others and talk over them. They may also take credit for group successes while downplaying the contributions of others, undermining the sense of collegiality and collective achievement in the organization.

Cynical Carl(le): The Constantly Critical and Pessimistic Personality

This personality manifests overtly critical tendencies, displaying a high degree of cynicism and skepticism. They have a proclivity to magnify perceived shortcomings and faults in organizational processes, openly expressing doubt regarding the likelihood of success of team endeavors. Generally risk-averse, they cloak their negative outlook under the guise of wanting to be "safe" and/or "careful." Adopting a "glass half empty" mentality, they tend to focus on problems rather than being solution-oriented.

Meddling Martin(a): The Excessively Involved and Nit-Picking Personality

This difficult personality exhibits a consistent tendency to interfere with the daily tasks performed by other team members, particularly those in subordinate positions. They closely monitor every step, always ready to intervene and rectify any perceived lapses in project completion. They tend to excessively focus on minor details that could easily be delegated to other team members, providing unsolicited and ill-timed critiques. Their quest to ensure that things unfold precisely as they envision renders them hyper-focused on trivial matters, making it difficult for them to see the big picture.

Prima Don(na): The Emotionally Volatile and Attention-Seeking Personality

This difficult personality disrupts the stability of the workplace by engaging in actions that introduce unnecessary drama and intrigue, diverting attention from the primary tasks at hand. With a penchant for being center stage, they strive to remain in the spotlight by displaying exaggerated emotional reactions to perceived offenses and trivial matters. They may possess lofty standards that are not in line with the expectations of a professional work environment. When their expectations are unmet, particularly if they hold a position of authority or high value, they are prone to throwing tantrums and expressing dissatisfaction.

Passive-Aggressive Paul(a): The Covertly Oppositional and Undermining Personality

This difficult personality frequently exhibits indirect dissent through negative body language, snide or sarcastic remarks, inappropriate humor, withholding relevant information, or agreeing to tasks but failing to complete them in a timely or satisfactory manner, leading to delays and frustrations. While they may not openly express opposing views or negative emotions, their actions and words generate hostility and hinder progress in the workplace. Passive-aggressive personalities often present a facade of agreeableness outwardly but behave in a manner that contradicts their apparent compliance.

Passive Pat(Ty): The Uncommunicative and Unresponsive Personality

On the passive end of the spectrum, the silent personality often abstains from active participation in team discussions and avoids sharing their opinions publicly, creating difficulties in collaborative decision-making processes. The inability or unwillingness to engage displayed by this personality type can indicate disengagement and a sense of detachment from the larger team. Consequently, their behavior can impede progress, as significant time may be dedicated to involving them or attempting to elicit their input before making important decisions, or worse still, they may be excluded altogether. This passive demeanor slows down the decision-making process and hampers the team's ability to move forward efficiently.

Mutinous Michael(a): The Instigating and Rebellious Personality

This personality openly defies rules and demonstrates a disregard for established organizational norms. They may hold the belief that rules do not apply to them or that rules are meant to be challenged and broken. This personality can be quite dangerous, insidiously causing anarchy and chaos in group settings. If they hold a position of relative authority, they can influence their peers and subordinates, resulting in the formation of factions within the workplace. This division undermines the creation of a harmonious work environment and negatively impacts team dynamics.

Understanding the Root Cause of the Problem(S)

Understanding Underlying Causes and Motivations for Difficult Behavior

In understanding difficult personalities, it is important to take into consideration the underlying factors and motivations that drive difficult behavior. It is only after one contemplates these root causes that one can effectively develop the skillset needed for management. The following are three main factors that influence the development of difficult personalities: intrinsic personality traits, extrinsic stressors, and prior experiences [4].

Intrinsic Personality Traits

Personality traits that make individuals successful clinicians can sometimes pose a liability to the group if not well-balanced. For example, excessive perfectionism can cause chronic stress, anxiety, and burnout, hinder creativity and innovation, and lead to conflicts and dissatisfaction within the team [6]. An excess of assertiveness may result in confrontational behavior and escalation of conflict, contributing to a climate of fear, anxiety, and stress among the healthcare team and negatively impacting patient care and job satisfaction. Finally, excessive self-criticism may pose challenges as individuals constantly second-guess themselves and may have difficulty with learning from mistakes due to feelings of guilt and inadequacy [7, 8].

Extrinsic Stressors

External stressors, such as high patient volume, staff shortages, and increased administrative burdens, impose a heightened workload on healthcare professionals, leading to chronic stress, fatigue, and burnout. Research demonstrates a correlation between stress and increased error rates in healthcare settings. These stressors undermine effective communication and collaboration within healthcare teams. The psychological and physiological consequences of stressors can exacerbate difficult personality traits in otherwise reasonable individuals. Therefore, it is crucial to contextualize challenging behaviors within the specific environmental and situational factors present. When healthcare professionals operate under elevated stress levels, their cognitive functioning, attention to detail, and decision-making capabilities may be compromised, potentially resulting in medical errors, delayed diagnoses, and suboptimal treatment outcomes. External stressors associated with managing difficult patients, witnessing patient suffering, and confronting ethical dilemmas can significantly impact emotional well-being. Compassion fatigue and emotional exhaustion among healthcare professionals diminish the capacity to provide attentive and empathetic care, thereby reducing patient satisfaction and eroding trust in the healthcare system [9].

Prior Experiences and History

Negative experiences can have a profound impact on the development of difficult personalities, as they contribute to short and long-term effects on well-being. Clinicians and trainees often endure emotional distress, guilt, and burnout as a result of challenging patient interactions and uncontrollable adverse outcomes.

Without proper debriefing and processing of these experiences, they gradually shape personalities and affect professional performance. Moreover, if a culture of negativity and toxicity persists within the organization, such as a blame-oriented atmosphere or a lack of open communication, individuals may develop reactive personality traits in response to the stressors they face. These traits can include passive aggression, unresponsiveness, and cynicism [10, 11].

Managing Difficult Behaviors/Personalities

Table 23.1: Types of Difficult Personalities and How to Manage Them

The following table details the different difficult personalities that are encountered in the workplace and specific management strategies [12–14].

Table 23.1 Management of difficult personalities in the workplace

Difficult personality	Management approach
Domineering Daniel(a): The assertive and controlling personality	**Promote equitable participation:** e.g., round-robin discussions or designated speaking turns to ensure everyone has equal opportunity to contribute and be heard **Set explicit boundaries**: Establish clear guidelines and expectations for communication and behavior to foster a respectful and inclusive environment **Offer individual feedback privately**: Address difficult behavior through one-on-one conversations, providing constructive feedback and guidance to help individuals understand the impact of their actions and encourage positive changes

(continued)

Table 23.1 (continued)

Difficult personality	Management approach
Cynical Carl(ie): The constantly critical and pessimistic personality	**Reframe challenges**: Encourage individuals to approach challenges as opportunities to offer potential solutions from alternative perspectives, fostering a problem-solving mindset **Spotlight positivity:** Recognize and celebrate achievements to cultivate a positive and motivating work environment with a sense of accomplishment and teamwork **Encourage constructive feedback:** Soliciting specific suggestions for improvement that take into account what is already working well to build upon existing strengths while providing opportunities for growth
Meddling Martin(a): The excessively involved and nit-picking personality	**Establish clear expectations early on:** Set clear roles, responsibilities, and project milestones from the outset to provide clarity and minimize confusion within the team **Foster trust:** Demonstrate confidence in the team's abilities and provide support, empowering them to take ownership of their tasks and contribute effectively **Open communication:** Encourage regular check-ins and updates at appropriate intervals to promote transparency, collaboration, and information sharing. This helps ensure that everyone is informed and aligned on progress, challenges, and any necessary adjustments
Prima Don(na): The emotionally volatile and attention-seeking personality	**Maintain composure:** Model and encourage a calm and composed demeanor, even in challenging situations, to promote a positive and professional atmosphere **Redirect focus**: Help individuals redirect their energy toward activities that align with team goals and priorities. This can help shift their mindset and channel their efforts in a more constructive direction **Provide guidance:** Offer support and guidance to help individuals develop self-awareness and understand the impact of their behavior. Provide resources, mentorship, or coaching opportunities to aid in their personal and professional growth

Table 23.1 (continued)

Difficult personality	Management approach
Passive-aggressive Paul(a): The covertly oppositional and undermining personality	**Encourage open communication:** Foster a safe and inclusive environment where team members feel comfortable expressing their thoughts, concerns, and ideas without fear of judgment or reprisal. This promotes transparency, trust, and collaboration within the team **Provide direct feedback:** Offer constructive feedback directly to individuals regarding the specific behaviors they display that undermine team morale and progress. Clearly communicate the impact of these behaviors and provide suggestions for improvement
Passive pat(ty): The uncommunicative and unresponsive personality	**Provide alternative communication channels:** Offer additional avenues for feedback, such as written submissions or smaller team meetings, to accommodate different communication preferences. This helps ensure that valuable input is captured **Solicit their feedback:** Engage in one-on-one conversations to actively seek input and insights from individuals who may be more hesitant to speak up in group settings. This allows for personalized communication and provides an opportunity to address any concerns or challenges they may have
Mutinous Michael(a): The instigating and rebellious personality	**Offer individual feedback privately**: Address difficult behavior through one-on-one conversations, providing constructive feedback and guidance to help individuals understand the impact of their actions and encourage change **Intervene early:** If initial feedback is not incorporated, corrective measures and interventions should be applied in order to discourage future negative actions **Enlist help:** If negative behavior continues despite corrective attempts, enlist the help of a senior partner, manager, and/or human resources

Self-Management for Managers: Managing Your Own Personal Reactions and Emotions

- Maintain composure: In emotionally charged situations, pause and take the time needed to approach conflict with a rational and measured mindset.
- Maintain Objectivity: Avoid personalizing difficult behavior by recognizing that they are not indicative of the individual's overall character or capabilities.
- Seek Support and Guidance: Utilize the resources of mentors, coaches, or colleagues who can offer objective insights and advice on managing difficult personalities.
- Monitor and Address Stress and Burnout: Recognize signs of personal stress and burnout, allowing time for self-care and rest to effectively lead from a position of strength.
- Request Feedback Often: Actively solicit feedback from team members, including both superiors and subordinates, to identify areas for personal growth and improvement.
- Learn Continuously: Enhance communication and conflict resolution skills by participating in workshops, seminars, and training programs aimed at professional development.
- Promptly Seek Assistance: Involve senior partners or higher-level management when persistent issues with challenging individuals pose risks to team safety or patient care.

Summary

The challenges posed by difficult personalities are not unique to the healthcare industry but can be encountered in various workplace settings. The solutions outlined earlier can be valuable for physicians and healthcare leaders in identifying and managing difficult personalities in their teams. By recognizing the diverse backgrounds and motivations of team members and understanding the underlying causes of challenging behavior, healthcare professionals can employ these strategies to foster a more positive work environment and improve patient outcomes.

SAGES Takeaway

- Certain personality traits that make individuals successful clinicians like perfectionism and candor can contribute to workplace conflict and disharmony if not recognized and regulated appropriately.
- While difficult personality traits are part of but do not define the entirety of a person's character, an understanding of the different archetypes can help isolate difficult behaviors so that they can be addressed effectively.
- Patient and clinician safety should always be paramount when addressing difficult personality traits and leaders should feel empowered to seek additional insistence if difficult behavior persists, despite initial corrective measures.

References

1. Porath C, Foulk T, Erez A. How incivility hijacks performance. Organ Dyn. 2015;4(44):258–65.
2. Pearson C, Porath C. On the nature, consequences, and remedies of workplace incivility: no time for "nice"? Think again. Acad Manag Exec. 2005;19(1):7–18.
3. Babchenko O, Scott K, Jung S, et al. Resident perspectives on effective surgical training: incivility, confidence, and mindset. J Surg Educ. 2020;77(5):1088–96.
4. Veyckemans F. The difficult colleague: about disruptive behaviors and narcissistic personalities. Pediatr Anaesth. 2021;31:6–7.
5. Gallo A. Getting along: how to work with anyone (even difficult people). Boston, MA: Harvard Business Review; 2022.
6. Corkin D, Yu S, Lindt S. Perfectionism, interpersonal problems, and stress generation: a short-term diary study examining cognitive-affective and behavioral pathways. Personal Individ Differ. 2017;116:67–72.
7. Cooper W, Spain D, Guillamondegui O, et al. Association of coworker reports about unprofessional behavior by surgeons with surgical complications in their patients. JAMA Surg. 2019;154(9):828–34.
8. Fast N, Chen S. When the boss feels inadequate: power, incompetence, and aggression. Psych Sci. 2009;20(11):1406–13.
9. Stecker M. Disruptive staff interactions: a serious source of inter-provider conflict and stress in healthcare settings. Issues Ment Heal. 2014;35:533–41.

10. Avesar M, Erez A, Essakow J, et al. The effects of rudeness, experience, and perspective-taking on challenging premature closure after pediatric ICU physicians receive hand-off with the wrong diagnosis: a randomized controlled simulation trial. Diagnosi. 2020;8(3):358–67.
11. Woolum A, Foulk T, Lanaj K, Erez A. Rude color glasses: the contaminating effects of witnessed morning rudeness on perceptions and behaviors throughout the workday. J Appl Psychol. 2017;102(12):1658–72.
12. Vukmir R. Disruptive healthcare provider behavior: an evidence-based guide. Springer International Publishing AG; 2016.
13. Santin B, Kaups K. The disruptive physician: addressing the issues. Bull Am Coll Surg. 2015;100(2):20–4.
14. Rosenstein AH. Managing disruptive behaviors in the health care setting: focus on obstetrics services. Am J Obstet Gynecol. 2011;204(3):187–92.

Dealing Effectively with Challenges

24

Abier A. Abdelnaby and Julie Ann Sosa

Introduction

There are a multitude of leadership challenges in 2023. These can include issues with personnel or other internal factors or external factors, to which leaders must react. Levels of unwellness and burn out in the work force are at an all-time high, and many of our colleagues are leaving healthcare altogether. Overcoming these obstacles is challenging but also provides opportunities, including the diversification of our surgical community and other overdue changes in the workforce to improve processes, and provides a greater sense of community among coworkers. Below, we will

A. A. Abdelnaby (✉)
Department of Surgery, Montefiore Medical Center, The University Hospital for Albert Einstein College of Medicine, Bronx, NY, USA
e-mail: aabdelnaby@montefiore.org

J. A. Sosa
Department of Medicine, Philip R. Lee Institute for Health Policy Studies, University of California San Francisco (UCSF), San Francisco, CA, USA

Department of Surgery, Philip R. Lee Institute for Health Policy Studies, University of California San Francisco (UCSF), San Francisco, CA, USA
e-mail: Julie.sosa@ucsf.edu

S. M. Johnson et al. (eds.), *The SAGES Manual of Strategy and Leadership*, https://doi.org/10.1007/978-3-031-62359-2_24

explore leadership challenges that may arise in any organization and provide tips for overcoming them.

Conflict in the Workplace

Employees and leaders may experience conflict that can cause disruptions and affect current and upcoming projects. Leaders seek to resolve issues to keep projects moving forward. This should involve first listening carefully and doing due diligence to establish the facts and to separate perceptions from reality, followed by speaking to each person involved in the conflict, offering solutions, revising current processes, and acting as a mediator so that the involved parties potentially can return to positive working relationships. When employees work together, they may have conflicting goals and workstyles. As a result, conflict is not uncommon. If you understand how to oversee conflict and interact with difficult people, you can turn potentially destructive forces into an opportunity for creativity and greater productivity. In informal conflict management, supervisors or employees may initiate a problem-solving process aimed at settling differences fairly, at an early stage, in an open manner, without retaliation, and as close in time as possible to the source of conflict. Informal conflict management may include mediation as a problem-solving strategy. When conflicts cannot be resolved through individual discussions, employees may initiate a formal complaint resolution process by filing a complaint or grievance. One good strategic approach for leaders today falls under the rubric of *Humble Inquiry: The Gentle Art of Asking Instead of Telling*, a book published first in 2013 by Edgar Schein [1]. The premise of the book is that "the partisan perspective outshouts the science" too often and "there is more actionable information in the details of what's really going on than in simply knowing what happened or what has changed." Therefore, leaders should inquire, listen, reflect, and only then act. Leadership comes from influence; in so doing, leaders move from the transactional to the personal [1].

Some tips for handling conflict in the workplace include:

Listen Carefully

- Listen to what the other person is saying instead of getting ready to react.
- Avoid interrupting the other person.
- After the other person finishes speaking, rephrase what was said to make sure you understand it.
- Ask questions to clarify your understanding.

Focus on Behavior and Events, Not on Personalities

- Say "When this happens ..." instead of "When you do ...".
- Describe a specific instance or event instead of generalizing.

Talk with All Involved Parties

- Ask the other person to name a time when it would be convenient to meet.
- Arrange to meet in a place where you will not be interrupted.

Identify Points of Agreement and Disagreement

- Summarize the areas of agreement and disagreement.
- Ask the other person if there is agreement about your assessment.

Modify your assessment until both of you agree on the areas of conflict.

Prioritize the Areas of Conflict

- Discuss which areas of conflict are most important for each of you to resolve.
- Develop a plan to work on each conflict, starting with the most important conflict.

Focus on the Future

- Set up future meeting times to continue your discussions.

Follow Through on Your Plan

- Stick with discussions until you have worked through each area of conflict.
- Maintain a collaborative, "let's-work-out-a-solution" attitude.

Build on Your Success

- Look for opportunities to point out progress.
- Compliment the other person's insights and achievements.

Congratulate each other when you make progress, even if it is just a small step. Your hard work will pay off when scheduled discussions eventually give way to ongoing, friendly communication.

Managing Up

What is managing up and why is it important?

Managing up is:

- Managing your relationship with your boss.
- Developing and cultivating a productive working rapport with your boss.
- Learning your boss's management, leadership, and communication styles and preferences.
- Increasing your awareness of your own work and communication style and preferences.
- Adapting and aligning the work styles of you and your boss to form a productive working relationship centered around mutual growth and understanding, work productivity, and career development.
- If we manage up successfully, we create a strong relationship with our supervisor that allows us each to have our work needs met and encourages each person to learn and grow. When managing up, it is very important to:
- NOT supervise or oversee your boss.
- NOT evaluate or judge your boss's management or leadership style.
- NOT change or develop your boss into a better manager or leader.

Not all leaders are created equally. Some have formal training, and some do not. In surgical residency, we do not receive formal leadership training, making it critically important to seek out training before you are in a leadership role. This can take the form of reading, attending courses and classes provided by professional academic and surgical societies and your institutions, as well as executive coaching, which in its best form is not intended just to remediate but rather to enhance leadership skills to make good leaders great. Some surgical leaders are more task oriented, while others are more relationship- and team-building-oriented. Some may be very present and attentive to our work, while others may encourage autonomy and a self-driven team.

Working Relationships with Difficult People

Listen Carefully

- Listen to what the other person is saying instead of getting ready to react.
- Avoid interrupting the other person.
- After the other person finishes speaking, rephrase what was said to make sure you understand it.

Be Honest and Direct

State your concern from your perspective, for example:

- I have a challenging time concentrating when...
- I cannot meet my deadlines if...
- It is hard for me to be positive when...

Avoid Blaming

Focus on the facts. Finding faults can prevent problem-solving.

Stay Focused

- Discuss particulars; avoid generalizing.
- Avoid getting sidetracked into discussing other problems.
- Keep bringing the conversation back to the concern you have stated.

Team Development and Teamwork

Without effective teamwork, productivity and quality of work will likely suffer, even with a group composed of multiple brilliant individuals. Likewise, without effective teams, a surgical department or organization will struggle to keep pace with the ever-changing demands of the field.

Multiple studies have shown that promoting good teamwork in the workplace will have positive effects on productivity, quality of work, creativity, innovation, and job satisfaction, all of which benefit the organization itself. In a recent study by Stanford, participants who were working on a team, as opposed to working alone persevered longer on difficult tasks, showed more interest and enjoyment in working on the tasks, required less self-regulatory effort to complete tasks, and generally performed better on the tasks. The participants who were part of a team even decided to do more tasks related to those performed in the study in a personal setting 1–2 weeks after the study [2].

Build Diverse and Inclusive Teams

First and foremost, it is important to focus on creating diverse teams rather than teams of all like-minded people. A group of people with diverse backgrounds and life experiences are more likely to bring diverse perspectives and ideas to the table. With more perspectives comes more thorough and inclusive decision-making. We tend to want to surround ourselves with people who think and act in ways that reflect our own thoughts and actions. While a group of like-minded individuals with similar backgrounds may get along well, we have to think about the bigger picture—Will they bring fresh ideas to the table? Will the team members challenge each other to tackle a project from all angles? Or will the team members be so agreeable that they produce ideas that do not get questioned or elaborated upon? If all team members think the same way, come from similar backgrounds, and have the same beliefs and opinions, the work that the team produces will likely be one-sided and less creative. However, if each team member has unique opinions, beliefs, and life experiences, they will likely produce work that reflects more creativity and innovation.

Clearly Define the Roles and Responsibilities of Every Team Member

When team members are unsure of their own tasks and responsibilities, it often creates tension within a team. It is important for each team member to know exactly what they are responsible for so that there is no overlap in projects. If multiple employees are working on the same task due to confusion in responsibility, invaluable time and team effort spent on the task will be wasted. Everyone should have responsibility for reaching the team goals as well as the tools and mutual support to obtain satisfactory results. Setting clear goals for each team member will help keep people aligned around their assigned tasks and responsibilities.

Build Trust Between Team Members

It is difficult to work productively with somebody who you do not trust. For this reason, trust is essential if you want to lead a successful team. Trust and respect between team members can flourish by doing something as simple as attending a happy hour together, participating in team-building activities, or simply eating lunch together [3]. It is important to encourage team members to interact with each other outside of their work; of course, this has become more challenging with the pandemic, where feelings of isolation prevail and more and more people have become inward facing toward their families and away and outside of the workplace Building trust will also likely increase employee morale and job satisfaction—work is more enjoyable when you enjoy the people you work with. In the end, finding the right balance of in person vs virtual activities is essential for faculty, learners, and especially staff colleagues, who have emerged as the most vulnerable members of our communities during the pandemic.

Encourage Frequent and Clear Communication

As the saying goes, communication is key! Though this sounds like basic knowledge, it is often passed over when analyzing how to improve teamwork in the workplace. We know that maintaining clear, frequent communication—especially with large and/or remote teams—is easier said than done. Clear and frequent communication will ensure that all team members are on the same page, leading to more accurate work being completed over a shorter timeline. Strong communication also helps to build trust between team members, thus improving the overall performance of the team. In the current era of digital health, it is also important not to overcommunicate, where information overload makes it more difficult for colleagues to triage important events from those that can be skipped.

Autonomy in Decision-Making

Trusting your team members to make their own decisions is important in building trust and improving teamwork. Oftentimes, if people do not have the autonomy and power to make decisions regarding their own work, they will begin to resent their work, thus hindering the work of the entire team. In order to keep team members engaged and working hard, it is important to provide all members with the freedom to make their own decisions.

Provide the Team with Learning Opportunities

Structuring Team Dynamics

If certain roles and/or responsibilities are not working out for some team members, it is important to make changes. You cannot be afraid to regroup and reassign tasks as necessary to improve the team dynamic. If team members are in roles in which they are not succeeding, this will negatively impact the entire team—in most teams, each person's work is dependent on the work of one or more other team members. Therefore, it is important to ensure that colleagues are in appropriate roles that will allow them to use the skills they have and unlock potential for themselves as well as the larger team.

Team Huddles/Meetings

Team meetings, however often they happen, should be used to plan, brainstorm, reflect, and share ideas. For example, they are an essential part of a "time out" in the operating room, to anticipate the challenges and equipment/materials needed for a case and then to debrief afterward about things that went well or did not go so well. They are frequently also used before or after clinics, to review the patients seen and the outstanding work that requires follow-up by different members. It is important to keep team meetings focused and useful in for efficiency to prevail. No matter how often teams meet, they should have a structured plan for each meeting. Circulating an agenda before a meeting so that colleagues can come prepared and avoid wasted time is helpful. Meetings are a time to focus on opportunities for collaboration, brainstorming, and creating a plan to move forward.

Diversity and Inclusion

Diversity and inclusion are two interconnected concepts—but they are far from interchangeable. Diversity is about representation or the make-up of an entity. Inclusion is about how well the contributions, presence, and perspectives of diverse groups of people are valued and integrated into an environment. Any environment, where many different genders, races, nationalities, and sexual orientations and identities are present but only the perspectives of certain groups are valued or carry any authority or influence, may be diverse, but they will not be inclusive. Historically, many departments of surgery have hired the exact same type of faculty members and learners over and over; for that reason, American surgery was populated largely by cis- white men for a very long time. The thinking was that if employee X is doing a great job and everyone gets along with them, then the smart thing to do must be to hire more people exactly like them. This strategy leads chairs or division and section chiefs to seek out faculty, residents, and fellow candidates who mirror their existing workforce. In this framework, they look for the same educational background and skill sets, source from the same narrow list of medical centers, and look for similar personality traits during interviews. As a result, a department or surgical team can come to look, think, and—to a degree—act almost exactly the same. Not only does this tend to result in a reduction in diversity of thought (among other aspects of diversity), but it can prevent the department or surgical team from realizing its true potential. Fresh new perspectives are necessary to bring forth bold innovative ideas, challenge long-standing inward looking thinking, and lead to innovation and discovery.

Here are a few strategies to consider:

- Build self-awareness around your biases. To create an inclusive work environment, you must first be comfortable recognizing situations in which your biases are most likely to negatively impact your decision-making or judgment.
- Practice active listening. In a culturally diverse workplace, successful chairs, section/division chiefs, and laboratory managers know how to interact with people who have different communication styles (verbal, nonverbal, written, or visual), approaches to problem-solving, and even methods of asking for help.
- Ensure equity in retention and promotion. Hold yourself accountable to your diversity, equity, and inclusion goals by tracking how merits and promotions are awarded on your team and within the larger school of medicine or healthcare system. Reviewing compensation and benchmarking it to local, regional, or national milestones is essential to retain and recruit the very best colleagues. When inequities are identified, it is essential to work explicitly on how to address them. At many public institutions like the University of California, salaries and compensation are publicly available, making it easier for

faculty members to raise concerns when inequities exist. Anticipating such and being proactive around remediating inequity is important.
- In so doing, it is essential to avoid falling back to the concept of "meritocracy," which is a principle in academic medicine that is unfortunately fraught with privilege.

When a leader demonstrates cultural competence, they show respect for cultural differences and recognize how those differences drive engagement, productivity, and innovation on their teams and throughout a department of surgery or school of medicine. Developing this level of fluency is not easy, and there is no finish line. It is a lifelong process of self-assessment and curiosity. Know that it starts at the top. While not impossible, it will likely prove difficult to gain traction on diversity initiatives without the expressed commitment from leaders to make a difference. If existing leaders do not acknowledge their own privilege or view their lack of diversity as a challenge, their demanding that colleagues focus on solving these challenging issues is unlikely to result in there being meaningful traction. The bottom line is that whatever your department chair or chief declares to be important is usually what everyone else will focus on. You cannot just wish diversity into reality; the work is hard, and it must be continuous, or change will not be durable. Recruitment should be ambitious, with goals that are aligned with those of a school of medicine or academic health system in order to gain momentum. Diversity, equity, and inclusion priorities should be stated, and there should be accountability for leaders. Search committees should be diverse; at the University of California San Francisco, every search committee should be made up of half women and/or underrepresented in medicine minorities. Holistic review should be deployed, and selection should be made based on a job description. All faculty members, staff, and learners should complete substantive unconscious bias training, and this could be bolstered for search committee members [4]. Allyship with affinity groups like the Association of Women Surgeons, the Society of Black Academic Surgeons, the Latino Surgical Society, the Society of Asian

Academic Surgeons, and the Association of Out Surgeons and their allies can help to identify a more diverse set of candidates. Also, it is important to keep in mind that for diversity, equity, and inclusion efforts to move forward in a meaningful and sustainable way, structural change will be required. This requires leadership, resourcing, and courage.

Benefits of diversity, equity, and inclusion initiatives:

- Higher productivity.
- Greater readiness to innovate.
- Increased ability to recruit a diverse talent pool.
- Higher faculty and staff retention.
- Less bias.
- Better organizational culture overall.

Leading Change in the Workplace

When change occurs in the workplace, it affects the ways our colleagues do their jobs. Change management is the systematic approach to handling the transformation of a department's policies, systems, or goals. Leadership facilitates change management by formulating strategies that ensure a smooth transition. Effective change management strategies take a variety of aspects into consideration to optimize the impact of a change before it has been implemented. Changes in the workplace can impact performance and outlook, so it is important to understand (and anticipate) the positive and negative outcomes that can occur. Change opens the door for opportunity but does not guarantee a good outcome. Surgeons—all of us - tend to resist change because we may feel we cannot adapt or that we will lose our relevance within our department or team. Change is also hard because it brings into conflict tensions between survival anxiety—where we know we need to change and evolve to survive in a changing world—and learning anxiety, which comes from the fact that to change, we need to unlearn and then relearn what we do; this requires significant energy and time, making it hard. But change is essential; a great published around the time of the pandemic is *Think Again:*

The Power of Knowing What You Don't Know by Adam Grant [5]. When change implementation goes wrong, it is often because of a lack of consideration for how the change affects the department or organization as a whole. Offering transparency, effective communication, and support at all levels can make for smoother transitions and happier colleagues. When managed poorly, changes implemented by an organization may cause:

- Communication breakdown: When a change is made without proper communication, colleagues may feel as if their input is irrelevant and become less likely to speak up in the future when it is important.
- Surgeon disengagement: When a department, division, or team does not properly assess how a change will affect its team members, they may feel leaders are being inconsiderate. Colleagues may become much less involved in department or division/section culture if they feel their well-being does not matter.
- Resistance to future changes: If changes have negatively affected colleagues, those may make them more hesitant to trust a leader. This can lead to negative behaviors and deficient performance [6].
- Less engagement: When there are major changes to tools or processes, it is natural to see a temporary decline in productivity; however, if employees are not trained properly, they may feel overwhelmed and give up. When managed effectively, change in the workplace may result in:

Employee skill growth: If your team's routine or your clinical practice has become stale, staff may not have a chance to grow and develop. Change can provide the opportunity to nurture new skills and specialties that help your department.

- **Improvement of morale:** Colleagues who see your team as ready to adapt to new circumstances may feel more confident about its future performance.
- **Opportunities for advancement**: Your department/division/section/lab may need to create new roles to facilitate changes

in the workplace, which means more opportunities for colleagues to advance.
- **Cultural development:** Good change management offers the chance for colleagues to speak up about their concerns regarding the status quo, which can facilitate cultural growth.

Most changes can be classified as one of the following:

- **Developmental changes**: Changes that are aimed at improving what the surgical team is currently doing. Adjusting existing skills, methods, metrics, and/or conditions are all types of developmental changes.
- **Transformative changes:** Plans to completely reshape the strategy, processes, and culture of your department, making a transformative change. These are usually in response to an unpredicted or extreme shift like the pandemic.
- **Transitional changes:** Replacing leadership is a transitional change. There are many effective strategies to choose from when it comes to workplace change management, and they all share common factors that increase the likelihood for success. Managing change in the workplace can be a daunting process for any surgical department or team, but by implementing these practices, you can create an effective strategy that makes it more likely that your goals will come to fruition.
  - **Clarify your goal:** Evaluate how your team is performing and what improvements need to be made for future success. Envisioning a clear picture of your goals is an essential step before creating an action plan. An executive coach can help to do this. Alternatively, coming together with your leadership team or the larger department via a retreat or facilitated process for forming strategy.
  - **Define the change:** Once you know what needs to change, try to categorize it. Changes can be defined by what aspect of your team they will impact, such as organizational, procedural, or cultural changes. Refine the language that you

use to describe the change you want so that it can be clearly conveyed to others. Communication is key!

- **Assess potential challenges:** Any significant changes in the workplace will have their own set of challenges. Sit down with departmental experts and stakeholders to discuss how your plans may impact their teams.
- **Create a roadmap:** Before implementing any changes, it is essential to create a plan that navigates where pain points can occur. Though creating an action plan can be daunting, you do not need to reinvent the wheel. Consider preestablished models, such as Lewin's change management model or Kotter's eight-step process for leading change [7].
- **Establish measurable goals**: Unless measurable goals are established, there is no objective way to monitor progress or identify success. Organize your action plan into smaller, more manageable goals, and then consider what metrics you will use to measure them.
- **Listen to feedback:** Create focus groups and seek feedback. Identify key players who have the respect of their coworkers and can articulate concerns from the perspective of faculty, staff, and learners.
- **Invest in training:** Training your deputies like section chiefs and directors as well as staff managers and chief/senior residents can give them the tools they need to confidently support teams through the adjustment period.
- **Foster transparency:** Openly providing information and updates about your plan helps to create a feeling of certainty within the workplace. Employees are likely to perform better if they have a clear understanding of what is going on and why it is happening.
- **Demonstrate patience**: It is important to keep a calm and confident demeanor during a challenging adjustment period. If a worst-case scenario does occur, remember that no one works well in a panic. React with a cool head, and your employees will likely do the same.
- **Reward satisfactory performance:** Rewarding employees who perform well during transitional periods can incentivize others to do the same. One option may be to offer

performance-based rewards to employees who eagerly embrace the changes you have made.

Conclusion

Dealing effectively with challenges is a skill that can help you cope with difficulties that may arise in the surgical workplace. In this chapter, we reviewed some strategies that will help you overcome those challenges and obstacles. If you have clear plans and goals, obstacles and challenges become much easier to handle, as they are no longer seen as chaotic and random. If you feel like you are facing a challenge you need to overcome, the first step toward the resolution should be **defining the problem**. Make sure all parties involved agree on the problem and participate in ways to resolve that problem. Trust and teamwork are keys to successful resolution of identified problems and conflict resolution. Team building and structuring are also key to success in the world of surgery. Identifying roles for team members helps them unlock individual strengths and increases self-esteem and positive attitudes. Implementing strategies that increase diversity and inclusion within departments of surgery can drive engagement, productivity, as well as critical innovation.

SAGES Takeaway

- Diversity and inclusion result in innovation and faculty retention.
- Open communication and teamwork can eliminate workplace conflict.
- Adapting and aligning the work styles of you and your boss to form a productive working relationship centered around mutual growth and understanding, work productivity, and career development.
- Team building and focusing on team dynamics is key to success in the workplace.

Disclosures JAS is a member of the Data Monitoring Committee of the Medullary Thyroid Cancer Consortium Registry supported by Novo Nordisk,

Astra Zeneca, and Eli Lilly. Institutional research funding was received from Exelixis and Eli Lilly.

References

1. Schein EH, Schein PA. Humble inquiry the gentle art of asking instead of telling. Berrett-Koehler Publishers; 2021.
2. TMA World. Stanford study demonstrates how collaboration and teamwork can dramatically improve productivity. TMA World; 17 Aug. 2021. https://www.tmaworld.com/2017/08/24/stanford-study-demonstrates-how-collaboration-and-teamwork-can-dramatically-improve/.
3. 8 Useful Ways to Enhance Teamwork in the Workplace. LumApps. www.lumapps.com/employee-experience/improve-teamwork-in-the-workplace/. Accessed 29 July 2023.
4. Hays-Thomas R. Diversity, equity, and inclusion in organizations. In: Managing workplace diversity, equity, and inclusion; 2022. p. 3–22. https://doi.org/10.4324/9780367808884-2.
5. Grant AM. Think again: the power of knowing what you do not know. Penguin Random House; 2023.
6. Kotter JP. Leading change: a conversation with John P. Kotter. Strategy Leadership. 1997;25(1):18–23. https://doi.org/10.1108/eb054576.
7. Bedard A. The 8-step process for leading change: Dr. John Kotter. Kotter International Inc.; 2023. www.kotterinc.com/methodology/8-steps/

Part VI

Leading Others—Engagement/ Consensus Building

Organizational Strategic Planning

25

Danny Mou, Jon C. Gould,
Deidra J. Sampson, and Edward Lin

Developing a Strategic Plan

Establish a Steering Committee

The development of a strategic plan begins with identifying the priorities of the organization. A steering committee should be created to lead this initiative. The steering committee should include relevant stakeholders of the overarching direction of the organiza-

D. Mou (✉)
Minimally Invasive Surgery, Department of Surgery,
Emory University, Atlanta, GA, USA
e-mail: danny.mou@emory.edu

J. C. Gould
Division of Minimally Invasive and Gastrointestinal Surgery,
Department of Surgery, Medical College of Wisconsin,
Milwaukee, WI, USA
e-mail: jgould@mcw.edu

D. J. Sampson
Emory Healthcare, Atlanta, GA, USA
e-mail: Deidra.Sampson@emoryhealthcare.org

E. Lin
Division of General and GI Surgery, Department of Surgery,
Emory University, Atlanta, GA, USA
e-mail: elin2@emory.edu

S. M. Johnson et al. (eds.), *The SAGES Manual of Strategy and Leadership*, https://doi.org/10.1007/978-3-031-62359-2_25

tion. For a department, this may include individuals within the department such as the department chair, division chiefs, clinical and research leaders, and administrative staff. The committee should also include more hospital systems-level members beyond the department who can assess the strategies from a systems perspective. These members may include vice-president (VP) and director-level executives in strategic planning and network development. Having this perspective is important as there may be similar initiatives in other departments. Awareness of this may prevent duplicative efforts within the same health system. Finally, if there are any external third-party consultants or strategists involved, they should be a part of the steering committee. These third-party members may not have specific institutional knowledge or a deep sense of the organization's culture, but they do bring with them experience from other similar organizations or have familiarity with regulatory or payor agencies (i.e., external forces), which may facilitate the strategic development process. The steering committee should have a clear place in the organization chart so that its relationships with other committees are well-defined (Fig. 25.1). When recruiting the steering committee, it is advisable to set a commitment duration, be it several months to a year, with expectations for attendance and workload (e.g., 1–2 h a week). The urgency and scope of the work at hand are reflected in the duration and workload. Very few strategic planning committees should last more than one year, with the implementation phase handed off to those who will execute the plans. The committee or its subcommittees should have executive sponsors who do not have to be the chairs but are present to maintain alignment with organizational purpose and goals. *The make-up of the steering committee members can come from different experience strata, and in our experience, two essential qualities make the most effective members. First, these members are trusted and have influence with their peers. Second, they have a track record of producing deliverables on time in prior tasks.*

After a steering team has been finalized, it is helpful to set a timeline for the series of meetings that will be needed to complete

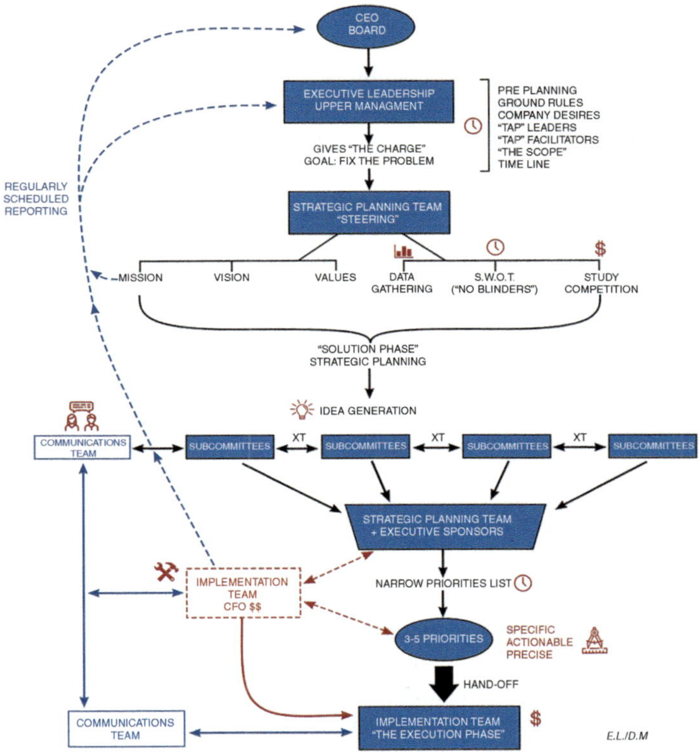

Fig. 25.1 Example of how a strategic planning team may fit into an institution's organizational chart. Solid line = direct relationships; Dotted line = indirect relationships; Clock = significant time requirement; Dollar = significant resource requirement. *CEO* chief executive officer, *CFO* chief financial officer, *XT* cross-talk, *SWOT* strengths, weaknesses, opportunities, threats

a strategic plan. This timeline often includes meetings for the kickoff event, developing the mission and/or vision statement, identifying market benchmarks, assessing the department's current state, setting near-term and long-term goals, and developing a tracking system for progress toward those goals.

Identify Strategic Priorities

One of the first steering committee meetings should be dedicated to identifying the organization's vision and mission statement. The vision is the state where the organization aspires to be. An example would be: "To be the nation's leading academic department of surgery." A mission statement is a summary of the organization's purpose, who it serves, and its long-term approach to realizing its goals. As an example, the mission statement for a major academic surgery department can be: "We are dedicated to providing high value, compassionate care to every patient through collaborative, team-based approaches, as we define the future of surgery through discovery and education." The vision and mission statements help guide the steering committee to prioritize initiatives that contribute most to those statements. When investing in major new initiatives, it is always wise to revisit the mission statement to ensure that these initiatives are in line with the mission statement.

Next, the steering committee should develop a consensus around long-term initiatives for the organization. This includes but is not limited to continued investment in existing areas of excellence, identifying areas of weakness that require more resources, or implementing new projects from scratch. Each of these initiatives should then be assigned a priority level. For example, a healthcare system that is suffering from severe clinical staff shortages and consequent financial hardship may need to address those issues before ensuring sufficient funding for research conferences. Conversely, if a healthcare system prioritizes becoming a leading academic medical center but is suffering from an exodus of talented physician researchers, then ensuring funding for research conferences becomes a more urgent matter. Oftentimes some of the priorities at the systems level have already been outlined by the hospital leadership such as the hospital chief executive officer (CEO) or board of trustees. For example, if hospital length-of-stay reduction is a healthcare systems-level priority, it is advisable to prioritize these initiatives at the department level. Doing so may not only demonstrate to the hospital leadership that the department is prioritizing their interests but also create opportunities for collaboration with the hospital system at large.

Each initiative should have a clear timeframe and scope. It is tempting to pitch lofty ideas that transform the status quo, but these ideas need to be realistic in terms of scope, time, and resources needed. These metrics should be agreed upon to minimize "scope creep" of projects, which is an indolent expansion of the scope of work over time. Long-term projects and projects that have multiple leaders over their lifespan are particularly at risk for scope creep, which can lead to significant wasted resources and frustration among team members.

Where Are We Now? The Organizational Environmental Assessment

Once a set of long-term strategic priorities is outlined, the steering committee should lead a comprehensive assessment of its organization. This environmental assessment evaluates the organization's current position through a combination of surveys, focus groups, interviews, and benchmarking exercises. It is critical that this internal assessment is as accurate as possible. All the techniques employed should optimize for honest feedback from the organization's members. Honest feedback may be difficult to elicit in a culture where employees do not speak up due to hierarchical norms or fear of retaliation. This culture needs to be corrected. Some techniques to promote honest feedback include making the surveys anonymous when possible. Focus groups and interviews should be conducted by third parties and kept anonymous when possible. Failure to elicit honest feedback has enormous consequences. It will result in an inaccurate picture of an organization's capabilities and shortcomings. With an inaccurate starting point, all subsequent strategies are at risk of failing.

The environmental assessment also evaluates the organization's current and historical performance trends and identifies strengths and weaknesses. It also assesses the existing macro trends to determine opportunities and threats. For example, an academic department historically has held a dominant market position, serving the majority of the regional market share. However, several other regional hospitals recently merged and have created a combined network that is now larger than the department, resulting in its significant loss of market share. This concerning development should prompt the department to prioritize competing with the newly merged hospital system, be it in expanding the existing referral network, improving efficiencies, and service offerings, or patient access.

Often, self-diagnosis will require time and budget to gather information through focused surveys, mass surveys, retrieve market analysis data, and accessing databanks. Multiple inputs are always best to understand the current state of the organization to avoid making decisions based on anecdotes or personal experience.

The result of the organization's environmental assessment should be a document that accurately outlines the organization's **s**trengths, **w**eaknesses, **o**pportunities, and **t**hreats. This outline (the SWOT analysis) will serve as the "starting point" for the organization (Fig. 25.2). It is also advisable for different members to be assigned to analyze each SWOT category so that the report outs are specific and clear. The SWOT analysis is only one way to diagnose your organization's current state. *There are many tools*

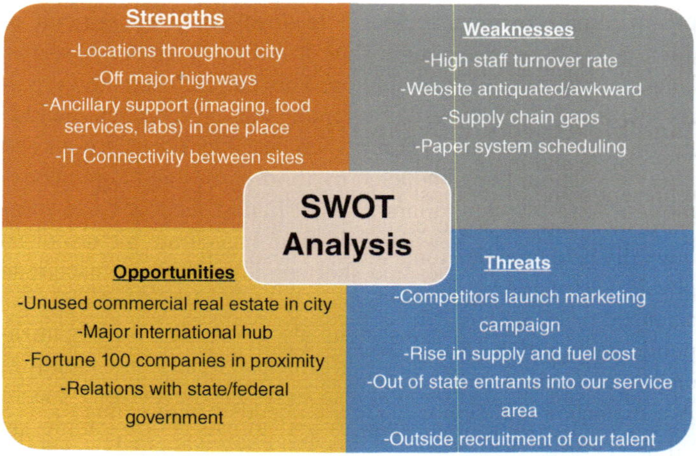

Fig. 25.2 Example of a strengths, weaknesses opportunities, threats (SWOT) analysis for a healthcare system

for self-diagnosis but all should be used to compare your organization to competitors or regulatory benchmarks (e.g., how are we doing compared to what is required of us or compared to our peers?)

Where Do We Want to Be? The Desired Future State

To determine what an organization wants to become, it is instructive to look at other best-in-class organizations. As an example, when a new department chair developed a strategic plan for the large academic department, she and her team performed a comprehensive analysis of leading departments that excelled in the tripartite mission of clinical, education, and research excellence [1]. Each of these areas was defined by objective metrics. Benchmark institutions were initially identified by eliciting the perspectives of clinicians, patients, students, and researchers. The clinical performance of these departments was ranked based on a combination of inpatient volume, average Case Mix Index (CMI), and the number of divisions that are nationally ranked in the US News and World Report. Research performance was evaluated by NIH funding and the alumni publication percentile. Finally, education performance was evaluated for the reputation of the residency per the Doximity Residency Navigator Tool and the size of the residency. The steering committee assessed its own performance along the same metrics and graphically displayed how they compared to the best-in-class institutions. This provides a compelling depiction of where they excel and where they can improve.

The steering committee observed from their research that leading departments focused their efforts on four areas: investing in people, clinical excellence, intentional research development, and financial profitability and autonomy. These areas were explored in more detail to reveal productive practices that are worthy of emulating. For example, leading departments invest in their people through formal programs to promote an inclusive, collaborative culture. Such programs include 360 feedback platforms, paid psychologists to coach clinicians, formal leadership development opportunities, formal interfaculty mentoring programs, and annual retreats. Formal career tracks have been developed to align with the research, clinical, and educational goals of the department. Given historical financial biases toward clinical output, some institutions implemented compensation models that reward research and teaching. Departments that lead in research were observed to physically colocate researchers near the operating rooms (ORs) to promote collaboration and optimize convenience. Some department chairs invested significantly in a small group of high-caliber investigators to generate tremendous academic output. Other department leaders pursued the strategy of hiring the best researchers and supporting them at the department level (not the divisional level) to ensure long-term and consistent support. For clinical excellence, leading departments catalyzed quality improvement (QI) projects by requiring each division to have at least three active QI projects at any given time. Other leaders scheduled regular meetings to identify clinical growth opportunities, updated the department website, and even invested in tailored teams to equip new physicians with marketing and strategy advice. Finally, financially successful departments often mandate division profitability, some with profit margin requirements. Other leaders explored alternative revenue streams such as philanthropic campaigns and business model restructuring. Several department chairs made the department finances available to each division on a monthly basis and provided financial training to the faculty.

From this best-in-class benchmarking exercise, many ideas and strategies will likely resonate with the steering committee. Seeing how other leading departments achieve their status minimizes “reinventing the wheel” for an organization. Beyond just understanding how other departments excel, it can be productive to reach out to relevant contacts there to ask about how they were so effective, lessons learned, and anticipated obstacles. A 30-min conversation can save months of work when talking to people who have achieved what an organization is attempting to achieve.

As the ideation process evolves, it is necessary to have regular check-ins with executive teams to assure alignment with organizational missions and goals. These usually take on the form of executive summaries and present unfinished work as the product takes shape.

It is natural for an organization to aspire to great heights. *The most difficult part of the strategic planning process is paring down the number of priorities and then ordering each priority by importance. This is when the leader has to steer the emotions and passions of the strategic planning team who have all labored over and taken over ownership of ideas for the last several months, fully understanding that it is impossible to tackle every initiative.* An indispensable aspect of this stage of ranking priorities should be listing out priorities and plotting them based on urgency, impact, and effort (including cost and resources). Team polling usually allows the entire team to rank each priority on these parameters to reach a comprehensive picture of what needs to be done and the cost of achieving them. High-cost-low-impact items can probably be eliminated from the next iteration of the poll. High-impact-high-cost priorities will depend on the urgency of the matter. The final work product of the strategic planning process should be a short list (three to five priorities), has actionable priorities, uses precise language that everyone understands, lists desired outcomes, has a delivery date, and is measured by numbers.

Executing the Strategic Plan

The strategic planning team and the execution team do not have to be the same personnel, and in fact, the skill sets are often different. However, key leaders and some staff overlap will be necessary for continuity and remaining true to the original priorities.

Once a set of strategic initiatives has been finalized by the steering committee, there are several important considerations to maximize the chance for success. These include identifying implementation leaders, finalizing the timeline and scope, developing a progress tracking system, and implementing a communication plan.

For each strategic initiative, the steering committee should identify a leader who will be responsible for the progress and ultimately the completion of the initiative. It is important that this leader not only possesses the qualifications and experience to fulfill this role but that he/she should also have enough time given his/her existing role in the department. There may be many qualified physicians to lead projects, but if they are clinically busy and have ongoing research projects, they may simply not be able to dedicate sufficient time to new initiatives. Thus, it may be necessary to internally fund positions to provide the necessary protected time for team leaders to effectively execute their projects.

As mentioned earlier, clearly defining the scope and timeline of new strategic initiatives is paramount. Each initiative should be impactful and meaningful but also realistic and time-bound. Clearly articulating these boundaries will minimize wasted or misdirected resources and facilitate subsequent progress evaluations.

A critical component of the successful execution of a strategic plan involves developing a rigorous progress-tracking system. Each strategic initiative needs to have a set of objective target metrics that once achieved, indicates that the initiative has succeeded. Between the starting point and these targets, there should be objectively measurable milestones—commonly the key performance indicator (KPI)—over the specified timeline. It should be emphasized that these milestones should be objectively measurable to prevent getting a subjective sense that a project is moving along when it is actually stalling. The leader of each initiative should be held accountable for meeting these milestones. It is advisable that these initiative timelines are developed by people with operational experience. Various tracking tools are available at the American Association of Medical College (AAMC) Strategic Planning Affinity Group website [2]. Our experience is that tasks involving consensus-building or collaboration among multiple different collaborators may often take longer than planned. For example, an initiative to launch an IT platform collecting clinical data across five divisions will require buy-in from many stakeholders ranging from division chiefs to physicians to nurses to medical assistants. Such an initiative will likely require significant time up front to build consensus among these team members prior to operationalizing. Periodic meetings should be scheduled to review the progress of the initiatives. After the launch of the strategic initiatives, the steering committee should anticipate making frequent adjustments to the timeline, resource allocation, and even scope. Being adaptable in real time is critical to completing strategic initiatives.

Finally, a communication plan is an important part of successfully executing a strategic plan. Relevant stakeholders for each initiative should be updated regarding the progress at regular intervals. Stakeholders may include faculty, hospital staff, hospital executives, philanthropists, politicians, and influencers. Progress updates should provide a cogent summary of tasks completed and the next steps. This is an effective platform to recognize team members who have put forth a lot of effort. It is also a good place to highlight successes to date, no matter how small, to motivate the team. Beyond regular communication, it is productive to have regular social events for teams to promote team member bonding outside of a work environment. There is strong evidence that these "teaming" exercises can significantly improve productivity and decrease burnout [3].

Lessons Learned

Having a linear series of steps to plan organizational strategy is reassuring, but anyone with experience leading organizations will be able to attest to the fact that executing these strategies is anything but linear. There will be constant surprises, unforeseen challenges, complaints, interpersonal conflicts, and many other obstacles that arise and threaten to doom the strategic initiatives. We have outlined some of the lessons learned in our experience. Industries where the climates change fast and often without warning, such as a major pandemic for healthcare organizations, need to move with more speed and precision than others.

Balance Vision with Practicality

Though it is always tempting to pursue initiatives with transformative impact, these projects need to be balanced by practicality, given time and resource constraints. This is where having experts with prior experience is critical. A hospital executive or department chair's vision may need to be adjusted to the realities of practical limitations. This "practicality" assessment is something that should be continuously assessed throughout each strategic initiative. This is important because some projects start off but encounter obstacles later on that may prompt re-scoping the original goals. An effective project leader should always have a sense of this and be able to both manage the project's team members and manage the expectations of his/her superiors. Strategic plans that fail are usually due to a deficiency in one of the following three items: talent, resources, and funds. When a project stalls, it is worth asking which of these key ingredients is missing and then addressing the deficiency. Leaders should keep in mind that when expertise or talent is lacking, outsourcing certain components of the project is a potential option. For every project, there is a point where giving more sources may not justify the investment into that project. We suggest that the steering committee should incorporate "circuit breakers" that alert the team when the return on investment of the initiative is becoming less than the original investment. Should this be the case, serious consideration should be given to stopping the project (e.g., exit ramp).

The Four P's Framework

In any organization, all the planning tends to distill down to developing **p**olicies that can be understood, creating **p**rocesses that can be followed, making appropriate use of the **p**hysical space, and mobilizing the **p**eople involved. Considering these 4 P's serve as the operational framework for moving an organization toward a goal.

Conclusion

Strategic planning is a critical step for an organization to realize its aspirations. It should objectively display where the organization currently stands, summarize its short-term and long-term goals, and outline how to achieve those goals. Strategic initiatives should be developed with both regulators and market competitors in mind. Each initiative should abide by all regulatory standards and ideally differentiate the organization from its competitors. Planning is usually done by one team who thinks strategically, while another team with specific skillsets takes over the execution. Poorly derived plans are difficult to execute and poor execution derails any good plan. Some have estimated that two-thirds of strategic plans fail ("shelved") because people lose sight of the intentions (i.e., the vision). In contrast, the best execution of strategic plans—the ones that do not get shelved—is measured by frequency of communication and re-communication, frequency of vision casting, broadcasting milestones that can be verified, open ownership of failures (which earns trust), low team turnovers, and completion ahead of schedule.

SAGES Takeaway

- Effective strategic planning requires a systematic, candid assessment of an organization's current state, creating a vision for the organization's future state and developing a plan to achieve that future state.
- The strategic plan should clearly identify and prioritize specific actionable goals with measurable endpoints.
- Understanding an organization's strengths, weaknesses, opportunities, and threats provides a helpful framework to guide strategic priorities.
- A strategic plan should make any deviations from the plan appear obvious so that they can be addressed promptly.

References

1. Kibbe MR, Buckio J. Developing and implementing a department of surgery strategic plan. Chapel Hill: University of North Carolina; 2018.
2. AAMC. Affinity group: strategic planning. https://www.aamc.org/career-development/affinity-groups/gip/strategic-planning. Accessed 11 May 2023.
3. Wisner PS, Feist HA. Does teaming pay off? Strategic Finance. 2001;82(8):58–64.

Achieving Effective Data Analysis and Research

26

Laura Fischer

Introduction

The core mission of the surgeon is to provide the highest quality of care for patients with surgical disease, which accounts for an estimated one-third of the global burden of disease [1]. In order to fulfill this mission, it is vitally important that surgeons continue to be leaders in the field of scientific research to develop a deeper understanding of the fundamental contributors to biologic disease. Although surgeon-scientists face significant challenges such as ever-increasing clinical and administrative demands, decreased funding opportunities [2], and insufficient protected time [2–4], surgeons stand at a critical crossroad between clinical experience and the basic science laboratory. Without the input, insight, and direction that surgeons can provide by virtue of direct patient interaction in the clinical setting, our scientific community runs the risk of performing scientific experiments that do not improve patient care and potentially waste valuable time and money.

L. Fischer (✉)
OU Health Metabolic & Bariatric Surgery Program, University of Oklahoma, Oklahoma City, OK, USA

Department of Surgery, University of Oklahoma, Oklahoma City, OK, USA
e-mail: laura-fischer@ouhsc.edu

S. M. Johnson et al. (eds.), *The SAGES Manual of Strategy and Leadership*, https://doi.org/10.1007/978-3-031-62359-2_26

Surgeon-scientists are uniquely positioned to provide highly specialized and innovative solutions to complex problems in healthcare [5].

Research Tracks

Basic Science

Basic science research, also called "bench research," aims to discover the underlying mechanisms behind biologic processes and disease [6]. This can encompass a variety of scientific disciplines, including biochemistry, biology, chemistry, physics, pharmacology, chemistry, physics, as well as behavioral and social sciences. Basic science research involves the development of hypothesis-driven experimental designs that can be tested, revised, and consistently replicated by others [6]. There are several areas of basic science research including the following: (1) in vitro studies which are experiments performed in a controlled laboratory setting, often using cells or tissue cultures as a substrate and focusing on mechanisms at the molecular or cellular level; (2) animal studies, often using mice or rats, to study biological processes and disease mechanisms in the context of a whole organism; and (3) computational models which use mathematical models to simulate complex biologic processes and make outcome predictions.

Translational

Translational research aims to move scientific discoveries from the "bench" laboratory to clinical care in order to improve healthcare delivery. At its most fundamental roots, basic science research is pure scientific discovery without explicit consideration of the practical implications; translational research tries to bridge this gap [7]. There are four phases of translational research: T1, "development of concepts and discoveries from basic science research through early phase clinical trials"; T2, "establishment of efficacy in humans and clinical guidelines"; T3, "implementation and dissemination of phase T2 research results"; and T4, "assessment of outcomes and effectiveness of clinical interventions in populations" [7]. Early translational research can be difficult to distinguish from basic science research, while late translational research overlaps significantly with clinical and outcomes research. Estimates of average time needed for a scientific discovery to be established in clinical care is currently between 17 and 24 years [7]. Translational research is critically important to accelerate the process of delivering new interventions, such as new cancer drugs or surgical devices, directly to the patients who need them.

Clinical and Outcomes

Clinical research, including a subset called outcomes research, is a term used to describe research studies analyzing clinical outcomes, such as morbidity, mortality, and quality of life following specific healthcare interventions in large cohorts of patients. The benefit of large populations studies is that they minimize selection and referral bias that are inherent in smaller, institutional studies [8] and they can help to answer research questions that are not amenable to randomized controlled trials (RCT) due to limitations of feasibility or ethics [8]. Outcomes studies can be complementary to RTCs as they can help to answer whether a particular finding from an RCT is generalizable to a larger population [8]. Some limitations to outcomes studies is that there is generally limited ability to control the quality and completeness of clinically relevant data in large, national databases or data derived from insurance companies or healthcare systems. Additionally, because outcomes studies do not have the rigorous control of other research methods, they are susceptible to bias; therefore, clinical inferences from study results should be made with caution [8]. However, despite these limitations, there are many examples where outcomes research has led to substantial improvement in the delivery of surgical care, such as the extensive, comprehensive improvement in quality and safety that the bariatric surgery community has produced over the past 20 years [9].

Quality Improvement

Quality improvement research is a fairly new branch of academic surgery that focuses on developing, instituting, and evaluating "systematic efforts to improve the value, quality, and safety of healthcare" [10]. Initial consensus guidelines for performing quality improvement (QI) research were published in 2008 [11] and a revised version in 2016 [10], termed "Standards for QUality Improvement Reporting Excellence" or "SQUIRE." These guidelines aimed to increase the completeness, precision, and transparency of QI research publications. QI research has dramatically changed the healthcare landscape by introducing systematic processes to improve quality and safety, in addition to measure the efficacy of the processes themselves. In particular, SQUIRE focuses on inclusion of key features such as "context" and "ethics" in study protocols, in order to better aid the interpretation and application of results. The key aspect of quality improvement research is the focus on the *study* of an intervention rather than the *performance* of an intervention. The focus of the study is not on the quality improvement per se but rather on whether the intervention was effective in achieving predefined goals [10]. Protocols for formal intervention testing to evaluate whether the intervention is associated with the observed changes and the overall impact of the intervention are the primary components of a QI project. Mechanisms for how the intervention did or did not achieve the observed changes, as well as theoretical mechanisms are included in the interpretation of the data analysis.

Getting Started

Developing a productive research career is challenging in today's academic healthcare landscape. Surgeon-scientists are often clinically busy with expectations to perform a certain volume of clinical work, making it difficult to devote the time and energy needed to perform valuable research. It is important to consider multiple factors in order to maximize efficiency and cost-effectiveness. The most vital characteristic of a first faculty appointment is a supportive environment with engaged and effective mentorship [12]. Trainees in search of a first faculty position should seek out surgery departments that have a track record for training and supporting young surgical investigators [12].

Negotiating a Research Package

During a job search, faculty can negotiate with the department of surgery for a research package. This generally includes some measure of salary support for the surgeon to spend a percent of time away from clinical, revenue-generating duties, financial support for laboratory materials and equipment, and salary support for research team members, such as post-doctoral students, laboratory technicians, and research coordinators. Research support through an academic department should be used as bridge funding to obtain preliminary data in order to be competitive for independent, extramural grants that will carry faculty's research projects forward [13].

Prior to entering into a contract negotiation, faculty candidates should carefully consider what factors are critical in order to reach their personal career goals and have job satisfaction. Decide ahead of time which factors are "deal-breakers" and which factors can be negotiated to acceptable alternatives [14]. Investigate what other faculty members have previously negotiated in order to understand what the standards are for the desired research field. It is important to be flexible, and remember that negotiating is working toward a common goal rather than competing against an adversary. There are often multiple options to create a win-win situation and creatively exploring all options can often lead to new opportunities [14]. It is imperative to be specific regarding details for requested items, e.g., clinical volume expectations, call schedule, financial support for research (time and allocation), call obligations, etc. If conflict arises, it is best to use objective data to argue a position based on merit and avoid becoming defensive or negative [14]. Above all, faculty candidates should be upfront and honest about their desires and expectations to ensure the negotiations ends with an employment situation that sets the surgeon-scientist up for academic success. Contract negotiation is discussed in more detail in preceding chapter.

As it relates to determining a research package, faculty candidates should carefully consider all associated costs for establishing a basic or translation science laboratory, associated personnel, and personal contract considerations. Departmental funding packages often include financial support for salary plus benefits for research assistants, laboratory technicians, research nurses, and coordinators as well as equipment and reagents. Faculty candidates should clearly delineate concrete needs; some examples include the following: (1) dedicated research space (whether independent or within a mentor's existing space), (2) access to research cores providing routine services (sample storage, sample processing, etc.), (3) access to specialized equipment and services, (4) access to collaborators, and (5) other support including grant writing assistance, IRB and grant management, and biostatistical support such as research design and statistical analysis [12]. While it is challenging to balance the needs of the laboratory with the needs of patients, "protected time" can be negotiated and confirmed with structured weekly scheduling that establishes quantifiable time during the work week that is dedicated to research. It is important to remember that many career-development grants require a commitment of 50–75% protected time for grant awardees. A minimum of 3–5 years should be supported to give the faculty member time to establish enough preliminary data to be competitive for independent extramural funding. Benchmarks should be clearly established for renewal or extension of departmental funding based on interim results [12] with the understanding that the current age for a surgeon to attain their first R01 is 45 and the average time to convert a K-award to an R01 is 5 years [12, 15–17].

Surgeon compensation is a complicated topic that is further challenged by an academic research role. National data, such as MGMA and AAMC, provide out-of-context salary data that is often inaccurate and does not take individual practice patterns or nonmonetary benefits into account [15]. In an academic setting, compensation is typically based on clinical productivity, administrative roles (e.g., chief quality officer), education (e.g., residency program director), and research [15]. There are many models for academic surgical compensation, and each faculty candidate should thoroughly investigate the percent contribution each category plays into the model and how a research role is financially supported, both at the time of the initial contract and in the future for contract renewal. Of note, the salary cap for surgeon compensation from the NIH is set at $203,700 per year; a number significantly lower than most surgeon salaries [15]. Gap compensation to cover the difference between the NIH component of salary and a fair market value surgeon salary should also be negotiated as part of a start-up package. For example, if a fair market value for a surgeon is $400,000 per year and they receive $100,000 for 50% research effort plus $200,000 for 50% clinical effort, then their compensation gap will be $100,000 [15].

Team Building

As the healthcare landscape has evolved, the importance of building a collaborative team has never been more important for establishing a productive research career. We can apply team-building models from business strategies to build effective research teams. The primary investigator (PI) is the leader of the team and is responsible for identifying and organizing the research strategies and goals that are best suited to the team [18, 19]. The PI is also responsible for evaluating whether the team members are executing the strategies effectively and whether or not the strategies helped the team meet their goals. The PI should carefully assess the background and experience of each team member to ensure their assigned tasks are appropriate distributed. For example, medical students who are interested in surgery may be effective at performing chart reviews for a retrospective analysis, while a research resident who is interested in an academic surgical career (and perhaps already has an MD-PhD) would be more effectively placed in a laboratory performing bench work.

As a surgeon-scientist, it is particularly important to establish research collaborations with MDs or PhD in other specialties to augment research creativity and capabilities. Multidisciplinary teams are now at the forefront of biomedical research; "No one person or one department or one lab is going to have all the tools they need to tackle the problem" [20]. For surgeons in particular, it can be extremely beneficial to establish relationships with PhD basic science researchers, whereby the surgeon can collect tissue and serum samples from patients to assist with basic science studies in the laboratory setting. Beyond the clear relationship between surgeons and basic scientists, relationships with computer programmers, mathematicians, biostatisticians, epidemiologists, biomechanical engineers, behavioral scientists, psychologists, nutritionists, physical therapists, and numerous other disciplines can create valuable connections that extend the limitations of what discoveries may be possible to new, uncharted territories. Some ways to meet and interact with potential collaborators are to attend conferences in their field, asking department heads who they think might be a good fit, and talking with grant funding managers who often have a broader view of research projects within the university setting [20].

Project Management

Project management models can be useful to maximize organization and efficiency in managing one or more research projects as a PI [19]. There are four stages in project management: (1) defining and organizing the project, (2) logistical planning, (3) management and tracking, and (4) evaluating outcomes [19]. The PI is often the leader in terms of defining the scope of a research project and defining the necessary tasks for completion. Tasks should be appropriately delegated to research team members and should set objective time, quality, and cost parameters that can be monitored. Careful planning a research project can help improve speed and efficiency and limit the need for repetitious or time-consuming work. The PI can assign team members to be responsible for a different part of a research project. Research projects can be broken down into various components, each with subtasks: developing the project research design, obtaining funding, obtaining ethics approvals, organizing and executing data acquisition, data analysis, and presenting and publishing results [19]. For practical use, items such as Gantt charts can be employed to track the various aspects of a research projects including deadlines, completion dates, and delays. File sharing is an important component of project management, and all team members should have a clear understanding of where and how data is collected and stored and how document management will be handled. Having a centralized location in the form of a "shared folder" on a university-based server or in the "cloud" for document and data storage can help to increase efficiency and reusability and reduce errors [19].

Research Funding

Obtaining funding is necessary to build a sustainable research program. Unfortunately, while the NIH budget has increased over $4 billion from 2006 to 2016, funding for surgical departments decreased by $three million per year in the same time period [21]. Surgeon-scientists are at a disadvantage compared with nonsurgical physicians as they have significant demands on their time to maintain a surgical practice, in addition to increasing administrative and regulatory obligations. Although there has been concern that surgeon-scientists have seen a decline in research funding, a recent study showed a significant increase the number of funded surgeons from 0.5% to 0.7% from 2010 to 2020, while funded non-surgeon physician-scientists declined from 2.2% to 1.6% in the same time period [22]. In 2020, surgeons held a total of $872 million in NIH funding [22]. It is helpful to have a comprehensive knowledge of potential funding sources and as well as which funding mechanisms are appropriate to the career stage of the primary investigator [13].

Apart from departmental support in the form of a "start-up" package, it is often the most feasible to obtain early career grants from the faculty's home institution or from national societies. Institutional funding can be offered on multiple levels (Department of Surgery, College of Medicine, University, Hospital, Cancer Center, etc.) and includes pilot grants and career-development awards that can be used to generate data that will be used to apply for large national funding through NIH or other organizations [13]. Surgical societies often offer career-development grants that can be used to complete pilot projects or supplement other institutional support. Additionally, the NIH offers loan-repayment grants to recruit and retain young faculty into biomedical research careers [13]. These grants can supplement other early-career grants in addition to establishing a relationship with the NIH.

Career-development awards offered through extramural organizations often focus explicitly on the feasibility and likelihood of the junior faculty applicant becoming an independent investigator as a result of the award. These awards should emphasize the mentorship relationship, institutional support, and rigorous research training plan. These grants should be structured to allow the early faculty applicant to obtain sufficient preliminary data to be competitive for larger extramural funding mechanisms. The NIH offers multiple K-series options such as the K08 which targets mentored scientists and the K23 which targets patient-oriented research [13]. K-awards are accompanied by strict requirements for protected time ranging from 50% to 75% [13] and may be restricted to faculty within a specific time period after completion of surgical training. The Veterans Administration (VA) system also offers similar substantial career-development awards with similar requirements.

K-awards are not required to achieve independent funding, and many surgeon-scientists have been awarded R01s without a preceding K-award [12]. In addition to the other career-development grants listed above, there are multiple alternative mechanisms for research funding that can be pursued. Private foundations also offer grants; however, these are typically targeted toward a specific disease process or patient population, so applicability may be limited [13]. Industry also frequently offers grant funding in order to promote the evaluation and adoption of new products. These grants can supply funding for a variety of studies; however, it is important to ensure appropriate contracts are established in advance to confirm research independence, ownership of data results, ownership of new products or inventions, and the ability to publish results freely without intervention or bias.

NIH R01 awards are one of the highest levels of independent research funding, typically covering a 3- to 5-year project time period supplying up to $250,000 per year. Many surgeon-scientists aspire to obtain R01 funding as part of an academic career. Smaller R awards are also available, such as R03 and R21 awards. These are shorter in covered time period and are for smaller funding amounts, suitable for pilot studies or secondary analyses [13]. Surgeon-scientists who are early in their research career and have never been awarded an R01 can apply for "Early-Stage Investigator" (ESI) status if they are within 10 years of completion of training or "New Investigator" (NI) status with the NIH. These statuses confer additional benefits in terms of access to exclusive funding lines, leeway in the grant review process, and time off for certain life events [13].

Effective Research Design

Study design selection is an essential factor necessary to provide unbiased answers to research questions [23]. Effective research is only possible when data is collected using valid scientific methods that are clear, rigorous, and reproducible and analyzed using the appropriate statistical test(s); otherwise, inferences may be subject to bias and error leading to incorrect conclusions. Each study design has a unique set of characteristics that determine its applicability to different experimental situations.

Study design can be broadly categorized into "experimental" (or "interventional"), where researchers control one or more of the study conditions, and "observational," in which the researchers do not control any study conditions [23]. Experimental study design is typically used to precisely compare one or more interventions and determine the relative efficacy and safety of the intervention in question. Experimental studies can be either uncontrolled or controlled depending on whether the study performs an intervention in isolation or compares the intervention of interest with an alternative or no intervention (placebo) [23]. Uncontrolled studies run the risk of overestimating the efficacy and magnitude of an intervention as any observed effect is attributed directly to the intervention.

There are several common types of controlled experiments: *randomized controlled trials (RCTs)*, historical controlled trials, crossover trials, and cluster group designs, among others. RCTs are often considered the "gold standard" for scientific methodology. An RCT is a type of parallel, controlled, experiment study in which the subjects are randomly assigned to one or more interventions in order to compare the outcome between groups. A control group which does not receive the intervention can be utilized to determine whether or not the observed outcome is due to the intervention. A "placebo-controlled" group is a control group where the study subjects assigned to the placebo intervention receive identical-appearing treatment but without the critical intervention factor being studied (e.g., an injection of saline rather than a study drug). RCTs are not feasible for diseases which have a low prevalence as the number of subjects needed to a see a difference between groups is large and this would require enormous amounts of time and funding. RCTs also need to be evaluated for ethical issues as it relates to the control group and whether or not withholding the intervention is within the standard of care [23].

Historically controlled studies are those in which the control group data is collected retrospectively from a similar group of patients who were treated in the past. As the historical data is often gathered *post hoc*, it can often be prone to bias and inaccuracies. Historical studies can be useful to compare new interventions with historical standards, although care should be taken when interpreting results. A *crossover study* is one in which the study subjects receive more than one treatment in different time increments, e.g., administering different chemotherapeutic agents to two groups and then switching the groups to the other agent at a specific time point. This allows investigators to study the effect of interventions both within groups and between groups.

Randomization is a study design technique that attempts to reduce selection and allocation bias by removing the subjects' and/or investigators' knowledge of whether or not they are receiving the experimental intervention [23]. Randomization provides balance between subject groups as unknown, or interrelated risk factors will have a similar distribution if the sample size is of adequate size. There are multiple methods to perform randomization. *Simple randomization* is the selection of a random group assignment at the time each subject is enrolled in the study. This can be done with a coin toss, randomly ordered cards, or a computer-generated algorithm [23]. *Block randomization* places subjects into groups based on predefined similarities to help streamline the logistics of administering a complex intervention. This can assist with keeping treatment group sizes similar but does not guarantee balance between risk factors [23]. *Stratified randomization* is a combination of block randomization into groups as well as performing in-group randomization to balance prognostic factors [23].

Blinding or *masking* is a study design technique that hides the assignment of treatment randomization from the study subjects (*single-blinded*), both the subjects and the investigators (*double-blinded*), or from the subject, investigators, and data analysts (*triple-blinded*). This is a useful strategy when the outcome measure of the intervention can be affected by this knowledge, e.g., symptom severity, as these subjective measures are highly susceptible to recall or reporting bias [23]. Sometimes, it is difficult to perform blinding, such as with the performance of a surgical intervention, and in other studies, it is not effective to consider blinding, such as studies that require subject participation (e.g., nicotine cessation). In double-blinded studies, a data review committee oversees the study and monitors for safety and efficacy. In a triple-blinded study, the data review committee is also blinded, so response to adverse events may be compromised [23].

An important aspect of study design is the careful avoidance of bias, which is a systematic error in the study design that leads to a deviation from the true analytic result [23]. *Bias* is a type of systematic error that comes from preconceived beliefs or ideas on the part of the investigators, study subjects, or data analysts that changes how they perform or report an assessment, measurement, procedure, or analysis [23]. *Selection bias* occurs when the study population is not representative of the larger population, leading to inaccurate inferences from the data analysis. *Assessment bias* is when the study participants are aware of what treatment intervention is being offered. *Information bias* occurs when study subjects provide information to the investigators that is significantly altered by preformed beliefs or ideas. *Recall bias* is when study subjects report inaccurate information due to the study tool, the timing of the data collection, or other factors that increase subjectivity. *Observer bias* occurs when the investigators do treat all study subjects equally. All forms of bias introduce error into the analytic model, thus decreasing the accuracy of results and potentially leading to incorrect inferences regarding clinical care recommendations.

The other major subset of research design includes observational studies, sometimes called a "natural experiment" as an intentional intervention is not being performed [23]. Observational studies are useful when experimental studies are logistically improbable or unethical. *Cohort studies* are observational studies that examine groups of patients who are classified by the presence or absence of an "exposure" (e.g., second-hand smoke), while *case-control studies* examine groups of patients who are classified by the presence or absence of a disease (e.g., lung cancer) [23]. Observational studies can be either retrospective (collecting data from events that have previously occurred) or prospective (collecting data in an ongoing fashion). The subject groups in observational studies are not randomized and so can exhibit a high-degree of selection bias. Selection bias in this type of study design leads to an imbalance of potential risk factors, or confounders, for a particular outcome measure. Confounders can either mask a significant association between an exposure or disease and an outcome of interest or make the association appear stronger than it truly is [23]. Observational cohort studies typically report their analytic results in terms of the "relative risk" of developing the outcome based on the presence or absence of the exposure or disease. Case-control studies report their results in terms of the "odds ratio" of having the disease as it relates to the risk factor of interest.

Writing a Successful Grant

Writing a successful grant is a critical skill necessary to obtain the research funding that can support a surgeon-scientist's academic career goals. However, obtaining grant funding has become increasingly difficult, so it is important to deliberately develop skills and seek out critical feedback in order to write a grant that can be successfully scored and funded.

A common mistake made by junior surgeon-scientists is not spending enough time on writing a grant [24]. A typical, successful NIH R01 award takes approximately 100–200 h of work spread out over many months [24]. Time needs to be included for all of the following tasks: reviewing relevant literature, compiling preliminary data, identifying and collaborating with coinvestigators, writing the proposal, developing a budget, obtaining letters of support and biosketches, performing appropriate editing and formatting, and seeking out critical feedback [24].

It is important to carefully read the "Request for Applications (RFA)" that accompanies funding opportunities. RFAs state the grant mechanisms funded by the award, instructions for eligibility criteria, and the type of projects the award is intended to fund [24]. The research project should match the funding agency's goals, and the scope of the project needs to match the grant mechanism and eligibility criteria [25]. Additionally, all grants have detailed instructions on page length, word limits, and formatting requirements; failure to comply with these regulations will likely lead to rejection [24].

The grant itself should be clearly written, visually pleasing, and as concise as possible [24]. Most grant reviewers will not have in-depth knowledge of the particular field covered by the grant application, so it is best for applicants to avoid abbreviations or scientific jargon that is hard to understand. Using clearly formatted sections with heading and subheadings can help the reviewer navigate the grant more easily. Bold text can be used to call attention to critical points. Figures, charts, and tables should be easy to understand and should avoid the use of very small fonts. Above all, it is critical to carefully review the grant application prior to submission to correct all typographical and grammar errors. Such errors suggest a lack of attention to detail that may cause a reviewer to question the applicant's thoroughness with regard to the proposed study.

The "Specific Aims" page is the foundation of a grant proposal and should carefully and specifically describe the aims of the intended study. The Specific Aims are often highly scrutinized by reviewers as it is used to generate overall impressions of the study [24]. It is important to avoid writing an overly ambitious grant. Keeping the grant application focused can help convince a funding agency that the primary investigator will be able to accurately test the stated hypothesis [24, 25]. It is also important to ensure that multiple specific aims are not interdependent. Each aim should be a self-contained project, such that no aim depends on the successful completion of any other aim [24].

After the Specific Aims are completed, the remainder of the grant should provide detailed information that explains how the Specific Aims will be successfully studied and analyzed. Detailed, yet concise, descriptions of the study methods are needed to convey enough information about the project that reviewers can determine whether the methods are sound and feasible; each component of the project needs to be described separately. A description of potential limitations of the methodology and alternative strategies should be included so that reviewers can assess a PI's ability to navigate unexpected events during the study [24]. For example, a PI should describe how they will address an inability to enroll enough patients to meet the requirements of a power analysis. A clear data analysis plan needs to be described with a list of statistical tests and why each test was selected. Finally, the grant should be completed in draft form no less than 3 months prior to the submission deadline to allow for enough time for coinvestigators and mentors to provide critical feedback and editing.

It is important to recognize that the majority of grant applications are rejected [24, 25]. Surgeon-scientists who achieve successful funding often apply and reapply for multiple funding mechanisms for the same project. There is evidence that the number of grant applications submitted by a surgeon-scientist correlates with the likelihood of achieving funding: surgeons who submitted ≥5 grants had almost 100% funding success, while surgeons who submitted only one grant had less than 20% success [2]. Grant writing is a skill that can be developed through deliberate practice and coaching. Although grant writing is challenging, with consistent practice and a supportive environment, one can learn to write an effective and successful grant.

Database Development

Proper development of a database is critically important to establish a quality research program. Gathering too much or too little information will impair statistical analysis and clinical interpretation of results, while poorly designed data fields will necessitate time-consuming post-collection data management. Prior to creating a database, the primary investigator (PI) should determine which data should be collected. It is important to establish a clear research hypothesis and project plan prior to building the database. Data elements should only be included in the database if they are needed to answer the research question. Elements that are typically needed in a research database include the following: (1) data needed for indirect record identification to assist with validation and correction, (2) primary and secondary outcomes, (3) eligibility criteria, (4) matching and/or stratification criteria, and (5) potential confounding factors [26]. It is important for the PI to work closely with a statistician during the development phase of a database to ensure that the design and collection algorithm leads to accurate, complete, and analyzable data at the end of the study.

Databases should be created using data management software that are confirmed to be HIPAA compliant by the researcher's healthcare employer. Some common software applications include RedCap, Excel, Google docs, Sharepoint, SPSS, and MS Access. Every database variable should have standard coding including the following factors: variable name (unique identifier for the variable), variable label (name that is viewed during data entry; often a shorter version of the variable name), variable type (numeric, text, date, time, etc.), variable length (allowed number of characters or digits after a decimal point), definition to explain the content of the variable, algorithm for derived or calculated variables, and any dependent relationships.

Data can be structured either chronologically (e.g., recording the time and date of sequential medication administrations) or thematically (e.g., recording categories of nicotine-use history: "never, former, current") [26]. In general, raw data should be collected to avoid loss of information. For example, one can record both "date of birth" and "date of surgery" instead of "age at surgery" as these data fields can then be used to calculate "age at surgery" in another data field. Then, both fields can be used in additional calculations, e.g., "age at adverse event." As much as possible, the data field should have limited and structured answer choices, e.g., "yes" or "no", "male" or "female", etc. Open-ended questions or data fields that rely on free text entries should be avoided as they cannot be statistically analyzed. Make sure all data fields have documented, consistent units of measurement to avoid confusion during data entry and analysis. It can be helpful to create a "coding guide," which delineates the structure and contents of the database for use reference [26].

The PI should then create a data management plan, which is essentially a "to-do list that details how one plans to collect, clean, store and share the products of their research" [26] so that the research team can work safely and efficiently. Data can be collected either retrospectively or prospectively. Retrospective data collection includes all data abstracted from the electronic or paper medical record prior to the time of the study. This collection can be performed via IT-led data requests or by individual person's entering a health record and abstracting the data one chart at a time. Prospective data includes any data that are created and collected after study initiation. Data can be collected using a "case report form," which is a structured document that allows for safe and efficient data collection by a multidisciplinary team [26]. The primary investigator should communicate clear guidelines for how the research team should deal with optional fields or missing data. For example, if a patient misses a follow-up appointment, the PI may request that the data field for that time point is not left blank but rather marked as a "missed" appointment, in order to clarify that the data field itself has been evaluated by the research time and not inadvertently left blank. All data downloads or manual data entry from the health record should be double-checked and edited for accuracy and completeness. This can be completed either at the time of data entry, during post-collection data processing, or at both time points.

After data collection, checks, edits, and post-collection processing has been completed and the database is confirmed complete, then all identifying information should be removed from the database to protect patient anonymity. If needed, a unique, anonymous identifier can be used to label individual patient data records. A separate, password-protected database can then house the unique record identifiers with the patient's identifying information such as name, date of birth, and medical record number for later retrieval.

Data Analysis

Biostatistics allow surgeon-scientists to effectively analyze their research results in order to make discoveries and inferences that can positively affect clinical care. "Statistical inference is the process of drawing conclusions about populations of interest" [27]. It is important for surgeons to have a basic understanding of common statistical tests so that they can be effective in designing their own research studies and in interpreting the results of others' work.

The primary investigator performing statistical analysis needs to decide what hypothesis the analysis is trying to test. For example, a scientist may be investigating whether administration of a drug (event) is related to a specific adverse outcome (exposure variable). The hypothesis may be that the event (drug administration) is associated with adverse outcome. Then, the "null hypothesis" states that the event (drug administration) is *not* associated the adverse outcome. Hypothesis testing using the statistical tests below is then used to determine whether the null hypothesis is true or false. The cutoff to determine whether a null hypothesis is false and can be rejected is usually set at 5% or less.

In hypothesis testing, one also needs to calculate the "power" of the analysis. The power is the probability of (correctly) rejecting the null hypothesis when it is false ($1 - \beta$) [27] (i.e., "true positive"). The power of a study is dependent on the effect size and the study sample size. Outcomes that are rare or have a very small measurable effect and smaller study populations lower the power of a study and make it more difficult to reject the null hypothesis. If the null hypothesis is incorrectly rejected when it is actually true, then this is considered a Type I error (i.e., "false positive," e.g., drug administration is reported as being significantly associated with an adverse outcome when they are actually not associated). The probability of a Type I error, α, also called the significance level, is often set at a predetermined value of <5%. A Type II error, β, is the probability of accepting the null hypothesis when it is actually false (i.e., "false negative," e.g., drug administration is reported as not being associated with the adverse outcome when they are actually correlated); thus, the power is the probability of avoiding a Type II error.

Descriptive Statistics

Descriptive statistics are often used as the first step of a statistical analysis (Table 26.1). These tests describe fundamental aspects of the study population and allow the reader to assess whether the study findings will be applicable to their own population of interest [27]. Some common descriptive tests include mean (average), standard deviation (spread around the mean), median (midpoint of a set of ordered numbers), range (spread), interquartile range (spread around the median), proportion (fraction of times an event (n) occurs in a population (N)), and incidence rate (frequency of an event (n) in a defined population (N) over a given period of time) [27]. While summary measures and proportions are informative and allow for easy interpretation of data, it is important to note that they can be misinterpreted without appropriate context and cannot be used to make inferences about statistical associations [27].

Inferential Statistics

Inferential statistics are used to interpret and make deductions about characteristics and associations in a study population (Table 26.2) [27]. The choice of statistical test used depends on the type of data being analyzed (categorical or continuous) and the research purpose (e.g., measure strength of association, calculate risk of an event occurring, calculate a confidence interval)

Table 26.1 Descriptive statistical tests [27]

Test	Definition	Detail
Mean	Average of a set of numbers (n)	$= (x1 + x2 + \cdots + xn)/n$
Standard deviation	Amount of spread around a mean	$= \sqrt{((\sum (n\text{-mean})^2/(n-1))}$
Median	Midpoint of a set of ordered numbers (n) such that half the numbers are above and half are below the median	= middle value of a set of n numbers (if n is odd) or mean of two middle values (if n is even)
Range	Overall spread of a set of numbers (n)	Lowest n–highest n
Interquartile range	Amount of spread around a median	25th percentile–75th percentile
Proportion	Fraction of times an event (n) occurs in a population (N), expressed as a fraction	$= n/N$
Percentage	Fraction of times an event (n) occurs in a population (N), expressed as a percent	$= (n/N) * 100$
Incidence proportion (risk)	Fraction of times an event (n) occurs in a population (N) over a specific period of time (t)	= (n during time period)/(N at beginning of time period)
Incidence rate	Frequency of new events (n) in a population (N) over a period of time	= (n during time period)/(total person-time ($N*t$))

[27]. These types of statistical tests make a series of assumptions about the data that need to be assessed prior to reporting results. Incorrect assumptions can make the statistical test results inaccurate and lead to invalid conclusions. There are several statistical applications that can be used to perform the tests described here, including IBM® SPSS® Statistics (IBM Corporation, Armonk NY), Stata® (StataCorp LLC, College Station TX), and R© (The R Foundation for Statistical Computing, Vienna, Austria).

Prior to performing an inferential statistical test, the researcher should first assess the data being analyzed in order to select the appropriate test. Continuous data refers to data that can change

Table 26.2 Inferential statistical tests

Test	Data type	Definition	Assumptions
T-test	Continuous	Comparison of two independent means	Normal distribution; homogeneity of variance; independence of observations
Paired *t*-test	Continuous	Comparison of two related means	Normal distribution; homogeneity of variance
Wilcoxon rank-sum	Continuous	Comparison of data distribution between two independent samples	Samples have similar-shaped distribution but do not need to be normally distributed; independence of observations
Wilcoxon signed rank	Continuous	Comparison of data distribution between to related samples	Symmetric distribution (mean = median)
ANOVA	Continuous	Comparison of ≥2 independent means	Normal distribution; homogeneity of variance; independence of observations
Kruskal-Wallas	Continuous	Comparison of ≥2 related means	Samples have similar-shaped distribution but do not need to be normally distributed
Binomial test	Categorical	Calculate a confidence interval or perform hypothesis testing for a sample proportion	Asymptotic normal distribution
Chi-square test	Categorical	Compare ≥2 independent sample proportions	Asymptotic normal distribution; independence of observations
Fisher's exact test	Categorical	Compare ≥2 independent sample proportions without asymptotic normal distribution	Independence of observations
McNemar's test	Categorical	Compare 2 related sample proportions	Asymptotic normal distribution
Stuart-Maxwell test	Categorical	Compare ≥2 related sample proportions	Asymptotic normal distribution

Pearson correlation	Continuous	Analysis of the linear association between two variables (x and y), without assumption of directionality; Correlation values range from −1 to 1 with 0 meaning "no correlation," −1 meaning –"strong negative correlation," and +1 meaning "strong positive correlation"	Association between x and y is linear; normal distribution of both x and y; homogeneity of variance across all pairs of x and y
Linear regression	Continuous	Analysis of the linear association between an outcome variable (y) and ≥1 exposure variables (x)	Association between x and y is linear; normal distribution of model residuals; constant model error variance for all values of x; independence of observations; no multicollinearity with multiple exposure variables
Logistic regression	Categorical	Analysis of the association between an outcome variable (y) and ≥1 exposure variables (x)	Association between log-odds of x and y is linear; asymptotic normal distribution of model parameters; constant model error variance for all values of x; independence of observations; no multicollinearity with multiple exposure variables
Log rank test	Categorical with time-to-event	Analysis of distribution of times until a binomial event (n) occurs; compare differences of time-to-event for independent groups	Independence of observations
Cox proportional hazards regression	Categorical with time-to-event	Analysis of distribution of times until an event (n) occurs and one or more exposures (x) are present; predict future risk of an event (n) based on ≥1 exposure variables (x)	Independence of observations; constant ratio of event hazards between two subjects

over time and has an infinite number of possibilities (e.g., age, weight, temperature, blood pressure). Categorical data refers to data that can be divided into unique groups (e.g., race/ethnicity, sex, whether or not an adverse outcome occurred). After data collection has been completed, categorical data is converted into integers in order to perform analysis. For example, for the sex variable, male can be coded as "0" and female coded as "1." All codes used should be clearly documented in the event post-collection cross-checking, error correction, or data editing is needed.

Various assumptions are made about the nature of the data when inferential tests are used. "Normal distribution" refers to the data being distributed symmetrically around the mean, which is zero, and the data will be more frequent near the mean than far away (Fig. 26.1) [28]. This is commonly called a "bell curve." The standard deviation of data with a normal distribution is 1. Many data sets are not normally distributed, and therefore, the tests that make these assumptions should not be used; instead, tests that are appropriate for "nonparametric" data are used, e.g., using Wilcoxon rank-sum instead of a *T*-test. Nonparametric tests have a robust ability to hand skewed data; however, they have less power to

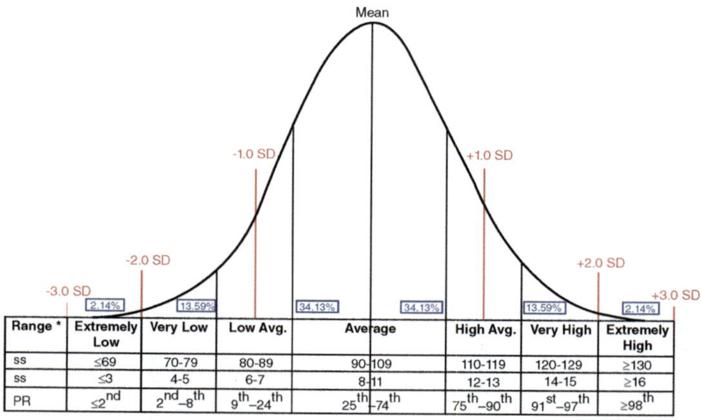

Range *	Extremely Low	Very Low	Low Avg.	Average	High Avg.	Very High	Extremely High
SS	≤69	70-79	80-89	90-109	110-119	120-129	≥130
SS	≤3	4-5	6-7	8-11	12-13	14-15	≥16
PR	≤2nd	2nd–8th	9th–24th	25th–74th	75th–90th	91st–97th	≥98th

*Range descriptions based upon WISC V descriptors.

Fig. 26.1 Normal distribution of a data set [28]

reject a null hypothesis due to the inability to assume a specific data distribution in the model. Statistical software applications typically have the functionality to test for normal distribution.

Many statistical tests also make the assumption that the two variables being compared are independent from one another. Variables may be correlated when they are looking at study samples that are clustered in one region (e.g., due to multiple clinical trials), when cohort patients are matched to control patients, or when multiple, longitudinal values are measured in the same study participant (e.g., blood pressure measured before and after a blood pressure medication is administered) [27]. Variables can also be correlated when each can potentially alter the magnitude of the other (e.g., BMI and presence of diabetes). In linear regression, this is called "multicollinearity," and it means that the outcome of interest can be predicted by more than one of the exposure variables (e.g., risk of myocardial infarction may be predicted by both BMI and the presence of diabetes). Multicollinearity can be addressed by removing one or more of the related exposure variables or combining them using known indexes. Correlated variables and multicollinearity introduces bias into statistical analysis and can lead to erroneous interpretation of results.

Presenting and Publishing

The first step in preparing the results of research study for presentation and publication is writing the abstract. An abstract is a comprehensive, concise, and stand-alone summary of a research project, including background information, project design, results, and conclusions. One of the primary aims of an abstract is to draw attention to a study, inviting the audience to learn more through a presentation or manuscript [29]. The abstract should accurately and clearly convey the primary results of the study so that a journal editor or conference program reviewer can ascertain whether the study will provide a valuable addition to their respective organization. It is vital that an abstract is critical: its conclusions should logically flow from the stated results and should not be over- or underestimated [29].

An abstract typically has four sections: introduction, methods, results, and conclusions. The introduction briefly describes relevant background information on the topic that explains its importance, highlights the current gap in scientific knowledge, and provides a rationale for why the study was performed. The introduction then concludes with the study's hypothesis and primary outcome measure. The methods section then describes the key steps for performing the study, including the study design, setting, subject sample size and sampling strategy, data collection, and an statistical plan for analysis (including a power analysis, when appropriate) [29]. The results section should include the most important findings of the study, presented as an objective, high-level summary [29]. The results section should clearly address the hypothesis of the study as described in the introduction and should report relevant statistical test results such as *P*-values, hazard ratios, and odds ratios. In qualitative research, the results should provide a descriptive summary of the research themes [29]. The conclusion should summarize and interpret the study results and provide implications for clinical relevance, if possible. Abstracts are generally used to submit research work to regional or national conferences for presentation. Presenting one's work allows for dissemination of new ideas and can generate excitement about a particular line of research inquiry.

The final stage of a research project is the preparation of a manuscript for peer review and publication. Academic work is evaluated on the number and quality of published manuscripts, as well as the "impact factor" of the journals where the researcher's body of work has been accepted. Journals with higher impact factors have a wider reach and are generally more competitive to gain acceptance. Many of the same suggestions for writing an abstract apply to writing a scientific manuscript, particularly as it relates to structure and organization. Manuscript writing, like grant writing, is a skill that can be learned with deliberate practice and seeking out critical feedback.

There are several types of manuscripts that have varying levels of complexity; however, most scientific research is published as an "original research" manuscript. The structure of most manuscripts follows the IMRAD scheme—introduction, methods, results, analysis, and discussion [30] which allows for a logical flow of information with regard to context, content, inferences, and conclusions. The introduction section provides context for the study, both in terms of the current state of the problem and "what are the gaps in our knowledge," and also presents the rationale for why the study is important [30]. The study hypothesis, specific aims, and the primary and secondary outcome measures should be clearly stated at the end of the introduction.

The methods section should explicitly and thoroughly describe how the study was performed as well as providing a rationale for how the study design was selected [30]. There are seven critical components of the methods section: (1) study setting, describing the area or setting where the experiment was conducted; (2) study design, identifying the type of study (e.g., cross-sectional, cohort, randomized controlled trial, etc.) and stating whether the appropriate study guidelines were followed; (3) sample size and sampling technique, stating the number of samples needed and how they were collected; (4) ethics approval, identifying the study approval body and proper collection of informed consent; (5) recruitment methods, stating the inclusion and exclusion criteria; (6) experimental details, an exhaustive description of the experimental details so that an independent researcher could recreate the same study and achieve identical results; and (7) statistical analysis, describing the statistical tests used in the analysis and any necessary information regarding significance cutoffs [30]. The methods section should focus on "how" the study was performed, while the results section focuses on "what" data was collected.

There are a variety of universal guidelines (Table 26.3) that can help researchers to perform and report different study designs in a transparent, reliable, and reproducible way [30, 31]. These reporting guidelines provide a checklist of recommended items that should be included in the manuscript and are specific to a study design [31]. For example, CONSORT (**Con**solidated **S**tandards **o**f **R**eporting **T**rials) applies to randomized controlled trials, PRISMA (**P**referred **R**eporting **I**tems for **S**ystematic Reviews and **M**eta-**A**nalysis) is used for systematic reviews and meta-analyses, and STROBE (**Str**engthening the **R**eporting of **O**bservational Studies in **E**pidemiology) is used for observational studies [31].

Table 26.3 Universal reporting guidelines [31, 32]

Study design	Reporting guideline
Randomized controlled trial	CONSORT
Animal preclinical trials	ARRIVE
Observational studies	STROBE
Systematic review	PRISMA
Meta-analysis	PRISMA
Qualitative research	SRQR, COREQ
Quality improvement studies	SQUIRE
Study protocols	SPIRIT, PRISMA-P
Diagnostic/prognostic studies	STARD
Prognostic studies	TRIPOD
Case reports	CARE
Clinical practice guidelines	AGREE, RIGHT
Economic evaluations	CHEERS
Artificial intelligence (AI) studies	MINIMAR

(Adapted from Ferreira JC et al. and https://www.equator-network.org/ [31, 32])

Most of the commonly used guidelines were developed by the EQUATOR Network (**E**nhancing the **Qua**lity and **T**ransparency **o**f Health **R**esearch), a "global initiative that seeks to improve the reporting quality of published health research globally." [31, 32]. Most high-impact, peer-reviewed journals now require that RCTs are written using the CONSORT guidelines and observational studies using the STROBE guidelines [31].

The results section is a summary of the data that was collected and the analytic results obtained from statistical testing. Results should be written in past tense without interpretation [30]. Lists of data should be presented in table form and should not be duplicated in writing in the results section. Typically, demographic data is reported first, followed by the results of descriptive statistical tests, and finally the results of inferential statistical tests.

The discussion section provided the authors' summary and interpretation of the findings within the context of the existing literature. The authors should aim to "fill in the gap" that was identified in the introduction [30]. The discussion should summarize the key results of the study and then provide both concordant and discordant comparisons with existing studies, making an effort to highlight the unique features of the study results. After a thorough interpretation is offered, the discussion section should then provide a thorough examination of the strength and weaknesses of the study, clearly delineating limitations to the study design and highlighting potential areas of bias and error. The conclusion is the final paragraph of the manuscript and should represent the key findings of the study, how the study adds to the literature, and provide "take-away" messages for the reader [30]. The conclusion can also state what future directions can or should be studied as results of the present study.

Writing a scientific manuscript can be a time-consuming, arduous process that requires time and effort to learn how to perform effectively. Many authors find that it is easiest to write the methods section first, as it is an objective description of the study design and execution [33]. The results section is often written immediately following the completion of data analysis, and this will logically flow into the compilation of the discussion section. The introduction is often written last [33]. Reference management software is extremely useful to allow for easy and efficient placement of reference into the body of the manuscript and auto-updating of the reference list when blocks of text are moved. Overall, writing with brevity and clarity and avoiding redundancy makes scientific writing easier to understand and will increase the chance of a successful publication [33].

There are some common mistakes to avoid that can help authors avoid rejection or requests for major revisions from journal editors [30]. It is important not to make the title too long or use jargon or abbreviations that would be unfamiliar to the general population. One should avoid making the abstract longer than the proscribed word count. The abstract should also not contain any information that is not included in the manuscript. The introduction should not omit citing publications that contradict the results of the manuscript as this raises concern for bias within the research conception and design. The methods should be thorough enough that the study can be replicate and the same results achieved by an independent researcher. It is important not to miss inclusions of vital information such as the study setting, inclusion/exclusion criteria, sample size and sampling technique, ethical clearance, an exhaustive description of the experimental methodology, and a thorough description of the statistical analysis used. The results section should avoid redundancy and overlapping information. It is important to review results and accompanying tables and figures for errors or missing values. The discussion section should avoid discussing results that are not statistically significant as "approaching significance." Additionally, the discussion section should never include new results that are not reported in the results section. Authors should be careful to avoid bias in their critical analysis of the data results and use a balanced scope of previously published work that both support and contradict the newly reported data. It is also critical to provide a thorough discussion of the limitations of the research design, data collection, and data analysis, so that the results can be interpreted in a fair and balanced way by the reader. The conclusion section should avoid overstating the results or suggesting clinical interventions that are not supported by the data.

In general, authorship should follow the International Committee of Medical Journal Editors (ICMJE) [34] and has important academic and financial implications. Authorship confers credits for the work performed but also implies accountability for methods and results. ICMJE suggests that authorship should be based on the presence of all four of the following criteria: (1) substantial contribution to the conception, design, acquisition, analysis, or interpretation of the study; (2) writing and critically reviewing the work for intellectual content; (3) final approval of the work prior to submission; and (4) agreement to accountable for all aspects of the work. All research team members who are included as authors should meet the above four criteria, and all team members who meet the above criteria should be included as authors. Participants in a research study who do not meet all four of the above criteria should be acknowledged.

It is good practice to determine who will be the first and last author of any publication prior to study initiation, so that clear roles and expectations can be established. Typically, the first author is the primary contributor to the conception and design of the project; they usually write the abstract and manuscript; and they present the study at conferences. The last, or "senior," author is generally the mentor or senior investigator on the study. The remaining authorship is ordered by level of decreasing contribution to the study [29]. The corresponding author is the author is who responsible for communicating with a journal publisher and performs the administrative tasks needed during the submission, peer-review, and publication process [34].

Research Mentorship

Maintaining the role of the surgeon-scientist in healthcare research requires ongoing education of the next generation. Becoming a successful surgeon-scientist requires intelligence, persistence, and creativity, but it also requires comprehensive education to learn necessary methodologic knowledge and skills [12]. Although the Accreditation Council for Graduate Medical Education (ACGME) requires residency programs to provide basic research curriculum, opportunities for scholarly activity, and allocation of appropriate resources, only 56% of surgery programs currently offer dedicated research time and 12% have mandated required research time [35]. There are multiple studies that show early exposure of residents to research opportunities increases the likelihood of pursuing an academic career. A national study looking at residents who participated in ≥1 year of designated GME research time (34.7% of all surgical residents in the cohort) had a significantly higher likelihood of a faculty appointment (31.1%) and nationally funded career grants (2.7%) [36]. Having a first author publication during general surgery residency increases the likelihood of pursuing an academic career (OR 1.25, 95% CI 1.0–1.5) [37]. Additionally, a higher number of publications completed during residency are associated with pursuing a specialty fellowship [37, 38].

There are multiple funding mechanisms for residents to pursue research during their training. Residents can be supported by training grants with a faculty member as the primary investigator and mentor. T-series grants through the NIH, such as the T32, are intended to train residents who are pursuing a specific surgical specialty [13]. The grant is obtained by a faculty member at the institution and the resident typically applies for grant support through local institutional mechanisms. F-series grants are awarded to individual trainee grant proposals for research salary and budgetary support during fellowship [13]. There are also many career-development grants offered through national societies that can be used to support the resident's salary during research years. These grants typically need to be submitted 6–12 months prior to the start of the academic year and often need the support of a faculty mentor who is also an active member of the society [13].

Mentorship for general surgery residents should be diverse and often consists of multiple individuals who provide guidance in different areas of career advancement [5]. Surgical departments and research faculty should establish clear guidelines and expectations for mentorship relationships. These rewarding relationship bridge into the trainees academic career and develop into lifelong, mutually beneficial interactions that can provide deep career satisfaction for both mentee and mentor.

Summary

Surgeon-scientists hold a unique position at the crossroad between the basic science laboratory and administering patient care in the clinical setting and their perspective can inform and guide research efforts to maximize benefits for patients. Building a successful research career requires dedication, drive, and persistence in addition to practical factors, such as funding, protected time, mentorship, and a supportive environment. With careful study and deliberate practice, surgical trainees and junior faculty can acquire the skills needed to establish a successful and sustainable academic research career. "Paying it forward" in terms of research mentorship can help to sustain the pipeline of productive surgeon-scientists in an ever-changing and challenging healthcare environment.

SAGES Takeaway

- Establishing a successful academic research career depends on multiple factors such as negotiating a supportive "start-up" package, identifying laboratory space and appropriate collaborators, building a research team, and securing research funding.
- Effective research design that is transparent, validated, rigorous, and reproducible is a fundamental component of the scientific method, allowing researchers to answer research questions in an unbiased manner.
- Database design, data collection, and data analysis are key components of effective research programs that require careful organization, planning, and execution.
- Presenting and publishing research results is the last step of a research project that allows a surgeon-scientist to share their work in a peer-reviewed setting and advance their academic career.
- Research mentorship is vital to engaging the next generation of surgical trainees and continue to support surgeons in research fields despite an ever-changing and challenging healthcare landscape.

References

1. Meara JG, Leather AJ, Hagander L, et al. Global Surgery 2030: evidence and solutions for achieving health, welfare, and economic development. Lancet. 2015;386(9993):569–624.
2. Keswani SG, Moles CM, Morowitz M, et al. The future of basic science in academic surgery: identifying barriers to success for surgeon-scientists. Ann Surg. 2017;265(6):1053–9.
3. Kibbe MR, Velazquez OC. The extinction of the surgeon scientist. Ann Surg. 2017;265(6):1060–1.
4. Hu Y, Edwards BL, Brooks KD, Newhook TE, Slingluff CL Jr. Recent trends in National Institutes of Health funding for surgery: 2003–2013. Am J Surg. 2015;209(6):1083–9.
5. Barker JC, Jalilvand A, Onuma A, et al. Facilitating success of the early stage surgeon scientist trainee: growing the surgeon scientist pipeline. Ann Surg. 2022;275(2):e334–44.

6. AAMC. Basic science. https://www.aamc.org/what-we-do/mission-areas/medical-research/basic-science. Accessed 15 Oct 2023.
7. Zarbin M. What constitutes translational research? Implications for the scope of translational vision science and technology. Transl Vis Sci Technol. 2020;9(8):22.
8. Brenneman FD, Wright JG, Kennedy ED, McLeod RS. Outcomes research in surgery. World J Surg. 1999;23(12):1220–3.
9. Hutter MM. Does outcomes research impact quality? Examples from bariatric surgery. Am Surg. 2006;72(11):1055–60. discussion 1061–1059, 1133–1048
10. Ogrinc G, Davies L, Goodman D, Batalden P, Davidoff F, Stevens D. SQUIRE 2.0 (Standards for QUality Improvement Reporting Excellence): revised publication guidelines from a detailed consensus process. BMJ Qual Saf. 2016;25(12):986–92.
11. Davidoff F, Batalden P, Stevens D, Ogrinc G, Mooney S, Group SD. Publication guidelines for quality improvement in health care: evolution of the SQUIRE project. Qual Saf Health Care. 2008;17(Suppl. 1):i3–9.
12. Goldstein AM, Blair AB, Keswani SG, et al. A roadmap for aspiring surgeon-scientists in today's healthcare environment. Ann Surg. 2019;269(1):66–72.
13. Gosain A, Chu DI, Smith JJ, Neuman HB, Goldstein AM, Zuckerbraun BS. Climbing the grants ladder: funding opportunities for surgeons. Surgery. 2021;170(3):707–12.
14. Nagaraj MB, Napier R, Ritter KA. Contract negotiations: a primer for surgeons. Financial Lectureship Series from the RAS-ACS Education Committee https://www.facs.org/media/xspexezz/final-contract-negotiation-primer.pdf. Accessed 18 Oct 2023.
15. Reiter AJ, Warner SG, Chen H, et al. Translating the value of the academic surgeon into salary, time, and resources. J Surg Res. 2023;285:A1–6.
16. Salata RA, Geraci MW, Rockey DC, et al. U.S. Physician-scientist workforce in the 21st century: recommendations to attract and sustain the pipeline. Acad Med. 2018;93(4):565–73.
17. Narahari AK, Mehaffey JH, Hawkins RB, et al. Cardiothoracic and vascular surgeons achieve high rates of K award conversion into R01 funding. Ann Thorac Surg. 2018;106(2):602–7.
18. Sterbenz JM, Nasser JS, Chung KC. Organizing a multidisciplinary research team: strategies, execution, and outcomes. Plast Reconstr Surg. 2019;143(3):951–61.
19. Swiatek PR, Chung KC, Mahmoudi E. Surgery and research: a practical approach to managing the research process. Plast Reconstr Surg. 2016;137(1):361–6.
20. Savage N. How team science extends your scope. Nature. 2018;556:S1–3.
21. Narahari AK, Mehaffey JH, Hawkins RB, et al. Surgeon scientists are disproportionately affected by declining NIH funding rates. J Am Coll Surg. 2018;226(4):474–81.

22. Demblowski LA, Busse B, Santangelo G, et al. NIH funding for surgeon-scientists in the US: what is the current status? J Am Coll Surg. 2021;232(3):265–74. e262
23. Lim HJ, Hoffmann RG. Study design: the basics. Methods Mol Biol. 2007;404:1–17.
24. Guyer RA, Schwarze ML, Gosain A, Maggard-Gibbons M, Keswani SG, Goldstein AM. Top ten strategies to enhance grant-writing success. Surgery. 2021;170(6):1727–31.
25. Harper L, Castagnetti M, Herbst K, et al. How to apply for a research grant: 10 tips and tricks. J Pediatr Urol. 2018;14(5):453–4.
26. Brembilla A, Martin B, Parmentier AL, et al. How to set up a database? A five-step process. J Thorac Dis. 2018;10(Suppl. 29):S3533–8.
27. Sebastiao YV, St Peter SD. An overview of commonly used statistical methods in clinical research. Semin Pediatr Surg. 2018;27(6):367–74.
28. Koziol LF, Beljan P, Bree K, Mather J, Barker L. The normal distribution of the bell-shaped curve. In: Large-scale brain systems and neuropsychological testing. Cham: Springer; 2016. p. 49–61.
29. Drury A, Pape E, Dowling M, et al. How to write a comprehensive and informative research abstract. Semin Oncol Nurs. 2023;39(2):151395.
30. Aga SS, Nissar S. Essential guide to manuscript writing for academic dummies: an editor's perspective. Biochem Res Int. 2022;2022:1492058.
31. Ferreira JC, Patino CM. Reporting guidelines: essential tools for manuscript writing in medical research. J Bras Pneumol. 2021;47(1):e20210057.
32. https://www.equator-network.org/. Accessed 19 Oct 2023.
33. Balch CM, McMasters KM, Klimberg VS, et al. Steps to getting your manuscript published in a high-quality medical journal. Ann Surg Oncol. 2018;25(4):850–5.
34. ICJME. Defining the role of authors and contributors. https://www.icmje.org/recommendations/browse/roles-and-responsibilities/defining-the-role-of-authors-and-contributors.html. Accessed 15 Oct 2023.
35. Brochu A, Aggarwal R. Research during general surgery residency: a web-based review of opportunities, structure and outputs. J Surg Res. 2018;223:149–54.
36. Andriole DA, Klingensmith ME, Fields RC, Jeffe DB. Is dedicated research time during surgery residency associated with surgeons' future career paths? A national study. Ann Surg. 2020;271(3):590–7.
37. Fladie I, Wise A, Carr M, et al. An evaluation of research publications for general surgery residents and its influence on the future pursuit of fellowship or academic career. J Surg Educ. 2023;80(3):352–9.
38. Wang H, Bajaj SS, Williams KM, et al. Early engagement in cardiothoracic surgery research enhances future academic productivity. Ann Thorac Surg. 2021;112(5):1664–71.

Leading Surgical Education Teams

27

Clarence E. Clark and Adrian G. Dan

Introduction

The term "doctor" originates from the Latin noun for teacher and the verb docere (to teach) [1]. Teaching the science and art of surgery has remained an integral and rewarding responsibility for surgeons over centuries. Passing down knowledge and skills amassed over careers spanning decades has been regarded as an honorable practice aimed at ensuring that new generations can master and further advance surgical principles.

Surgery, as a profession, is highly multifaceted. While technical and medical aptitude are the centerpieces of our responsibilities, the role of the "teacher" stands as one of the most crucial aspects. Surgeons are also recognized as natural leaders. It is

C. E. Clark
General Surgery Residency Program, Dignity Health System, Chandler, AZ, USA

Department of Surgery, Creighton School of Medicine, Phoenix, AZ, USA

A. G. Dan (✉)
Weight Management Institute—Bariatric Care Center, Akron, OH, USA

Akron City Hospital Campus, Akron, OH, USA

Northeast Ohio Medical Universities, Rootstown, OH, USA
e-mail: dana@summahealth.org

S. M. Johnson et al. (eds.), *The SAGES Manual of Strategy and Leadership*, https://doi.org/10.1007/978-3-031-62359-2_27

inherent in our nature to exhibit qualities necessary to command and lead operating room teams through challenging situations. In the educational setting, guiding independent surgeons and surgical trainees introduces an additional layer of complexity that requires a distinct set of leadership skills.

At the institutional level, surgical educators act as gatekeepers to the realm of autonomous surgical practice for burgeoning surgical trainees. Accrediting bodies such as the Accreditation Council for Graduate Medical Education (ACGME) and the Fellowship Council (FC) identify local leaders as program directors (PDs), associate program directors (APDs), chairpersons, and program coordinators/managers. This list may extend to clerkship directors, committee chairs, rotation directors, simulation champions, and core faculty. On the regional and national scales, surgical societies and accrediting bodies may appoint individuals with known interest, expertise, and passion for education to serve in roles such as surgical training committee chairs, course directors, educational event moderators, accreditation committee reviewers, and meeting program chairs, among many others.

For the purposes of this chapter, we will explore the domains that can impact educational groups on both the local (institutional) and regional (societal) levels. We will discuss concepts of leadership to consider and leadership skills critical for effectively guiding educational teams in various facets of surgical education governance. Initially, we will examine factors and strategies that influence a leader's behavior and ability to establish a work environment conducive to effective education at the graduate level. We will define the characteristics of effective leaders and link these traits to leadership styles that assist in various institutional and multi-institutional scenarios. Lastly, we will summarize the key concepts to contemplate when leading such educational teams effectively.

Factors Influencing Educational Leaders

Both seasoned and novice surgical educators find themselves navigating a complex web of influences that shape the planning and implementation of effective training programs at both local and national levels. These influences can be categorized into various factors, encompassing organizational dynamics, associates, direct reports, job demands, supervisors, environmental threats, and environmental opportunities. The following section delves into these influential elements and the intricate interplay that defines their impact.

Organizational factors encompass aspects of healthcare systems or national societies that set the direction and atmosphere for training programs operating under their umbrella. The trajectory is often guided by institutional and societal missions, overarching visions, and both short- and long-term goals. Program directors (PDs) must harmonize their awareness with these elements to guide existing programs or those in the process of initiation. Mission statements should be in sync with the institution's role in the community, as they significantly influence the program's cultural backdrop. These statements serve as cultural beacons and should be readily accessible to all personnel within the program. At a local level, oversight from Graduate Medical Education ensures the alignment and adaptation of these factors as the healthcare landscape evolves. On a broader scale, oversight may be facilitated by boards or executive councils of specialty societies and accrediting bodies that sponsor educational activities.

Associates encompass faculty members, rotation directors, clerkship directors, and simulation champions who collaborate closely with PDs to deliver daily educational programs to learners. These educators play a hands-on role in imparting skills and mentoring trainees. They contribute to committees such as the program evaluation committee (PEC) and clinical competency committee (CCC), and they hold a prominent presence at pivotal conferences like morbidity and mortality and journal clubs. Their influence extends to the program's clinical practices, serving as mentors to house staff and medical students. As a result, their input toward the PD and the overall program proves pivotal in crafting comprehensive surgical educational endeavors. In scenarios involving multi-institutional educational events, associates may be volunteer surgical faculty from various institutions, united by their shared interest in education and identified as such by societal leaders and committees.

Direct reports consist of house staff and program administrators. In societal programs, direct reports may encompass junior faculty and society support staff. These individuals serve as the lifeblood of the program, offering feedback to PDs and associates while actively participating in patient care delivery. The performance of these direct reports reflects the program's efficacy and the leadership it embodies.

Job demands, or the responsibilities tied to one's clinical practice, exert an indirect yet substantial influence on the PD. Institutions and accrediting bodies establish the time PDs should allocate to administrative duties versus clinical productivity. Managing these factors often entails striking a balance that optimizes effectiveness in both domains, a task demanding careful evaluation. Regular discussions with supervisors are imperative for preventing burnout and minimizing errors that could affect both the program and clinical practice outcomes. Societal programs are often steered by volunteer directors and faculty who must juggle their institutional clinical and administrative responsibilities while contributing to national endeavors.

Supervisors often encompass department chairpersons and the designated institutional officer (DIO), overseeing all graduate medical education training programs. For others, these supervisors might include training committee chairs, societal leaders, and leadership committees. Consistent interactions with these leaders are essential to ensure alignment of goals, personal growth, and mentorship, regardless of the educator's experience.

Environmental threats refer to external forces that may influence decisions made by PDs, healthcare systems, and professional societies. Factors such as local and regional training programs, healthcare systems within one's market, community demographics, and global pandemics/epidemics fall into this category. PDs must routinely assess these threats with input from supervisors and organizational/societal leadership. While these situations often manifest as challenges or crises, they inherently hold opportunities for innovation and strategic pivoting, necessitating recognition and proactive response from surgical educators.

Environmental opportunities are advantageous forces that can augment the efficacy and outcomes of a training program. PDs should proactively identify these factors, capitalizing on fleeting opportunities as they arise. Examples encompass local philanthropic engagement, provision of services to underserved communities, collaboration with neighboring programs in specialized fields, sharing of educational resources and expertise across programs/societies, pursuit of research prospects, and integration of emerging technologies. These opportunities often surface within the realm of graduate surgical education.

When these forces harmoniously interact, the leader and program influenced by them operate optimally. Moreover, leaders who adeptly comprehend these domains can enhance themselves through strategic approaches and personal development, cultivating the qualities commonly associated with effective leadership.

Leading Regional and National Societal Educational Teams

Beyond the confines of institutional surgical residency and fellowship programs, educational teams are assembled by universities, accrediting bodies, and national specialty societies to create courses, conferences, and materials. Regional and national teams wield the power to efficiently develop programs and pool faculty expertise, facilitating the education of surgical trainees across a broader geographical scope, even extending globally. This paradigm is particularly significant within highly specialized fellowship training programs, where limited class sizes or solitary fellows might engage with a handful of faculty members at their respective institutions. In such cases, the opportunity to leverage the teaching prowess of surgeons worldwide becomes invaluable.

Participation in these initiatives should be seen as a mark of professional esteem and an avenue for serving as a volunteer leader on behalf of the professional community. The leader's personal ambitions should be secondary to those of the society or the educational endeavor. Their focal point lies in maximizing available resources and the collective expertise of the group, thereby ensuring the optimal education of individual trainees. Their charge encompasses fostering the growth and advancement of individuals at every tier—be it medical students, residents, fellows, junior attendings, or senior faculty members. Meticulous oversight of budget allocation and delegation of teaching responsibilities is essential, underpinned by transparency and adherence to principles of merit, equity, inclusion, and diversity. The overarching ethos should be one of selflessness, grounded in judicious and equitable leadership. Simultaneously, it should offer ample avenues for all participants to further their own professional aspirations. This involves strategic succession planning as current leaders transition to new roles, paving the way for emerging leadership to infuse novel ideas and amplify the accomplishments of their predecessors.

Characteristics of Effective Leaders

Leadership is a multifaceted concept that can be influenced by both the culture of the group and the attributes of the leader. While the traditional hierarchical model of surgical residency training, as established by William Halsted in the United States, emphasizes a structured approach, regional and national educational endeavors often assemble teams composed of leaders from various institutions who possess similar qualifications and surgical education experience. In such scenarios, leading by committee consensus and ensuring active involvement from the entire group becomes paramount. Leaders typically emerge based on their contributions and evident dedication to teaching. Their ability to inspire and influence their team hinges on their capacity to engender respect and effect change. Achieving this requires the integration of senior members, mentorship for junior faculty, and responsiveness to trainees' needs, fostering a collaborative drive toward shared objectives.

The actions and choices made by leaders of programs or initiatives wield significant influence over the trajectory of the respective projects. These individuals must continually self-evaluate and seek feedback to ensure their effective engagement within their environment. Numerous positive attributes enhance the impact of an effective leader, and some of these characteristics are outlined below.

In their 2017 book, *The Leadership Challenge*, Kouzes and Posner identify three crucial attributes of a leader: honesty and truthfulness, forward-looking vision, and the ability to inspire [2]. Numerous other attributes can be categorized within these broader themes.

- **Honesty and Truthfulness:** Leaders who uphold ethics and standards serve as exemplars for their peers and direct reports. Authenticity empowers them to navigate challenging decisions for the program's direction. The mentorship provided by a PD who operates with truthfulness within a framework of fundamental fairness is invaluable to associates and trainees alike, fostering a functional and cohesive program. A leader's integrity significantly influences their capacity to inspire and influence. Transparency in matters and decision-making within the program is also crucial, as a consistent application of rules and bylaws underscores unbiased program administration.
- **Forward Thinking:** This trait drives programs forward, particularly in the face of evolving technology and societal changes. PDs exhibiting this quality often participate in local, regional, and national surgical and surgical education societies. Such leaders adeptly navigate environmental challenges and seize opportunities, ensuring their program remains relevant within the local and national contexts. Navigating change requires an open mind, preparedness, and a willingness to explore innovative solutions. For instance, the use of videoconferencing technology for educational content delivery during the initial months of the COVID-19 pandemic showcases the agility associated with forward thinking.
- **Inspirational:** Leaders who inspire evoke pride and optimism among their direct reports, associates, and future trainees. Visionaries can conceptualize and foresee attainable goals for the program before others can discern them. Effective communication of this vision motivates direct reports to channel their collective efforts toward a shared objective. This trait, when embodied by a PD, extends its impact beyond the healthcare system, facilitating the recruitment of house staff and faculty members.

Table 27.1 Characteristics of effective leaders

Honesty/ truthfulness	Forward thinking	Inspirational	Emotional intelligence	Competence
Fair	Visionary	Courageous	Reflective/ wise	Accountable
Trustworthy	Intelligent	Charismatic	Empathetic	Organized
Inclusive	Adaptable	Motivational	Attentive	Capable
Transparent	Progressive	Dedicated	Understanding	Decisive
Timely	Optimistic	Communicator	Modest/ humble	Resilient
With integrity	Creative	Empowering	Patient	Self-reliant
Unbiased	Pioneering	Hopeful	Gracious	Skillful

Numerous other attributes contribute to effective leadership and can be subcategorized within these three main themes (Table 27.1). The authors also highlight two additional overarching categories: emotional intelligence and overall competence.

Certain qualities warrant further exploration due to their significance in the realm of surgery:

- **Emotional Intelligence:** This expansive category encompasses qualities such as wisdom, which is challenging to quantify yet vital in effective leadership. Attributes like reflection, patience, attentiveness, and empathy foster relatability and inclusivity, engendering a more cohesive environment.
- **Humility and Modesty:** A trait not often associated with surgeons, ***modesty*** signifies maturity and self-assuredness. It fosters an uplifting atmosphere for associates and direct reports. A hint of self-deprecation can even denote confidence, bridging the gap between leadership and direct reports. Those spearheading programs and collective educational initiatives should adopt the role of servant leaders, ensuring that the project's objectives surpass any individual participant's aspirations.
- **Clinical and Technical Competence:** Demonstrating relevant surgical expertise is crucial for leading a successful surgical program. Administrative leadership also necessitates the strategic application of the aforementioned characteristics. Competence also aligns peers and trainees, bolstering the program and cultivating autonomous surgeon leaders recognized by healthcare systems at local, regional, and national levels.

Conversely, leaders should be mindful of attributes that can hinder effective leadership and work toward rectifying them. Self-reflection and 360-degree feedback from supervisors, associates, and direct reports are essential in identifying and correcting detrimental traits. Negative attributes encompass narcissism, sarcasm, aggression, confrontational behavior, self-centeredness, self-promotion, prejudice, bias, exclusivity, disorganization, tardiness, inattention, untrustworthiness, unreliability, criticism, difficulty, ambiguity, inconsistency, and deceitfulness.

Leadership Styles to Consider

Enhancing leadership skills can be achieved through formal courses offered by universities and professional societies, such as Fellowships in Academic Medical Education (FAME) programs and the American Society for Metabolic and Bariatric Surgery (ASMBS) Leadership Academy for fellows and junior attendings. Comprehensive curricula provide a thorough education in leadership principles that cannot be substituted. It is crucial to underscore that this chapter cannot replace a formal leadership curriculum, which is strongly recommended. Refining leadership skills is a continuous process of learning that spans a lifetime. When applying leadership skills within institutional training programs, two organizational leadership styles have proven effective in driving decision-making: task behavior and relationship behavior.

Task behavior takes various forms, including goal setting, alignment, establishing timelines, directing, and controlling. PDs establish goals at both the program and rotation levels. Input from rotation directors and faculty is essential before engaging the Program Evaluation Committee (PEC) and the Graduate Medical Education (GME) office for oversight. Goal setting allows the PD to synchronize faculty, residents, and the institution with the program's vision, fostering harmonious collaboration. Timelines are pivotal throughout the academic year, particularly when introducing or revising program or resident/fellow goals. Timelines also guide the PD and coordinator when contemplating service expansion, adjusting program size, or collaborating with other institutions for care delivery. On the ground level, directing and controlling learners ensures the faithful execution of program and society goals, with consistent reassessment for future planning.

Relationship behavior serves as the adhesive for managing personnel. This behavior entails asking questions, providing support, coaching, listening to understand, and furnishing feedback to direct reports, associates, and supervisors. Within training programs, PDs often gather information from the PEC, comprising faculty and resident representatives. Feedback from the PEC informs the PD and GME about changes that optimize resident and fellow training. Transitioning effectively from asking questions to offering support necessitates adept listening skills, enabling leaders to comprehend the concerns and solutions of their peers and trainees. Ultimately, feedback based on resident training outcomes—such as case volume, rotation experiences, program satisfaction, and budget management—empowers the PD to furnish substantive input to faculty, institutions, and trainees, steering the program's course.

Team Growth and Effective Teamwork

At the intermural or societal levels, the dynamics of teamwork among equally qualified volunteer educators and the strategies fundamental for team growth demand consideration. A key leadership task entails sustaining the engagement of the entire team and ensuring effective collaboration. Establishing clear guidelines for team communication, decision-making, and progress assessment is essential. Tools such as the Situation-Background-Assessment-Recommendation (SBAR) framework and Goals/Objectives can foster transparency and enhance communication among individuals from diverse regions. The team's objective can be conveyed through a mission statement, and team member roles should be clarified to cultivate robust working relationships.

Working groups undergo distinct stages of team growth. An initial honeymoon phase characterized by high morale might give way to periods of discord, loss of focus, and interpersonal conflicts. It falls to the leader to nurture a sense of unity and mutual trust among team members. The cultivation of shared goals and a constructive exchange of ideas creates an environment conducive to productivity and high performance.

Adaptability in Teaching Modalities and Resources

Surgical education has its historical foundations deeply rooted in the traditions of residency training. Emerging from Halsted's principles and evolving through the influence of accreditation bodies over the decades, this paradigm has traditionally combined a rotational preceptorship model with an organized, validated programmatic curriculum. Key elements of this traditional approach encompassed practices such as morbidity and mortality conferences, journal club literature reviews, extensive hours of resident duty, textbook-based review sessions, and the familiar adage "See one, do one, teach one." Nonetheless, the advent of new technologies has brought forth changes to this conventional training paradigm, propelling it toward further evolution in the future.

Several environmental factors have wielded transformative influence over surgical residency and fellowship programs in recent decades. These include the impact of medicolegal pressures, work hour restrictions, heightened patient scrutiny, the rise of super-specialization, increased administrative responsibilities for faculty, and the advent of technological advancements. These factors have given rise to adjuncts for surgical training and, in some cases, have replaced traditional teaching modalities. The concept of fellowship training, aimed at refining skills in specific surgical specialties, has gained popularity, often accompanied by the creation of best practice guidelines, typically sponsored by national societies or accrediting bodies. Factors like consumer demand and medicolegal pressures have also curtailed autonomy in residency, delaying opportunities for trainees to achieve proficiency in advanced surgical procedures until their fellowship training. Educational leaders need to recognize the dynamic catalysts of this evolving environment and adapt their programs to ensure trainees receive comprehensive educational experiences.

The surge in technological advancement, however, has also opened doors to modernizing surgical education and achieving new levels of efficiency in response to the aforementioned pressures. Traditional didactic activities in surgical training have evolved through computer-based programs, simulation platforms, and video conferencing. Institutions nationwide now have the capacity to pool their resources and expertise, facilitating the sharing of high-quality didactics in a cost-effective and convenient manner. The swift embrace of such technologies has transformed the methods of surgical education. Video-based learning of surgical procedures has empowered trainees to master the intricate steps of an operation before stepping into the operating room. Surgical simulators, particularly for robotic, laparoscopic, and endoscopic techniques, have enabled trainees to attain technical competency and proficiency outside the clinical setting. Web-based resources and lecture series have redefined the role of traditional weekly conferences. In many aspects, technological advancements have greatly benefitted surgical education and should be embraced by surgical educators. As new technologies continue to emerge, such as virtual reality (VR) and artificial intelligence (AI), the potential for their utilization in education is practically limitless. The capacity of programs to adapt to and even pioneer such novel training modalities often begins with the willingness of educational leaders to explore and endorse their use.

The involvement of local leaders in national societies is equally important, as their contribution to materials and content garners the confidence and credibility of local faculty members and trainees. Leaders who excel in teaching at the institutional level are often selected to participate in and direct such collective educational endeavors. Ensuring diverse representation among individuals who are experts in the specific field can be facilitated by the group or society's diversity, equity, and inclusion (DE&I) committee. The authors' experience attests that this approach leads to stronger and higher-quality educational programs [3].

Equally vital is the selection and mentorship of junior faculty members, considering the phenomenon of imposter syndrome. This psychological phenomenon involves high achievers experiencing self-doubt and fearing exposure as frauds, despite objective measures of their accomplishments [4]. Seasoned leaders of educational initiatives must play a role in building the confidence of junior faculty who are eager to teach and share their insights with trainees [5]. On the other hand, individuals lacking ample or current practice experience may be guided toward alternative contributions.

Summary and SAGES Takeaway

Surgical educators and leaders play a vital role in training residents, fellows, and practicing surgeons. These leaders are subject to various factors that impact their roles both at local and national levels. The development of leadership skills is paramount for effective team building. Encouraging formal leadership training courses for leaders of educational teams is crucial, as they equip faculty with the essential skills and strategies for effective leadership. The adaptability to pivot teaching methods and harness novel technologies is indispensable for enhancing the impact of educational programs. To gain followers and establish leadership credibility, leaders must foster an inspirational environment that motivates faculty and trainees to actively participate in educational efforts. By harnessing the collective contributions of faculty in a synergistic manner, educational leaders can create high-quality educational initiatives that reflect resonant and inspirational leadership.

References

1. "Origin of the word Doctor" Oxford Languages.
2. Kouzes James M, Posner BZ. The truth about leadership: the no-fads heart-of-the-matter facts you need to know. 1st ed. Jossey-Bass A Wiley Imprint; 2010.
3. Rosenkranz KM, Arora TK, Termuhlen PM, Stain SC, Misra S, Dent D, Nfonsam V. Diversity, equity and inclusion in medicine: why it matters and how do we achieve it? J Surg Educ. 2021;78(4):1058–65. https://doi.org/10.1016/j.jsurg.2020.11.013.

4. Bhama AR, Ritz EM, Anand RJ, Auyang ED, Lipman J, Greenberg JA, Kapadia MR. Imposter syndrome in surgical trainees: clance imposter phenomenon scale assessment in general surgery residents. J Am Coll Surg. 2021;233(5):633–8. https://doi.org/10.1016/j.jamcollsurg.2021.07.681.
5. Choron RL, Manzella A, Teichman AL, Cai J, Schroeder ME, Yao M, Greenberg P. The impact of surgical boot camp on medical student confidence and imposter syndrome. J Surg Res. 2023;283:872–8. https://doi.org/10.1016/j.jss.2022.11.013.

Managing Superiors and Your Team

28

Mai Al Khadem and Mujjahid Abbas

Introduction

In a critical environment of a surgical setting, effective leadership and management play a vital role in forming a unified team and achieving positive outcomes. Effective leadership requires a level of emotional intelligence and soft skills to see the big picture and envision the future. This allows the team to be goal-driven, motivated, and focused. While leadership is a critical component in surgeons' skillset, management acts as a distinct element. It is important to understand that leadership is different from management. While both terms are used interchangeably, they are distinct from one another. The skills and expertise used to navigate leadership are separate from management. Leadership involves change on a larger scale, emphasizing innovation and fostering personal and organizational growth. Management entails coordinating tasks, ensuring efficiency, and focusing on operational execution and resource allocation to achieve established goals. A physician can play one or both roles at an institution, although one might be

M. Al Khadem · M. Abbas (✉)
Bariatric Division, Department of Surgery,
University Hospitals Cleveland Medical Center, Case Western Reserve University School of Medicine, Cleveland, OH, USA
e-mail: Mai.alkhadem@uhhospitals.org; Mujjahid.abbas@uhhospitals.org

S. M. Johnson et al. (eds.), *The SAGES Manual of Strategy and Leadership*, https://doi.org/10.1007/978-3-031-62359-2_28

suited to be a leader but not a manager, and vice versa. Typically, physicians that seek immediate gratification and find satisfaction in managing the day-to-day tasks are better suited as managers. However, physicians who aspire to change the future of an organization on a larger scale tend to be effective leaders [1].

Fundamentals of Team Management

This chapter focuses on management of your juniors and superiors on the team. However, management is in fact divided into self-management and team management. To succeed in both, one must have an optimal level of emotional intelligence (EI). Emotional intelligence was first defined in 1990 as "the subset of social intelligence that involves the ability to monitor one's own and other's feelings and emotions, to discriminate among them, and to use this information to guide one's thinking and actions" [2]. The authors described that the emotions of oneself is important to appraise and express to others in a verbal and a nonverbal method. Equally important is the perception of emotions of others and the empathy exhibited toward them. The four elements of EI that were later described were self-awareness, social awareness, self-regulation, and relationship management [3, 4]. One must strive to have an accurate self-assessment, confidence, and sufficient emotional control. While dealing with others, one must strive to have empathy and organizational insight and be skillful in conflict management.

Foundations of team management include building a united team, formulating strategies, stress management, and flattening the hierarchy. These foundations are mostly extrapolated from the aircraft industry. Serious and fatal aircraft accidents occurred due to the failure of the copilot to challenge the captain. In some instances, the copilot would be hesitant to speak up despite realizing something might be wrong. The industry, later, made changes to allow any crew member to challenge one other, without fear of retribution. Formal Crew Resource Management training programs were established, which created a safety culture, attentiveness to human error, and a need for trustworthiness

[5]. Unfortunately, the hierarchy is still steep in the healthcare field, especially in a surgical specialty [6]. We know that patient complications can result from poor or lack of communication [7]. In a cross-sectional survey measuring attitudes relating to error, stress, and teamwork among operating room staff compared to airline cockpit crew, 97% of pilots rejected steep hierarchies, but only 55% of consultant surgeons did [8]. While the study is limited, it was observed that medical staff find it difficult to discuss errors without fear of retribution. During that period of time, the World Health Organization Surgical Safety Checklist was created, and it has been successful in improving patient outcomes in anesthesia and surgery [9]. The checklist is typically reviewed by multiple team members prior to commencing the operation. This can be a junior attending or a circulating nurse. Therefore, anyone will have the opportunity to speak up. This might aid in leveling out the hierarchy in the surgical field.

Leadership Styles

Management leadership styles were divided into six main styles. The styles are listed in the following paragraph. Goleman emphasized that a successful leader is one who uses different styles in various situations [10].

1. **Coercive Style:** It is the most controlling, where a top-down approach is followed. The manager orders the employees to execute tasks without question. Employees are not encouraged to share their opinions. Strict compliance is required with little room for error. It is expected that employees will be dissatisfied, leading to a high turnover rate and resentment. It is natural to expect that this style might not be successfully used in an organization; however, it is useful in settings where decisions need to be executed quickly. Specifically, this style yields best results when directing large teams and unskilled employees. Emergency situations would be an appropriate platform to use this style [10].

2. **Authoritative Style:** The leader is a visionary, who inspires staff by explaining the goals and vision of the organization. Once staff are inspired, they can execute the tasks using their creativity and skills. Managers give their staff regular positive or negative constructive feedback during this process. The employees are generally more satisfied and motivated since they understand the overall vision and take responsibility for their own actions. It is important to know that not all managers can be genuinely inspiring to their team members, so this style cannot be forged. As a downside, staff who are more experienced than the manager might see the leader as an overbearing one with little influence on the team [10].
3. **Affiliative Style:** Managers use this style with the focus on the staff's emotions and morale. There is an ample amount of positive feedback throughout the day-to-day tasks. The goal is to increase the bond among the staff members which eventually translates into improved performance and innovation. While this can increase job satisfaction especially in those who favor autonomy, productivity might decrease and the outcomes of the projects can suffer. Team members can become complacent if all they receive is positive feedback without correcting areas that require improvement. This style should not be used alone [10].
4. **Democratic Style:** This style is used by managers who do not have ideas of where to start or how to solve a problem. Managers ask their employees to generate ideas and share thoughts. They provide the employees with the opportunity to be creative. This allows members to form a close bond with the managers since they feel heard. However, this style can be time-consuming, especially when a consensus is not made. In some circumstances, this can lead to escalating conflicts and endless meetings. This type of manager would not like to make a formal decision him/herself [10].
5. **Pacesetting Style:** The manager sets an exceedingly high standard and embodies it. If the team members require direction or feedback, the manager takes over the tasks. Any staff member who falls behind gets punished or replaced. This style leaves no room for creativity, flexibility, innovation, or trust.

The morale drops among the organization, which leads to a high turnover rate. While it is normal to think that this type of style should not be used, it is helpful, especially when the staff are highly skilled and self-driven. They follow and personify the manager so their productivity is high [10].

6. **Coaching Style:** Managers guide their team members to focus on long-term development despite transient failures. The focus is on promoting growth and talent from within the organization as opposed to recruiting new employees. This is useful in organizations with a competitive market, where it might be expensive to hire new employees. However, short-term projects might be left unattended on the expense of long-term development. This type of style is most useful when the employee knows his/her weakness and wants to be coached to improve his/her performance [10].

Goleman studied the effect of the aforementioned styles on the six drivers of climate: flexibility, responsibility, standards, rewards, clarity, and commitment [10]. The authoritative style yielded the most positive impact on climate, followed by the affiliative, democratic, and coaching styles. The more styles a manager masters, the better the climate and performances one can expect. It is important to remember that as healthcare professionals, we are leaders from the first day we start medical school. Our vision and thought process varies at different levels in medical education. A study conducted in Canada by Saxena et al. examined the preferred styles that leaders at different levels would utilize [11]. The authors divided the medical education leaders into first-level (limited responsibility, i.e., medical students/residents), middle-level (wider responsibility, i.e., coordinators, curriculum chairs, program directors), and a senior-level (highest responsibility, i.e., deans and associate deans). The most frequently used leadership style by the first-level leaders was the democratic style, followed by coaching. The middle-level leaders chose coaching as their preferred leadership style. The senior leaders did not have a preferred style and instead used multiple styles. The second phase of the study involved interviewing the senior-level leaders. Results showed that some senior leaders would resort to using the pace-setting style, especially with physicians who are difficult to engage. Interestingly, five out of eight senior leaders did not use coaching or affiliative styles.

It was believed that a successful leader is an effect of one's personality solely, but this concept has been discredited. It has been demonstrated that EI grows with age [4]. However, it is not enough to rely on life experiences to improve one's EI and, consequently, management skills. In the modern world, it is believed that a leader can reach his/her potential through behavior modification, practice, and education. In the study by Ford et al., the performances of trauma team leaders improved with didactic teaching and practice simulations [12]. In his article, Goleman described the methods used to change an executive's social intelligence to improve her relationships with her team members and higher-ups and land a promotion [13]. In this article, the executive went through a 360-degree evaluation by an organizational psychologist and senior consultant. According to her peers and managers, the executive had a lack of empathy and adaptability and had poor skills at managing conflicts. She would not recognize the different social cues when a team member is reacting negatively. She was blunt when dealing with managers but did not know when to back off. She subsequently was coached by one of the socially intelligent leaders in the organization. The executive's behavior and performance changed drastically with reported improved satisfaction from her peers and managers. She went from losing her job to being promoted, increasing the annual sales, and was later made president of a multibillion-dollar company [13].

Managing Up

The idea that we can manage "upwards" is probably an uncommon concept to grasp, especially in the healthcare setting and, more closely, a hierarchical surgical setting. This concept was established in 1980, by the business world. Managing upwards means "being the most effective employee you can be, creating value for your boss and your company" [14]. In medicine, the mentor and mentee relationship is a perfect example of when the junior manages the senior. To start this mentorship, it is important for the mentee to self-reflect and identify what his/her goals are [15]. The mentee should be able to express his/her preferred communication style, expectations, and values [16]. Once the mentee conducts the self-assessment, he/she should find a mentor who can cultivate the relationship. It is an effective way to meet with different individuals and provide documents (i.e., curriculum vitae) that showcase your previous work, prior to choosing a mentor. By speaking to individuals across the department, one can get recommendations [16]. Communication styles matter to both mentor and mentee [15]. While certain individuals might prefer quarterly face-to-face meetings, others might favor more frequent, weekly meetings. It is also important to note that underrepresented minorities in academia might now be able to find a compatible mentor easily. That being said, it is often helpful to have a mentor from a diverse background who might have different perspectives and thought processes [16]. For sure, this helps in career and network development [17]. Also, ensuring that the mentee has realistic expectations and goals that would align with what the mentor has to offer is helpful. Making sure that these expectations are revised on a regular basis will go a long way [18]. It is key to be proactive when it comes to this type of relationship by setting yourself up for success. Prepare and brainstorm ideas to make the most out of your meeting and save the mentor's time [18]. Part of being proactive is keeping up with regular meetings with the mentor. Therefore, understanding both your preferred communication styles helps in maintaining your interactions [18]. Modeling professional behavior is critical when it comes to the mentor-mentee relationship. One can be friendly but should avoid being intrusive in asking about the mentor's personal life [18].

Similarly, in a managerial role, an individual can "manage up" his/her superiors. An important factor to take into consideration is the work style [19].

Four main types were described [19–21]:

1. **Logical or the advancer:** This individual will be efficient, analytical, and focused when it comes to achieving goals. Such a person might be perceived as insensitive and indifferent. To manage such a manager, be brief and concise as opposed to being casual when conversing with them. Also, it is wise to bring ideas and solutions to the table. It is best practice not to oppose them in public. The goal is to accomplish tasks as quickly and efficiently as possible.
2. **Detail-oriented or the evaluator**: This individual values precision and accuracy. In general, he/she is rigid and critical. To manage this type of manager up, come prepared and be attentive to the process. You might think the process is too detailed or redundant, but that does not matter when it comes to this type of manager.
3. **Emotionally-oriented or the harmonizer**: This individual cares about his/her team's harmony and collaboration. The team's satisfaction and wellness are a priority. To manage up this manager, aim to communicate openly and be synergistic with the rest of the team. Being supportive to your team members goes a long way with this type of manager.
4. **Idea-oriented or the energizer**: This individual thinks of the big picture and the direction of the team/organization. They are innovative and yearn for risks. They might be perceived as impatient or reckless. To manage this manager, ride on the same boat and be optimistic regarding his/her novel ideas. Show devotion, synergy, and loyalty to the overall vision.

The Challenging Boss

Managing your boss means that you might need to give feedback [22]. If your relationship with your boss does not have trust, it is not advised to give unsolicited advice, even if you have the best intentions. The best approach is to avoid giving feedback, unless you were requested to do so. Nevertheless, you can inquire if he/she desires feedback when the time seems proper. This is appropriate specifically in situations where you are working on a particular project together. When giving feedback, it is vital to remember to focus on the issue at hand, again, with the best intentions. No matter how constructive your feedback is, it will be limited because of your narrow perspective. You cannot imagine the entire burden or demands your boss has. Therefore, focus on what you hear and see rather than presuming you understand the entire situation. Now, it is expected for your boss to become defensive, even if he/she did ask for the feedback. When that happens, it is helpful to remind him/her that you were asked to do so. Attempting to reword your feedback might be useful. Also, knowing the topics that are off-limits to your boss is critical. This aids in avoiding conflict or forming a crack in the relationship. As always, if unsure about the outcome of providing feedback and how it might affect you, then it is better to avoid it altogether. The stakes can be too high to risk your job or the quality of your relationship with your boss. As you can see, you require a certain level of emotional intelligence to evaluate and expect your boss's reaction to your feedback. On the other hand, a receptive boss, one with a high level of emotional intelligence, is more likely to appreciate your feedback, even when unsolicited. Their ability to manage their emotions and remain open to a different perspective can lead to constructive dialogue and growth within the workplace. When we possess a high level of understanding, we become more empathetic toward a difficult or a challenging boss. When we understand that everyone, including our boss, has their own strengths and weaknesses and that these manifest in diverse ways, we become equipped to handle difficult situations.

If the situation is serious enough, where the team or organization will suffer and it is believed that feedback is necessary, a 360-degree feedback is warranted. This 360-degree, or multisource, feedback is an anonymous method of providing feedback. It serves as a review process that measures a physician's performance [23]. It was demonstrated that feedback does improve leadership and that feedback from the bottom up is preferred when delivered anonymously [24].

As noted, it is not simple to be a manager of a junior or a superior employee. In a healthcare setting, where the hierarchy is usually steep, the acronyms "PACE" and "CUS" were developed to gain attention when faced with this steep hierarchy [6]. **P**robe: Question the decision. **A**lert: Be more decisive. **C**hallenge: Directly challenge the decision. **E**mergency: Ask for help. **C:** I am Concerned. **U:** I am Uncomfortable, or this is unsafe. **S:** I am Scared. As we can see, managing a senior colleague who might cause detrimental harm to a patient is a separate skill to acquire, especially when the outcomes can be devastating.

Lastly, it is not unusual that individuals in the healthcare setting might face a toxic boss. There are signs of toxicity that we should learn to identify and recognize. A person who has no interest whatsoever in what people have to say can behave in a noxious manner. Another worrisome sign is the lack of empathy and failed recognition when "firing" someone. There is usually an air of distrust among the team where each person is looking out for "who is going to backstab me next." Individuals can feel humiliated and coerced, especially those who are more junior and vulnerable. It is not surprising that toxic bosses act similar to a typical bully. They gain satisfaction when they push others around and allow them to feel smaller. They usually exhibit a malignant and controlling behavior with lack of flexibility in communication. In these cases, to save yourself from the negative effect and, ultimately, the organization as a whole, it is your responsibility to report this individual to people that can exhibit change, including terminating this toxic boss. Usually, there will be multiple reports of misconduct that will, eventually, push this individual out of the organization [25].

Conclusion

In summary, surgeons should not only harness the knowledge and technical abilities for patient care. With the modern advances and larger, more complex teams and organizations, it is imperative that the surgeon identify his/her own personal qualities, work style, and level of emotional intelligence. Subsequently, the surgeon should work on developing these skills, ideally, with the support of a mentor. Providing and receiving feedback aids in the progress of these skills and abilities. Therefore, possessing an open communication style with all team members aids in fostering a relationship that advances the projects at hand and the organization as whole.

SAGES Takeaway

- Leadership is a soft skill that every surgeon or surgeon-in-training should work on developing throughout their career.
- Leadership and management are two distinct entities with different skills required to execute successfully.
- A competent leader should aim to possess more than one leadership style to be used in various settings.
- Managing superiors is just as important as managing juniors on a team.
- One of the ways to handle a challenging or a toxic boss is performing a 360-degree feedback.

References

1. Dye CF. Physicians in management vs. leadership positions. Understanding the difference between the two is critical to success. Healthc Exec. 2014;29(5)
2. Salovey P, Mayer JD. Emotional intelligence. Imagin Cogn Pers. 1990;9(3):185–211. https://doi.org/10.2190/DUGG-P24E-52WK-6CDG.
3. Goleman D. Emotional intelligence. Bantam Books; 1995.
4. Mayer JD, Caruso DR, Salovey P. Emotional intelligence meets traditional standards for an intelligence. Intelligence. 1999;27(4) https://doi.org/10.1016/S0160-2896(99)00016-1.
5. Reynard J, Reynolds J, Stevenson P. Professional culture. In: Practical patient safety. Oxford University Press; 2009. p. 247–62. https://doi.org/10.1093/med/9780199239931.003.0008.
6. Green B, Oeppen RS, Smith DW, Brennan PA. Challenging hierarchy in healthcare teams—ways to flatten gradients to improve teamwork and patient care. Br J Oral Maxillofac Surg. 2017;55(5):449–53. https://doi.org/10.1016/j.bjoms.2017.02.010.
7. Manser T. Teamwork and patient safety in dynamic domains of healthcare: a review of the literature. Acta Anaesthesiol Scand. 2009;53(2):143–51. https://doi.org/10.1111/j.1399-6576.2008.01717.x.

8. Sexton JB, Thomas EJ, Helmreich RL. Error, stress, and teamwork in medicine and aviation: cross sectional surveys. BMJ (Clin Res Ed). 2000;320(7237):745–9. https://doi.org/10.1136/bmj.320.7237.745.
9. Haugen AS, Sevdalis N, Søfteland E. Impact of the World Health Organization surgical safety checklist on patient safety. Anesthesiology. 2019;131(2):420–5. https://doi.org/10.1097/ALN.0000000000002674.
10. Goleman D. Leadership that gets results. Harv Bus Rev. 2000;78(2)
11. Saxena A, Desanghere L, Stobart K, Walker K. Goleman's leadership styles at different hierarchical levels in medical education. BMC Med Educ. 2017;17(1):169. https://doi.org/10.1186/s12909-017-0995-z.
12. Ford K, Menchine MDM, Burner ME, Arora MS, Inaba MDK, Demetriades MDD, Yersin PDB. Leadership and teamwork in trauma and resuscitation. Western J Emerg Med. 2016;17(5) https://doi.org/10.5811/westjem.2016.7.29812.
13. Goleman D, Boyatzis R. Social intelligence and the biology of leadership. Harv Bus Rev. 2008;86(9):74–81. 136
14. Gabarro JJ, Kotter JP. Managing your boss: a compatible relationship with your superior is essential to being effective in your job. Harv Bus Rev. 1980;58(1)
15. Han AY, Gentle CK, Stefanopoulos S, Burneikis T, Lipman JM, French JC. Managing up: approaching mentoring from a Mentee's perspective. J Surg Educ. 2022;79(6):e161–5. https://doi.org/10.1016/j.jsurg.2022.07.004.
16. Jackson VA, Palepu A, Szalacha L, Caswell C, Carr PL, Inui T. "Having the Right Chemistry": a qualitative study of mentoring in academic medicine. Acad Med. 2003;78(3) https://journals.lww.com/academicmedicine/fulltext/2003/03000/_having_the_right_chemistry___a_qualitative_study.20.aspx
17. Manuel SP, Poorsattar SP. Mentoring up: twelve tips for successfully employing a mentee-driven approach to mentoring relationships. Med Teach. 2021;43(4):384–7. https://doi.org/10.1080/0142159X.2020.1795098.
18. Lee SP, Mcgee R, Pfund C, Branchaw J. "Mentoring Up": learning to manage your mentoring relationships. In: The mentoring continuum: from graduate school to tenure; 2015.
19. Tate C. Differing work styles can help team performance. Harv Bus Rev. 2015; https://hbr.org/2015/04/differing-work-styles-can-help-team-performance
20. Abbajay M. Managing up: how to move up, win at work, and succeed with any type of boss. Wiley; 2018.
21. Wahab RA, Brown A, Vijapura C, Mahoney MC. "Managing Up": cultivating relationships with practice leaders. J Breast Imaging. 2022;4(2) https://doi.org/10.1093/jbi/wbab097.
22. Gallo A. Managing up: how to give your boss feedback. Harv Bus Rev. 2010;

23. Donnon T, Al Ansari A, Al Alawi S, Violato C. The reliability, validity, and feasibility of multisource feedback physician assessment: a systematic review. Acad Med. 2014;89(3) https://doi.org/10.1097/ACM.0000000000000147.
24. Gauly J, Court R, Currie G, Seers K, Clarke A, Metcalfe A, Wilson A, Hazell M, Grove AL. Advancing leadership in surgery: a realist review of interventions and strategies to promote evidence-based leadership in healthcare. Implement Sci. 2023;18(1) https://doi.org/10.1186/s13012-023-01274-3.
25. Gunderman RB. Seven signs your boss is toxic. J Am Coll Radiol. 2015;12(10) https://doi.org/10.1016/j.jacr.2015.01.011.

Goal Implementation 29

Judy Chen

What you will learn: This chapter covers critical skills that leaders must have for goal implementation and how to develop these skills and implement them.

Overview

We are all goal-oriented people—no one accidentally becomes a physician. But having goals, especially large life-defining goals, is different from professional and project-based goals. Many of us identify what we want to accomplish or how we could be better at our jobs, but creating an actionable plan is difficult and requires mindful planning. These sections will discuss critical steps to successfully implementing goals as individual professionals and as leaders [1].

J. Chen (✉)
Department of Surgery, University of Washington School of Medicine, Seattle, WA, USA
e-mail: jycm@uw.edu

S. M. Johnson et al. (eds.), *The SAGES Manual of Strategy and Leadership*, https://doi.org/10.1007/978-3-031-62359-2_29

Strategy for Individual Goal Implementation

Goal Implementation is the process of intentionally organizing actions to reach a desired objective [2]. Be truthful with yourself about your ability to accomplish this. Setting goals for yourself is different than setting goals for a team. So, when facing a new project or position in life, begin by understanding what your own overarching aim and tasks are. Whether you're applying goal implementation to improve your skills or to address new challenges, be considerate of what can be defined as success, failure, or even something in between. In addition, consider how to monitor, evaluate, and adjust your goals as you progress. Goal implementation is an iterative process and is critical to promoting effective changes over the course of a career [1].

The most important step is the first: identify the vision underlying your goal [1]. What are the facts, values, and purpose behind the goal? What will success look like? Have a realistic and reasonable definition of success based upon and tethered to the vision of your goal. Work backward from your goal, vision, and definition of success to list objectives with clear, achievable parameters. A list of objectives allows for measurement of progress and performance. Unclear objectives can create failure before your opportunity for implementation arrives. Do not set objectives that are impossible to reach. Having realistic expectations will keep you from feeling overwhelmed or outmatched. Your objectives should also be meaningful, as tasks can become burdensome without the result desired. The most detrimental end point is not to take the opportunity to learn but for the process of goal and action planning.

After understanding your inspiration and ideal performances, understand the steps needed to achieve your goal [3]. Imagine the ease of cooking with a well-written, well-conceived recipe. This ability to organize a plan can be written as an outline, drawn out with figures and graphics, or any organizational design that suits you. Examples in quality projects often include the PDCA method (plan-do-check-act/adjust), also known as the Shewhart cycle [4]. Set aside the time to find organizational tools to make your planning smoother, easier, and less challenging. Within the steps, be open to being flexible and adjust as needed, since achieving goals is not just following the recipe. Goal implementation needs the organization of a blueprint to lay a path toward success. You must monitor, evaluate, and adjust your plans toward the ultimate goal you envisioned.

You will experience both successes and failures, so identify possible barriers and insights that can affect the execution of your plan to achieve your objectives. Create an action plan with clear steps to define your approach [3]. Your action play should account for all deliverables, tasks, resources, and resource needs. Create a realistic timeline, considering your experiences and circumstances [3]. Identify milestones for each objective. Listing the objectives is essential in defining success with clear achievable parameters. If it is not clear, this may create failure before that implementation even happens.

If you're looking at career changes or advancement in regard to goal implementation, the outcome of your work is important to understand. As highlighted above, it is the overarching vision that drives what success means for you. The outcomes can hinge on both success and failures but acknowledge that there are other benefits such as goals that stretch you. Stretch goals can be characterized by two variables, difficulty and novelty [5]. The difficultly of goals asks you to go beyond current capabilities and performance. The novelty of goals requires new approaches to achieve the desired outcome. These types of stretch goals should propel you to move out of your comfort zone if used in goal implementation.

In summary, there are essential ingredients for goal implementation. It is defined by the original vision and requires mindfulness. Goals must be SMART [3, 6] (specific-measurable-attainable-result oriented-time defined) with clear outlines, check-ins, and techniques to optimize accountability. Barriers, risks, assessments, roles, and responsibilities will need to be anticipated for successful implementation. Goal implementation requires thinking, doing, deciding, planning, and producing a strategy that accomplishes the initial goal envisioned. These activities involve many tools and have different specificities. In the end, the process of goal implementation and defining targets for yourself creates value for yourself, your team, and your organization.

Strategy to Lead in Goal Implementation

As a leader or manager, performance is based on what is accomplished through others, often as a team. For team management and leadership, much of the strategic framework for goal implementation is the same, but every step requires effective communication, active listening, and the ability to rally a team behind a shared goal [7].

As an individual setting a goal, you're the only person who needs to understand your vision. As a leader, you must be able to explain it to the team you need to achieve it. Whether you find the introspective work for individual goal implementation to be torture, or you find the collaborative, extroverted work of managing others to be equally unpleasant, you're a physician and must do both. Every attending physician leads a team. You may lead a team of office support staff, a team of medical personnel, a team of other physicians, or, perhaps, all three. This requires strong skills in leadership and management: thoughtful, effective delegation; personal and team-based organization; developing your emotional intelligence to understand professional relationships; and creating clear communication [5].

As a leader or manager, performance is based on what is accomplished through others, often as a team. Thus, setting goals for a team is different than setting goals for yourself. The performance and success need to have a clear understanding of resources and collaboration by each team member. A leader must clarify how work is accomplished and understand the limitations of the team. It is important to consider building realistic expectations in any goal implementation plan.

One way many of us stumble when first becoming leaders is that we think of communicating as providing information *to* other people. "Was my presentation a success? It must have been: I explained everything very clearly." But explanation and presentation are specific communicative tools and can be inappropriate for the unstructured or conversational manner of many team communications. The basis of effective communication *with*—and not just *to*—your team is creating clear and honest channels for communication. If your team is unable or unwilling to communicate clearly and honestly with you, then the project could hit avoidable obstacles you did not know about and could not plan for. For team members, their performance and success are accomplished through individual actions. So, understanding their limitations, such as having the busy schedule clinicians often do, is important to delegating work, setting timelines, and setting up your team members for success.

To understand how to be successful, your team members need to understand your vision. But, especially for busy team members, they want actionable steps and a clear process [3]. By providing a clear set of reasonable expectations, your team gets a roadmap to success as your vision defines it. The word "work" is full of expectations. Provide clear outlines, set check-ins, and create opportunities to optimize accountability. Provide clear tasks. Progress is so difficult if there is no vision or inspiration. We've all been on teams, in trainings, or in presentations that lack a clear purpose and leave us asking, "What was that about? Why did I need to be here?" Avoid these moments by providing a set of reasonable expectations, enabling your team to progress toward your shared goal.

To set reasonable expectations, assign team roles, and designate responsibilities, you must understand your team member's capacity to work and succeed. Utilize interpersonal skills to develop your team members' potential. Interact positively to create and sustain relationships needed to navigate obstacles. A strong team requires interpersonal trust, and strong teams can create solutions to unforeseen problems because each member of the team is empowered to act independently and professionally toward your shared goal. The success of every person on the team depends on the results of others, so create a team culture where members are inspired to provide maximal productivity because they share the team's goal or are motivated to help each other succeed.

Believe in your team's ability to have the capacity to improve. The development of the team requires your flexibility to implement strategic thinking and change management. Draw upon experience—whether your own or that of your team members—to provide leadership, guidance, and inspiration. For each team member, consider how frequent or formal check-ins or progress updates must be. A new team member might appreciate frequent, formal check-ins where they can ask questions and get advice. An experienced team member may need no more than an occasional, informal conversation. Understand your team member's needs to be able to gauge specific and meaningful progress.

Being effective is being insightful and open to consistent accountability to ensure the plan is moving forward with regular check-ins and updates [3]. Consider how your team is progressing toward their objectives and be willing to adjust to having success versus chaos. If there are unforeseen changes, your action plan may need to change and shift, but not to the detriment of the goal. Adaptability promotes understanding when obstacles are encountered. In tough scenarios, setbacks can be uncomfortable. But change can be a benefit when a leader champions it and sets an example to help the team manage in an intentional and strategic way. Do so by considering the strengths, weaknesses, opportunities, and threats presented by the obstacle. This can minimize challenges that may appear overwhelming. Thinking strategically to generate solutions is a tool for leadership in successful goal implementation. After each obstacle has been navigated, reflect and debrief how the process went without publicly making a judgment or laying blame.

For specific communications within your team, your leadership sets the tone [7]. That tone is essential to establishing clear and open channels of communication. Encourage active engagement to ensure shared understanding and interests. Establish a safe and open environment. Doing so ensures your teams' needs are met because questions can be asked without fear and answered in depth. When running meetings, take simple measures to invite dialogue and discussion, but in a frame that allows the meeting to be kept on target. Whoever is leading the meeting—it does not always need to be you, especially if the topic is on a subject where a team member is responsible—should have created an agenda for it and identified the meeting's propose. For meetings and other communications where tasks are established, be sure to use closed-loop communication to ensure all team members understand their responsibilities, the expectations, and the timeline.

The benefits of goal implementation can foster growth and mindset. The process includes how leaders can provide direction and sense of purpose, as well as motivate behavioral changes. It is essential to clarify how work is accomplished and identify resources and collaborations needed. There is accountability for specific outcomes, and this can foster alignment within groups and ultimately a culture of achievement.

References

1. Drucker PF. The practice of management. New York: HarperCollins; 1954.
2. Favaro K. Defining strategy, implementation, and execution. Harv Bus Rev. 2015;3
3. Management by Objectives (MBO)—Aligning objectives with organizational goals (mindtools.com).
4. Tague NR. Plan-do-study-act cycle. In: The quality tool box. 2nd ed. ASQ Quality Press; 2005. p. 390–2.
5. Lee, Grace. How to implement goals across your organization with the Asana way of change. The Workback October 8, 2020.
6. SMART Goals—how to make your goals achievable (mindtools.com).
7. Stettner M. Leadership and management. In: The new manager's handbook. 24 Lessons for mastering your new role. McGraw-Hill; 2003.

Part VII

Leading Systems—Learning Local Context

Managing Human Resources and Organizational Talent

30

Joon K. Shim and Ian S. Soriano

Learning Objectives

1. Learn strategies to recruit, identify, develop, and retain organizational talent.
2. Discuss negotiation strategies from both sides of the table to achieve personal and institutional objectives.
3. Understand the benefits of physician talent management.

Introduction

Management is defined as (1) the act or art of managing or conducting something (such as a business) and also refers to (2) the collective body of those who direct (or manage) an enterprise [1]. Healthcare management refers to the group of individuals who provide leadership and direction to organizations that deliver personal health services, and to divisions, departments, units, or services within those organizations [2].

J. K. Shim
Bassett Healthcare Network, Cooperstown, NY, USA
e-mail: joon.shim@bassett.org

I. S. Soriano (✉)
Department of Surgery, University of California San Francisco, San Francisco, CA, USA
e-mail: Ian.soriano@ucsf.edu

S. M. Johnson et al. (eds.), *The SAGES Manual of Strategy and Leadership*, https://doi.org/10.1007/978-3-031-62359-2_30

As healthcare organizations expand through growth, including mergers and acquisitions, the importance of having a pipeline of physician healthcare leaders to lead various aspects of the healthcare organization who have the same cultural beliefs becomes imperative. Through external hiring or internal development, the identification, promotion, and retention of these individuals should be proactive rather than reactive.

The International Hospital Federation has defined five core competencies for healthcare leaders. In this chapter, we will focus on human resource management, including organizational talent, which is a key component of business competency [3].

Human Resource Development

Human resources can play a key role in surgery by improving the work environment, which will help retain talent in the organization. Effective policies can also help cultivate and enhance skills, which can achieve larger talent management goals. Policies including assistance in increasing productivity through marketing and staff support in alignment with a surgeon's goals will increase job satisfaction, enable surgeon's ability to maintain their quality of patient care and increase downstream revenue.

The human relations approach (HRA) recognizes that surgeons may be motivated by a range of factors, not only by financial reward [4]. So, if a leader or manager takes a step back, how does an organization focus on the importance of the person in human resources? Research from Gallego-Losada et al. shows the framework of strategic human resource management, which is based on the resource-based view of the firm. Their work highlights the uniqueness of the workers' competencies for organizational success, as well as individual commitment, skills, and knowledge [4]. Human relations approach was a precursor to the discipline of human resource management that we know today. Job satisfaction is seen as a key factor in encouraging staff to accomplish organizational goals. In essence, this theory supports the importance of the person, their values, and their social interactions within an organization such as the department of surgery. The human relations approach is a management theory that truly emphasizes the importance of human beings in organizations [4]. In a sense, it is personal and it emphasizes leaning into emotions, feelings, and social needs as considerations to improve productivity and job satisfaction.

The human relations approach originated from the Hawthorne studies in the 1920s and 1930s [5]. The Hawthorne studies found that productivity was not solely determined by physical working conditions or financial incentives but also by social and psychological factors [6]. The human relations approach emphasizes the importance of open communication, employee involvement, and the creation of a supportive work environment to improve motivation, job satisfaction, and productivity. It also recognizes the role of management in providing guidance, support, and encouragement to employees to help them reach their full potential. A low-hanging fruit for creating a supportive work environment for surgery would be one in a morbidity and mortality conference, where surgeons feel comfortable speaking up, asking questions, and making mistakes without fear of being ridiculed or punished. In the operating room, psychological safety is essential for effective teamwork, as it allows team members to communicate openly and honestly, which is critical for patient safety.

The role of the manager and leader usually involves interacting with human resources, either with the organization department itself or with human resource practices. There are several assumptions underpinning the practice of human resource management. Human resource management is founded on the belief that an organization's performance is based on the structures in place for the workers: for example, policies and systems (i.e., equality and diversity policy, training, performance appraisal, and more). Human resource management aims to maximize productivity and minimize staff turnover [7]. But it's easier said than done.

How does a department of surgery design a position of a surgeon within human resource management? It is the process of deciding the aspects, roles, and responsibilities of a particular position of employment within an organization. It is wise for a job to be designed in such a way that aids organizational productivity and also the satisfaction of the incumbent, likely resulting in longer-term retention. It's the personalized approach that may be effective in this case. There are several factors that influence job design. Hyde et al. explored the facets of job design necessary within the National Health Service in the British system [6], including how the workers will interact with the technology available to them and how technology can be used to improve productivity and job satisfaction.

In surgical departments, human resource plays a crucial role in making sure that the department has a skilled and diverse workforce to meet the demands of patient care. Leaders and managers in surgery work closely with surgeons, nurses, anesthesiologists, and other healthcare staff to identify staffing needs and to develop strategies to recruit and more importantly retain talent. It starts with having accurate job descriptions, holistic interviews, and reference checks. Once the newly hired surgeon begins their role, it's prudent to make sure there is a thoughtful orientation and training. Initially, there should be robust management and support of the surgeon's performance. Benefits, payroll, and any grievances and concerns should be addressed early on as part of inclusivity. This is part of creating a positive work environment that truly promotes surgeons' engagement and job satisfaction, which can ultimately lead to better patient outcomes.

One may want to consider a thoughtful process of selection techniques in hiring and retaining surgeons. Some departments assess a surgeon's skill in a hands-on setting, that is, they may have them join in cases prior to employment, if possible. They may also visit them at their home institutions to see them perform cases, too. There are several assessments for personality traits such as one's risk for tolerance of ambiguity and ability to handle stress. This seems a bit controversial, but there may be considerations for this in the future. In the end, the selection technique may depend on the specific needs of one's organization. It's prudent to use a variety of techniques to get a well-rounded assessment of each candidate. One of the questions one may consider is how a candidate is able to communicate effectively with patients and other members of the healthcare team. Another important aspect may be how one is compassionate and has a strong commitment to patient care.

Negotiating Organizational Talent

Organizational talent management and negotiation are how employers recruit and develop a workforce that is as productive as possible and likely to stay with their organization long term. When implemented strategically, this process can help improve the overall performance of the department's business and ensure that it remains competitive. The question that leaders and managers must ask themselves is - how dose one attracts, retains, and develops talented surgeons within an organization? How does one develop and implement strategies to do so?

Before hiring new talent, it will be prudent to assess the current needs of the organization and then address the future needs of the organization. A department of surgery can identify skill gaps and potential opportunities for growth and development. Some considerations include identifying potential areas of growth in which surgical services and specialties have the potential for expansion with regard to patient demand, market competition, and staffing needs. What new technologies should be invested in when recruiting specialized surgeons and collaborating with other departments? Partnering with the c-suite, an essential component of success would be implementing efficient scheduling systems with regard to operating times and clinic, optimizing patient flow and improving patient outcomes through quality improvement initiatives. Reviewing patient satisfaction surveys and clinical outcomes along with financial metrics will provide information to identify areas of opportunities for further improvement within an organization.

Based on this needs assessment, the organization can develop a talent strategy that outlines the specific action plan to attract, retrain, and develop talented employees. It may start with recruitment efforts. Faculty development programs and retention strategies such as flexible work arrangements or employee recognition programs. It will also be important to do research and understand the market value of the talent an organization is seeking to set realistic expectations and avoid mismatches with overpayment and underpayment. An organization must evaluate itself to see if surgeons may work part-time or less than full-time equivalent (FTE) to accommodate personal or family responsibilities [8]. Some organizations have considered surgeons sharing a full-time position with another surgeon, splitting responsibilities, and workload. Some surgeons have sought out opportunities to work remotely for administrative tasks such as charting, research, and education. Academic and community hospitals have offered flexible scheduling options, such as staggered start and end times or ability to work compressed work weeks. And, rather than continuing medical education days, some surgeons may be able to take extended leave for personal or professional development, which is a sabbatical to conduct research or pursue advanced training.

To attract and retain top talent, it will be important to create a compelling employee value proposition that differentiates the organization from its competitors. Why would one surgeon choose one organization over the other? Does the organization provide competitive salaries and benefits? Are there opportunities for career advancement? Is there a positive work environment? Creating a positive work environment in surgery can help to improve job satisfaction, reduce burnout, and improve patient outcomes. Civility and promoting a culture of respect by all staff members, regardless of their role or level of experience, will foster true professionalism [9]. Leaders within the department of surgery can encourage teamwork and collaboration by providing opportunities for communication and feedback. By building a learning environment, it will provide opportunities for continuing education and professional development. Prioritizing a safe and supportive environment by ensuring that the physical environment itself is clean, well-maintained, and free of hazards will promote health. By incorporating ergonomic principles into the design and operation of the surgical environment and equipment, surgical departments can reduce the risk of injury and strain for the surgical team, while also improving patient outcomes and efficiency in the operating room [10]. This will lessen stress and burnout for surgeons.

Building a strong employer brand can help attract top talent to the organization. This involves creating a positive image of the organization as an employer, which may include highlighting the organization's values, missions, and culture. An organization's commitment to delivering high-quality care, prioritizing patient safety, and fostering a supportive work environment will help create a positive image of the organization. In smaller rural areas, engaging with the community through outreach programs, educational events, and other initiatives can help to build awareness and trust in the surgery department and its organization. This can also help to identify potential patients and referral sources.

To attract and retain a talented workforce in surgery, it will be prudent to create a diverse and inclusive workplace culture. This will involve implementing policies and programs that promote diversity and inclusion, such as training programs, employee resource groups, and mentoring programs. An organization should implement inclusive hiring practices to seek and attract surgeons from diverse backgrounds [11]. An organization can try to achieve this by posting job openings on diverse job boards, actively recruiting candidates from underrepresented groups, and conducting blind curriculum vitae reviews to reduce the impact of unconscious bias. By providing training and education to staff members on cultural competency, unconscious bias, and diversity and inclusion, these actions can also help in recruiting and retaining a talented workforce in surgery. As mentioned by Massick and others, the patient-clinician race and ethnic concordance have been associated with improved patient outcomes, higher patient satisfaction, and greater treatment plan compliance among racial and ethnic minority patients who receive care from physicians who share a similar diverse background. Diverse teams also lead to more innovation, discovery, and better science [11].

It's important to measure and evaluate the success of talent negotiation strategies. This can be done through employee engagement surveys, turnover rates, and performance metrics. These elements will help to identify areas of success and areas of improvement. Failure to prioritize and negotiate talent management can lead to a loss of high-potential surgeons in the organization.

Understanding Talent Management

Talent management is defined as the process of attraction, development, and preservation of working people of increased abilities, skills, and knowledge with the goal of increasing productivity, effectiveness, and quality of their services, which is vital to survival and the organizations' competitive advantage [12, 13]. At its heart, it is simply a matter of anticipating the need for human capital and then setting out a plan to meet it [14].

The significance of physician talent management in healthcare has significant benefits. One study showed that hospitals with the most clinician involvement in management affairs performed 50% higher on drivers of performance, such as the effectiveness of overall management, performance management, and leadership compared with hospitals with little clinical leadership [15]. Physicians represent a "high value-added, difficult to replace" group of professionals within healthcare organizations [16]. In addition, studies have shown reduced clinical errors and mortality rates, shorter lengths of stays, and reduced costs [17–19]. Furthermore, healthcare organizations will need to develop specific talent management strategies for women who are the largest growing group in medicine, with approximately 50% of students and 46% of trainees [20].

Unfortunately, most organizations do not have a programmatic approach to developing organizational talent, but often what passes as leadership development in some hospitals and medical schools is a hodge-podge of classes and lectures lacking coherence, logical progression, comprehensiveness, and relevance presented on a variety of leadership and administrative topics. The episodic nature of the instruction is rarely successful in developing effective physician-leaders [21].

In a systematic review of various programs geared toward developing physician leaders, the following elements were found to be most effective: (1) conducting a needs and gap analysis with relevant stakeholders to inform the selection of the program's desired outcomes; (2) selecting the desired outcomes for the program including enhancing self-awareness, self-efficacy, and leadership knowledge, skills, and behaviors; (3) selecting explicit goals for the program that are aligned with organizational strategy or priorities and are linked directly to the desired outcomes and the evaluation framework; (4) selecting the participants intentionally based on their suitability to fill the needs and gaps identified during step one; (5) selecting the program structure, content, faculty, and developmental activities using an outcomes-based design that are included specifically according to their intended efficacy in facilitating the achievement of the desired outcomes; (6) devising an evaluation framework for the program overall, for individual activities, and for participants to include subjective and objective data at the individual level, as well as metrics pertaining to organizational impact and benefit to patients outcomes; (7) conducting a barriers assessment of organizational cultural factors that may hinder the achievement of desired outcomes and attempting to circumvent or remove them by incorporating "training transfer" or application of learning strategies; and, lastly (8), ensuring that the principles of adult learning or principles of leadership development have been addressed in the program design [22].

One such program was initiated by the Department of Surgery at The Ohio State University Wexner Medical Center over a decade ago. The Talent Management and Leader Development Academy (TMALDA) was created for surgeons who desired specific training for administrative and leadership roles not just within the department but at the medical school, hospital, and organizational level. Due to the success of the surgically oriented program, this was expanded into the Faculty Leadership Institute (FLI) and offered to all faculty members of the university. While other physician leaders became exposed to an MBA-type curriculum, the TMALDA curriculum included topics on (1) change management, (2) team building, (3) stress/burnout and lifestyle issues, and (4) healthcare law, while including common MBA topics such as financial management, leadership, and strategic planning and vision [21].

It is imperative that surgical departments evaluate potential hires not only for clinical, research, and teaching skills but also for leadership roles, both within and outside the department. In addition, once these physician leaders have been identified, provide them with the necessary training and education to fulfill these roles.

SAGES Takeaway

- Healthcare management, including talent management and succession planning, is key to the long-term success of healthcare organizations.
- Negotiating talent management should include stakeholders within and outside the department to be more strategic and optimize institutional resources.
- The skills and knowledge needed to become a highly effective physician-leader are unique to the field that should be obtained in a dedicated, structured curriculum focused on clinician-administrators.

References

Management

1. "Management." Merriam-Webster.com Dictionary, Merriam-Webster, https://www.merriam-webster.com/dictionary/management. Accessed 12 May 2023.
2. Thompson JM, Buchbinder SB, Shanks NH. An overview of healthcare management. In: Buchbinder SB, Shanks NH, editors. Introduction to health care management; 2012. p. 1–16.
3. Stefl ME. Common competencies for all healthcare managers: the healthcare leadership alliance model. J Healthc Manage. 2008;53(6):360–74.

Human Resources Development/Negotiating Organizational Talent

4. Rodriguez-Sanchez JL, Gonzales-Torres T, Montero-Navarro A, Gallego-Losada R. Investing time and resources for work-life balance: the effect on talent retention. Int J Environ Res Public Health. 2020;17(6):1920.
5. Ozgur O. Human resource theory: from Hawthorne experiments of mayo to groupthink of Janis. Global J Hum Resource Manage. 2016;4(1):95–110.
6. Ogbonnaya C, Babalola M. A closer look at how managerial support can help improve patient experience: insights from the UK's National Health Service. Hum Relat. 2021;74(11):1820–40. https://doi.org/10.1177/00187267209388.
7. Mathisen J, Nguyễn T, Jensen J, Rugulies R, Rod N. Scans J. Work Environ Health. 2021;47(6):456–65.

8. Hingstman L, de Jong J, Heiligers P, Hingstman L. Part-time and full-time medical specialists, are there differences in allocation of time? BMC Health Serv Res. 2006;6:26.
9. Smith C, Purcell L, Charles A. Cultural competence, safety, humility and dexterity in surgery. Curr Surg Rep. 2022;10(1):1–7.
10. Schulssel A, Maykel J. Ergonomics and musculoskeletal health of the surgeon. Clin Colon Rectal Surg. 2019;32(6):424–34.
11. Massick S, King K, Pawlik TM. Practical approaches to Foster diversity in surgical faculty recruitment. JAMA Surg. 2022;157(11):981–2. https://doi.org/10.1001/jamasurg.2022.3119.

Understanding Talent Management

12. Wood P. Continuing professional development in higher education: a qualitative study of engagement in the field of nursing and midwifery. J Enhanc Learn Teach. 2008;4:508.
13. Ahmed HK. The impact of talent management on the competitive advantage in the organizations. In: Proceedings of the 37th ISERD International Conference, Abu Dhabi, United Arab Emirates, 2–3 April 2021; 2021.
14. Cappelli P. Talent management for the twenty-first century. Harv Bus Rev. 2008;86(3):74.
15. Castro PJ, Dorgan SJ, Richardson B. A healthier health care system for the United Kingdom. McKinseyQuarterly.com; February 2008.
16. Lewis RE, Heckman RJ. Talent management: a critical review. Hum Resource Manage Rev. 2006;16(2):139–54.
17. Husebø SE, Akerjordet K. Quantitative systematic review of multi professional teamwork and leadership training to optimize patient outcomes in acute hospital settings. J Adv Nurs. 2016;72(12):2980–3000. https://doi.org/10.1111/jan.13035.
18. Rosenman ED, Shandro JR, Ilgen JS, Harper AL, Fernandez R. Leadership training in health care action teams: a systematic review. Acad Med. 2014;89(9):1295–306.
19. Mountford J, Webb C. When clinicians lead. McKinsey Q. 2009:1.
20. American Association of Medical Colleges. Physician specialty data book. Washington, DC: American Association of Medical Colleges; 2012.
21. Satiani B, Sena J, Ruberg R, Ellison EC. Talent management and physician leadership training is essential for preparing tomorrow's physician leaders. J Vasc Surg. 2014;59(2):542–6.
22. Geerts JM, Goodall AH, Agius S. Evidence-based leadership development for physicians: a systematic literature review. Soc Sci Med. 2020;246:112709.

31 Leading Systems: Assessment, Innovation, and Sustainability

Shukri H. A. Dualeh, Brian T. Fry, and Dana A. Telem

Introduction

Leading a healthcare system is a multifaceted endeavor that demands a diverse skill set. It necessitates dynamic interpersonal skills, a high degree of emotional intelligence, and, occasionally, a significant amount of courage. While a singular, universally accepted definition of a "system" remains unclear, when viewed through the lens of healthcare, a healthcare system encompasses more than just the assets, including support staff and management, required for patient care. It also entails a central, cohesive mission that resonates throughout the entire system. The alignment of a system's mission, vision, and core values is pivotal in striving toward a shared objective.

For instance, let's consider a large academic healthcare system as an example. This healthcare system's mission "to advance health to serve Michigan and the world" is accompanied by a vision where their "discoveries change care," ultimately leading to their "care changes lives" [1]. Moreover, they uphold a set of core values such as caring, inclusion, integrity, and teamwork [1]. While an academic institution may place emphasis on being a leader in medical

S. H. A. Dualeh (✉) · B. T. Fry · D. A. Telem
Department of Surgery, University of Michigan, Ann Arbor, MI, USA
e-mail: shukrid@med.umich.edu; dtelem@med.umich.edu

S. M. Johnson et al. (eds.), *The SAGES Manual of Strategy and Leadership*, https://doi.org/10.1007/978-3-031-62359-2_31

education and cutting edge research, a nonacademic system may focus on building relationships and serving the surrounding community. The core values of that system may be based on specific needs of patients at the individual level or be guided by overarching faith-based principles [2]. There is no one set definition on what a hospital system is and how different systems may have difference priorities. Understanding these differences are not only essential for effective and purposeful leadership but also for supporting functional aspects and driving necessary changes. Furthermore, regardless of what type of system you are leading, consistent evaluation and innovation are imperative for maintaining sustainability.

Our shared core values serve as the binding force for all members within the healthcare system. Beyond merely valuing diversity, fostering a culture of inclusion is paramount. This involves creating an environment that fosters equitable opportunities for growth and achievement. Upholding the utmost integrity should be complemented by a culture that empowers individuals at all levels to voice their thoughts and concerns. Ultimately, the large task of managing a large healthcare system effectively hinges on collaboratively working toward a common goal, which lies at the heart of successful healthcare delivery and is an absolute requirement for effective leadership.

In this chapter, we will discuss how to leverage models of quality improvement and implementation science to systematically and effectively shape leadership approaches and explore novel techniques that elevate leadership skills, including participation in a leadership development program and the facilitation of opportunities for team members to assume leadership roles. Finally, we will focus on how, once you have a successful approach to leadership, you can take the steps you need to sustain this success.

Assessment

Using a Quality Improvement Approach to Leadership

When Donabedian introduced his conceptual model for evaluating healthcare quality, it primarily found application within the clinical context to gauge the quality of healthcare delivery [3].

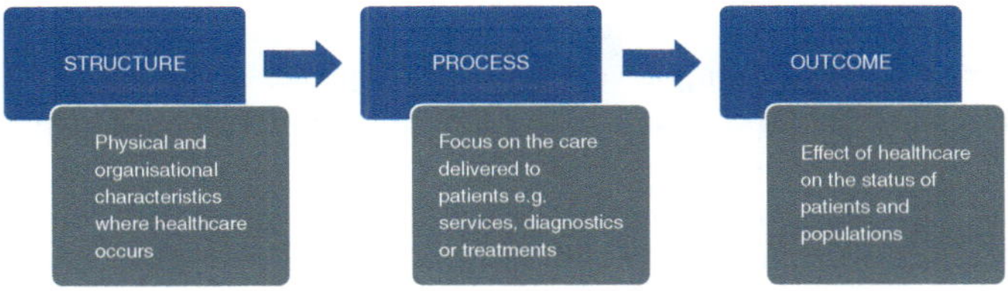

Fig. 31.1 Donabedian model for quality improvement [4]

This model established a framework for measuring and enhancing the quality of care by examining three key components: structure, process, and outcomes (Fig. 31.1) [4]. Drawing parallels between patient care and leadership, these components offer a valuable lens through which to assess and quantify the effectiveness of your leadership. The concept of structure measures was initially conceived as an input metric, emphasizing the essential services and resources required for delivering optimal care. These encompassed elements such as hospital infrastructure, financial resources, staffing, and equipment. On the other hand, process measures delineate how healthcare systems function to provide care to patients, encapsulating every step from the initial patient interaction with the healthcare team to the actual delivery of care. Meanwhile, outcome measures serve as indicators of the ultimate results emanating from the interplay between the established structures and operational processes. In the context of hospitals and networks tending to surgical patients, traditional outcome metrics encompass parameters like 30-day mortality rates, post-operative complications, length of hospital stays, 30-day readmission rates, and the need for reoperations.

When assessing quality improvement from a leadership perspective, the same triad of structures, processes, and assessment methodologies proves invaluable in fostering effective leadership. Structures, in this context, encompass the organizational framework within which your leadership is exercised. This may entail leading a team responsible for daily patient rounds, directing the activities within the operating room, or overseeing an entire section as a chief or department as a chair. Understanding the hierarchies and reporting structures—whether to the chair, dean, or president—provides a crucial foundation. Process measures, in the leadership realm, delve into the prerequisites essential for you to not only be a proficient leader. A few examples of process measures include ensuring attendance at a weekly morbidity and mortality conference, enforcing thorough clinic and operative notes that are submitted in a timely fashion, and keeping up to date on necessary certifications. Spending time assuring the completion of even mundane processes measures for you and your team provides time to devote to providing resources for good outcomes.

The third aspect of the Donabedian model focuses on outcomes. If the desired outcome of your leadership is to cultivate productive surgeon-scientists, it becomes imperative to supply them with resources, such as protected research time, laboratory facilities, and research personnel. On the other hand, if your goal is to nurture clinically adept surgeons, considerations would gravitate toward optimizing surgical scheduling and operation room resources to accommodate an increased caseload. Another illustration of leadership outcomes is the retention of faculty and staff. When the essential resources for ensuring the productivity, engagement, and job satisfaction of faculty and staff are accessible, the retention rate becomes a reliable metric for assessing this. In essence, the application of Donabedian's model to the sphere of leadership offers a comprehensive framework to gauge and enhance the quality of your leadership endeavors. Just as it aids in optimizing healthcare delivery, this model can guide you in establishing the foundational structures, refining processes, and ultimately achieving outcomes aligned with your leadership objectives.

How Can We Apply the Principles of Implementation Science to Leadership?

In addition to the Donabedian model, implementation science offers a structured framework to effectively translate leadership strategies, principles, and initiatives into tangible practice. There are multiple frameworks that can be applied to research and real-life implementation of evidence-based practices, but there are a few core principles that can be used to frame leadership strategies. Here, we will focus on (1) understanding the context and defining the problem, (2) establishing pertinent stakeholder engagement, and (3) implementing solutions and evaluating outcomes.

First, it's important to comprehend the environment in which these strategies will unfold. By doing this, you'll be able to gain a deep grasp of factors, such as team dynamics, organizational culture, and external influences, that can impact the trajectory of leadership initiatives. This contextual understanding provides the foundation for customizing your approach to seamlessly align with the unique needs and challenges of your team or organization. It will also facilitate the transparent identification of barriers and facilitators of change. There must be avoidance of a "one-size-fits-all" strategy of problem solving and instead focus on forming multifaceted, theory informed solutions. The next pivotal step involves meticulous planning. This involves delineating explicit goals, charting actionable steps, pinpointing key stakeholders, and judiciously allocating resources. By proactively engaging stakeholders and consistently involving them, you foster a culture of support and inclusivity. This process not only ensures that your team feels acknowledged but also cultivates a sense of investment in your overarching vision and mission.

Undoubtedly, the next essential step is the continuous monitoring and evaluation of your leadership endeavors, both quantitatively and qualitatively. This dynamic feedback loop can take the form of soliciting insights from all team members and leveraging data to drive informed decision-making, thus facilitating the evolution and optimization of your strategies. With insights garnered, you can then proceed to implement evidence-based interventions that have demonstrated efficacy. Embracing an assessment-driven approach goes beyond mere problem identification. It calls for a deliberate exploration of past setbacks, transforming them into invaluable lessons for learning and advancement.

Many of the concepts discussed above bear a resemblance to a Type 3 effectiveness-implementation hybrid design model. According to Curran et al., this model involves "testing an implementation strategy while simultaneously observing and gathering information on the clinical intervention's impact on relevant outcomes" [5]. There are occasions when it becomes necessary to implement a leadership strategy even without complete assurance of its effectiveness. In certain circumstances, the urgency of action outweighs the risks associated with indecision or inaction. This approach is particularly valuable in times of uncertainty and when there is minimal risk in implementing a strategy. By integrating these fundamental principles of implementation science into your leadership strategies, you establish the groundwork for sustainable and transformative change. Your leadership becomes a force that not only persists but also thrives in the face of challenges, resulting in lasting positive outcomes.

Innovation and Sustainability

Leadership Development Programs

Constantly assessing and reevaluating the efficacy of leadership is important, but equally vital is staying well-informed of novel and innovative strategies to leadership. Another avenue of innovation, along with incorporating implementation science, involves enrolling in a comprehensive leadership development program that extends its benefits to everyone within your sphere. Whether they belong to your clinical or research team, each team member can learn valuable insights and tools to become a proficient leader. Irrespective of one's official title, the lessons and approaches can be universally applicable.

The purpose of a leadership development program is to prepare surgeons for the many roles that they will take on in their careers. The program can be tailored to distinct levels, such as a resident leadership development program, an early career counterpart, and a dedicated track for mid-career and senior surgeons. Recognizing the distinct needs of surgeons at various career stages ensures targeted guidance and support. For optimal impact, these programs should be thoughtfully spread throughout the year and organized around well-defined themes, such as improving culture, fostering innovation, and how to handle difficult discussions. An effective program hones in on the bedrock principles of leadership—navigating team dynamics and resolving conflicts—through collaborative case-based discussions and seminars conducted by co-faculty, higher-tier leaders, and executive coaches [6]. This platform not only facilitates the collective examination of challenges encountered within teams but also fosters cross-subspecialty relationships, enriching the learning experience. Integral to the program is a holistic evaluation approach, encompassing 360° assessments from peers and supervisors, as well as anonymous written feedback. Investing in an executive coach, either personally or asking for resources from your supervisors, can intentionally aid in identifying problem areas and give you the tools to appropriately approach situations and develop a personal improvement plan.

Collectively, a robust leadership development program spans key domains, such as leadership essentials, team dynamics, business acumen, and contextual understanding (Fig. 31.2) [6]. This multifaceted approach equips surgeons with a comprehensive toolkit to not only excel in their surgical and research roles but to also lead with efficacy, enrich team dynamics, and contribute to the larger organizational mission.

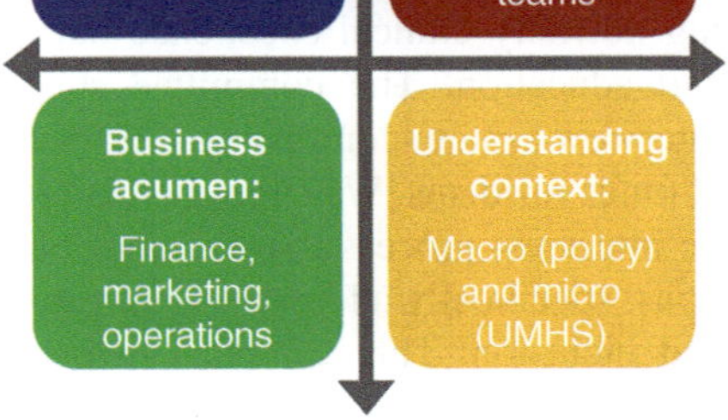

Fig. 31.2 Competency model for leadership development program. (Adapted from UMHS, Ref. [6])

Prioritizing Diverse Recruitment Efforts

Another pivotal facet of effective leadership within systems is the deliberate emphasis on recruiting and retaining a team that encompasses diversity. The United States continues to become more diverse, and with that, unfortunately, has come the widening of healthcare disparities. The responsibility of prioritizing diversity of thought, experience, background, and culture rests squarely upon hospital systems and leadership committees. Although medical schools have made strides in diversifying their student bodies, this diversity tends to diminish as one progresses through advanced specialty training and academic pathways. An alarming statistic illustrates that over 90% of 787 division chiefs were male, with only 4% being Black and 2.5% Hispanic [7]. This trend is mirrored in program director and chair positions. Furthermore, a substantial majority, around 89%, of hospital chief executive officers identify as White [8]. A team boasting a varied array of skills, backgrounds, and education can markedly amplify its capacity for problem-solving and foster cultural humility. Beyond this, the incorporation of purposeful antiracism initiatives and a commitment to enhancing cultural competence ae imperative in safeguarding the mission of sustaining a workforce rich in diversity.

One example of an initiative to prioritize and increase the diversity work force is by intentionally starting a faculty recruitment committee that is committed to hiring the best people. The goal should be to attract and retain faculty members from diverse backgrounds, encompassing race, ethnicity, gender, religion, sexual orientation, and age, who share a common mission of delivering not only clinical excellence but also excellence in research and education. The committee should have a comprehensive interview system comprising members from both the faculty and at times residents. We strongly recommend incorporating a holistic interview process that includes tailored attribute-based questions, specifically addressing key values such as diversity, equity, and inclusion. This approach helps identify individuals whose fundamental values align with the core principles and culture of the department, contributing to a more diverse and inclusive academic environment. To ensure objectivity, a set of standardized scoring criteria is utilized to reach a consensus on the top candidate. Already established leaders empower the faculty recruitment committee to play a pivotal role in selecting the most suitable candidates.

Fostering a Culturally Competent Environment

To enhance cultural humility within a diverse work environment, implementing a cultural complications curriculum is a great avenue. This innovative approach tackles a range of intricate clinical and cultural challenges, whether they involve patients or members of the healthcare team [9, 10]. Several surgery departments across the nation have already adopted this curriculum, which mirrors the structure of the traditional morbidity and mortality conference. The morbidity and mortality conference is an esteemed practice that is vital to surgical quality improvement. These conferences tend to have high attendance as they are often mandatory for accreditation purposes. To ensure the broadest participation and knowledge dissemination, cultural complications curriculum works best when seamlessly integrated into regularly scheduled morbidity and mortality conferences. If advertised as a separate conference, typically those who exhibit greater cultural competence are the ones who are self-motivated to attend. This inclusive approach benefits individuals who may not actively seek out this information but are exposed to it in the regular weekly morbidity and mortality conferences.

Within the cultural complications curriculum, the same structure and principles are applied to cases involving breakdowns in culturally inclusive communication or events misaligned with the desired work culture. These conferences have played a pivotal role in fostering an environment that prioritizes improving the daily experiences of individuals from historically marginalized groups. Incorporating cultural discussions within a formal, largely mandatory conference setting encourages engaged conversations and collaborative problem-solving. A key takeaway from the success of this curriculum is the provision of evidence-based data, highlighting the critical importance of addressing cultural complications in creating an open and inclusive workplace culture.

Providing Others Opportunities for Leadership

One critical part of effective leadership involves the recognition and cultivation of leadership opportunities for those around you. Members of your own team may show interest toward assuming greater responsibilities and seek enhanced leadership exposure. Making leadership opportunities, such as vice chair positions, clinical service line leads, or institute heads, can offer individuals a platform to demonstrate their dedication and leadership skill while concurrently affording you, as the leader, the means to uphold accountability and incrementally expand roles. This allows delegation of tasks that will move everyone forward and give team members valuable face time for learning from your expertise and providing you with an avenue to impart the essentials of team maintenance and influential leadership.

To this end, instituting a regimen of regular check-ins and making yourself available and approachable is vital. These interactions serve to promptly pinpoint any challenges that may arise, thereby laying the groundwork for tailored solutions and the seamless early implementation of necessary changes. This not only gives insight into the person's aptitude for resolving conflicts and addressing systemic issues but also shows leadership potential. Creating opportunities for leadership can hold immense potential and not only serve as professional development but can encourage your team members to stay engaged and work toward collective dedication to the shared mission.

Sustainability

Efforts to enhance the healthcare system inevitably encounter challenges and necessitate iterative cycles of reevaluation. Once a leadership approach has been implemented, proven effective, and reevaluated, it becomes essential to maintain what is working. Whether it involves leadership development programs, securing executive coaches, or purposefully focusing on diverse recruitment efforts, the rigor and intentionality must be an ongoing process to ensure long-term success. Building a culturally competent environment is not an overnight accomplishment but rather a consistent process of trial and error. This adaptability and willingness to reevaluate the needs of your health system or team are crucial as the environment evolves. It is imperative to continue prioritizing holistic leadership and active listening.

Conclusion

The leadership of a healthcare system is a multifaceted challenge that demands a diverse skill set, encompassing dynamic interpersonal skills, emotional intelligence, and courage. The essence of a healthcare system goes beyond its assets and incorporates a cohesive mission, vision, and core values that resonate throughout. The mission and values may vary between academic and nonacademic systems, reflecting their unique priorities and objectives. Regardless of the type of system, consistent evaluation and innovation are crucial for sustainability. The core values, fostering inclusion, and empowering individuals are the structure of effective leadership in healthcare. This chapter has explored the use of quality improvement and implementation science models to shape leadership approaches, develop leadership skills, and sustain successful leadership approaches. Emphasis on the importance of collaboration and a shared vision is at the heart of healthcare delivery and effective leadership.

SAGES Takeaway

- Effective healthcare leadership demands a diverse skill set, including interpersonal skills, emotional intelligence, and courage, and centers around a cohesive mission, vision, and core values that resonate throughout the entire system.

- Leadership strategies should be assessed using models like Donabedian's, which examine structures, processes, and outcomes, and implementation science principles to guide leaders to establish foundational structures, refine processes, and achieve outcomes aligned with leadership objectives.
- Engaging stakeholders and continuous evaluation offer a structured framework for translating leadership strategies into tangible practice, enabling sustainable and transformative change.
- Innovation in leadership involves participation in comprehensive leadership development programs tailored to different career stages, fostering diverse recruitment efforts, creating culturally competent environments, and creating opportunities for leadership within the team.

References

1. Welcome to Michigan Medicine. Michigan Medicine. https://www.uofmhealth.org/about. Accessed 9 Oct 2023.
2. Trinity H. Our mission, vision and values. https://www.trinityhealthmichigan.org/about-us/mission-and-values. Accessed 10 Oct 2023.
3. Donabedian A. Evaluating the quality of medical care. 1966. Milbank Q. 2005;83(4):691–729. https://doi.org/10.1111/j.1468-0009.2005.00397.x.
4. Creighton S. Avedis Donabedian: the creator of the Donabedian model of care. https://blog.lifeqisystem.com/avedis-donabedian. Accessed 31 Oct 2023.
5. Curran GM, Bauer M, Mittman B, Pyne JM, Stetler C. Effectiveness-implementation hybrid designs. Med Care. 2012;50(3):217–26. https://doi.org/10.1097/MLR.0b013e3182408812.
6. Leadership Development Program—Surgery—Michigan Medicine. Surgery. Published 14 Sept 2020. https://medicine.umich.edu/dept/surgery/michigan-promise/leadership/leadership-development-program. Accessed 29 Sept 2023.
7. Kassam AF, Taylor M, Cortez AR, Winer LK, Quillin RC. Gender and ethnic diversity in academic general surgery department leadership. Am J Surg. 2021;221(2):363–8. https://doi.org/10.1016/j.amjsurg.2020.11.046.
8. American College of Healthcare Executives. Increasing and sustaining racial/ethnic diversity in healthcare management. Healthc Exec. 2011;26(5):104–7.
9. To Err is Helpful. Cultural Complications. https://www.culturalcomplications.com. Accessed 28 Sept 2023.
10. Harris CA, Dimick JB, Dossett LA. Cultural complications: why, how, and lessons learned. Am J Surg. 2021;221(3):609–11. https://doi.org/10.1016/j.amjsurg.2020.09.002.

Accountability and Effective Communication

32

Juan S. Barajas-Gamboa

Introduction

In the ever-evolving landscape of modern medicine, the significance of accountability and effective communication cannot be overstated, especially in the realm of surgery [1]. As a discipline that inherently involves high stakes, complex team dynamics, and intense pressure, surgery demands not only technical proficiency but also a strong foundation in these softer skills. This chapter aims to delve into these critical aspects, unpacking their meanings, implications, and applications in the surgical environment [2, 3].

Accountability in surgery is a multifaceted concept, encompassing responsibility for both actions and outcomes, adherence to ethical standards, and a commitment to continuous learning and improvement [4]. In a field where decisions can have life-altering consequences, the importance of accountability becomes paramount. It's not merely about personal responsibility; it extends to creating a culture where every team member feels accountable for patient care and safety [5].

Effective communication, on the other hand, serves as the linchpin of successful surgical teams. It's about more than just

J. S. Barajas-Gamboa (✉)
Department of General Surgery, Cleveland Clinic Abu Dhabi, Abu Dhabi, United Arab Emirates

S. M. Johnson et al. (eds.), *The SAGES Manual of Strategy and Leadership*, https://doi.org/10.1007/978-3-031-62359-2_32

exchanging information; it's about ensuring clarity, understanding, and collaboration in high-pressure situations [6]. In the operating room, where every second counts and every action carries weight, the ability to communicate clearly and efficiently can be the difference between success and failure [7].

This chapter seeks to explore these concepts in depth, offering insight into how they intertwine and impact the surgical field. Through this exploration, we aim to equip academic surgeons, physicians, and those in training with the knowledge and tools to lead with accountability and communicate with efficacy. We will examine historical perspectives, current challenges, and future directions, anchoring our discussion with practical examples and case studies. By the end of this chapter, readers should have a thorough understanding of why these skills are indispensable and how they can be fostered and implemented in their own practice.

In the following sections, we will first define and dissect each concept individually and then demonstrate how they seamlessly integrate to form the bedrock of effective surgical leadership and team dynamics. We will also discuss the role of mentorship and leadership in cultivating these skills, and provide strategies to overcome common barriers.

Embarking on this journey, we hope to provide a comprehensive guide that not only informs but also inspires. Let us begin by exploring the concept of accountability in the surgical context and understanding its roots, relevance, and ramifications (Fig. 32.1).

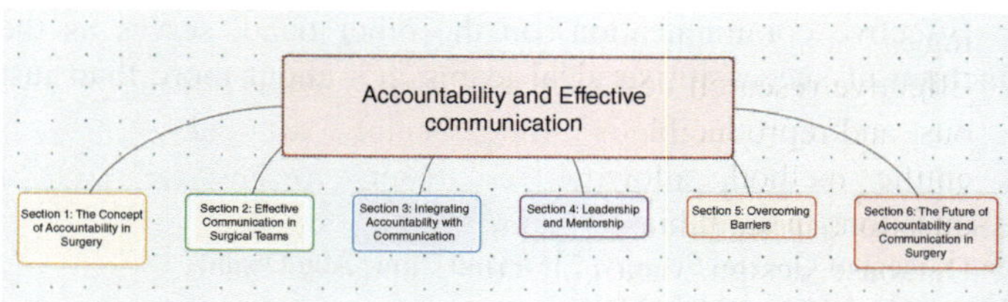

Fig. 32.1 Distribution of sections

Section 1: The Concept of Accountability in Surgery

Definition and Importance

Definition in a surgical context: Accountability in surgery encompasses more than just the responsibility for the outcomes of a surgical procedure. It represents a comprehensive commitment to ethical practice, patient safety, and continuous professional development. In this context, it involves a surgeon's obligation to uphold the highest standards of care, to acknowledge and learn from mistakes, and to foster an environment of trust and transparency [8].

Importance for patient safety, team dynamics, and clinical outcomes: The essence of accountability in surgery is intrinsically linked to patient safety. A surgeon's accountability ensures that every step, from preoperative planning to postoperative care, is executed with the utmost diligence and care [9]. This commitment not only protects patients but also builds a foundation of trust within the surgical team, enhancing collaboration and communication. In doing so, it significantly contributes to improved clinical outcomes. When surgeons and surgical teams embrace accountability, they create a culture of continuous improvement, where learning and growth are integral parts of daily practice [10].

Historical Perspective

The concept of accountability in surgery has evolved significantly over time. Historically, the focus was primarily on individual skill and success rates. However, as the medical field progressed, the scope of accountability expanded to include ethical considerations and systemic responsibilities [11].

Early developments: In the early days of surgery, accountability was a personal affair, closely tied to the surgeon's reputation. Surgical outcomes were often seen as a direct reflection of a surgeon's skill [12].

Shift toward systemic accountability: With advancements in medical knowledge and technology, the concept of accountability in surgery began to shift. The introduction of surgical standards, ethical guidelines, and regulatory bodies marked a new era, where accountability extended beyond individual surgeons to the systems and processes in which they operate [13].

Current Challenges

In modern surgical practices, implementing accountability faces several challenges:

Complex surgical environments: Today's surgical environments are more complex than ever. The integration of advanced technology and the increasing complexity of surgical procedures have made maintaining accountability more challenging. Surgeons must not only be skilled practitioners but also adept at managing sophisticated equipment and staying abreast of the latest developments [14].

Cultural and institutional barriers: Cultural norms within surgical teams and institutions can sometimes impede accountability. Hierarchical structures might discourage junior staff from speaking up, while a lack of transparency can create environments where errors are hidden rather than addressed openly [15].

Balancing accountability with learning from errors: One of the most significant challenges in modern surgery is creating a balance between being accountable for errors and using those errors as learning opportunities. There is a fine line between fostering a culture of accountability and creating a fear of reprisal that can inhibit learning and improvement (Fig. 32.2) [16].

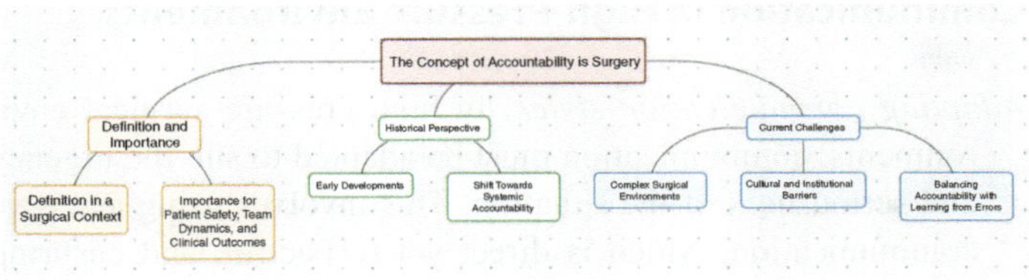

Fig. 32.2 The concept of accountability in surgery

Section 2: Effective Communication in Surgical Teams

Basics of Effective Communication

The four pillars of effective communication: Effective communication within surgical teams is built upon clarity, accuracy, brevity, and timeliness. Each message should be clear and unambiguous, accurate with no room for misinterpretation, as brief as necessary to reduce cognitive load, and timely to ensure relevance to the task at hand [17].

Listening as a core component: Active listening is equally as important as speaking. It involves full attention to the speaker, understanding the message, and responding appropriately. In the surgical setting, this ensures that all team members are on the same page and that important information is not overlooked [18].

Verbal and nonverbal communication: The effectiveness of communication also lies in the balance between what is said and what is conveyed through nonverbal cues like body language and tone of voice. In surgery, where team members are often masked and focused on the procedure, nonverbal cues become even more critical [19].

Communication in High-Pressure Environments

Adapting communication styles: In high-pressure surgical environments, communication must be adapted to suit the urgency and seriousness of the situation. This involves using assertive communication, which is direct yet respectful, and ensuring that critical information is prioritized [20].

Situational awareness: All team members must maintain situational awareness, which includes an understanding of the procedure, the roles of each team member, and the current status of the patient. This awareness informs the communication process, ensuring that it is relevant and appropriate to the context [20, 21].

Stress and communication: Stress can significantly impact communication. It is important to understand how stress affects one's ability to communicate and to employ strategies to manage stress in order to maintain clear and effective communication [21].

Tools and Techniques

Standardized communication protocols: Surgical teams often employ standardized communication protocols such as SBAR (Situation, Background, Assessment, Recommendation) to ensure that every message is structured and complete [22–24].

Checklists and briefings: Preoperative briefings and surgical safety checklists are critical tools for ensuring that all team members are informed and that key safety checks are communicated before the procedure begins [22–24].

Debriefing for continuous improvement: Postoperative debriefings provide an opportunity for the surgical team to discuss what went well and what could be improved, fostering an environment of continuous learning and improvement in communication practices (Fig. 32.3) [22–24].

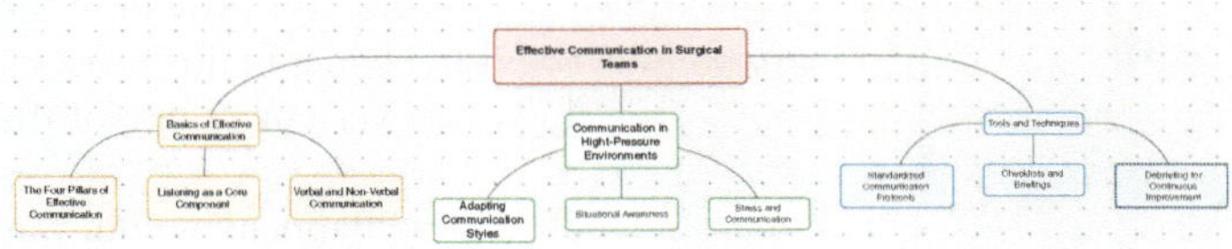

Fig. 32.3 Effective communication in surgical teams

Section 3: Integrating Accountability with Communication

Linking the Two Concepts

The symbiotic relationship: Accountability and communication are interdependent, each reinforcing the other. A culture of accountability is sustained by open, clear, and honest communication, while effective communication is essential for maintaining accountability. When communication fails, accountability can falter, leading to errors and decreased team morale. Conversely, when accountability is not emphasized, communication may lack the necessary assertiveness and clarity needed in high-stakes surgical environments [25, 26].

Establishing a framework for integration: To integrate accountability with communication, a framework that includes clear expectations, defined roles, and mutual respect must be established. Within this framework, communication is the method through which accountability is expressed and upheld. Surgeons and surgical teams should communicate not just facts and observations but also the rationale behind decisions, fostering a deeper understanding and shared accountability (Fig. 32.4) [27].

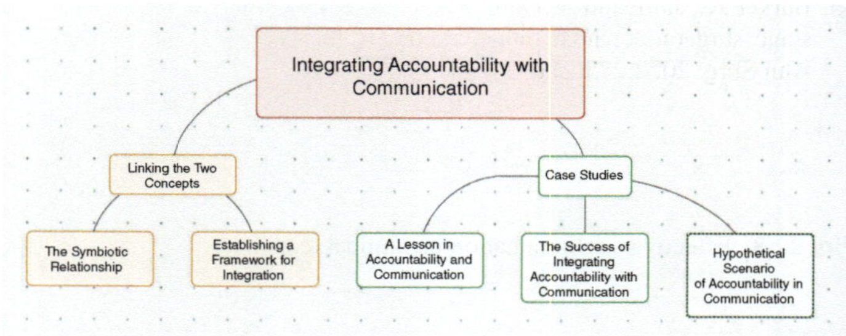

Fig. 32.4 Integrating accountability with communication

Case Studies

Case study	Description
A lesson in accountability and communication	A surgical team encountered complications during a complex procedure. Due to a lack of clear communication, team members were unaware of a critical step being missed. Postoperative review revealed that although the lead surgeon was aware of the mistake, they failed to communicate this effectively to the team. This case study highlights the consequences of poor communication on accountability and patient outcomes. It also demonstrates the importance of debriefing sessions where open discussion can lead to process improvements.
The success of integrating accountability with communication	In another scenario, a surgeon openly communicated a near-miss that could have led to significant patient harm. By doing so, they not only took responsibility but also encouraged a culture where such admissions are seen as learning opportunities rather than failures. This transparency led to the implementation of new safety checks and a team approach to accountability, demonstrating how effective communication can enhance the practice of accountability.
Hypothetical scenario of accountability in communication	Imagine a situation where a surgical instrument count after a procedure indicated a missing item. Instead of assigning blame, the team communicated to retrace their steps, leading to the discovery of the item misplaced in the operating room. This scenario illustrates how accountability, paired with clear and nonjudgmental communication, can resolve potential patient safety issues without creating a culture of blame.

Section 4: Leadership and Mentorship

Role of Leadership in Promoting Accountability and Communication

Leadership as the cornerstone of culture: Leadership within surgical teams plays a crucial role in establishing and maintaining a culture of accountability and communication. Leaders set the tone for openness and transparency, creating an environment where team members feel empowered to speak up, share concerns, and contribute to the decision-making process. This involves not only verbal encouragement but also leading by example, where leaders themselves demonstrate the behaviors they wish to instill in their teams [28, 29].

Implementing systems and processes: Effective leaders facilitate the implementation of systems and processes that support accountability and communication. This includes clear reporting structures, feedback mechanisms, and regular team meetings to discuss outcomes and areas for improvement. By prioritizing these systems, leaders can ensure that accountability and communication are not just aspirational concepts but are embedded in the everyday operations of the surgical team [29].

Navigating challenges and conflict: A key aspect of leadership is the ability to navigate challenges and conflicts that may arise. Leaders must be adept at conflict resolution, ensuring that any disagreements or issues are addressed constructively, without compromising the team's ability to communicate effectively or hold one another accountable [30, 31].

Mentorship and Training

Mentorship as a vehicle for cultural transmission: Mentorship is an essential tool for transferring the values of accountability and communication to the next generation of surgeons. Through one-on-one guidance, mentors can provide personalized advice and feedback, helping mentees understand the nuances of these concepts and how they are applied in clinical practice [32].

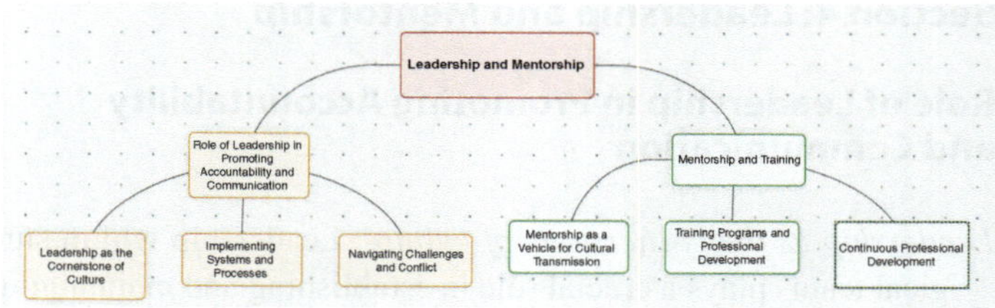

Fig. 32.5 Leadership and mentorship

Training programs and professional development: Structured training programs that focus on developing leadership, accountability, and communication skills are vital. These programs should include practical exercises, such as simulations and role-playing, to allow surgeons to practice these skills in a safe and controlled environment [33].

Continuous professional development: Leaders and mentors should encourage continuous professional development in accountability and communication. This includes providing opportunities for learning through conferences, workshops, and seminars, as well as encouraging self-reflection and lifelong learning (Fig. 32.5) [34].

Section 5: Overcoming Barriers

Common Barriers to Accountability and Communication

Recognizing the hurdles: In surgical practice, common barriers to accountability and communication can stem from hierarchical team structures, varied communication styles, and the high-stress nature of the work. These barriers can impede the flow of critical information and hinder the establishment of a culture where accountability is a shared value [35].

Hierarchical and cultural obstacles: Hierarchical structures can create environments where junior team members may feel reluctant to speak up, and cultural differences may lead to misinterpretations or misunderstandings. These elements can disrupt accountability by preventing issues from being promptly and effectively addressed [36].

Resource limitations and systemic constraints: Often, systemic constraints such as resource limitations, administrative burdens, and time pressures can compromise the ability of surgical teams to maintain clear communication and accountability. Under these conditions, crucial steps may be overlooked or errors may not be communicated, out of fear or perceived lack of time to address them properly [36, 37].

Strategies to Overcome These Barriers

Fostering a culture of openness: A key strategy to overcome barriers is to foster a nonpunitive culture of openness, where every team member feels empowered to share insights or concerns without fear of retribution. This involves regular team-building exercises and the establishment of clear protocols that encourage speaking up [36, 37].

Training and standardization: Investing in regular training that focuses on communication skills and accountability practices can equip team members with the tools they need to overcome these barriers. Additionally, implementing standardized communication protocols can help ensure consistency and clarity in high-pressure situations [38].

Leveraging technology: Technology can also play a role in bridging communication gaps. For example, digital checklists and real-time reporting systems can enhance accountability and ensure that all team members are informed and in agreement on critical patient care decisions [39].

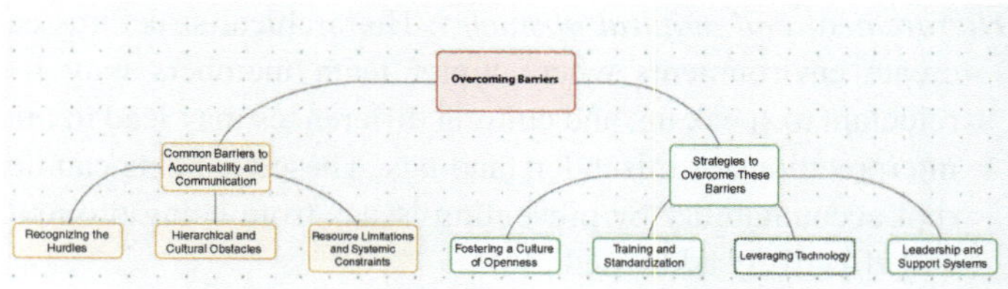

Fig. 32.6 Overcoming barriers

Leadership and support systems: Leadership support is essential in overcoming barriers to accountability and communication. Leaders must actively work to dismantle hierarchical barriers, promote inclusivity, and provide support systems that allow for error reporting and process improvement without fear of negative consequences [40].

Continuous evaluation and adaptation: Finally, continuous evaluation of communication and accountability processes is necessary. Teams should regularly assess their effectiveness in these areas and be willing to adapt their strategies to address any identified issues. This might involve debriefings, feedback sessions, and quality improvement initiatives (Fig. 32.6) [39, 40].

Section 6: The Future of Accountability and Communication in Surgery

Emerging Trends

Technological advancements: The integration of advanced technology in surgical practice is shaping the future of how accountability and communication are managed. Innovations such as electronic health records, telemedicine, and AI-assisted diagnostics are enhancing the ways in which information is shared and how responsibilities are defined and tracked [41].

Interdisciplinary collaboration: Emerging trends point toward increased interdisciplinary collaboration, breaking down traditional silos between different specialists. This collaboration necessitates the development of shared languages and protocols to ensure seamless communication and accountability across diverse teams [41].

Patient-centered models: The shift toward patient-centered care models emphasizes the importance of including patients as active participants in their own care. This approach requires clear communication and shared accountability between patients and surgical teams, potentially leading to better outcomes and higher patient satisfaction [41, 42].

Continuous Improvement

Quality improvement initiatives: The surgical field is seeing an increased emphasis on quality improvement initiatives that rely heavily on accountability and communication. These initiatives often involve continuous monitoring, data analysis, and feedback loops that foster a culture of ongoing learning and adaptation [42].

Training and education: Continuous improvement in accountability and communication also relies on evolving training and educational methods. Simulation-based training, interactive learning modules, and continuing professional development courses are being increasingly used to enhance these skills among surgical teams [43].

Policy and protocol evolution: As insights into the best practices for accountability and communication grow, policies and protocols are evolving to incorporate these findings. This dynamic process ensures that surgical practices remain at the cutting edge of patient safety and care quality (Fig. 32.7) [43, 44].

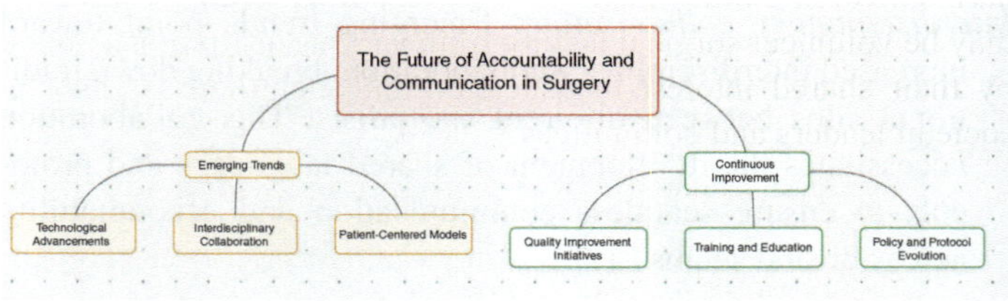

Fig. 32.7 The future of accountability and communication in surgery

Conclusion

This chapter has embarked on a comprehensive journey through the intricate relationship between accountability and effective communication within the surgical field, uncovering the layers of complexity and interdependence that define this dynamic. From the foundational definitions to the visionary future trends, we have explored the multifaceted nature of these concepts and their critical importance in the realm of surgery.

SAGES Takeaway

- Accountability as a Foundation: Accountability is essential for patient safety and the integrity of surgical teams, encompassing both individual actions and systemic practices.
- Primacy of Effective Communication: Clear, timely, and precise communication is crucial for the functionality of surgical teams, especially under high-pressure conditions.
- Synergy of Concepts: The integration of accountability and effective communication is critical for effective surgical leadership and optimal team performance.
- Leadership and Mentorship Role: Leaders and mentors are key in instilling a culture that values and upholds accountability and communication within surgical teams.
- Navigating Challenges: Identifying and overcoming barriers to accountability and communication is necessary for progress, alongside adapting to emerging trends for continuous improvement.

References

1. Ohlinger J, Brown MS, Laudert S, Swanson S, Fofah O, CARE Group. Development of potentially better practices for the neonatal intensive care unit as a culture of collaboration: communication, accountability, respect, and empowerment. Pediatrics. 2003;111(4 Pt 2):e471–81.
2. Battié R, Steelman VM. Accountability in nursing practice: why it is important for patient safety. AORN J. 2014;100(5):537–41. https://doi.org/10.1016/j.aorn.2014.08.008. Epub 2014 Oct 25.
3. Mansour D, Sayeed Z, Padela MT, McCarty S, Tonnos F, Silas D, Mostafa G, Yassir WK. Accountable operating room teams. Orthopedics. 2021;44(4):e463–70. https://doi.org/10.3928/01477447-20210618-01. Epub 2021 Jul 1.
4. Schneller ES, Wilson NA. Professionalism in 21st century professional practice: autonomy and accountability in orthopaedic surgery. Clin Orthop Relat Res. 2009;467(10):2561–9. https://doi.org/10.1007/s11999-009-0836-4. Epub 2009 Apr 18.
5. Whittemore AD. The competent surgeon: individual accountability in the era of "systems" failure. Ann Surg. 2009;250(3):357–62. https://doi.org/10.1097/SLA.0b013e3181b28c93.
6. Garrett JH Jr. Effective perioperative communication to enhance patient care. AORN J. 2016;104(2):111–20. https://doi.org/10.1016/j.aorn.2016.06.001.
7. Lima JC, Intrator O, Wetle T. Physicians in nursing homes: effectiveness of physician accountability and communication. J Am Med Dir Assoc. 2015;16(9):755–61. https://doi.org/10.1016/j.jamda.2015.02.018. Epub 2015 Apr 7.
8. Marrone SR. Perioperative accountable care teams: improving surgical team efficiency and work satisfaction through interprofessional collaboration. J Perioper Pract. 2018;28(9):223–30. https://doi.org/10.1177/1750458918788975. Epub 2018 Jul 23.
9. Teunissen C, Burrell B, Maskill V. Effective surgical teams: an integrative literature review. West J Nurs Res. 2020;42(1):61–75. https://doi.org/10.1177/0193945919834896. Epub 2019 Mar 10.
10. Boysen PG 2nd. Just culture: a foundation for balanced accountability and patient safety. Ochsner J. 2013;13(3):400–6.
11. Ellaway RH. Trust, but verify. Adv Health Sci Educ Theory Pract. 2023;28:1363. https://doi.org/10.1007/s10459-023-10306-y. Epub ahead of print.
12. Iacono MV. The culture of accountability. J Perianesth Nurs. 2013;28(2):107–9. https://doi.org/10.1016/j.jopan.2013.01.002.
13. Wachter RM. Personal accountability in healthcare: searching for the right balance. BMJ Qual Saf. 2013;22(2):176–80. https://doi.org/10.1136/bmjqs-2012-001227. Epub 2012 Aug 31.

14. Duthie EA. Accountability: challenges to getting it right. J Patient Saf. 2018;14(1):3–8. https://doi.org/10.1097/PTS.0000000000000161.
15. Zeller JL, Fontanarosa PB. Shared accountability, appropriateness, and quality of surgical care. JAMA. 2009;302(14):1590–1. https://doi.org/10.1001/jama.2009.1495.
16. Bell SK, Delbanco T, Anderson-Shaw L, McDonald TB, Gallagher TH. Accountability for medical error: moving beyond blame to advocacy. Chest. 2011;140(2):519–26. https://doi.org/10.1378/chest.10-2533.
17. Raper SE, Gupta M, Okusanya O, Morris JB. Improving communication skills: a course for academic medical center surgery residents and faculty. J Surg Educ. 2015;72(6):e202–11. https://doi.org/10.1016/j.jsurg.2015.06.008. Epub 2015 Jul 14.
18. Gillespie BM, Chaboyer W, Longbottom P, Wallis M. The impact of organisational and individual factors on team communication in surgery: a qualitative study. Int J Nurs Stud. 2010;47(6):732–41. https://doi.org/10.1016/j.ijnurstu.2009.11.001. Epub 2009 Nov 27.
19. Little P, White P, Kelly J, Everitt H, Gashi S, Bikker A, Mercer S. Verbal and non-verbal behaviour and patient perception of communication in primary care: an observational study. Br J Gen Pract. 2015;65(635):e357–65. https://doi.org/10.3399/bjgp15X685249.
20. O'Daniel M, Rosenstein AH. Professional communication and team collaboration. In: Hughes RG, editor. Patient safety and quality: an evidence-based handbook for nurses. Rockville, MD: Agency for Healthcare Research and Quality; 2008. Chapter 33. Available from: https://www.ncbi.nlm.nih.gov/books/NBK2637/.
21. Creswick N, Westbrook JI, Braithwaite J. Understanding communication networks in the emergency department. BMC Health Serv Res. 2009;9:247. https://doi.org/10.1186/1472-6963-9-247.
22. Sacks GD, Shannon EM, Dawes AJ, Rollo JC, Nguyen DK, Russell MM, Ko CY, Maggard-Gibbons MA. Teamwork, communication and safety climate: a systematic review of interventions to improve surgical culture. BMJ Qual Saf. 2015;24(7):458–67. https://doi.org/10.1136/bmjqs-2014-003764. Epub 2015 May 22.
23. Gillespie BM, Chaboyer W, Murray P. Enhancing communication in surgery through team training interventions: a systematic literature review. AORN J. 2010;92(6):642–57. https://doi.org/10.1016/j.aorn.2010.02.015.
24. Mendick N, Young B, Holcombe C, Salmon P. How do surgeons think they learn about communication? A qualitative study. Med Educ. 2015;49(4):408–16. https://doi.org/10.1111/medu.12648.
25. Mills P, Neily J, Dunn E. Teamwork and communication in surgical teams: implications for patient safety. J Am Coll Surg. 2008;206(1):107–12. https://doi.org/10.1016/j.jamcollsurg.2007.06.281. Epub 2007 Sep 17.
26. Tørring B, Gittell JH, Laursen M, Rasmussen BS, Sørensen EE. Communication and relationship dynamics in surgical teams in the

operating room: an ethnographic study. BMC Health Serv Res. 2019;19(1):528. https://doi.org/10.1186/s12913-019-4362-0.
27. van Dalen ASH, Swinkels JA, Coolen S, Hackett R, Schijven MP. Improving teamwork and communication in the operating room by introducing the theatre cap challenge. J Perioper Pract. 2022;32(1–2):4–9. https://doi.org/10.1177/17504589211046723.
28. Swiggart WH, et al. Promoting professionalism and professional accountability. In: Viera AJ, Kramer R, editors. Management and leadership skills for medical faculty and healthcare executives. Cham: Springer; 2020. https://doi.org/10.1007/978-3-030-45425-8_13.
29. Grimshaw J, Baron G, Mike B, Edwards N. How to combat a culture of excuses and promote accountability. Strategy Leadership. 2006;34(5):11–8. https://doi.org/10.1108/10878570610684793.
30. Walker A, Ko J. Principal leadership in an era of accountability: a perspective from the Hong Kong context. Sch Leadersh Manag. 2011;31(4):369–92. https://doi.org/10.1080/13632434.2011.606269.
31. Men LR, Stacks D. The effects of authentic leadership on strategic internal communication and employee-organization relationships. J Public Relat Res. 2014;26(4):301–24. https://doi.org/10.1080/1062726X.2014.908720.
32. Norris S, Sitton S, Baker M. Mentorship through the lens of servant leadership. NACTA J. 2017;61(1):21–6.
33. Hairston-Green DY, Smith LS. Accountability, growth, and excellence: mentorship through the AGEs. In: Proceedings of the New Mexico Mentoring Institute, developmental networks: the power of mentoring and coaching; 2016. p. 1275–8.
34. Ruiz JP, Gurel P, Olds WH, Bankston A, McDowell GS. Inspiring and ethical mentorship in STEM: a meeting highlighting need for engagement, incentives, and accountability. PeerJ Preprints. 2019;7:e27474v1. https://doi.org/10.7287/peerj.preprints.27474v1.
35. Quill TE. Barriers to effective communication. In: Lipkin M, Putnam SM, Lazare A, Carroll JG, Frankel RM, editors. The medical interview. Frontiers of primary care. New York: Springer; 1995. https://doi.org/10.1007/978-1-4612-2488-4_8.
36. Dickson D. Barriers to communication. In: Long A, editor. Interaction for practice in community nursing, Community health care series. London: Palgrave; 1999. https://doi.org/10.1007/978-1-349-14757-1_5.
37. Hartley BR, Elowitz E. Barriers to the enhancement of effective communication in neurosurgery. World Neurosurg. 2020;133:466–73.
38. Weller J, Boyd M, Cumin D. Teams, tribes and patient safety: overcoming barriers to effective teamwork in healthcare. Postgrad Med J. 2014;90(1061):149–54. https://doi.org/10.1136/postgradmedj-2012-131168.

39. Nakagawa S, Fischkoff K, Berlin A, Arnell TD, Blinderman CD. Communication skills training for general surgery residents. J Surg Educ. 2019;76(5):1223–30.
40. Callahan ME, Brant EB, Mohan D, Norman MK, Arnold RM, White DB. Leveraging technology to overcome the "scalability problem" in communication skills training courses. ATS Sch. 2021;2(3):327–40. https://doi.org/10.34197/ats-scholar.2020-0164PS.
41. Aragues A, et al. Trends and challenges of the emerging technologies toward interoperability and standardization in e-health communications. IEEE Commun Mag. 2011;49(11):182–8. https://doi.org/10.1109/MCOM.2011.6069727.
42. Peteet JR, Witvliet CV, Glas G, et al. Accountability as a virtue in medicine: from theory to practice. Philos Ethics Humanit Med. 2023;18:1. https://doi.org/10.1186/s13010-023-00129-5.
43. Kumar H, Morad R, Sonsati M. Surgical team: improving teamwork, a review. Postgrad Med J. 2019;95(1124):334–9. https://doi.org/10.1136/postgradmedj-2018-135943.
44. Bearman M, O'Brien R, Anthony A, Civil I, Flanagan B, Jolly B, Birks D, Langcake M, Molloy E, Nestel D. Learning surgical communication, leadership and teamwork through simulation. J Surg Educ. 2012;69(2):201–7.

33 Educational Opportunities in Strategy and Leadership

John R. Romanelli

Surgeons are natural leaders. We have to command an operating room, get a team working in concert to provide optimal patient care, lead a team of trainees when in a teaching setting, and run a clinical practice. That said, there are many aspects of leadership that are foreign to physicians and are largely concepts that are not taught in a medical school curriculum or surgical residency. As a result, additional education is often helpful as surgeons begin to become leaders in their own organizations.

The first place a surgeon should look to for leadership training is internally—at one's own organization. Many healthcare organizations offer educational opportunities designed to develop a new generation of future leaders, and it is important to identify these programs and take advantage of them when offered. For example, my employer (Baystate Health) offers a Physician Leadership Academy (PLA), which I had the fortune to participate in during the 2016–2017 academic year. This course was held off-site (to prevent clinical distractions) every other Friday over a period of 6 months. Acceptance to the course was by invitation only and required the granting of time by the Department Chair for each candidate. Physicians of all disciplines participated in the course, and

J. R. Romanelli (✉)
Department of Surgery, University of Massachusetts Chan Medical School—Baystate Medical Center, Springfield, MA, USA
e-mail: John.Romanelli@baystatehealth.org

S. M. Johnson et al. (eds.), *The SAGES Manual of Strategy and Leadership*, https://doi.org/10.1007/978-3-031-62359-2_33

diversity of specialty was paramount to the success of our working groups. Many topics were covered, such as compensation, financial planning, difficult conversations, healthcare policy, strategic planning, and diversity, equity, and inclusion. Each participant was required to "pitch" a project and, once accepted by the PLA mentors, worked in small groups to hone the concepts, develop implementation strategies, receive critical feedback, and then make a presentation to the entire group at the end of the course. Approximately 50% of the projects were ultimately implemented, and many were quite successful. The alumni of the academy participate in quarterly virtual sessions with hospital leadership to keep us engaged and learning. Newer programs such as a "Division Chief Leadership Bootcamp" are being implemented to reinforce topics learned in the PLA. As a sign of the program's success, PLA alumni often go on to chair hospital-level committees or serve in other leadership functions, including a Department Chair.

Several surgical societies offer leadership curricula that are usually available for its members with an application and nomination process. The American College of Surgeons (ACS) offers a course called "Surgeons as Leaders" [1]. Designed for both academic and community surgeons, the course is taught over a 3-day period of time and features content such as the following: leadership challenges, dealing with microaggressions and leading difficult personalities, leading through and sustaining change, building and maintaining team effectiveness, leading oneself, and the arts and principles of leadership. This course is open to 60 participants, requires an application and commitment to attend, offers CME credit for attendees, and has priority consideration for members of the ACS.

A multi-society effort in 2022 that may be repeated in the future was the Promising Leaders Program [2], which was created by the Society of University Surgeons (SUS), the Society of Black Academic Surgeons (SBAS), the Society of American Gastrointestinal and Endoscopic Surgeons (SAGES), the Eastern Association for the Society of Trauma (EAST), and the Society for Surgery of the Alimentary Tract (SSAT). This program was designed for six individuals who, by race, ethnicity, gender, sexual orientation, or any other personal identification, are an underrepresented voice in academic surgery [2]. The program was designed for surgeons at the academic rank of assistant or associate professor who were at least 7 years out from the end of their training. The program, spaced out over 2 years, consisted of professional coaching, as well as attendance at three leadership courses: the SUS Leadership Agility Program, the EAST Leadership Development Workshop, and the SUS Mid-Career Academic Surgery Professional Development Course. The cost of the course was covered 50% by the societies, with the expectation of matching awards from the surgeons' institutions. It remains to be seen if this will be offered in another 2-year cycle at the time of the writing of this chapter.

SAGES also has an award available to members who have completed residency and/or fellowship and are in good standing in the society. The SAGES Foundation Excellence in Medical Leadership Award enables an individual to attend a 7-day program that will push the way they think deeply about change within themselves and their organization as a high potential leader in the medical world [3]. The purpose of this scholarship is to optimize one's impact in the medical industry so they can deliver sustainable results driven by their greatest capabilities and purpose as a leader by exposing one SAGES member to the leading minds in leadership development, strategy, management, and execution [3].

One popular course for surgeons is the Brandeis Health Leadership Program (BHLP) in Health Policy and Management [4]. The BHLP is sponsored by seventeen surgical societies, including SAGES, ACS, EAST, and the American Surgical Association, along with many other subspecialties and/or regional societies. The course, led by Dr. Jon Chilingerian and Dr. Stuart Altman, is an immersive 7-day course where the course attendees live at the school and attend lectures and workshops all day and then retire to do coursework in the evenings. Sample program topics include the following: US health policy, economics and financing, individual and group decision-making, managing clinics and the care process, effective leadership styles, managing change in complex systems, conflict negotiation, and financial literacy for physician leaders [4]. The course typically admits 30–35 attendees and has surgeons from all disciplines and from all parts of North America interacting to work and learn together.

Harvard also has a course for leadership development for physicians in academic health centers, which is held on-site over a 2-week period [5]. This program is designed for physicians who are not yet chairs of clinical departments, covering topics such as understanding the responsibilities and tasks of leaders in complex institutions, relevant concepts and techniques in key management disciplines, methods of analyzing problems and identifying critical questions, and increasing effectiveness in formulating and implementing change.

BHLP or Harvard graduates sometimes go on to study with the same faculty in an MBA program to further their education. There are other MBA programs designed specifically for physicians, such as the Kelley School of Business in Indiana, the University of Tennessee Haslam College of Business, Auburn University Raymond J. Harbert College of Business, or the University of Texas–Dallas. These programs range from 1 to 2 years and are obviously a more substantial cost and time commitment to complete.

SAGES Takeaway

- Surgeons are natural leaders in healthcare and face leadership challenges beyond clinical expertise, necessitating additional education.
- Internal programs, like Baystate Health's Physician Leadership Academy, offer tailored training for surgeons to develop essential leadership skills within their organizations.
- Surgical societies, including ACS and SAGES, provide specialized leadership courses, addressing challenges, diversity, and team effectiveness.
- Collaborative efforts, like the Promising Leaders Program, focus on underrepresented voices, offering coaching and leadership courses for academic surgeons.
- The Brandeis Health Leadership Program and Harvard's program equip surgeons with knowledge of health policy, management, and leadership, with potential pathways to further education through MBA programs.

References

1. ACS Surgeons as Leaders—ACS. facs.org. Accessed 4 Sept 2023.
2. Promising Leaders Program—Society of University Surgeons (SUS). sus-web.org. Accessed 11 Sept 2023.
3. The SAGES Foundation Excellence in Medical Leadership Award. Accessed 11 Sept 2023.
4. Brandeis Health Leadership Program (BHLP) in Health Policy and Management—The Heller School. Accessed 11 Sept 2023.
5. https://execed2.sph.harvard.edu/leadership-development-for-physicians-in-academic-health-centers?_gl=1*18f51wv*_ga*MTAwMTc3MzUzMS4xNjk0NzAzNzY3*_ga_J4XYGFMG9Z*MTY5NDcwMzc2Ni4xLjAuMTY5NDcwMzc2Ny41OS4wLjA. Accessed 14 Sept 2023.

Part VIII

Leading Systems—Building an Efficient System/Organizational Structure

Building an Effective Administration

34

Terrence Fullum and Robert B. Lim

Introduction

Building an effective administration in surgery requires skills in leadership, organization management, and an appreciation for business. Effective leadership involves developing a strategy that outlines organizational goals and objectives, evaluates deliverables/outcomes to track progress, and implements operational plans.

When developing an effective administration in surgery, leaders must also consider the unique challenges this specialty presents. Surgery involves unique risks and rights, a need for effective communication among all stakeholders, compliance with continually changing regulations and standards, and, of course, the challenging mission of providing high-quality healthcare in a complicated patient population.

T. Fullum (✉)
Department of Surgery, Howard University College of Medicine, Howard University Hospital, Washington, DC, USA
e-mail: tfullum@Howard.edu

R. B. Lim
Wake Forest University, Atrium Health Carolinas, Department of Surgery, Charlotte, NC, USA
e-mail: robert.lim@atriumhealth.org

S. M. Johnson et al. (eds.), *The SAGES Manual of Strategy and Leadership*, https://doi.org/10.1007/978-3-031-62359-2_34

Surgeons who become healthcare administrators must be enthusiastic individuals who strive to improve healthcare systems/processes and the patient experience. Essential skills and qualities of a successful healthcare administrator include:

- Business administration
- Communication
- Understanding of patient care
- Quality assurance and quality improvement

While utilizing these skills and qualities, the ability to organize is a core competency required to be successful in achieving effective goals and completing projects on time. Effective administration begins with a shared mission statement and vision throughout the organization. This communication then translates into all functions related to the management systems and business processes underlying clinical care. The objective of this chapter is to discuss the systems and processes required to build an effective administration in surgery.

The Need for a Clear Mission and Vision

Most clinicians did not go to medical school and finish residency to become an administrator. The most important aspect of a surgeon's practice remains providing timely and quality patient care [1] and, not surprisingly, performing surgery [2]. Leadership and administrative tasks will always be a part of any surgical practice. With high rates of burnout and an average work week of 64 h, the ability to provide quality care can be challenging. The goal of any business or product line is to be profitable, while that of clinicians' is to obtain quality patient outcomes. These two goals can fundamentally oppose one another. Ideally, hospital leadership and clinicians would have similar goals when it comes to patient care, but sadly, this is not always the case.

Having a clear mission, whether in a single operating room, a university-level department, or an entire healthcare organization (HCO), can be a unifying effort to resolve conflict or to obtain resources. A clear mission defines the overall purpose and objective of an HCO. Moreover, surgeons, who perceive receiving support to achieve a mission, are more likely to contribute to the mission [3].

Forming a mission can be done based on the current needs and gaps in care of the HCO, like improving upon surgical outcomes from vascular surgery. Or it can be set to a higher, more encompassing goal like improving access to care and quality of care for an entire state. This can be decided by a hospital leader, but it can also be dictated by local community needs or even a state or region's needs. Whatever it is, it should be a clear and concise statement.

Vision is the desirable state one would be in to achieve the mission. For instance, if the mission were to provide high-quality and reliable surgical care, the vision could be that each surgeon is aware of 100% of their outcomes and works continuously to make improvements based on those outcomes. The strategy would include the plans and mechanisms one would use to achieve the vision. In this case, a strategy is that each surgeon takes part in a monthly review of their outcomes where goals are created, discussed, and monitored by the surgeon and the surgical leaders with the goal of improving processes of care. This is the basis for the American College of Surgeons quality improvement programs like the National Surgical Quality Improvement Program (NSQIP) and Metabolic and Bariatric Surgery—Accreditation Quality Improvement Program (MBS-AQIP).

To form a vision, the leader or leadership should evaluate its assets and determine what other resources might be needed to achieve the mission. Using those resources and assets or by acquiring new ones, a vision can be creating to achieving the mission. So, for instance, if the goal were to improve access to care, the leadership may identify hurdles from insurance companies or that patients have a difficult time making an appointment. The vision then could be that all patients would not only be able to make an appointment online or have easy access to an appointment clerk via the phone that patient would be put in touch with a payment specialist to help navigate their insurance approval. The strategies to achieve this vision then would be to improve the

HCO's online presence and make its navigation easy. The HCO would also then track how its patients make appointments and where any gaps remain, or insurance hurdles remain.

As an effective administrator one should expect change over time in many aspects of medical care. The mission and vision must be flexible and adaptable as the surgical world transforms. It is critical that leadership provides an updated mission and vision when changes occur. The mission and vision will then help identify priorities. Providing quality medical care is paramount but the cost of care is also a moving target that must be managed. When building an effective healthcare administration, the team should consist of members who have expertise and who can lead their department in achieving the goals of the priorities set forth by the mission and vision. Each member of the team should also be aware of the work of the other members to achieve the common goal. This requires engaging all members of the team for the leadership's vision to translate into organized practical work. This concept also works to eliminate redundancy and disparate workloads. This is known as the learn management philosophy [4]. With all members of the team involved and interacting, the HCO can work toward system and process improvement rather than changes coming solely from an autocratic leadership mandate.

Priorities of Effective Administration in Surgery

The military's organization is an example of involving an administrative team to succeed in a mission. The commanding officer will build a support staff with each member of the staff focused on one aspect of leading a team. In the United States Army, a brigade commander is typically in charge of 3000–5000 soldiers, each of whom works for a team that makes up the brigade. Typically, there are combat arms teams, like an infantry or armor battalion, and several support teams, like engineer, signal, and supply companies. To lead and control his or her team, the brigade commander forms a staff of 6–7 people, each with a designed role that helps manage the entire brigade. These roles usually include personnel management, supply and support, training, and intelligence

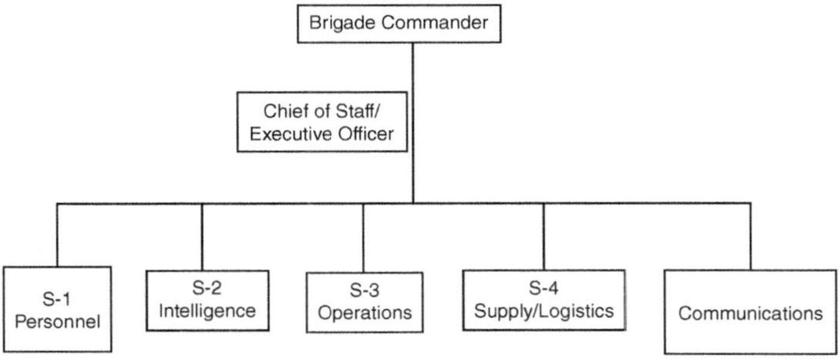

Fig. 34.1 *Brigade Commanders Staff/Headquarters company*: each position assists the commander in achieving the mission. They are also responsible for providing the resources and personnel so that the battalions within the brigade have what they need to succeed in their missions

(see Fig. 34.1). Similarly, effective HCO leadership will include an administrative team that manages the priorities of healthcare (see Fig. 34.2).

Primarily, efficient administration will facilitate better communication between healthcare personnel. A smooth system is one that reduces confusion and is more efficient. Smooth systems for information sharing and coordination, including an efficient scheduling system, help save time and energy, allowing personnel to focus on providing better patient care and take on other more critical tasks throughout the course of the surgery.

Second, with effective administration, hospitals and other healthcare facilities can better manage their resources. Hospital administrators can use their administrative skills to reduce unnecessary costs and make the most of the available resources. This can result in more cost-effective surgeries and reduce the risk of expensive errors.

Third, effective administration can improve patient safety. Having well-thought-out strategies, detailed planning, and strong coordination between staff and healthcare personnel can minimize the possibility of errors and ensure that everything runs accordingly.

Finally, successful administration can lead to increased patient satisfaction and improved outcomes for surgeries. Adequate and

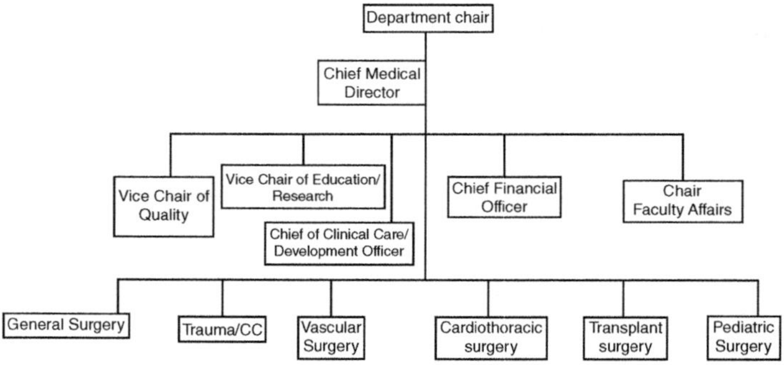

Fig. 34.2 *Department Administration example*: as with the military's organization, this department chair's administrative staff (made up of the vice chairs of quality, education, and research, along with the chiefs of clinical care, finances, and faculty affairs) is structured to assist the department chair to make sure the mission and vision are met and the sections of surgery to ensure they have the resources to be successful. A similar structure can be utilized at the hospital level, which would have several departments, or within a section, which may have several physicians. In this example, the chair could create or eliminate certain staff positions based on the mission. A department that does not train residents or fellows may not have a need for a vice chair of education, for example

timely administration can allow for safer operations, better availability of resources, more reliable scheduling, and better coordination with other medical staff. At a lower level, the department chief may try to take on all these roles, but that would likely take away from their clinical practice. He or she should probably disperse one or two of these tasks to others, so they can be more efficient, and others can be more involved in the practice. This would allow a leader to focus on the priorities of healthcare.

These priorities include:

- Best practices of healthcare
- Clinical care and delivery
- Regulatory requirements
- Cost management
- Personnel behavior

There is often an overlap and conflict among these priorities, but they need to be addressed individually and collectively for an organization to be successful. The application of these priorities depends on what level the administrator is overseeing. For instance, the needs and resources of a healthcare system like the Veterans Administration (VA) would be different in scope for an administrator than that of a four-person private practice surgical group. However, as one of the omnipresent goals of healthcare is to provide quality healthcare, these priorities can be utilized but with a different vision and different strategies to achieve similar goals. Let us review and give examples for each priority.

- *Best practices*—From the National Institute of Health, best practices are health practices, methods, interventions, or techniques based on high-quality evidence to obtain improved patient and health outcomes [5]. An administrator should focus on ensuring that the best practices are used and the resources to provide the best practices are available. In a hospital, this position would set the standards for clinical outcomes. Typically, this person would be the chief medical officer. Within this area, a leader could also have another position based on their HCO's more specific goals. In academic institutions, for instance, there may be a vice chair of research, who oversees the research mission, and a vice chair of education, who oversees the education goals of the HCO.
- *Clinical care and delivery*—This area deals with assuring that surgeons have what they need to provide quality care and that patients have access to care. Resources needed include professionally trained personnel, quality equipment and technology, and care pathways or the standardization of medical services like blood transfusion protocols. The second critically important aspect is making sure that patients have dependable and easy-to-navigate access to quality care. Patient navigation systems that frequently touch the patient along their journey from initial consultation, through the preop process, the surgical experience, and recovery, i.e., the patient experience will help ensure the overall success of the program.

- *Regulatory requirements*—An HCO will need to monitor and manage its surgical outcomes to maintain compliance with local and national standards. These standards should be met regardless of patient factors by adjusting resources to maximize the skill set of the providers. All process improvements need to be continuous and fluid. The HCO must comply with the regulations and standards required to run the hospital. This would include the standards of the Joint Commission for Accreditation of Hospital Organizations (JCAHO). Within a department, this would be the role of the vice chair of quality.
- *Cost management*—An HCO cannot run without effective fiscal management. The idea of "no margin, no mission" is alive and well in today's post-pandemic economy. While not the primary goal of healthcare, a sound financial margin is needed for an HCO to be successful and to grow. Effective cost management includes everything from day-to-day surgical operations to an efficient and effective revenue cycle management team, recruitment of outstanding providers, reducing the length of stay and patient throughput, and the value analysis of capital purchases. Cost management also extends into the community to improve access to care (transportation, preop surgery clinic) and to support research for better medical care (best practices). In the hospital setting, the chief operating officer and the chief financial officer would be the administrator assigned to these duties along with the surgeon-in-chief who provides the academic surgeon's point of view.
- *Personnel management*—This administrator is responsible for the management of the organization's healthcare providers (nurses and physicians) and supporting staff. This administrator is often the point person for the inevitable conflicts that arise within an HCO. In academic practice, this person would be responsible for the growth and professional development of the personnel, as well as including academic promotion. This role is often shared by several administrators since personnel are from a diverse pool of occupations and responsibilities. Administrators who may share these responsibilities include chair of faculty affairs, chief nursing officer, chief people officer, office of general counsel, chief of human resources, and sometimes union officials.

Conclusion

Administrative efficiency is essential for successful healthcare organizations. This is particularly true in the field of surgery. A clear mission and vision are the essential first steps and a requirement for focus and purpose. Once aligned, an effective administration can help ensure the smooth functionality of the operations, improve quality, reduce costs, and streamline processes.

Overall, once a sharp vision and mission are established, the benefits of implementing an effective administration in surgery include improved coordination and communication between medical personnel, improved transparency and precision in the performance of procedures, and improved patient outcomes. This leads to increased patient satisfaction, which provides an increasingly competitive opportunity in the marketplace. The result is often a positive margin and a greater opportunity to serve the community.

SAGES Takeaway

- A clear, overriding mission and vision are key.
- Vision priorities should be divided into tasks led by support staff. Communication among the support staff is vital to success.
- Healthcare visions should focus on patient safety, outcomes, and cost.
- Change will occur and leaders should be able to adapt the mission and vision to that change.
- Leaders should also anticipate unprofessional or poor behavior to occur, and a plan should be in place to address those issues.

References

1. Ahmed N, Conn LG, Chiu M, Korabi B, Qureshi A, Nathens AB, Kitto S. Career satisfaction among general surgeons in Canada: a qualitative study of enablers and barriers to improve recruitment and retention in general surgery. Acad Med. 2012;87(11):1616–21.
2. Holzer E, Tschan F, Kottwitz MU, Beldi G, Businger AP, Semmer NK. The workday of hospital surgeons: what they do, what makes them

satisfied, and the role of core tasks and administrative tasks; a diary study. BMC Surg. 2019;19(1):112.
3. Mache S, Vitzthum K, Klapp BF, Groneberg DA. Improving quality of medical treatment and care: are surgeons' working conditions and job satisfaction associated to patient satisfaction? Langenbeck's Arch Surg. 2012;397(6):973–82.
4. Aij KH, Teunissen M. Lean leadership attributes: a systematic review of the literature. J Health Organ Manag. 2017;31(7–8):713–29.
5. Ten Ham-Baloyi W, Minnie K, van der Walt C. Improving healthcare: a guide to roll-out best practices. Afr Health Sci. 2020;20(3):1487–95.

Navigating an Academic Career in Surgery

35

Shaneeta M. Johnson, Juan S. Barajas-Gamboa, Aaron M. Alford, and Susan Pories

Academic Pathways

Academic surgeons (AS) play a crucial triple role in clinical practice, education, and research, constituting an essential segment of the academic and healthcare workforce. By combining expertise from all three domains, they have the opportunity to enhance the well-being of patients, improve surgical education, and advance scientific goals [1]. The nature of their work is broad-ranging and

S. M. Johnson (✉)
Department of Surgery, Morehouse School of Medicine, Atlanta, GA, USA

Satcher Health Leadership Institute, Morehouse School of Medicine, Atlanta, GA, USA
e-mail: shajohnson@msm.edu

J. S. Barajas-Gamboa
Department of General Surgery, Cleveland Clinic Abu Dhabi, Abu Dhabi, United Arab Emirates

A. M. Alford
Department of Surgery, Morehouse School of Medicine, Atlanta, GA, USA

S. Pories
Department of Surgery, Rutgers New Jersey Medical School, Newark, NJ, USA

S. M. Johnson et al. (eds.), *The SAGES Manual of Strategy and Leadership*, https://doi.org/10.1007/978-3-031-62359-2_35

demands deep commitment to the mission. The commitment will vary depending on individual's career stage, role, and interests, as well as the healthcare, academic and wider social systems [2]. The roles held by AS yield benefits on multiple fronts: individuals find satisfaction and professional diversity, patients receive the advantages of top-tier research in actively engaged institutions, and institutions themselves gain from the transferable skills, financial contributions, and extensive professional networks of AS. Pursuing an academic career in surgery is a dynamic journey that offers countless opportunities for growth, innovation, and impact. Understanding the different positions within the academic territory is crucial for any aspiring surgeon seeking to navigate this landscape effectively [3].

The common academic positions, their definitions, along with a general ranking based on the typical progression within an academic medical career are explained below:

1. *General surgery intern/resident*: After graduating from medical school, physicians enter a residency program. Residents who are interested in academic careers should be counseled to start working on research collaborations and publications early in their residency, in order to be competitive for fellowships and subsequent leadership positions.
2. *Fellow*: Some surgeons choose to pursue additional training after residency in a specific surgical subspecialty. This period of specialized training is called a fellowship. Most fellowships are competitive and a track record of research and publications as a resident will help in obtaining these opportunities.
3. *Instructor/clinical instructor*: After completing training, AS can take on teaching roles at medical schools or hospitals. They often supervise medical students and residents in clinical settings. If at all possible, collaboration with an ongoing research project or development of their own projects should be encouraged, with a goal of producing publications and obtaining grant support. It is important to align any research or education efforts with clinical interests to assure seamless integration of goals and establish a reputation in one's field. For

instance, if the surgeon's passion is colorectal surgery, research and publications should focus on colorectal disease as well. Most importantly, a reputation for clinical excellence should be established.

4. *Assistant professor/clinical assistant professor*: At this stage, AS are expected to be actively involved in teaching, research, and clinical care. This is the time to start establishing a local and regional reputation by serving on hospital committees as well as reaching out into the community via city and state surgical chapters and associations. As an example in Boston, there is a Boston Surgical Society and Massachusetts Chapter of American College of Surgeons. It is also useful to network within other specialties to broaden your reach, so the Massachusetts Medical Society is another option for involvement, giving talks, and serving on committees. Often surgeons are underrepresented in medical societies, and their input and opinions are valued. It is important to produce publications because most academic institutions will not promote individuals who do not publish. If possible, first or last authorship should be pursued because this demonstrates true involvement and responsibility for the project. Books and chapters do not carry the same weight as peer-reviewed publications.
5. *Associate professor/clinical associate professor*: This is a mid-career faculty rank. AS at this level have typically demonstrated excellence in clinical care, education, and research. They may start to take on more administrative responsibilities and establish a national as well as international reputation and presence via involvement in national surgical societies.
6. *Professor/clinical professor*: Professors are at the top of the academic hierarchy. They have usually made significant contributions to their field through research and are recognized experts. They often take on leadership roles in their departments or institutions, such as division chief, department chair, or dean.
7. *Department chair/division chief*: This is a senior administrative role where an AS oversees an entire department or a specific division within a department (e.g., general surgery, gastrointestinal surgery).

8. *Dean/associate dean*: Deans are the top academic administrators in a medical school. They are responsible for the overall functioning of the medical school, including education, research, and clinical programs.
9. *Medical school dean/university provost*: In some cases, a dean of a medical school may rise to a higher administrative position within the university, such as a provost. This role involves overseeing academic programs across the entire institution.

Rankings within the academic hierarchy can vary based on both country and institution. Furthermore, AS may also engage in healthcare administration, policy-making, or public health roles, which may not always align seamlessly with this hierarchy [4, 5].

How to Navigate the Academic Leadership Ladder

Embarking on a career in academic surgery is a journey that presents a multitude of opportunities for professional growth. Aspiring AS seeking to ascend the academic leadership ladder must embrace a strategic and deliberate approach [6]. The first step involves excelling in clinical practice and establishing a solid foundation in research. Demonstrating proficiency in both fields not only establishes credibility but also lays the groundwork for potential leadership roles. Engaging in collaborative research projects, contributing to publications, and presenting findings at conferences are essential steps in building a strong academic portfolio [7].

Active involvement in professional organizations and societies within the field of general surgery is another key facet of ascending the academic leadership ladder. Joining committees, participating in educational initiatives, and taking on leadership roles within these organizations not only foster networking opportunities but also showcase dedication to advancing the field. It also provides a platform for interacting with like-minded peers and mentors, allowing for the exchange of ideas and the cultivation of lasting professional relationships [8]. It is important to choose wisely with regard to committee roles, making sure the goals of the committee align with personal interests and that you have the time and passion to deliver meaningfully and substantially on any projects you are responsible for.

Mentorship plays a pivotal role in career advancement in academic surgery. Seeking out experienced mentors who have successfully navigated the academic leadership ladder can provide invaluable guidance and insight [9]. A mentor can offer personalized advice, facilitate networking opportunities, and provide candid feedback on career decisions. Additionally, mentors can serve as advocates or sponsors, endorsing individuals for leadership positions and helping them navigate the complexities of academic institutions.

Demonstrating effective leadership within one's clinical practice and research endeavors is the cornerstone of ascending the academic leadership ladder [10]. Taking on roles such as division chief, program director, or departmental committee chair showcases an individual's capacity to lead and manage. Moreover, active involvement in educational initiatives, such as teaching medical students, residents, and fellows, underscores a commitment to academic excellence. Building a reputation for excellence in clinical care, education, and research endeavors paves the way for progression into higher levels of leadership within the academic surgical community [11]. Research today does not require a basic science lab or grant support to get started. It is always possible for surgeons to partner with a basic scientist and provide tissue for research or enroll patients in clinical trials. Outcomes research or curriculum design and medical education research are other options for establishing a reputation in research without the requirement of a wet lab.

Educational Leadership Roles

Program director (PD): As the cornerstone of the educational pathway, PDs oversee the training and development of surgical residents and fellows. They meticulously design and implement educational curricula, ensuring compliance with accreditation standards. PDs serve as mentors, providing guidance and support to trainees as they navigate their educational journey [12].

Medical student clerkship director: Responsible for overseeing the surgical education of medical students, clerkship directors play a crucial role in shaping the early experiences of future surgeons. They coordinate clinical rotations, develop curriculum content, and assess student performance during surgical clerkships.

Director of surgical education: This position focuses exclusively on the educational aspects of surgical training. Directors of surgical education play a critical role in curriculum development, assessment, and faculty development. They work closely with PDs to implement effective teaching methodologies and foster a culture of continuous learning.

Vice chair for education: This pivotal role involves the strategic leadership of educational programs within the department. The vice chair for education collaborates closely with program directors, ensuring the seamless execution of residency and fellowship programs. They spearhead initiatives to enhance the quality of education, represent the department in educational committees, and advocate for essential educational resources.

Administrative Leadership Roles

Vice chair (clinical affairs): This role focuses on the clinical operations of the department, ensuring the delivery of high-quality patient care. The vice chair for clinical affairs oversees patient safety initiatives, quality improvement programs, and workflow optimization within clinical settings [13].

Vice chair (research): Leaders in this position drive the research agenda within the department. They guide faculty in securing research funding, foster collaborative research endeavors, and promote a culture of scholarly activity. The vice chair for research plays a vital role in elevating the department's research profile.

Vice chair (administration): Responsible for the administrative functions of the department, the vice chair for administration handles budgeting, resource allocation, and strategic planning. They ensure efficient utilization of resources and facilitate the operational excellence of the department.

Assistant/associate dean (faculty affairs): This position focuses on the development and management of faculty within the academic institution. Assistant/associate deans for faculty affairs oversee recruitment, appointment, promotion, and professional development of faculty members.

Assistant/associate dean (student affairs): Responsible for the well-being and educational experiences of medical students, these deans oversee aspects such as career advising, student support services, and extracurricular activities.

Leadership Pathways

There are several pathways for an academic leadership pathway. One path is that of program director or division chief followed by the vice-chair and finally department chair roles. Another pathway is the decanal pathway. In this route, the leader would be promoted to assistant or associate dean, then senior associate dean, followed by dean and/or president and CEO [14].

Balancing Paths for Optimal Leadership

Combining roles in multiple pathways can provide a well-rounded perspective for effective leadership in academic surgery. Through the cultivation of expertise in education and administration, the complexities of the academic surgical landscape can be navigated with proficiency and vision by aspiring leaders [15].

Importance of Relationships and Networking

In the world of academic surgery, the adage "it's not what you know but who you know" holds a profound truth. A successful journey toward leadership in general surgery is characterized by the cultivation of meaningful relationships and the establishment of a robust professional network [16].

Collaborative endeavors: An environment of collaboration and shared knowledge is fostered by building strong relationships within the academic surgical community. These relationships extend beyond casual interactions; they encompass mentorship, sponsorship, coaching, collaborative research projects, and joint educational initiatives. Avenues for intellectual discourse and the exchange of innovative ideas are opened through engagement with colleagues, both within and beyond one's immediate department. This collaborative spirit not only enriches individual pursuits but also elevates the collective standard of care and research in the field [17, 18].

Mentorship and guidance: A cornerstone of professional development is the establishment of mentor-mentee relationships with experienced academic surgeons. Seasoned mentors offer invaluable guidance, sharing their wealth of knowledge, experiences, and perspectives. They provide insight into navigating the intricacies of academia, from securing research funding to managing teaching responsibilities. Additionally, mentors serve as advocates or sponsors, endorsing their mentees for leadership opportunities and offering constructive feedback to aid in personal and professional growth. It is important to remember that these relationships are two way streets and making sure that mentee expectations are clear and met consistently will be helpful to the mentor [19].

Access to opportunities: A well-nurtured professional network serves as a gateway to a plethora of opportunities. This may encompass invitations to speak at conferences, collaborations in influential research endeavors, or participation in leadership development programs. Engaging with peers and leaders in the field in meaningful way exposes one to diverse perspectives and emerging trends, broadening both knowledge and influence [20].

Visibility and recognition: Active participation in professional societies, conferences, and workshops is essential in establishing a visible presence in the academic surgical community. It provides a platform to showcase expertise, share research findings, and contribute to discussions shaping the future of surgery. Through these engagements, individuals can garner recognition for their contributions, positioning themselves as thought leaders in their respective domains [21].

Long-lasting impact: The relationships forged and networks cultivated in the journey toward academic surgery leadership extend beyond personal achievements. They lay the foundation for a legacy of collaborative research, innovative clinical practices, and the mentorship of future generations of surgeons. As one ascends the leadership ladder, these connections become conduits for continued growth, impact, and the advancement of surgical care and education [22].

In essence, the development of relationships and networking is not just a supplementary aspect of academic surgery leadership; it is a cornerstone. The bonds created and the collaborations forged are not only professionally and personally enriching but also essential for propelling the field forward into new realms of excellence and innovation [23, 24].

Balance Between Internal and External Relationships

In the demanding field of academic surgery, academic surgeons face a perpetual challenge in balancing internal and external relationships. We navigate a complex terrain of clinical duties, research commitments, and external professional engagements. Achieving the right equilibrium between these domains is not only crucial for career progression but also for personal well-being [25].

Internal Relationships

In the crucible of clinical responsibilities, an academic surgeon's relationships with colleagues, nurses, and support staff are essential. Effective collaboration and communication within the clinical setting are vital. Engaging in open dialogue, actively listening, and fostering a culture of mutual respect can go a long way in fortifying these internal relationships. Resolving conflicts harmoniously, whether they arise from differences in approach or resource allocation, is equally pivotal. By establishing a harmonious clinical environment, AS can cultivate a strong foundation for their professional endeavors [25].

The world of academic surgery is intimately entwined with research and academic collaborations. Building and sustaining successful research teams requires a delicate balance of skill sets and personalities. Nurturing relationships with research collaborators, ranging from experienced faculty to budding students, is a dynamic process. It demands clear communication, shared expectations, and a collective commitment to the research mission. The impact of their research endeavors can be amplified by fostering an environment of intellectual exchange and mutual support by academic surgeons [26].

Teaching and mentorship form the linchpin of an AS's legacy. Guiding students and trainees toward excellence requires more than just didactic instruction. Effective mentoring involves setting clear goals, providing constructive feedback, and igniting a passion for learning. Empowering learners to take ownership of their education is a transformative process. It involves instilling confidence, fostering critical thinking, and nurturing a thirst for knowledge. Balancing teaching commitments, alongside clinical and research duties, necessitates astute time management and a strategic approach to curriculum design [26].

External Relationships

External relationships form a vast landscape beyond the confines of one's institution. Strategic networking within the professional community is not merely a pursuit of personal advancement but a means of contributing to the collective body of knowledge. Identifying key contacts, attending conferences, and engaging in online platforms are all avenues to establish meaningful connections. AS can leverage external relationships to bolster their research and clinical impact by actively participating in the broader discourse of their field.

Collaborations that transcend institutional boundaries can yield groundbreaking discoveries and innovations. Selecting compatible collaborators and institutions requires a discerning eye for shared vision and complementary expertise. Effectively communicating and coordinating across different organizations demands not only technological proficiency but also a keen understanding of the nuances of interinstitutional collaboration. AS can amplify the scope and reach of their contributions by navigating the intricacies of external partnerships [27].

However, the pursuit of external opportunities must be tempered with a judicious approach. Prioritization is key. Not every invitation or collaboration aligns seamlessly with one's career trajectory or academic interests. Strategic discernment is required to invest time and energy, where it will yield the greatest return. Balancing external commitments with the core responsibilities of clinical practice and research necessitates a shrewd evaluation of the potential benefits and potential trade-offs.

Strategies for Balance

Time is the most precious resource in the life of an AS. A methodical approach to time management is nonnegotiable. Conducting a thorough time audit can illuminate areas of inefficiency and guide the allocation of resources. Time-blocking techniques, such as the Pomodoro method, provide a structured framework for maximizing productivity. The Pomodoro technique is a simple time management system using a timer to break work into 25-min intervals punctuated by short breaks using a timer, then taking a longer break after four work times [28]. By honing their time management skills, AS can optimize their output without succumbing to burnout [29].

Effective communication is the linchpin of success in the AS's multifaceted role. Advocating for oneself, whether in negotiating workload or setting boundaries, requires a blend of assertiveness and diplomacy. Constructive feedback is equally pivotal, both in giving and receiving. A culture of open dialogue fosters continuous improvement and strengthens professional relationships.

The rigors of academic surgery demand a holistic approach to self-care. Physical, mental, and emotional well-being are inextricably linked to professional success. Prioritizing regular exercise, balanced nutrition, and adequate sleep is foundational. Moreover, building resilience to navigate the inevitable stresses of the profession is a learned skill. Techniques such as mindfulness, meditation, and stress-reducing practices can fortify an academic surgeon's mental and emotional well-being [30]. Taking time away from work to recharge and enjoy family, friends, exercise, hobbies, or just fun and downtime is essential.

Achieving a National Presence

In the dynamic landscape of academic surgery, establishing a national presence is a crucial step toward advancing both personal career goals and the broader field of surgical science. This section delves into the significance of attaining a national profile and outlines strategic approaches to accomplish this milestone [31].

Importance of Achieving a National Presence

Knowledge dissemination and influence: A national presence allows academic surgeons to disseminate their research findings, clinical expertise, and innovative practices on a broader scale. This dissemination contributes to the advancement of surgical knowledge and practice, influencing the direction of the field.

Collaborations and networking: A national platform provides opportunities to forge collaborations with esteemed peers, researchers, and institutions. These connections facilitate the exchange of ideas, collaborative research endeavors, and the creation of multidisciplinary teams to tackle complex surgical challenges [32].

Advocacy and policy influence: A prominent national profile positions academic surgeons as thought leaders capable of influencing healthcare policies and advocating for advancements in surgical care. Their expertise becomes instrumental in shaping policies that affect surgical practice, education, and research.

Mentorship and educational impact: A national presence affords academic surgeons the platform to mentor and educate the next generation of surgical leaders. Their influence extends beyond their immediate institution, impacting a broader spectrum of students, residents, and fellows.

Recognition and career progression: A well-established national and international reputation garners recognition from peers, institutions, and professional organizations. This recognition can lead to various opportunities for career progression, including academic promotion, collaborations, leadership positions, prestigious awards, and invitations for keynote presentations at national conferences.

Strategies to Achieve a National Presence

Active involvement in professional organizations: Joining and actively participating in relevant surgical societies and associations at the national level provides opportunities for networking, presenting research, and contributing to the larger surgical community [32]. It is important to choose these commitments carefully so that they relate to your personal goals and that you can contribute in a meaningful way without becoming overwhelmed with commitments.

Publishing high-impact research: Publishing in reputable, peer-reviewed journals with a wide readership enhances visibility and credibility. Consistent publication of high-impact research solidifies one's reputation as a thought leader in the field.

Speaking engagements and conference presentations: Presenting research findings, innovative techniques, and clinical insights at national conferences and symposia elevates visibility and establishes expertise. It also fosters connections with like-minded professionals.

Engagement in collaborative research initiatives: Actively participating in multi-institutional or inter-disciplinary research projects fosters collaboration and enhances visibility on a national scale. It demonstrates a commitment to advancing surgical science beyond individual institutional boundaries.

Advocacy and policy involvement: Engaging in advocacy efforts and participating in committees related to surgical care, education, and research at the national level allows for direct involvement in shaping policies that impact the field [33].

Mentorship and educational leadership: Offering mentorship and sponsorship to trainees and junior faculty on a national scale, through programs, workshops, or virtual platforms, establishes a legacy of leadership and extends one's influence in surgical education.

Utilizing social media and online platforms: Leveraging social media, academic platforms, and professional networking sites allows for the dissemination of ideas, engagement with a broader audience, and participation in relevant discussions [34]. Social media engagement can be treacherous as well so it's best to stay strictly professional and avoid posting any identifiable clinical or hospital information on these platforms. Disagreements are best handled in person rather than on X (Twitter), Facebook, or Instagram.

Staying current with emerging trends: Keeping abreast of the latest advancements, technologies, and debates in the field ensures that AS remains at the forefront of surgical knowledge and contributes meaningfully to national conversations [35].

The academic surgeon can proactively establish a robust national presence through the adoption of these strategies. In doing so, not only are their own careers advanced but also a significant contribution is made to the progress and evolution of academic surgery on a broader scale [36].

Tips for Success

Navigating an academic career in surgery can be challenging and the pathway to leadership is not always intuitive. Developing an academic career is a skill that can be learned and should be taught during the formative years of surgical training. However, developing into an academic surgeon is not a one-size-fits-all track. To ascend in surgical academics, the aspiring leader must demonstrate certain desirable qualities. Although not a panacea, clearly defined traits will position you to be promoted to the next level.

In contradistinction, select habits may need to be avoided when attempting to climb the academic ladder. Along the way, there are pitfalls and snares to avoid.

Appropriate Selection of Academic Endeavors

A common mistake when seeking to advance in the academic universe is focusing on tasks that have limited value for promotion to professorship. Rewriting and retooling a set of guidelines that have been established, reestablished, and agreed upon by a committee for the third time during the last academic year may not be a valuable use of your time. The pursuit of perfection and unanimous agreement on guidelines is not a realistic approach to collaboration in academics and life. Sometimes, shared understanding and agreed-upon concessions are necessary to advance policy. Understanding that your *truth* is not always *the truth* is critical in collaboration. Redoubling efforts to make others see things "your way" can be counterproductive and create duplicity among colleagues. Therefore, spending large periods of time on limited-value tasks is a pitfall to avoid while navigating a career in academics.

Effective Time Management

Time management begins with organizational skills. We are all very familiar with being told, "If you did not write it down, then it did not happen." This is especially true in medicolegal documentation but also applies to time management. Our brains are wired to become fuzzy with an increasing list of tasks. Given the seemingly Sisyphean tasks faced as a physician on the track to advancement, a workaround to this conundrum is to create a to-do list with specific assignments that can be reasonably accomplished.

Creating a list of tasks allows a record-keeping system in which items can be crossed out. Furthermore, crossing out a task liberates space in the mind's eye, allowing further focus on the remaining tasks. It allows maintenance of a bird's-eye view, which can easily be converted to a magnified view of the tasks remaining on the to-do list.

Emotional Intelligence

Emotional intelligence can be a difficult but crucial trait to master. A person's ability to manage their feelings so that those feelings are expressed appropriately and effectively are tenets of emotional intelligence. There are four components of emotional intelligence: self-awareness, self-management, social awareness, and relationship management [37]. Underdevelopment of these characteristics can potentially hinder academic advancement. For instance, a junior faculty member with excellent motivation who lacks social awareness may be perceived as lacking the ability to relate to colleagues productively. A faculty member who lacks the ability to hold crucial conversations with learners, colleagues, or staff may be perceived as having poor relationship management skills. Ultimately, this lack of development can lead to stagnation on the academic ladder. Developing emotional intelligence is fundamental to success and its absence can lead to failures regardless of medical knowledge.

The Importance of Meeting Deadlines

Academic advancement to the next level can be seen as validation of value and confirmation of trust to remain consistent in productivity. The inability to meet deadlines can negatively impact the reputation of a faculty member and raise questions about the ability to complete trusted tasks in a timely manner. Once a reputation has been damaged, it can be difficult to repair and lead to stagnation in academic advancement. It is better to take on fewer, less complicated tasks and take them to completion than to say yes to everything and then fail to deliver.

Choosing Wisely

Saying yes too often can be a difficult habit from which to depart. Several drivers may make someone feel compelled to frequently agree to tasks. A reason for this sentiment may be that faculty wants to be perceived as being a "team player" or collegial. Faculty may also be driven by the perceived benefits of completing the next task. Faculty may also hold personal beliefs or biases from past experiences of not agreeing to tasks frequently enough. Regardless of the motivation for agreeing to participate in every project, committee, lecture, and delegation, there may be benefits in respectfully declining to take on more responsibilities. Tactfully declining to agree to all requests may help prevent faculty burnout and moral injury. In addition, a task you can't take on may be an opportunity you want to pass on to a mentee. Respectfully declining but suggesting a colleague or mentee is a form of active sponsorship.

Effective Communication

It is important to establish bidirectional communication of your expectations and vision with the department chair and institutional leadership. There is no substitute for clear and transparent goals regarding academic responsibilities. Not having a clear understanding of academic responsibilities can lead to losing focus on the matter at hand and ultimately produce a vain attempt at advancement.

Development of Leadership Skills

Effective leaders take the time and effort to develop skills such as mastery of visioning, communication, change management, emotional intelligence, team building, business skills, personnel management, and systems thinking.

Important Competencies of an Academic Leader

There are many important qualities and competencies for an academic leader. While many leaders may possess several of these qualities naturally, many develop and nurture these qualities and competencies through various means. Avenues to develop these competencies include executive and leadership coaching, educational courses, as well as formal and informal mentorship.

The purview and responsibilities of an academic leader require knowledge and expertise to effectively lead the clinical, research, and educational enterprise as well as manage the day-to-day functions of the organization. Some of the required skills are managerial rather than true leadership skills, and some may be delegated but will need attention nonetheless.

Budgeting and Finance

A strong understanding of the financial status of the program, institute, or department is essential to ensure the longevity and stability of the organization. Knowledge of research funding avenues, clinical revenues, grants, as well as state and federal funds are essential to the growth of the academic arena. Strong finance and operations administrators and relationships with the financial leadership of the organization are key. While not mandatory for assuming these leadership roles, a master of business administration degree or educational courses in finance, administration, and operations are helpful for the academic leader.

Accreditation

The education provided by medical institutions is governed by national accrediting bodies. The Liaison Committee on Medical Education (LCME) governs the medical curriculum of accredited medical schools within the United States and Canada [38]. This voluntary process provides a quality assurance of the medical education provided by the medical institutions [38]. Similarly, graduate medical education in the United States is overseen by the Accreditation Council for Graduate Medical Education (ACGME) [39].

The academic leader must be familiar and competent with accreditation guidelines to ensure the stability and growth of educational programs. Necessary resources to support the educational and other initiatives within the academic program must be accurately identified and procured effectively. The academic leader must possess organizational and forward-thinking skills to ensure that needs, concerns, and strategic initiatives are effectively addressed.

Strategic Planning

Strategic planning is an essential competency of an effective academic leader. The ability to cast vision, obtain resources, and facilitate growth is essential to the well-being of the academic organization. This skill is often attained through mentorship, education, and collaboration. Effective strategic planning requires the ability to fully understand the needs of the organization and its constituents as well as the strengths, weaknesses, and future growth endeavors. Appropriate metrics and a framework for accountability of the attainment of proposed metrics are essential within the proposed strategic plan. A key component of effective strategic planning is an alignment of the leader's purview with the overall strategic plan of the organization and attaining buy-in both upstream and downstream. The leadership, as well as the faculty and staff of the academic arena, must identify and own the strategic plan and its vision to ensure success collectively. A strong leader possesses vision skills, creativity, effective communication skills, superb listening skills and is not afraid to fail [40].

Management of Human Talent/HR Competencies

Human talent is the most important asset of any organization. Physician talent is also a high-cost item for academic institutions. Effective management of human talent by the academic leader requires many skills, including effective recruitment, the ability to retain talent, performance assessment, and termination of faculty and staff when necessary. Leaders are required to function in many roles including a guide, support, visionary, disciplinarian, and even a coach for faculty or staff requiring assistance to attain performance goals. Managing talent effectively requires active listening skills and the ability to provide encouragement for faculty to work on improved performance and skills acquisition when needed. Faculty and staff career and personal development models and opportunities are essential to improve the forward growth of the institution. The effective leader possesses skills of effective communication, accountability, delegation of tasks, and effective management of human talent regarding faculty compensation and development.

Systems Thinking

The ability to work collaboratively at multiple levels within the organization is an important tenet of leading within an academic setting. The institutional goals and direction are guides for the academic leaders at all levels within the organization. The effective leader is able to envision how their programs, initiatives, and directives impact the overall organization and drive change within the institution. They understand the organizational culture and work to ensure a culture that is appropriate for improving and expanding the institution's reputation.

Team management and team building are essential for the academic leader who must ensure that appropriate surgical, administrative, and operational teams are built and nurtured to drive forward the mission of the academic program or institution.

Fundraising

A common requirement for academic leaders is the knowledge and expertise to bring funds to the academic department or institution. These funds are utilized for programmatic initiatives, clinical directives, operations, research, and educational opportunities within the academic setting. This skill of attracting and obtaining donors and donations is often unfamiliar to a new academic leader and is therefore attained over time and with practice. There are strategies to maximize funding opportunities for academic leaders such as whom to target with asks and also curating carefully which initiatives to highlight for support. Institutional offices such as the Office of Institutional Advancement, Office of Alumni Affairs, and Office of Philanthropy can be strong partners for the academic leader in this space.

Communication

Strong, frequent, and clear communication is a stronghold of any effective academic leader. The leader must be a role model of excellent communication, available, honest, transparent, and trustworthy. Bidirectional communication is key to the effective relay of information and ensuring that all parties are in alignment with understanding and direction. A strong leader also understands the importance of "managing upstream." Regular communication and alignment with organizational leadership are effective means of ensuring the forward movement of initiatives and programs. It is also important to ensure that leadership is aware of the accomplishments, challenges, and forward growth of the leader's area of responsibility. In addition to strong communication skills, effective and active listening skills are paramount for the academic leader. The leader encourages open communication by demonstrating the willingness to listen actively to staff, faculty, and trainees ("I want my people to tell me the things that I need to know"). In this vein, open and frequent communication should be encouraged.

Dealing with the Difficult Resident or Faculty Member

In the ever-evolving landscape of general surgery, navigating challenging interactions with residents and faculty members is a hallmark of effective leadership. These encounters, while demanding, present opportunities for growth, collaboration, and ultimately, a more cohesive surgical team [41, 42].

Addressing Difficult Residents

Encountering a resident who presents challenges requires a proactive and empathetic approach. The initial step is to arrange a private meeting, selecting a setting that ensures confidentiality and encourages open discourse. By setting this tone of privacy, it allows the resident to feel more comfortable expressing their concerns and viewpoints [43].

During the conversation, it is imperative to adopt an active listening stance. Give the resident the space to articulate their perspective without interruption. This not only demonstrates respect for their opinions but also provides valuable insights into their perceptions of their role and interactions within the team.

Following this, the feedback provided should be specific and focused on observable behaviors. For instance, if there are concerns about communication style, providing examples of specific instances allows for a clearer understanding. Additionally, it's crucial to elucidate the potential impact of these behaviors on patient care, team dynamics, and their own professional growth.

A collaborative approach should be taken when establishing expectations and a developmental roadmap. Encourage the resident to take an active role in formulating goals, ensuring they have a sense of ownership in their professional progress. This approach not only addresses immediate concerns but also fosters a culture of accountability and continuous improvement within the surgical team [43]. Depending on the situation, additional resources, such as professional counseling, coaching, general health evaluation, or assistance with addiction, may be helpful.

Managing Challenging Faculty Members

A strategic and respectful approach is essential when engaging with a challenging faculty member. Emphasize mutual respect and a shared commitment to the department's success during private meetings with faculty members. By acknowledging their invaluable contributions to the program and highlighting their expertise, you establish a foundation of respect for their experience and knowledge [44].

While addressing specific behaviors or concerns, it is crucial to utilize "I" statements to express how these issues impact the broader team, patient care, and the educational environment. This approach focuses on the tangible consequences of behavior, steering the conversation toward solutions rather than blame [44].

Furthermore, collaborative problem-solving is key. Invite their input on strategies for improvement, ensuring they feel invested in creating a more harmonious work environment. This involvement not only demonstrates respect for their expertise but also fosters a sense of ownership in building a positive and productive professional setting.

Maintaining Documentation and Seeking Support

Thorough documentation is a linchpin in the process of addressing difficult interactions. It serves as a reference point for future discussions and ensures accountability for agreed-upon action plans. Consistency in documenting progress updates is equally important, providing a clear record of any positive changes or areas that still require attention [45].

If challenges persist, seeking guidance from departmental leadership or utilizing institutional resources for conflict resolution can provide additional support. Involving higher authorities with a neutral perspective can help navigate complex situations, offering an objective viewpoint and facilitating constructive resolutions [46].

By incorporating these tailored strategies, you empower yourself to not only address challenges directly and constructively but also to foster a culture of growth and accountability within your surgical team [47]. This, in turn, contributes to a more cohesive and effective healthcare environment, ensuring the continued success of the general surgery program [48].

Strategies and Challenges for Women and Minorities

While there has been an increase in the percentage of women matriculating and graduating from medical school and matriculating into residency programs, there have been few advances in academia for women and minorities. The percentage of women faculty in medical schools remains low, and the number of female faculty at each academic rank decreases as the rank increases. AAMC data demonstrated that in 2023, medical school applicants were 56.6% women, while women comprised 54.6% of total enrollment in 2023–2024. The racial and ethnic breakdown for medical school matriculants was 51% White, 29% Asian, 13% Hispanic, 10% Black, 1% American Indian or Alaska native, and less than 1% Native Hawaiian or other Pacific Islander [49]. As of 2023, 27% of medical school deans were women and 18% were URIM [50, 51].

With regard to clinical department chairs, 23% were women in 2023 [52]. Only 8% of surgery chairs were women, and there were only four African-American female surgical chairs [52, 53].

Similarly, there are disparities in residency matriculation and graduation rates and decreased representation in NIH funding and leadership roles [54, 55]. While black male medical students accounted for 3.1% of the national student body in 1978, they represented only 2.9% in 2019 [56]. Without the four HBCU medical schools, that percentage would be 2.4% [56]. Native Americans accounted for less than 1% of the medical student body in 2019 [56]. While African-Americans account for 30% of the US population and the Latinx population account for approximately 18%—they account for 5% and 4% of our physician population [57].

Especially worrisome is the high residency attrition rate for female and URIM trainees. In a study by Haruno et al., overall attrition rate among all specialties was 6.9% [58] Female residents had a significantly higher relative risk (RR) of than their male counterparts. URiM residents were at significantly higher RR for attrition than non-URiM residents. The highest attrition (10.6%) rates were in Black/African-American residents.

While the causes for the disparities in representation within academia are multifactorial, they include biases, lack of mentorship, lack of role models, and publication gap [59, 60]. Strategies to increase representation and retention include engagement with recruitment and pathway programs, mentoring programs, sponsorship, involvement in representative organizations (e.g., Association of Women Surgeons, Society of Black Academic Surgeons, Society of Asian Academic Surgeons, Latino Surgical Society, the Association of Out Surgeons and Allies, Association of American Indian Physicians), and professional accountability to formulate guidelines to improve representation within academia. Mentorship programs include those offered by the Association of Women Surgeons, American College of Surgeons, and Southern Surgical Leadership Development Program, among others.

Interim to Permanent

The interim academic role has several benefits as well as challenges. As an internal candidate to the position, the interim role allows the leader to assess the work demands, institutional/departmental resources, additional attributes of the position, and how they might assimilate into the role. The interim candidate has developed a reputation within the institution and relationships with key stakeholders in their immediate area and beyond. The leader serving in the interim role has earned the respect and belief that they are capable of fulfilling the position and its duties effectively.

However, the interim role also carries significant challenges. Often, the leader has assumed the interim role in addition to their previous roles, responsibilities, and duties. Thus, the addition of this role may further extend their responsibilities and potentially jeopardize their ability to lead and manage within the position effectively. When accepting an interim role, it is important to negotiate for a budget and protected time in order to manage the additional responsibilities and meet expected goals.

Navigating the transition from interim to permanent requires beliefs and resources. While in the interim role, it is important to perform the job as if you are in the permanent role. This interim role allows an opportunity to demonstrate the strengths that you bring to the position. Additionally, the interim leader has been appointed to advance the unit rather than tread water, so utilize your role to implement initiatives and enhance the growth of the unit.

Show you passion for the job and belief in the organization's mission. Demonstrate this passion in your dedication to the job, communication downstream and upstream, and attentiveness to the growth of the unit. Finally, above all, be true to yourself.

Helpful Resources for the Academic Leader

There are many resources which may prove helpful to the academic leader. These include:

Mentorship

Formal and informal mentorship are important for the academic leader. Mentorship has been shown to improve performance, result in promotion sooner, and result in decreased levels of burnout [61]. Mentorship can occur via both formal and informal methods. Many surgical organizations offer formal mentorship programs such as the American College of Surgeons, Association of Women Surgeons, American Surgical Association, and Southern Surgical Association, among others. These programs often follow a standardized format and are geared toward specific groups of leaders, such as mid-career surgeons, early-career surgeons, and aspiring surgical leaders. The aspiring academic leader should also avail themselves of informal mentorship both internally at their institution as well as externally outside of their organizations with mentors who can guide and advise on leadership development.

Programs

Leadership development programs for academic leaders are of significant value to leaders for improvement or gaining skills. Some of these programs include:

Executive Leadership in Academic Medicine (ELAM) Program
American College of Surgeons: Surgeons as Leaders: From Operating Room to Boardroom Course
American College of Surgeons: Surgeons as Educators Program
Southern Surgical Association: Leadership Development Program
American Association of Medical Colleges: Early Career Faculty Development Courses
American Association of Medical Colleges: Mid-Career Faculty Development Courses
Harvard Surgical Leadership Courses
American College of Surgeons Academy of Master Surgeon Educators
Association of Surgical Education: The ASE Surgical Education and Leadership Fellowship (SELF)
Harvard Leadership Development for Physicians
Physician Leadership Academy

Additional Resources Include Textbooks, Audiovisual Materials, and Degree/Certificate Programs

Brandeis Heller School of Policy and Management Surgeons as Leaders Program
Brandeis Heller School of Policy and Management Executive MBA for Physicians
Crucial Conversations: Tools for Talking When Stakes Are High, Patterson, Grenny et al.
What Got You Here Won't Get You There, M. Goldsmith
The Five Dysfunctions of a Team, P. Lencioni
Leadership in Surgery, M. Kibbe, H. Chen
Higgins et al. Surgical Chairs Playbook, American College of Surgeons, 2023
Association of Women Surgeon: Navigating Your Surgical Career, 2nd edition, 2023

Conclusion

Navigating an academic career and reaching a leadership position requires possession and/or attainment of specific skills and expertise. There are many pathways to pursue an academic career however all require dedication and skill to attain. The academic surgeon should ensure diligent pursuit of skills necessary to ensure a successful career.

SAGES Takeaway

- There are many pathways to attain an academic career including administrative, research, educational, and decanal pathways.
- The academic surgeon must navigate internal and external relationships and develop a robust national presence to ensure continued ascension of the career ladder.
- Avoid pitfalls such as ineffective time management, inappropriate selection of academic endeavors, poor emotional

intelligence, failure of effective communication, and misalignment with goals and vision of leadership.
- The successful academic leader's competencies include strategic planning, management of human talent, budgeting, accreditation, effective communication, and systems thinking.

References

1. Raine G, Evans C, Uphoff EP, Brown JVE, Crampton PES, Kehoe A, Stewart LA, Finn GM, Morgan JE. Strengthening the clinical academic pathway: a systematic review of interventions to support clinical academic careers for doctors and dentists. BMJ Open. 2022;12(9):e060281. https://doi.org/10.1136/bmjopen-2021-060281.
2. Brown JVE, Crampton PES, Finn GM, Morgan JE, Project Team. From the sticky floor to the glass ceiling and everything in between: protocol for a systematic review of barriers and facilitators to clinical academic careers and interventions to address these, with a focus on gender inequality. Syst Rev. 2020;9(1):26. https://doi.org/10.1186/s13643-020-1286-z.
3. Campion MW, Bhasin RM, Beaudette DJ, Shann MH, Benjamin EJ. Mid-career faculty development in academic medicine: how does it impact faculty and institutional vitality? J Fac Dev. 2016;30(3):49–64.
4. Mayowski CA, Norman MK, Proulx CN, Hamm ME, Martin MK, Zellers DF, Rubio DM, Levine AS. Evaluation of two longitudinal faculty leadership training programs: behavioral change and institutional impact. J Health Organ Manag. 2022 (ahead-of-print). https://doi.org/10.1108/JHOM-03-2022-0088.
5. Steinert Y, Naismith L, Mann K. Faculty development initiatives designed to promote leadership in medical education. A BEME systematic review: BEME guide no. 19. Med Teach. 2012;34(6):483–503. https://doi.org/10.3109/0142159X.2012.680937.
6. Maykel JA. Leadership in surgery. Clin Colon Rectal Surg. 2013;26(4):254–8. https://doi.org/10.1055/s-0033-1356727.
7. Barnes T, Rennie SC. Leadership and surgical training part 1: preparing to lead the way? ANZ J Surg. 2021;91(6):1068–74. https://doi.org/10.1111/ans.16685. Epub 2021 Apr 7.
8. Barnes T, Rennie SC. Leadership and surgical training part 2: training toolkit for leadership development during surgical training. ANZ J Surg. 2021;91(6):1075–82. https://doi.org/10.1111/ans.16777. Epub 2021 Apr 7.

9. Gabram SG, Espat NJ, Jacobs LM, Macleod JB, Rozycki GS. Academic careers in surgery: the many paths from which to choose. J Surg Educ. 2007;64(1):27–35. https://doi.org/10.1016/j.cursur.2006.08.011.
10. Greenfield LJ. Challenges to academic surgery: are we recruiting the best and brightest? Bull Am Coll Surg. 2000;85(3):21–4.
11. Butch L. Mentorship program designed to advance women in academic surgery. Bull Am Coll Surg. 2009;94(10):6–10.
12. Ford HR. Mentoring, diversity, and academic surgery. J Surg Res. 2004;118(1):1–8. https://doi.org/10.1016/j.jss.2004.01.018.
13. Souba WW. Mentoring young academic surgeons, our most precious asset. J Surg Res. 1999;82(2):113–20. https://doi.org/10.1006/jsre.1999.5596.
14. McCord JH, McDonald R, Sippel RS, Leverson G, Mahvi DM, Weber SM. Surgical career choices: the vital impact of mentoring. J Surg Res. 2009;155(1):136–41. https://doi.org/10.1016/j.jss.2008.06.048. Epub 2008 Aug 13.
15. Goldstein AM, Blair AB, Keswani SG, Gosain A, Morowitz M, Kuo JS, Levine M, Ahuja N, Hackam DJ, Basic Science Committee of the Society of University Surgeons. A roadmap for aspiring surgeon-scientists in today's healthcare environment. Ann Surg. 2019;269(1):66–72. https://doi.org/10.1097/SLA.0000000000002840.
16. Luc JGY, Stamp NL, Antonoff MB. Social media in the mentorship and networking of physicians: important role for women in surgical specialties. Am J Surg. 2018;215(4):752–60. https://doi.org/10.1016/j.amjsurg.2018.02.011. Epub 2018 Feb 16.
17. Taylor CA, Taylor JC, Stoller JK. Exploring leadership competencies in established and aspiring physician leaders: an interview-based study. J Gen Intern Med. 2008;23(6):748–54. https://doi.org/10.1007/s11606-008-0565-5. Epub 2008 Mar 8.
18. Yang P, Diaz A, Chhabra KR, Byrnes ME, Rajkumar A, Nathan H, Dimick JB. Surgical leadership competencies for navigating hospital network expansion. J Surg Res. 2023;283:76–83. https://doi.org/10.1016/j.jss.2022.10.014. Epub 2022 Nov 11.
19. Champion C, Bennett S, Carver D, El Tawil K, Fabbro S, Howatt N, Noei F, Rae R, Haggar F, Arnaout A. Providing mentorship support to general surgery residents: a model for structured group facilitation. Can J Surg. 2015;58(6):372–3. https://doi.org/10.1503/cjs.004315.
20. Lang M, Keenan L. Canadian medical faculty senior leaders: what skills do they need? Leadersh Health Serv (Bradf Engl). 2022 (ahead-of-print). https://doi.org/10.1108/LHS-03-2022-0023.
21. Lee TC, Reyna C, Shah SA, Lewis JD. The road to academic surgical leadership: characteristics and experiences of surgical chairpersons. Surgery. 2020;168(4):707–13. https://doi.org/10.1016/j.surg.2020.05.022. Epub 2020 Jul 11.

22. Ocho ON, Wheeler E, Rigby J, Murphy GT. Core competencies and challenges among nurses transitioning into positions of leadership—a Caribbean perspective. Leadersh Health Serv (Bradf, Engl). 2021 (ahead-of-print). https://doi.org/10.1108/LHS-03-2021-0014.
23. Gonzalo JD, Ahluwalia A, Hamilton M, Wolf H, Wolpaw DR, Thompson BM. Aligning education with health care transformation: identifying a shared mental model of "new" faculty competencies for academic faculty. Acad Med. 2018;93(2):256–64. https://doi.org/10.1097/ACM.0000000000001895.
24. Lieff SJ, Baker L, Poost-Foroosh L, Castellani B, Hafferty FW, Ng SL. Exploring the networking of academic health science leaders: how and why do they do it? Acad Med. 2020;95(10):1570–7. https://doi.org/10.1097/ACM.0000000000003177.
25. Bleier JI, Kann B. Academic goals in surgery. Clin Colon Rectal Surg. 2013;26(4):212–7. https://doi.org/10.1055/s-0033-1356719.
26. Seymour V. The human-nature relationship and its impact on health: a critical review. Front Public Health. 2016;4:260. https://doi.org/10.3389/fpubh.2016.00260.
27. Columbus AB, Lu PW, Hill SS, Fields AC, Davids JS, Melnitchouk N. Factors associated with the professional success of female surgical department chairs: a qualitative study. JAMA Surg. 2020;155(11):1028–33. https://doi.org/10.1001/jamasurg.2020.3023.
28. Biwer F, Wiradhany W, Oude Egbrink MGA, de Bruin ABH. Understanding effort regulation: Comparing 'Pomodoro' breaks and self-regulated breaks. Br J Educ Psychol. 2023;93(Suppl 2):353–67. https://doi.org/10.1111/bjep.12593. Epub 2023 Mar 1. PMID: 36859717.
29. Welten VM, Dabekaussen KFAA, Hill SS, Columbus AB, Lu PW, Fields AC, Reich AJ, Davids JS, Melnitchouk N. Leadership styles among female surgical department chairs. J Gastrointest Surg. 2022;26(8):1776–80. https://doi.org/10.1007/s11605-022-05403-z. Epub 2022 Jul 6.
30. Huber-Lang M, Neugebauer E. The dual role of academic surgeons as clinicians and researchers—an attempt to square the circle? Patient Saf Surg. 2011;5:16. https://doi.org/10.1186/1754-9493-5-16.
31. Rosengart TK, Mason MC, LeMaire SA, Brandt ML, Coselli JS, Curley SA, Mattox KL, Mills JL, Sugarbaker DJ, Berger DA. The seven attributes of the academic surgeon: critical aspects of the archetype and contributions to the surgical community. Am J Surg. 2017;214(2):165–79. https://doi.org/10.1016/j.amjsurg.2017.02.003. Epub 2017 Feb 20.
32. Meer E, Hughes BD, Martin CA, Rios-Diaz AJ, Patel V, Pugh CM, Berry C, Stain SC, Britt LD, Stein SL, Butler PD. Reassessing career pathways of surgical leaders: an examination of surgical leaders' early accomplishments. Am J Surg. 2021;222(5):933–6. https://doi.org/10.1016/j.amjsurg.2021.04.012. Epub 2021 Apr 16.

33. Hughes BD, Butler PD, Edwards MA, Pugh CM, Martin CA. The Society of Black Academic Surgeons CV benchmarking initiative: early career trends of academic surgical leaders. Am J Surg. 2020;219(4):546–51. https://doi.org/10.1016/j.amjsurg.2020.01.047. Epub 2020 Jan 27.
34. Sanfey H, Gantt NL. Career development resource: academic career in surgical education. Am J Surg. 2012;204(1):126–9. https://doi.org/10.1016/j.amjsurg.2012.04.001.
35. Sanfey H, Boehler M, DaRosa D, Dunnington GL. Career development resource: educational leadership in a department of surgery: vice chairs for education. Am J Surg. 2012;204(1):121–5. https://doi.org/10.1016/j.amjsurg.2012.04.003.
36. Sanfey H, Hollands C. Career development resource: promotion to associate professor. Am J Surg. 2012;204(1):130–4. https://doi.org/10.1016/j.amjsurg.2012.04.004.
37. Goleman D. Emotional intelligence: why it can matter more than IQ. London: Random House Publishing Group; 2012.
38. LCME. https://lcme.org/about/. Accessed 28 Oct 2023.
39. ACGME. https://www.acgme.org/. Accessed 28 Oct 2023.
40. Clary B, Inabnet W, Kuo P. Chapter 5: Strategic planning: an essential tool for achieving success. In: Higgins R, Matthews J, Rosengart T, Wong S, editors. Surgical chairs playbook. Society of Surgical Chairs, American College of Surgeons; 2023.
41. Mrkonjic L, Grondin SC. Introduction to concepts in leadership for the surgeon. Thorac Surg Clin. 2011;21(3):323–31. https://doi.org/10.1016/j.thorsurg.2011.04.001.
42. Nes E, White BAA, Malek AJ, Mata J, Wieters JS, Little D. Building communication and conflict management awareness in surgical education. J Surg Educ. 2022;79(3):745–52. https://doi.org/10.1016/j.jsurg.2021.11.014. Epub 2021 Dec 21.
43. Ang M. Advanced communication skills: conflict management and persuasion. Acad Med. 2002;77(11):1166. https://doi.org/10.1097/00001888-200211000-00034.
44. Fahy AS, Mueller C, Fecteau A. Conflict resolution and negotiation in pediatric surgery. Semin Pediatr Surg. 2021;30(5):151100. https://doi.org/10.1016/j.sempedsurg.2021.151100. Epub 2021 Sep 5.
45. Wolfe AD, Hoang KB, Denniston SF. Teaching conflict resolution in medicine: lessons from business, diplomacy, and theatre. MedEdPORTAL. 2018;14:10672. https://doi.org/10.15766/mep_2374-8265.10672.
46. Lee L, Berger DH, Awad SS, Brandt ML, Martinez G, Brunicardi FC. Conflict resolution: practical principles for surgeons. World J Surg. 2008;32(11):2331–5. https://doi.org/10.1007/s00268-008-9702-x.
47. Sexton M, Orchard C. Understanding healthcare professionals' self-efficacy to resolve interprofessional conflict. J Interprof Care. 2016;30(3):316–23. https://doi.org/10.3109/13561820.2016.1147021.
48. Druckman D, Wagner LM. Justice and negotiation. Annu Rev Psychol. 2016;67:387–413. https://doi.org/10.1146/annurev-psych-122414-033308. Epub 2015 Aug 13.

49. AAMC. New AAMC data on diversity in medical school enrollment in 2023. 2023. https://www.aamc.org/news/press-releases/new-aamc-data-diversity-medical-school-enrollment-2023.
50. AAMC. US Medical School Deans trends, type and race ethnicity. 2023. https://www.aamc.org/data-reports/faculty-institutions/data/us-medical-school-deans-trends-type-and-race-ethnicity.
51. AAMC. US Medical School Deans trends, type and gender. 2023. https://www.aamc.org/data-reports/faculty-institutions/data/us-medical-school-deans-trends-type-and-gender.
52. AAMC. Faculty Roster US Medical School Faculty. 2023. https://www.aamc.org/data-reports/faculty-institutions/report/faculty-roster-us-medical-school-faculty.
53. Association of Women Surgeons. https://www.womensurgeons.org/page/FemaleSurgeryChairs.
54. Berry C, Khabele D, Johnson-Mann C, Henry-Tillman R, Joseph KA, Turner P, et al. A call to action: Black/African American women surgeon scientists, where are they? Ann Surg. 2020;272(1):24–9.
55. Keshinro A, Frangos S, Berman RS, DiMaggio C, Klein MJ, Bukur M, et al. Underrepresented minorities in surgical residencies: where are they? A call to action to increase the pipeline. Ann Surg. 2020;272(3):512–20.
56. Morris DB, Gruppuso PA, McGee HA, Murillo AL, Grover A, Adashi EY. Diversity of the national medical student body—four decades of inequities. N Engl J Med. 2021;384(17):1661–8.
57. AAMC. Diversity in medicine: facts and figures 2019. 2019.
58. Haruno LS, Chen X, Metzger M, et al. Racial and sex disparities in resident attrition among surgical subspecialties. JAMA Surg. 2023;158(4):368–76. https://doi.org/10.1001/jamasurg.2022.7640.
59. Stadler DJ, Ibrahim H, Cofrancesco J Jr, Archuleta S. Fixing the leaky pipeline: tips to promote gender equity in academic medicine. Asia Pacific Scholar. 2021;6(4):1.
60. Escobar N, Keshinro A, Hambrecht A, Frangos S, Berman RS, DiMaggio C, et al. A call to action to train underrepresented minorities in surgical subspecialties and fellowships. J Am Coll Surg. 2023;237(1):109–16.
61. Gotian R. How to develop a mentoring team. Forbes; 2020.

Further Reading

Kennedy GE, Bergstresser SL, Rakestraw SL, Novak Z, Corey B, Chen H, Sutzko DC. Does chair of surgery gender influence divisional or residency program director gender diversity? J Surg Res. 2021;267:224–8.

Keshinro A, Butler P, Fayanju O, et al. Examination of intersectionality and the pipeline for black academic surgeons. JAMA Surg. 2022;157(4):327–34. https://doi.org/10.1001/jamasurg.2021.7430.

Organizational Change Management in HealthCare

36

Sivamainthan "Siva" Vithiananthan

Introduction

In contemporary healthcare, spanning the past 25 years, we find ourselves amidst an unprecedented era of transformation and changes. These changes have indelibly reshaped the practice of medicine. For physicians, these transformations transcend mere professional shifts; they demand unwavering dedication to medical excellence while concurrently mastering the intricate art of change management.

For example, our journey through the healthcare landscape over the past quarter-century has been a testament to seismic changes instigated by technological innovations, evolving patient dynamics, and a push toward a commitment to value-based care. For surgeons, it is not merely a matter of choice but a compelling imperative to comprehend and adeptly navigate this ever-evolving terrain.

Let's explore some transformative shifts, each representing a pivotal facet of the new healthcare reality:

S. S. Vithiananthan (✉)
Department of Surgery, Cambridge Health Alliance, Harvard Medical School, Cambridge, MA, USA
e-mail: svithiananthan@cha.harvard.edu

S. M. Johnson et al. (eds.), *The SAGES Manual of Strategy and Leadership*, https://doi.org/10.1007/978-3-031-62359-2_36

- **Technological advances**: Groundbreaking technologies such as robotic-assisted surgery, catheter-based surgery, and telemedicine have revolutionized medicine. Rapid progress in diagnostic technology based on artificial intelligence will change how we practice medicine in the next few years. Those physicians who adeptly harness these innovations gain a distinct competitive edge, delivering state-of-the-art care to their patients. As minimally invasive surgeons, SAGES members are well aware of these changes.
- **Empowered patients**: The role of patients in shaping their healthcare decisions has undergone a profound transformation. Physicians must now cultivate exceptional communication skills and wholeheartedly embrace shared decision-making to meet the evolving expectations of their patient populations. A patient-directed approach to cancer care and technology has changed our approach to many disease processes.
- **Value-centric paradigm**: The conventional fee-for-service model is shifting toward a value-focused approach emphasizing cost-effectiveness and outcomes. Surgeons are entrusted with the responsibility of prioritizing high-quality care, cost-efficiency, and fostering interdisciplinary collaboration. Historical RVU or volume-based compensation is changing to a value-based payment model for many surgeons.
- **Changing demographics**: Aging populations and a surge in chronic illnesses have substantially amplified the demand for medical care and riskier procedures. Physicians must adapt their practices to cater to the unique healthcare needs of elderly patients grappling with complex medical conditions.

While these are some of the many transformational changes, the range, depth, and speed of change vary in almost every field of medicine. They are too numerous to analyze in this chapter.

In this dynamic backdrop, the art of change management transcends being a mere skill; it emerges as an indispensable necessity. Change management empowers physicians to deftly navigate ambiguity, instill adaptability, and proficiently lead healthcare teams in the swiftly evolving sphere of modern medicine. Recently, there has been an intense focus on physician burnout.

Not embracing or keeping up with change are some of the causes identified leading to significant physician burnout.

This chapter reviews foundational change management principles, underscoring their profound relevance to physicians, especially surgeons. By exploring tangible real-world surgical case examples and illustrative case studies, these change management principles are applied to healthcare so that physicians can leverage these principles to instigate positive transformations, elevate patient outcomes, and excel in the ever-fluctuating world of modern medicine.

Types of Changes

Changes can come in various forms. The concepts of **reactive** and **proactive** change in organizational management are fundamental distinctions that highlight an organization's approach to addressing challenges and opportunities [1].

Reactive Change

Reactive change occurs when organizations make alterations in response to external events or pressures after they have already affected the organization.

Closing a performance gap: This refers to the difference between the current state or performance ("what is") and the expected or necessary state or performance ("what should be"). Reactive change is about responding to discrepancies, often problems or challenges, that have already surfaced.

Examples: Implementing measures after a lost specimen in the operating room or responding to higher wound infections or longer lengths of hospital stay.

Proactive Change

Proactive change is initiated by the organization itself, based on foresight, anticipation, or the ambition to improve rather than in response to external pressures.

Closing an opportunity gap: This is about recognizing potential enhancements or opportunities for the organization and bridging the divide between the present state ("what is") and a potentially more favorable future state ("what could be"). The emphasis is on seizing opportunities before they become imperatives.

Examples: Launching a new wound care center based on market research, implementing a groundbreaking ambient electronic record documentation method to improve efficiency and decrease physician burnout, or hiring surgeons with advanced MIS skills in anticipation of future needs.

In essence, while **reactive** change is about responding to problems or pressures already arising, **proactive** change is about anticipating future needs or challenges addressed in the strategic plan. Both approaches are essential in different scenarios, but balancing the two often leads to a more resilient and agile organization.

Any proactive change requires planning, hard work, and, more importantly, alignment with the group/institutional priority. In any academic institution or community hospital, every 5 years or so, the leadership establishes a strategic plan after studying the market, speaking to its clients (patients, researchers, etc.), and going through a SWOT analysis. Various committees study and analyze the institution's **S**trengths, **W**eaknesses, **O**pportunities, and **T**hreats during this process. Ultimately, the strategic plan is adopted by the board of governors as the guide for growth in the next 3–5 years. There will be milestones to be met in this process, and senior leadership sponsors will oversee various pillars of the strategic plan.

Most major change management process happens within this context. To implement change, a thoughtful process is required. Emotions of anxiety and fear are common; inertia is powerful and needs to be overcome through a multistep process that generates enough power and motivation to overcome these negative human and system issues.

To understand change management, we will look at some successful processes described by thought leaders in the next section.

Models to Help with Change Management

Kotter's Model

Provides a systematic, step-by-step approach to change. By following this eight-step model, organizations can anticipate and address challenges before they become obstacles [1, 2].

Bolman and Deal's Four Frames [3]

Managers can view problems and solutions from multiple perspectives. Leaders can craft more comprehensive and effective change initiatives by understanding and addressing change from all four frames. While Kotter's model provides a pathway to implement change, Bolman and Deal's model offers lenses through which to understand the complexities of organizations. By combining insights from both, leaders can be better prepared to drive successful change initiatives.

Kotter's Change Management Model Through the Lens of a Surgical Environment [2]

1. Establish a sense of urgency: Understanding the critical need for change is paramount. One needs to identify potential threats and develop scenarios to see what the future might look like if these threats materialize.
2. Create a guiding coalition: Change isn't a solitary endeavor. Forming a group with enough power and vested interest can guide the change, making it a collective effort.
3. Develop a vision and strategy: Clarity on the change's destination and how to get there can guide efforts and keep the team cohesive.
4. Communicate the change vision: Regular, clear, and impactful communication of the vision ensures everyone understands and is aligned.
5. Empower broad-based action: Remove barriers. Empower people to act, foster an innovation environment, and acknowledge the initiative.

6. Generate short-term wins: Celebrating small victories en route to the larger goal provides motivation, offers a sense of achievement, and reduces cynicism.
7. Consolidate gains and produce more change: Change is a continuous process. Use the credibility gained from early wins to tackle bigger challenges and drive deeper change.
8. Anchor new approaches in the culture: Lasting change means ensuring that the new approaches become a part of the very DNA of the organization's culture.

As a surgeon leader looking at change management, understanding and embedding Kotter's principles can guide a structured and effective transformation. While benefiting the patients, this transformation ensures every surgical team member's growth, development, and well-being. In elaborating on these steps, Table 36.1 offers a clear and structured roadmap for surgical leaders seeking to initiate and sustain change within their surgical environments regardless of the change they wish to make.

Bolman and Deal's Four Frames Model: A Lens for Surgical Leaders

Another useful tool in instituting change management is Bolman and Deal's four frames [3]. This model offers a unique perspective on change by providing four distinct lenses to view and address organizational issues, particularly in the context of change (Table 36.2).

By understanding and adeptly integrating insights from all four frames, surgical leaders can artfully craft a comprehensive approach to change. This ensures that the organization's tangible and intangible aspects are thoroughly addressed and go beyond what is obvious and immediately visible.

A case study on introducing a new technology is discussed using Kotter's eight steps, and Bolman and Deal's four frames are discussed later in the chapter.

Navigating Change with Bridges' Principles: The Emotional Journey

Change is an ever-present companion in our personal and organizational lives. Heraclitus, a Greek philosopher, described "what is constant is change." However, navigating change often entails tra-

Table 36.1 Kotter's eight steps in the context of healthcare change management

Kotter's step	In-depth description for novice surgical leader	Surgery-specific healthcare example
1. Establish a sense of urgency	Before you can drive change, everyone needs to understand why it's crucial. As a leader, you'll want to highlight the immediate problems. Make sure to use tangible data and compelling narratives to make the need for change visceral	Example: "We've seen an uptick in post-operative infections; this isn't just a statistic. We had three open wounds and wound vacs in patients in 1 month. We need to act now"
2. Create a guiding coalition	Change isn't a one-person job. You must identify and rally key individuals who bring diverse perspectives, skills, and influence to the cause. This team will be the nerve center of your change initiative, offering guidance and advocating for the change throughout the surgical department	Example: "Let's form a 'surgical excellence team' comprising senior surgeons, house staff, OR nurses, and floor nurses. Everyone has a unique vantage point on how we can improve"
3. Develop a vision and strategy	This is about painting a clear picture of the future. What does a successful change look like? What path will lead us there? Ensuring that the vision is specific, achievable, and inspiring is essential	Example: "Imagine a surgery team where post-op infectious complications are the rare exception, not the norm. To get there, we must introduce standardized wound closure techniques, closing trays, train OR and surgical teams with recurring training modules, and regular meetings reviewing our data"
4. Communicate the change vision	Communication is more than just broadcasting; it's about ensuring understanding and buy-in at all levels. Regularly share updates, success stories, and even setbacks, fostering an environment of transparency and engagement	Example: "Every 2 weeks, we'll have a 'surgical ID rounds" where we discuss our improvements, challenges, and share feedback. And I'm always open for one-on-one conversations if anyone has ideas or concerns"

(continued)

Table 36.1 (continued)

Kotter's step	In-depth description for novice surgical leader	Surgery-specific healthcare example
5. Empower broad-based action	Give people the tools, training, and autonomy they need to make changes. Address any barriers to change, whether they are outdated processes or skeptical team members, or lack of resources	Example: "Starting next week, we're rolling out a new in-service on standard wound closures, wound care bundle, and maintaining closing trays. We've also set aside IT resources to update order sets for the timing of antibiotics, create a wound care bundle to improve patient outcomes"
6. Generate short-term wins	Progress can be slow, but celebrating small victories can keep morale high. These wins prove that the change is working and helps build momentum	Example: "Last week, we had no post-op infections at all. That's fantastic! Let's acknowledge those successes and learn from what went right." post it in the resident work room and in the OR lounge
7. Consolidate gains and produce more change	Early successes are just the beginning. Use the momentum from short-term wins to tackle bigger challenges and drive deeper change.	Example: "Our wound infection rates have dropped, which is great! Let's focus on further reducing SIRS, surgical wait times and enhancing our post-op patient education"
8. Anchor new approaches in the culture	For change to stick, it has to become "the way we do things around here." that means ensuring new practices are deeply embedded in training, processes, and the overall culture of the surgical department	Example: "Every new member (resident/RN) joining our surgical team will go through our updated training module. We'll have an annual 'surgical QI day' to strengthen our commitment to continuous improvement"

Table 36.2 Bolman and Deal's four frames

Bolman and Deal's frame	Description	Surgery-specific healthcare example
1. Structural frame	This frame focuses on the architecture of the organization: Its roles, responsibilities, policies, and procedures. How are things organized, and how do they function? It's about designing clear structures that match the organization's goals	Example: "Our surgical team has ten operating rooms, but they are often booked simultaneously, leading to long waiting times. By reorganizing our scheduling system and defining roles more clearly, we can maximize efficiency and reduce patient wait times"
2. Human resource frame	People are at the heart of every organization. This frame emphasizes understanding the needs, skills, and relationships of those in the organization. It's about aligning the organization's needs with those of the individuals	Example: "Our surgical team is feeling burnout due to too many overnight calls. By understanding their needs, we can restructure schedules, add middle-level providers for first call, and offer better sleeping facilities so that they're not only rested but also motivated and cared for"
3. Political frame	Organizations have power structures, and this frame is about understanding those dynamics. Who holds power? What are their interests? It's about negotiating, forming alliances, and managing conflicts for productive outcomes	Example: "Different surgical teams compete for the same laparoscopic instruments/robot time. By recognizing these political dynamics, we can negotiate equitable resource distribution and perhaps advocate for more funding or resources together rather than in competition"
4. Symbolic frame	Every organization has a culture built on rituals and ceremonies, stories, and symbols. This frame looks at these symbols' meanings and how they shape behavior. It's about shaping culture and fostering motivation	Example: "Every time we successfully complete a month with >90% first case on-time starts we celebrate with a 'surgical success day,' reinforcing our commitment to excellence and recognizing the team's hard work. It becomes a symbol of our dedication and unity"

versing a process of **transition**—a journey. William Bridges, a distinguished expert in change management, devised a model that accentuates this journey's psychological and emotional facets during times of change [4].

Transition fundamentally diverges from mere change. Change is a situational shift—an alteration in workforce size, a strategic adjustment, or a modification in reporting structures—all tangible "changes." Transition, however, represents a psychological realignment process encompassing three distinct phases that individuals navigate when grappling with change. It commences with an ending—a moment where individuals must relinquish their former reality and identity. Without genuinely concluding the past, embarking on a successful new beginning remains elusive.

Following the conclusion phase, individuals enter the second stage of transition: the neutral zone. This resembles uncharted territory. The neutral zone signifies a period and a state wherein old behaviors and attitudes fade away, and individuals lie dormant as they prepare for a fresh direction. While this phase poses risks for organizations, it presents an opportune environment for innovative ideas and experiments to flourish.

Only after traversing through these initial two transition phases can individuals effectively engage in the third phase: commencing anew, infused with renewed vigor, a fresh sense of purpose, a reinvigorated perspective, and an altered self-image.

Bridges' Transition Model: An Overview

Bridges' transition model [5] comprises three pivotal stages: **ending**, **neutral zone**, and **new beginning**. These stages facilitate a deeper understanding of the psychological and emotional dimensions accompanying transition during change.

Ending: The Farewell to Familiarity

The ending stage signifies the recognition of the need to bid farewell to established routines and the accompanying complex emotions. It is a phase where individuals grapple with the loss of the familiar and confront the enigma of the future.

Relevant emotions: During the ending stage, individuals traverse a turbulent terrain of emotions, including:

- **Resistance**: People may instinctively resist change due to the necessity of relinquishing the comfort of the known. Fear of the unknown or attachment to well-established routines can induce resistance.
- **Anxiety**: The uncertainty that accompanies change can lead to anxiety. Individuals may harbor concerns about their capacity to adapt or fret about the repercussions of impending alterations.
- **Nostalgia**: A poignant sense of loss and nostalgia for how things used to permeate this stage often. People frequently reminisce, sometimes idealizing it.

Example: Consider an organization on the brink of implementing a state-of-the-art technology system to streamline operations. In this ending stage, employees may wrestle with apprehension about parting with their well-practiced processes and tools. Resistance to change may emerge, and concerns about how the new system will affect their daily work can be palpable.

Neutral Zone: Embracing Ambiguity and Igniting Creativity

The neutral zone unfolds as a realm of ambiguity and exploration. It is where individuals confront uncertainty and experiment with novel possibilities. While discomfort and anxiety may persist, this stage also fosters sparks of creativity and innovation.

Relevant emotions: Within the neutral zone, emotions often form a complex tapestry, encompassing:

- **Frustration**: The terrain of experimentation may be strewn with obstacles and challenges, leading to frustration as individuals grapple with uncharted territory.
- **Confusion**: The inherent ambiguity of the transition phase can spawn confusion regarding roles, processes, and expectations.
- **Excitement**: Amidst the challenges, some individuals may experience excitement as they begin to perceive the creative potential and innovative prospects that change offers.

Example: Continuing with the technology system implementation, the neutral zone becomes the canvas upon which employees explore the new system's capabilities. Challenges and roadblocks may emerge, inducing moments of frustration and confusion. However, certain employees may need to find innovative ways to leverage the system to enhance their work processes during this stage.

New Beginning: The Embrace of Change

The new beginning stage signifies the acceptance of change and the seamless integration of novel practices into daily routines. It is characterized by heightened confidence, a sense of purpose, and a resolute commitment to the new way of doing things.

Relevant emotions: As individuals transition into the new beginning stage, emotions tend to metamorphose into:

- **Confidence**: Successful adaptation breeds confidence in individuals. They start to believe in their ability to navigate the changing landscape competently.
- **Motivation**: The positive outcomes and benefits of the change become motivating factors, propelling individuals forward with newfound energy.
- **Commitment**: A profound commitment to the new way of conducting affairs takes root, aligning individuals with the evolving landscape.

Example: In the new beginning stage of the technology system implementation, employees have adapted and excelled in using the new tools and processes. Confidence permeates the workforce as they recognize the tangible benefits of the change. Consequently, their work becomes more efficient, embracing the change as a positive stride toward progress.

Why Transition Matters in Change Management

Transition is not a mere byproduct of change but a vital journey aspect. Individuals and organizations must traverse the transition's emotional and psychological terrain to embrace change wholeheartedly. Overlooking the human aspect of change can trigger resistance, diminish morale, and potentially lead to the failure of change initiatives.

Understanding Bridges' transition model is instrumental for surgical leaders embarking on change endeavors. Recognizing that their team members will experience emotions and challenges throughout the transition can equip leaders with the empathy and insight necessary to guide their teams. It is about acknowledging that change is not just a series of steps and procedures but a profoundly human experience.

Two "C"s and Four "P"s of Communication of Change

In the transition period during change, a change leader must communicate very clearly. More time should be spent on "why" (problem) rather than "how" (solution) to be effective in change management. Bridges describes change communication with 2 C's and 4 P's [5].

The leader should maintain a connection with the team affected by the change and show concern for their adjustments and sacrifices.

1. **Purpose**: This refers to the need for a clear and compelling reason behind the change. People must understand why the change is happening and how it will benefit them and the organization.
2. **Picture**: After implementing the change, people need a clear vision or mental image of the future. A vivid and positive picture helps individuals to align their efforts and actions with the desired outcome.
3. **Plan**: A detailed plan outlines the steps and actions required to transition from the current state to the desired future. It provides a roadmap for how the change will be executed.
4. **Part**: The "part" in Bridges' model emphasizes the importance of involving and engaging people in the change process. It recognizes that individuals must actively participate in the change rather than be passive recipients.

Resisting Change: Why Do People Resist Change?

Change often meets widespread resistance. This resistance to change takes various forms, from passive reluctance to outright rebellion. Effective leaders must equip themselves with the tools to comprehend this resistance's predictable and universal sources and devise strategies to navigate it successfully. Here are the ten most prevalent sources of resistance to change identified by Rosabeth Moss Kanter from Harvard Business School [6].

1. Loss of control: Change can disrupt one's sense of autonomy and control, leading to discomfort. Leaders can mitigate this by involving those affected in the change process, granting them a sense of ownership.
2. Excess uncertainty: People resist change when it feels like navigating uncharted territory. To overcome this, leaders must provide a sense of safety, a clear, inspiring vision, and well-defined processes and timelines.
3. Surprise changes: Sudden, imposed decisions are met with resistance. Leaders should avoid secrecy and introduce changes gradually, seeking input along the way.
4. Overwhelming differences: Change inherently brings something new, but excessive differences can be disorienting. Leaders should minimize unrelated changes and maintain familiarity where possible.
5. Loss of face: Change often signifies a departure from the past, making those associated with the previous version defensive. Leaders can help maintain dignity by acknowledging the past and emphasizing the evolving landscape.
6. Concerns about competence: People resist change when it makes them feel inadequate. Leaders should provide reassurance through information, education, training, mentors, and support systems.
7. Increased workload: Change typically requires more effort, leading to overload. Leaders should recognize and reward the hard work of change participants and their families.
8. Ripple effects: Change affects not only the immediate area but also distant stakeholders. Leaders should consider all affected parties and collaborate with them to minimize disruptions.
9. Past resentments: Historical grievances can resurface when change is needed. Leaders should consider gestures to address past issues before moving forward.

10. Real threats: Change can bring real pain, such as job loss or financial impact. In such cases, leaders should be honest, transparent, fast, and fair in their approach.

While leaders cannot always eliminate the discomfort associated with change, they can reduce it. Understanding the sources of resistance is the initial step toward finding effective solutions. Feedback from those resisting change can also prove valuable in refining the acceptance process.

Case Study

Let's look at using some of the principles we discussed earlier in a familiar case study that surgeons are often asked to undertake:

Background *You are the new surgical director at a community hospital ("MIS Hospital") competing with academic medical centers for surgical patients. In your assessment as the only trained MIS surgeon, the hospital you are championing brings Robotic surgery technology to a hospital that has been doing open surgery. You feel this technology will give you a competitive edge. Your hospital receives additional funding from the government for taking care of underinsured or Medicaid patients. However, recent budget cuts will be affecting that share of the funding. In the recently concluded Strategic plan for the next 5 years, upgrading technology and providing up-to-date care locally was one of the main strategic goals for the hospital. Due to the financial effects of the pandemic, you start the year with concern for a tight budget.*

A Case Study for Promoting New Robotic Surgery at "MIS Hospital"

Change Proposal and Rationale

As we navigate the dynamic healthcare environment, MIS Hospital faces the challenge of competing with academic health systems (AHS) to sustain and expand our market presence. Our longstanding commitment to "up-to-date care for the community" remains steadfast, but it is essential to reinvigorate our in-patient surgical volume and explore new surgical opportunities. This shift is particularly crucial as government subsidies face a shortfall due to budget cuts, necessitating a strategic pivot.

As the newly appointed director of surgery, you propose introducing robotic surgical technology across subspecialties such as urology, thoracic, gynecology, general, and bariatric surgery. Our surgical offerings predominantly consist of routine procedures, limiting patient choices and resulting in a decline in surgical volume as patients seek care elsewhere. The adoption of robotic technology aims to modernize our surgical portfolio by converting existing open and laparoscopic procedures and introducing new surgeries, including solid organ and bariatric procedures. This change aligns perfectly with our new strategic initiative, which emphasizes "up-to-date care for all patients locally" and champions innovation and in-patient surgical volume growth.

At present, MIS Hospital faces challenges in fulfilling its surgical mission. Internal and external stakeholders perceive our hospital as needing help delivering its full potential. With a paradigm shift toward robotic surgery, you aim to overcome these perceptions and win over key stakeholders, including primary care physicians (PCPs) and patients. Robotic surgery offers a pathway to providing excellent and up-to-date care to all members of our local community, regardless of their ability to navigate complex AHS systems. Additionally, it bolsters our internal capacity and healthcare innovation efforts, attracting a younger generation of technologically savvy surgeons to build our future.

In addressing these challenges, we must maintain our patient-focused, multilingual, navigable system that sets us apart. This exceptional patient experience is vital for retaining our patient base positioning us as leaders. An external challenge revolves around the potential cost-prohibitive nature of acquiring robotic technology, a concern that must be carefully considered.

Stakeholders

The proposed change impacts a range of stakeholders, including patients, surgeons, operating room (OR) staff, primary care physicians (PCPs), and the hospital leadership, comprising department chiefs, administration, and the board of directors. Conflicting views are expected to emerge from these stakeholders, reflecting a natural resistance to change driven by fear of loss and uncertainty.

Looking through Bolman and Deal's lens, from a structural perspective, concerns will likely revolve around insurance coverage and surgeon credentials. Patients may fear that machines, rather than surgeons, will perform their surgeries. In the human resources frame, questions about credentialing criteria and the potential for poor outcomes and negative press may arise among physicians and administrators. Politically, non-surgeon stakeholders, particularly PCPs, may need help allocating capital expenditure and its impact on other funding needs. Seasoned surgeons may be concerned about losing their referral sources, and symbolically, all stakeholders may worry about the message this investment sends to taxpayers, given our reliance on state and city waivers.

On the supportive side, younger surgeons, already trained and privileged for robotic surgery, align with the structural frame. In the human resources frame, patients, PCPs, and surgeons recognize the benefits of robotic surgery, including reduced pain, quicker recovery, fewer transfusions, and improved outcomes. Leadership supports the move for minimally invasive surgery, leading to shorter hospital stays and lower readmission rates. The political frame aligns with surgeons aiming to level the playing field with larger academic centers, stem outmigration, and attract new patients. Symbolically, robotic surgery puts MIS Hospital on the map as a technologically advanced surgical destination, enhancing our surgeons' and hospital's reputation.

Implementation Strategy

You could follow John Kotter's eight-step change management process and Bolman and Deal's four frames as guides to engage stakeholders effectively to bring about successful change. Following are some potential strategies using these frameworks.

Creating a Sense of Urgency

The leadership and key decision-makers within the organization have recognized the imperative need for swift changes to transition towards robotic technology (RT) within a planned

6–12-month timeframe. It is essential not to extend this process over multiple budget cycles, as it could lead to complications, hinder adaptation across all surgical divisions, and lead to tech-savvy surgeons leaving the hospital. Identifying divisional RT champions, securing leadership support, and establishing fair credentialing criteria are crucial aspects framed within a structural perspective. Emphasizing the urgency, especially concerning impending changes in governmental funding mechanisms, must be communicated effectively during strategic planning sessions, leadership meetings, departmental gatherings, informal discussions, and newsletters. To fill open positions, recruiting new graduates, whose experience has been mostly in RT in urology and gynecology, adds to the urgency and must be communicated.

Creating a Powerful Guiding Coalition

Success in this initiative requires the formation of a coalition among the surgical departments that are RT advocates and gaining the support of other department chiefs, notably the chief of primary care and family medicine. Listening to and addressing the concerns of all stakeholders, including non-surgeons who might have reservations about resource reallocation, is paramount. The human resource framework can be utilized to build a coalition around objectives like reducing length of stay (LOS), decreasing readmissions, and enhancing patient satisfaction scores, ultimately contributing to increased hospital revenue. Meeting one-on-one with each department chief is vital to discuss how implementing RT within the Accountable Care Organization (ACO) framework can prevent patient outmigration and strengthen the healthcare system. A comprehensive training program should be established for surgeons and OR staff worried about adapting to RT. Surgeons seeking to extend their clinical careers can be encouraged to adopt RT for its ergonomic benefits. Creating a robotic core team consisting of surgeons, anesthesia personnel, and OR staff will foster camaraderie and identity transformation as they transition to this innovative platform.

Creating a Vision

The organization's new strategic planning initiative has created a compelling vision statement: "Current Care to the Community, Locally." The introduction of robotic technology represents a tangible embodiment of excellence and current care. This project aims to transition from open surgery and limited-service scopes to more advanced, outcome-oriented, patient-centric surgical services. Demonstrating the viability of this vision is essential. Overcoming initial skepticism about the "strange machine" can be achieved by showcasing the robot through live demonstrations. All staff, including surgeons and leadership, should have the opportunity to experience the robot's 3-D visualization, AI capabilities, ease of training, and straightforward setup process. Pre- and post-surveys can be instrumental in persuading leadership and hesitant stakeholders to embrace the change. Involving patients in sharing their success stories through news outlets and social media will reinforce the vision of excellence. Celebrating milestones such as the first hundred cases, naming the robot, and incorporating visual elements in the lobby will underscore the program's significance and visibility. It's vital to listen to stakeholders' concerns and challenges throughout this process and proactively address them.

Communicate the Vision

Effective communication of the vision is critical for its acceptance and adoption. Ensuring all employees understand and align with the new strategic direction is essential. The vision should be articulated clearly and consistently throughout the organization. Communication strategies may include newsletters, meetings, workshops, and targeted discussions.

Removing Obstacles

The primary obstacle in this initiative may be the substantial upfront capital cost in millions for purchasing the robotic technology. Alternative financing options such as leasing and philanthropic support should be explored to mitigate this challenge. Demonstrating the return on investment (ROI) within 3 years through a robust business plan can help garner primary care providers (PCPs) and organizational leadership support. Collaboration with union leaders to establish a "robot group" is essential due to unionization in the nursing sector. Developing and hiring robotic-trained surgeons and OR staff from the outset will ensure a smoother transition and early success. Addressing concerns related to the learning curve and temporary loss of productivity should involve discussions with anesthesia, PCPs, surgeons, and leadership. Establishing fair, widely accepted privileges documents for each department is also crucial. Forming a robotic steering committee comprising all stakeholders can facilitate obstacle removal and the adoption of best practices.

Generate Short-Term Wins

Creating short-term wins involves a pilot period, completing primary cases without complications, celebrating the first 25 cases, and evaluating the results. Achieving milestones like the first robotic prostatectomy and same-day robotic complex hernia repair within the initial 6 months demonstrates the organization's capability in robotic surgery. Celebrating the completion of nearly 100 robotic cases very quickly signifies the program's success, attracting and retaining young surgical talent in urology and gynecology and expanding services in thoracic and general surgery. Allocating protected robotic time within the OR schedule is crucial, and recognizing the contributions of OR staff through employee appreciation forums is essential.

Consolidate Gains

A deliberate and thoughtful approach during the initial phase is vital to ensure a safe transition and minimize complications. Assigning the most experienced RT surgeons to perform initial cases as everyone becomes familiar with the technology is a prudent step. Regular debriefing sessions within the robotic steering committee should focus on maintaining quality outcomes and continuous improvement. Building a dedicated "robot team" of trained nurses and introducing a robotic coordinator to the OR can facilitate the transition process and accelerate acceptance. Sharing outcomes with stakeholders is an effective means of garnering continued support.

Institute Change

After 18 months, with multiple services and surgeons comfortable with RT-based surgery and complex cases being performed, robotic technology will become an integral part of the organization's culture and identity. Discussions about acquiring additional robotic units can occur when robot utilization reaches 60–70%. Further investment in high-tech-based surgery, such as an orthopedic robot, will create the hospital's reputation synonymous with "current and cutting-edge care." Continued recruitment of surgeons and OR staff, along with the presence of an RT nurse coordinator, will be instrumental in coordinating services. RT will become a routine topic of conversation, solidifying this change within the organization's culture.

Conclusion

The introduction of robotic surgery at MIS Hospital marks a significant leap forward in the hospital's mission to provide up-to-date care locally in surgical care for our community. Your aim is to position yourselves as leaders in minimally invasive surgery through effective change management strategies, robust communication, coalition-building, and careful navigation of obstacles. With a shared vision and commitment to exceptional patient outcomes, you can surmount challenges and usher in a new era of surgical innovation at MIS Hospital.

Embracing Change: A Surgical Leader's Guide

Drawing upon the framework, real-world examples, and the case study detailed above, this chapter offers a synthesized roadmap for surgical leaders poised to lead their teams through transformative change. In closing, this guide has illuminated the critical importance of embracing change as a surgical leader in the dynamic landscape of modern medicine. We hope that the insights, strategies, and frameworks shared herein empower surgical leaders to navigate change with wisdom, empathy, and unwavering dedication to the highest standards of patient care. By embracing change, surgical leaders have the unique opportunity to shape the future of healthcare, ensuring that it is defined by excellence, innovation, and compassionate leadership.

SAGES Takeaway

- Surgical leaders must keenly understand the evolving healthcare landscape, marked by technological advancements, empowered patients, a value-centric paradigm, and changing demographics.
- Change management is not an option but an imperative for surgical leaders. It equips them with the tools to navigate ambiguity, instill adaptability, and lead healthcare teams effectively in the ever-evolving sphere of modern medicine.
- Kotter's eight steps, Bolman and Deal's four-frame model, and Bridges' transition model serve as invaluable frameworks for surgical leaders in orchestrating change. These models offer structured approaches for initiating, navigating, and ensuring the sustainability of change initiatives.
- Kotter's eight steps provides a step-by-step guide for change implementation, ensuring that every aspect of the process is carefully considered and executed. This model is adaptable to diverse surgical settings and offers a clear roadmap for novice surgical leaders.
- Bolman and Deal's four-frame model empowers surgical leaders to view change through four distinct lenses, addressing their organizations' structural, human resource, political, and symbolic aspects. By comprehensively understanding these dimensions, leaders can craft more effective change strategies.
- Bridges' transition model underscores individuals' emotional and psychological journey during change. Recognizing the ending, neutral zone, and new beginning stages is essential for surgical leaders to guide their teams effectively through the human dimension of change.
- Change management is not solely about processes and procedures; it is fundamentally about understanding and addressing the human experience of change. Surgical leaders must be empathetic, communicative, and adaptable, fostering an environment where team members can embrace change with confidence and commitment.

References

1. Kotter J. Leading change. Harvard Business Review. 23 Oct 2012.
2. Palmer I, Dunford R, Buchanan D. Managing organizational change: a multiple perspectives approach. 3rd ed. McGraw-Hill Higher Education; 2017. ISBN: 978-0073530536.
3. Bolman LG, Deal TE. How great leaders think: the art of reframing. 6th ed. Jossey-Bass; 2014. ISBN: 9781118140987.
4. Bridges W. Getting them through the wilderness: a leader's guide to transition. William Bridges Associates; 2006.
5. Bridges W. Managing transitions. William Bridges Associates; 2012.
6. Kanter R. Top ten reasons people resist change. Harvard Business Review. 25 Sept 2012.

Strategic Thinking and Leadership

37

Shaneeta M. Johnson

Basics of Strategic Thinking

Strategic thinking is seeing the big picture and developing a plan to achieve long-term goals. It requires the ability to think critically, analyze information, and make sound judgments. Strategic leaders are able to inspire and motivate others to work toward a common goal, adapt to change and manage uncertainty.

Strategic thinking is essential for navigating the complexities of today's organizational environment. It empowers individuals and organizations to envision and plan for a desired future. This capability goes beyond planning; it involves a deep understanding of the interconnections within and outside an organization and the foresight to anticipate how changes in one area can impact others.

Critical thinking is a cornerstone of strategic thinking. It allows leaders to sift through a wealth of information, differentiate between relevant and irrelevant data, and identify underlying patterns and opportunities. This analytical process is crucial for making informed decisions that align with long-term objectives.

S. M. Johnson (✉)
Department of Surgery, Morehouse School of Medicine, Atlanta, GA, USA

Satcher Health Leadership Institute, Morehouse School of Medicine, Atlanta, GA, USA
e-mail: shajohnson@msm.edu

S. M. Johnson et al. (eds.), *The SAGES Manual of Strategy and Leadership*, https://doi.org/10.1007/978-3-031-62359-2_37

However, Strategic thinking is not a solitary exercise. It requires engaging with others, pooling collective insights, and challenging assumptions to refine strategies and approaches. This collaborative aspect underscores the importance of communication skills for strategic leaders, enabling them to articulate their vision and rally their teams around shared goals.

Adaptability and resilience are also vital traits of strategic thinkers. The ability to pivot strategies in response to emerging threats or opportunities is invaluable. This agility ensures that the organization remains competitive and relevant even in the face of change.

Strategic leadership also involves vision casting, inspiring, and motivating others; thereby imbuing teams with purpose and encouraging them to meet and exceed expectations. By fostering a culture of innovation and excellence, strategic leaders can cultivate an environment where everyone is committed to achieving collective ambitions.

Strategic thinking is a multifaceted skill set that combines vision, analysis, collaboration, adaptability, and inspiration. It ensures long-term success and enables leaders and organizations to navigate the challenges of an ever-changing world with confidence and purpose.

Key critical skills that are essential for strategic thinking and leadership are listed below (Table 37.1).

Table 37.1 Key skills for strategic thinking and leadership

Critical thinking
Problem-solving
Decision-making
Communication
Teamwork
Leadership
Adaptability
Resilience
Vision casting
Change management

Leadership vs. Management

Leadership and management, while often discussed in the same context, encompass distinct skills and functions essential for effective organizational leadership. Leadership is "the art of mobilizing others to want to struggle for shared aspirations" [1]. Leadership is fundamentally about inspiring and motivating people toward a shared goal. It is setting a vision, getting others to align with that vision, and building relationships to foster a culture where everyone thrives.

In a multicontinental survey conducted by Kouzes and Posner, the four most admired characteristics of leaders were found to be honesty (89% of respondents), being forward-looking (71%), inspiring (69%), and competent (68%) [1]. This suggests that people value leaders who are not only visionaries but also grounded in their ethical stance and ability to inspire trust and confidence.

Management, in contrast, is defined by the concrete aspects of running an organization or a team. It involves planning, organizing, setting goals, delegating tasks, and monitoring progress. The role of a manager is to ensure that the day-to-day operations are aligned with the broader objectives of the organization. This requires a different set of skills than leadership, focusing more on efficiency, process, and the ability to execute plans effectively.

While both leadership and management are critical for the success of an organization, they serve different purposes. A good leader may not necessarily be a good manager, and vice versa. Leadership is about setting direction and inspiring people, while management is about efficiently executing plans and maintaining order. Effective organizational leadership often requires a blend of both sets of skills to navigate the complexities of leading an organization.

Differences between leadership and management:

- **People vs. Tasks: Leadership focuses on people, while management is about tasks**. Leaders focus on building relationships and motivating people, while managers focus on planning and organizing work.

- **Future vs. Present: Leadership plans for the future, while management focuses on the present**. Leaders set a vision and chart a course for the future, while managers focus on ensuring the day-to-day operations run smoothly.
- **Change vs. Stability: Leadership is about change, while management is about stability**. Leaders are change agents who drive innovation and progress, while managers maintain the status quo and keep things running smoothly.

Ultimately, both leadership and management are essential for any successful organization. A good leader can inspire and motivate people to achieve great things, while a good manager can ensure that the organization runs efficiently and effectively.

Leadership Styles

There are many different leadership styles and tools to evaluate and instruct on effective leadership and management skills. There is no one perfect or singular style of leadership. Instead, influential leaders may utilize multiple leadership styles and skills. Two examples of leadership styles are the situational leadership model and rational vs. relational leadership styles.

Situational Leadership Model

- The situational leadership model is a method for assessing a situation and the leadership style necessary for optimum results. It suggests an approach to leadership or management of a given situation based on the leader's leadership style and the performance readiness of the team member [2]. The model begins with the identification of the specific job, task, or activity and then an assessesment of the current performance readiness of the individual or team. This performance readiness is rated from R1 (unable and insecure or unable and unwilling) to R4 (able and confident and willing). Next, the leader's leadership style is assessed based on the relationship and task behaviors of the leader. Relationship behavior explains the engagement and relational skills of the leader, while task behavior focuses on the completion of the task being performed. The leadership style is matched to the performance readiness of the individual. Significantly, performance readiness may change, and there can be progression or regression in readiness [2].

Rational vs. Relational Leadership

Leadership styles may vary on a spectrum from rational leadership styles to relational leadership styles. The concept of relational leadership has been a subject of theoretical exploration for several decades [3]. Despite the efficacy of both approaches, they present distinct methodologies and outcomes.

Rational leadership is underpinned by logic, reason, and objectivity, privileging efficiency and productivity. It leans heavily on data-driven decision-making, prioritizing clear, concise communication and task orientation. This approach excels in scenarios demanding swift decision-making, promoting fairness and impartiality, and fostering a culture of accountability and high performance. Nevertheless, it may be perceived as detached or impersonal, potentially suppressing creativity and innovation, and could result in diminished employee engagement.

In contrast, relational leadership values the cultivation of strong interpersonal relationships and a supportive work atmosphere. It highlights empathy, encourages open communication and active listening, and centers on meeting the needs of team members, alongside motivating and inspiring them. This style tends to enhance team cohesion and productivity, boost employee engagement and satisfaction, and encourage an environment ripe for innovation and creativity. However, it might require significant time investment, present challenges in aligning individual needs with organizational goals, and prove challenging to scale in larger organizations.

Leaders Shape Organizational Culture

Organizational culture is an essential aspect of any company, encompassing the collective norms, values, expectations, and beliefs of its members [4, 5]. This culture is so pivotal that Peter Drucker famously remarked, "Culture eats strategy for breakfast" [6], emphasizing that the fabric of an organization's culture can overshadow and outwit even the most meticulously crafted strategies.

Culture plays a critical role in shaping not just the day-to-day operations but also an organization's long-term success, effectiveness, vision, and achievements. It is the underpinning foundation that influences how employees interact, make decisions, and, ultimately, how they contribute toward the organization's goals.

Leadership is at the heart of cultivating and maintaining this culture. The actions, behaviors, and decisions of an organization's leaders set a powerful example, establishing the standard for what is considered acceptable and desirable within the organization. As such, leaders have a profound impact on molding the organizational culture, and in steering the organization toward its strategic objectives.

A robust organizational culture offers a significant strategic advantage. It acts as a unifying force, aligning the organization's goals with the personal values and objectives of its members. This alignment boosts morale and engagement and fosters a sense of belonging and loyalty, which can significantly enhance productivity and innovation. Establishing a strong organizational culture is covered in further detail within another chapter of this text.

Leadership Skills for Effective Leadership

An effective leader must possess a comprehensive skill set that includes emotional intelligence, time management, the ability to cast a compelling vision, strategic planning capabilities, and adeptness at managing resistance. These skills are essential for guiding an organization with strategic leadership and a clear vision.

Emotional Intelligence

Emotional intelligence is an essential skill for leaders, facilitating the cultivation of robust relationships, adept conflict management, and fostering a positive workplace atmosphere. Leaders with high emotional intelligence are distinguished by their capacity to recognize and comprehend their own emotions and those of others, drive themselves and their teams forward, forge resilient relationships, communicate with clarity and empathy, resolve conflict, and engender a positive work environment.

At the heart of emotional intelligence lies self-awareness—the understanding of one's own emotions and their influence on behavior and interactions. Next, effective self-management is necessary, ensuring leaders can regulate and express their emotions and behaviors constructively. Social awareness equips leaders with the sensitivity to grasp and empathize with the emotions of others. This facet of emotional intelligence is instrumental in nurturing an environment of mutual respect and understanding. Finally, relationship management is the ability to build and maintain healthy relationships. This means communicating effectively, resolving conflict, and working collaboratively with others.

Time Management

Time management is crucial in enhancing the efficiency and effectiveness of leadership and management. For surgeons and their organizations to succeed, it is essential to prioritize tasks, delegate responsibilities, and organize workflows. This trio of skills ensures that both immediate and long-term goals are met, optimizing patient care and operations. The ability to manage time effectively not only contributes to the achievement of organizational objectives but also plays a pivotal role in improving the workflow for the surgical team, leading to improved job satisfaction and patient outcomes. The significance of developing strong time management skills is explored in depth in additional chapters of this text, providing readers with a comprehensive understanding of its impact on surgical leadership and management success.

Vision Casting

Leaders have access to a variety of tools to assess the organizational landscape and formulate strategic plans. Among these, the SWOT analysis stands out as a widely used tool, enabling leaders to evaluate the organization's strengths, weaknesses, opportunities, and threats. Understanding the organization's competitive advantage and key success factors is crucial. Another valuable framework is the McKinsey 7-S model, which focuses on achieving organizational alignment through seven key elements: strategy, structure, systems, shared values, skills, style, and staff. Together, these tools provide a comprehensive approach for leaders to navigate the complexities of strategic planning.

SWOT Analysis

The SWOT analysis is a comprehensive tool that facilitates the assessment of an organization's strengths, weaknesses, opportunities, and threats. Conducting a SWOT analysis is a crucial phase in grasping the organization's present circumstances, paving the way for strategic planning and vision formulation. By identifying and understanding the opportunities, weaknesses, and threats, leaders can craft strategies that leverage their organization's strengths and mitigate their vulnerabilities.

Stakeholders

Assessing key stakeholders is a critical step for leaders in formulating their strategic plans. It's crucial to identify stakeholders who possess influence, credibility, social capital, in-depth historical knowledge, and potentially aligned objectives. These individuals could be part of the internal organizational structure or external entities. Furthermore, their positions may vary across different levels of leadership hierarchy. Recognizing and understanding the dynamics of these stakeholders are essential for the strategic planning process.

Science of Persuasion

Persuasion is more than just an art; it is a strategic capability fundamental to leadership effectiveness. It is the ability to convince others to change their beliefs or actions. Renowned psychologist Robert Cialdini delineates persuasion as a science, unveiling its underlying principles that leaders can effectively leverage [7]. This skill is indispensable in a leader's toolkit, not merely for envisioning a future but for rallying team members around that vision, securing their commitment, and guiding them toward its realization. Cialdini describes six principles behind the science of persuasion:

1. Principle of Liking: People like those who like them—Find commonalities and offer praise.
2. Principle of Reciprocity: People repay in kind—Praise, gifts, and other tangible or intangible offerings have an influential effect.
3. Principle of Social Proof: People follow the lead of similar others.
4. Principle of Consistency: People align with their clear commitments—Thus, make these commitments public and voluntary.
5. Principle of Authority: People defer to experts—Demonstrate your expertise.
6. Principle of Scarcity: People want more of what they can have less of—Offer unique benefits and exclusive information [7].

Cialdini's principles equip leaders to craft compelling arguments, foster genuine buy-in, and drive collective action toward shared goals. Through understanding and applying these foundational elements, leaders can enhance their persuasive impact to impact the implementation of their vision.

Strategic Planning

Effective strategic plans are essential for pinpointing long-term aims and outlining the roadmap to reach them. This includes identifying and assessing opportunities and threats as well as developing and implementing strategies to capitalize on opportunities and mitigate threats. Key elements of strategic planning include:

- **Vision**: What is the long-term vision for the organization? What do you want to achieve?
- **Mission**: What is the purpose of the organization? What value do you provide to patients and key stakeholders?
- **Values**: What are the core values of the organization? How do you want to operate?
- **Goals**: What are the specific goals that you want to achieve? How will you measure success?
- **Strategies**: What are the strategies that you will use to achieve your goals? How will you execute your plans?
- **Resources**: What resources do you need to implement your strategies? How will you allocate your resources?

Strategic planning is a dynamic process requiring leaders to be agile, flexible, and ready to adjust strategies in response to changing circumstances.

Dealing with Resistance

Challenges, such as difficult personnel, misalignment with organizational or team strategic vision, resentment, and disgruntlement, can severely disrupt an organization's strategy and culture. Leaders must embrace strategic thinking to address these potentially destabilizing situations effectively. Mastering the art of navigating challenging conversations and fostering accountability is vital for maintaining alignment within the organization. Douglas Stone, the coauthor of the bestselling book *Difficult Conversations: How to Discuss What Matters Most*, suggests that these challenging discussions encompass three distinct conversations [8]. According to Stone, approaching these conversations with a standardized methodology—understanding the factual basis of the disagreement and recognizing how one's emotions and one's identity are affected—is essential [8]. These discussions should evolve from difficult to learning conversations, highlighting the importance of curiosity about the other person's viewpoint and encouraging all participants to consider alternative perspectives [8]. For a leader, possessing strong communication skills is non-negotiable. Stone emphasizes, "When you need to convey a tough message, your primary duty is to be clear" [8].

Effective leadership is pivotal in steering an organization toward its objectives, vision, and projects. A crucial aspect of this leadership involves holding team members accountable for their responsibilities and actions. This accountability ensures that each member understands their role and the expectations placed upon them, promoting a culture of responsibility and commitment.

Managing team members effectively is another crucial component. This involves assigning tasks, setting expectations, and providing the necessary support and resources for team members to achieve their goals. Effective management also includes offering constructive feedback, recognizing achievements, and addressing any issues or challenges that may arise promptly. Through such practices, leaders can foster a motivated and cohesive team capable of overcoming obstacles and driving the organization's progress.

Systems Thinking

Critical thinking by leaders is essential for an organization's vision and sustainability. Put succinctly, "Leaders are organizational architects…fitting the pieces of the organization together to guide the behavior of people" [9]. A thorough grasp of the organization's strategy and competitive edge is crucial for accurately assessing its strategic advantage. These elements are pivotal in shaping the organization's vision and gauging its success in achieving its goals. This understanding facilitates an insight into how the organization can optimally position itself for peak profitability. It is imperative to identify and analyze the key success factors that confer a competitive advantage upon the organization and implement strategies to bolster these factors.

There are several models for system thinking and evaluating organizational dynamics, including the Mckinsey 7-S framework:

Organizational Alignment: Mckinsey 7-S Framework (Adapted from Bradach [9])

The McKinsey 7-S model is based on the interrelatedness of organizational elements that contribute to its effectiveness. An in-depth understanding of these elements is necessary to gain an understanding of the organization's effectiveness.

1. *Strategy*: This element evaluates the methods of achieving competitive advantage for the organization. It reviews the key strengths, strategic priorities, and sources of sustainable advantages of the organization.
2. *Structure*: Structure is a vital element of this model and allows the leader to organize and group activities and reporting relationships. It focuses the team's attention on the desired product or output.
3. *Systems*: This refers to the processes and procedures utilized for management, such as organizational culture systems (e.g., Performance measurement and reward), planning, budgeting, resource, human resources, and management systems.
4. *Staffing*: This element evaluates the approach to recruitment and retention. It evaluates the people of the organization and their competencies.
5. *Skills*: Skills refer to the competencies in the organization that provide a strategic advantage, e.g., the people, management practices, systems, and technology within the system.
6. *Style*: The leadership style of the organization's leaders, as well as the culture and operating style of the organization, is important and impacts how people work and interact with each other.
7. *Shared Values*: The organization's shared values are core values that act as guiding principles and are deeply meaningful and valued to the organization.

Collective Intelligence

The study of individual intelligence has provided significant insights, revealing its correlation with crucial outcomes in life, such as academic achievement, professional success, and longevity [10]. However, the concept of collective intelligence diverges from individual intelligence, focusing on the cognitive abilities of a group as a whole [11]. Woolley and colleagues define collective intelligence as the observed capacity of a group to perform across a variety of tasks, where a group's success in one task predicts its ability to succeed in others [11]. Intriguingly, the collective intelligence of a group does not hinge on the average or highest individual intelligence within the group. Instead, it is positively associated with factors such as the group's overall social sensitivity, a higher proportion of female members, and a more equitable distribution of participation in discussions. Conversely, it is negatively associated with a lack of variability in conversational turn-taking [11] underscoring the need for parity in speaking within meetings.

Change Management

Change management, a necessary ability for leaders and organizations, particularly within the healthcare sector, is centered around the effective management and implementation of change. Given that change is a constant element in healthcare organizations—driven by technological advancements, policy shifts, and evolving patient needs—mastering change management is vital. John Kotter's strategic framework for managing change initiatives offers a structured approach to navigating this complex landscape [12]. The steps of this framework are:

1. *Establish a Sense of Urgency*: This initial step involves recognizing the need for change and creating a compelling case that convinces stakeholders of the immediate necessity for action.
2. *Form a Powerful Guiding Coalition*: Requires assembling a group of influential individuals with the right mix of skills,

power, credibility, and commitment to lead the change effort. This coalition works as a team to guide the organization through the change process.
3. *Create a Vision*: A clear and compelling vision serves as a roadmap for change. It articulates a future state better than the status quo, providing direction and inspiration. This vision should be easy to understand, communicate, and remember.
4. *Communicate the Vision*: Communication is vital in gaining buy-in. This step involves using every channel and opportunity to communicate the new vision and strategies to stakeholders, answering their questions and addressing concerns, thereby building support and minimizing resistance.
5. *Empower Others to Act on the Vision*: Removing obstacles and empowering people to execute the vision is crucial. Changing structures, systems, or policies that undermine the change vision or providing the necessary training and resources to enable people to contribute to the change effort may be required to ensure success.
6. *Plan for and Create Short-term Wins*: Planning for and achieving short-term wins provide evidence that efforts are paying off, helping to build momentum, motivate stakeholders, and silence naysayers.
7. *Consolidate Improvements and Produce More Change*: Building on the momentum of early wins, this step leverages gained credibility to change systems, structures, and policies that do not fit the vision and to ensure that the change process is seen as dynamic and adaptable.
8. *Institutionalize New Approaches*: The final step is to anchor the changes in corporate culture. This involves ensuring that the new behaviors are deeply rooted in social norms and shared values, making them sustainable. It demonstrates the effectiveness of new approaches, behaviors, and attitudes that have improved performance and embeds these changes into the organization's identity (Adapted from Kotter [12]).

This framework provides a roadmap for initiating, managing, and sustaining change and emphasizes the importance of leadership and collective action in making change effective and enduring in healthcare organizations. Change management is further explored in other chapters within this text.

Resources

Many resources are available for surgical leaders to strengthen their leadership, management, and strategic thinking skills. These include:

Degrees/Programs

1. Promising Leaders Program (Society of University Surgeons, Society of American Gastrointestinal and Endoscopic Surgeons, Society of Black Academic Surgeons)
2. Brandeis Heller School of Policy and Management Executive MBA for Physicians
3. Executive Leadership in Academic Medicine (ELAM) Program
4. American College of Surgeons: Surgeons as Leaders: From Operating Room to Boardroom Course
5. American College of Surgeons: Surgeons as Educators Program
6. Southern Surgical Association: Leadership Development Program
7. American Association of Medical Colleges: Early Career Faculty Development Courses
8. American Association of Medical Colleges: Mid-Career Faculty Development Courses
9. Harvard Surgical Leadership Courses
10. American College of Surgeons Academy of Master Surgeon Educators
11. Association of Surgical Education: The ASE Surgical Education and Leadership Fellowship (SELF)
12. Harvard Leadership Development for Physicians
13. Physician Leadership Academy
14. Brandeis Heller School of Policy and Management Surgeons as Leaders Program

Books and Audiovisual Materials

Crucial Conversations: Tools for Talking When Stakes are High, Patterson, Grenny et al.

What got you here won't get you there, M. Goldsmith

The Five Dysfunctions of a Team, P. Lencioni

Leadership in Surgery, M. Kibbe, H. Chen

Surgical Chairs Playbook, American College of Surgeons, Higgins et al., 2023

Association of Women Surgeon: Navigating Your Surgical Career, 2nd edition, 2023

SAGES Takeaway

- Strategic thinking is a critical skill for the surgical leader.
- Leadership and management serve unique purposes; leadership motivates others toward a shared vision, whereas management is concerned with accomplishing specific tasks.
- Understanding personal leadership styles is essential to maximize the effectiveness of leadership.
- Mastery of strategic planning and organizational alignment is essential for leadership to be truly effective.
- The ability to harness collective intelligence and effectively manage change is also vital for the success of the surgical leader.

References

1. Kouzes JM, Posner B. The leadership challenge. Wiley; 2016.
2. Hersey P. Situational leadership: a summary. Center for Leadership Studies Inc; 2006.
3. Maritsa E, Goula A, Psychogios A, Pierrakos G. Leadership development: exploring relational leadership implications in healthcare organizations. Int J Environ Res Public Health. 2022;19(23):15971. https://doi.org/10.3390/ijerph192315971.

4. Chalmers R, Brannan GD. Organizational culture. In: StatPearls [Internet]. Treasure Island, FL: StatPearls Publishing; 2022. PMID: 32809378.
5. McShane SL, Von Glinow MA. Organizational behavior and theory. McGraw-Hill; 2018.
6. Engel, J. Why does culture 'eat strategy for breakfast'? Forbes. 2018. https://www.forbes.com/sites/forbescoachescouncil/2018/11/20/why-does-culture-eat-strategy-for-breakfast/?sh=5631065e1e09. Accessed 21 Apr 2024.
7. Cialdini R. Harnessing the science of persuasion. Harv Bus Rev. 2001.
8. Christensen K. Difficult conversations: how to address what matters most. Rotman Mag. 2011;2011:22–7.
9. Bradach J. Organizational alignment: the 7-S model. Harvard Business School; 1996.
10. Deary I. Looking down on human intelligence: from psychometrics to the brain. Oxford Academic; 2000. https://doi.org/10.1093/acprof:oso/9780198524175.001.0001.
11. Woolley AW, Chabris CF, Pentland A, Hashmi N, Malone TW. Evidence for a collective intelligence factor in the performance of human groups. Science. 2010;330(6004):686–8. https://doi.org/10.1126/science.1193147.
12. Kotter J. Leading change, why transformation efforts fail. Harv Bus Rev. 2007.

Good Governance 38

Karenia Landa and Jacob A. Greenberg

Introduction

Governance has been defined by the World Health Report 2007 as "ensuring strategic policy frameworks exist and are combined with effective oversight, coalition-building, the provision of appropriate regulations and incentives, attention to system-design, and accountability" [1]. Health governance varies among each institution, organization, and individual. Within an institution, governance may refer to the formal or informal rules that guide behavior [2]. Good governance in healthcare has been difficult to measure within healthcare systems but critical to their success. Although there have been several components of governance previously described by other organizations, the United Nations Development Programme (UNDP) governance principles have been widely recognized. These principles include participation and consensus orientation, strategic vision, responsiveness, effectiveness and efficiency, accountability, transparency, equity and inclusiveness, intelligence, ethics, and rule of law [3]. Recognizing and applying this set of principles in healthcare has allowed for an analytical framework through which their effectiveness

K. Landa · J. A. Greenberg (✉)
Duke University in the Division of Minimally Invasive Surgery, Durham, NC, USA
e-mail: Karenia.landa@duke.edu; Jacob.greenberg@duke.edu

S. M. Johnson et al. (eds.), *The SAGES Manual of Strategy and Leadership*, https://doi.org/10.1007/978-3-031-62359-2_38

could be measured and established across many institutions. Furthermore, they lay the foundation for establishment of a fair and inclusive environment for all members of the healthcare team and the broader organization. In this chapter, we will discuss each principle of governance and its relevance in leading a successful health organization.

Governance Principles

Participation and Consensus Orientation

The principle of participation is critical to the success of an institution or practice. All members should feel comfortable and empowered to voice their opinions. In order to allow for fair participation, the organization should have systems in place that allow for each member to communicate their concerns in either a public or private manner [1, 2]. Public forums can include but are not limited to open meetings, citizen juries, public workshops, public health reporting, consensus conferences, and citizen advisory committees [4–6]. These allow for the presentation and discussion of the information affecting all members of an organization. Private forums could include satisfaction surveys [7]. The ability for team members to privately voice concerns without fear of retribution or adverse consequences is critical to ensuring that all voices can be heard within an organization. These strategies could be utilized to endorse feedback; however, it is of upmost importance, to ultimately have consensus on the best interest of the group.

Strategic Vision

Just as important as participation, having a strategic vision for the entire organization allows for its members to clearly understand goals moving forward. A vision should be based on the understanding of cultural and social complexities that are pertinent to the group [2]. Each goal should be clearly defined, measurable, actionable, and timely, and its importance to the overall vision should be determined [8]. Strategic visions should be updated every few years to account for the completion of goals, creation of new ones, and changes in the institution or its environment. It is also important for national organizations to account for local or regional variations amongst their branches. While the entire organization will want to align with the overall vision and strategic plan, there will likely be local and regional differences that require individual branches to focus on certain aspects, where they may have the greatest impact and ability to move their branch and the organization forward.

Responsiveness

Once the stakeholders have identified goals for their organization, responsiveness to their concerns must be assessed in a timely manner. Responsiveness is difficult to quantify and is perceived differently by each member of the organization [5, 9]. The World Health Organization (WHO) previously proposed the development of categorical surveys in order to best assess this principle [7]. Ideally, performance monitoring tools could be consistent across many organizations. This would facilitate members of an organization to assess their internal and national responsiveness as compared to other systems. Unfortunately, such reporting frameworks have not been validated. Prior to acquisition of the data, members should understand how the data will be analyzed, who will have access to results, and, most importantly, how it will aid in responsiveness to future issues within the organization [8]. In order for an organization to succeed in this domain, it remains critical that their strategic vision and plan is crafted in such a way that the goals are measurable through internal means.

Effectiveness and Efficiency

An organization must hold their leaders accountable to perform their functions effectively. There should be a clear understanding of how the performance of each leader is measured and reported

[10]. Accurate job descriptions, complete with defined goals and performance review metrics, should be clearly stated and put in place for all leadership positions within an organization. Yearly goals should be set at the beginning of each fiscal year, and leaders within an organization should be held accountable to meet these metrics or have plans for remediation/replacement should they fail to do so.

Accountability

Accountability has been previously defined as "the relationship based on the obligation to demonstrate and take responsibility in light of agreed expectations" [10]. In an organization, accountability is not only important within its members but also the organization's stakeholders. Commonly cited markers of strong accountability within an organization include existence of independent watchdog committees that can provide oversight of power, access to key representatives within the organization, transparent rules about codes of conduct and financial accounts, and self-audit through groups within the organization [9]. Accountability not only allows for active involvement of the members but also establishes lasting relationships and partnerships within other institutions that allow for the growth of the organization [7].

Transparency

Transparency can be defined as "public knowledge of the policies of the organization and confidence in its intentions" [11]. In a system of good governance this principle is required for the process of policy making to be clearly known to the members of the organization as well as the public. Lack of transparency could lead to corruption. Corruption is the abuse of public office or trust for private gains. In an organization, disclosure of key information, (i.e. financial reports, performance information, conflicts of interest, significant foreseeable risk factors, promotions), making public accounts verifiable and the ability to debate topics that influence its members, have been correlated with higher accountability and trust among its members [1, 12].

Equity and Inclusiveness

All members of an organization must be included in decision-making regardless of age, gender, ethnicity, educational backgrounds, religions, and social status [4, 13]. Equal representation and participation in policymaking within the organization are crucial to promote equity and inclusiveness. It has been shown that diversity among team members enhances productivity, team communication, and employee retention, both of which enhance the clinical and financial outcomes of an institution [13, 14]. Some ways in which an institution can assure that equity is established can be through guidelines for leaders within the organization (i.e., assuring inclusion of junior and senior members as well as underrepresented minorities in committees, sensitivity and diversity training for all members of the organization, and rewarding collaborative efforts rather than competition among members) [14]. Most importantly, all members of the organization should feel empowered to voice concerns about equity and fostering an inclusive environment of the institution if those were to arise.

Intelligence

Intelligence is required for all members and participants of an organization as it allows for informed decision-making. Three broad categories have been proposed to ensure adequate intelligence within an organization: First, understanding the current and future trends in health care, i.e., health system outcomes, organizational challenges, vulnerable groups, coverage schemes, etc.; second, understanding the role of each member within the organization; lastly, understanding the measurements of performance and how they affect change within the organization [9]. Intelligence allows for members of an organization to analyze and disseminate information that aligns with the principles and the vision of the organization [2].

Rule of Law

The underlying application of this principle is fairness and instituting the law equally among all members of an organization. The rules within an organization should be accessible and transparent. The system of laws should be enforced regardless of a member's standing within the organization. There should also be a system in place for appeals.

Applying Principles of Good Governance to Surgery

Thus far, we have highlighted the principles of good governance and provided broad definitions for its key aspects. It is easy to see how these principles can be applied to various domains of surgery, to include surgical teams in the operating room, departments of surgery, and to national and international surgical societies. Each of these domains are filled with opportunities to implement the principles of good governance for improvements in patient care as well as institutional and societal performance.

Good Governance in the Operating Room

There is likely no single domain more important to the daily professional life of a practicing surgeon than the operating room (OR). While the goal of any operation should be to provide the highest quality care for the patient undergoing the procedure, the OR is a unique environment with multiple key stakeholders. The creation of a high-performing team within this environment is not always easy nor successful, but utilizing some of the principles of good governance espoused above can help to transform the OR into a more effective, efficient, and safer place to provide care.

In his article on building high-performance teams in the operating room, Harry Sax identified several practical interventions that can improve team dynamics and increase efficiency and performance that are directly aligned with the principles of good governance [13].

1. Establish clear expectations for team member behaviors and orient new team members to institutional goals and culture [13]. Early inclusion of new team members can help decrease turnover and improve team performance.
2. Align incentives with desired behaviors [13].
3. Create multidisciplinary process improvement teams coupled with an expanded morbidity and mortality conference [13]. By engaging all team stakeholders in this process, a culture of safety and quality improvement can be created rather than a culture of blame.
4. Solicit active feedback to suggestions for change from team members [13]. Every team member should be empowered to make suggestions and to "stop the line" when safety concerns arise.
5. Establish friendly competition between teams to improve global performance [13].
6. Rapidly and consistently address disruptive behavior [13]. There should be an anonymous means for reporting said behavior, and actions must be taken to mitigate said behavior when it is present.
7. Hire for attitude, train for aptitude [13]. By focusing on traits like emotional intelligence and situational awareness in new hires, your organization will bring in talent that can then be molded to your institutional needs through training.
8. Identify informal leaders, even if they are not in leadership positions [13]. By highlighting those that consistently model exemplary behaviors at all levels, institutional culture can shift to reflect these leaders' values and behaviors.
9. Assure that there is institutional support for team-building initiatives with prompt responses to identified issues [13].

Good Governance in Surgical Departments

Similar to an operating room, a department of surgery is a complex organization with multiple, and sometimes competing, goals and priorities. Departments that focus on the principles of good governance will likely be able to overcome many of the challenges of modern healthcare. Chairs of surgical departments should enact leadership structures and policies in keeping with the principles of good governance in order to improve departmental function within the health system. Creation of a strategic plan, providing a vision for the departments' goals, enabling all members of the department to voice their opinions, aligning incentives with desired behaviors and strategic goals, and creating a culture of equity and inclusion, is increasingly critical to departmental success in modern healthcare. Training initiatives, such as the inclusion of cultural competency curricula [14], opportunities for faculty leadership training and executive coaching, and a focus on development of faculty across all domains of professionalism, can help to create a high-performing team within a department of surgery.

Good Governance in Surgical Societies

Surgical societies serve multiple functions for their members. Whether they are focused on clinical subspecialties, academic interests, social travel or dining clubs, or regional/institutional organizations, surgical societies represent an opportunity for professional networking, advancing surgical science, and improving clinical care. While many organizations have bylaws that date back to the time of societal creation, the demographics of surgery have changed dramatically since the inception of many if not most of these organizations. Societal leaders should update bylaws and strategic plans to help navigate the current and future demographics of surgeons and allow for greater diversity, equity, and inclusion within the leadership and membership of their organization. Following the principles of good governance can help foster these changes and improve the experience of surgical societies for their membership.

Conclusion

The principles of good governance are crucial to create successful and highly functioning teams and organizations. Not one out of the nine principles have proven to be superior to another when it comes to predicting success of an institution. Enactment of all the principles encourages a cohesive, inclusive, and diverse environment that ensures their members are valued and heard.

SAGES Takeaway

- Health governance involves strategic policy frameworks, effective oversight, and accountability, emphasizing participation, consensus, vision, responsiveness, efficiency, transparency, equity, inclusiveness, intelligence, and rule of law.
- Key principles of good governance include clear communication, aligned incentives, active feedback, accountability mechanisms, transparency, inclusiveness, and adherence to the rule of law, crucial for successful healthcare organizations.
- Applying these principles in operating rooms enhances team dynamics and patient care. In surgical departments, strategic planning, cultural competency initiatives, and faculty development are crucial.
- Enacting all these principles ensures cohesive, inclusive healthcare environments, valuing and empowering members, contributing to the success of healthcare institutions.

References

1. Barbazza E, Tello JE. A review of health governance: definitions, dimensions and tools to govern. Health Policy. 2014;116(1):1–11.
2. Siddiqi S, Masud TI, Nishtar S, Peters DH, Sabri B, Bile KM, et al. Framework for assessing governance of the health system in developing countries: gateway to good governance. Health Policy. 2009;90(1):13–25.
3. United Nations Development Programme. Governance for sustainable human development: a UNDP policy document [Internet]. 1997. http://magnet.undp.org/policy/chapter1.htm.

4. Kickbusch I, Gleicher DE. Governance for health in the 21st century. WHO Regional Office for Europe; 2012.
5. Islam M. Health systems assessment approach: a how-to manual. Version 2.0. 2007. www.healthsystemassessment.org.
6. Ritsatakis A, Järvisalo J. Opportunities and challenges for including health components in the policy-making process. In: Health in all policies. World Health Organization; 2006. p. 145.
7. WHO. Health systems governance: toolkit on monitoring health systems strengthening. Geneva: World Health Organization; 2008.
8. Smith PC, Anell A, Busse R, Crivelli L, Healy J, Lindahl AK, et al. Leadership and governance in seven developed health systems. Health Policy. 2012;106(1):37–49.
9. Travis P, Egger D, Davies P, Mechbal A. Towards better stewardship: concepts and critical issues. Geneva: World Health Organization; 2002. p. 5.
10. Edgar L, Marshall C, Bassett M. Partnerships: putting good governance principles in practice. Ontario: Institute on Governance Ottawa; 2006.
11. Agere S. Promoting good governance: principles, practices and perspectives, vol. 11. Commonwealth Secretariat; 2000.
12. Fernando AC. Corporate governance: principles, polices and practices, 2/E. India: Pearson Education; 2011.
13. Hecht EM, Wang SS, Fowler K, Chernyak V, Fung A, Zafar HM. Building effective teams in the real world from traps to triumph. J Am Coll Radiol. 2023;20(3):377–84.
14. Gomez LE, Bernet P. Diversity improves performance and outcomes. J Natl Med Assoc. 2019;111(4):383–92.

Creating Opportunities for Tomorrow's Leaders in Surgery

39

S. D. Schwaitzberg and Nargis Hossain

Introduction

There is an ongoing national effort to transform postgraduate surgical education. For more than 100 years, the surgery resident training model has relied primarily on Halsted-era methods of mentorship and clinical apprenticeship, which provide a fund of knowledge and skill development in surgical techniques and graduated responsibility. The training environment has since evolved dramatically, and the surgeon's work is increasingly distributed across a variety of settings, creating both opportunities and challenges. Yet the surgeon trainees of today must also be equipped to step into a chaotic and evolving healthcare landscape. We are facing rapid technological development, societal change, and the potential for health system transformation: preparing residents to encounter these challenges may be beyond the scope of the traditional 5-year residency training structure, apart from a topical lec-

The value of acquiring durable credentials and experiences during surgical training.

S. D. Schwaitzberg (✉) · N. Hossain
Department of Surgery, University at Buffalo Jacobs School of Medicine and Biomedical Sciences, The State University of New York, Buffalo, NY, USA
e-mail: schwaitz@buffalo.edu

S. M. Johnson et al. (eds.), *The SAGES Manual of Strategy and Leadership*, https://doi.org/10.1007/978-3-031-62359-2_39

ture here and there, but the development of cadres of surgical leaders to steer us into the future is nonetheless critical if we are to keep up with the pace of change.

The typical trajectory of surgery training has evolved since the current 5-year residency model took shape 40 years ago with the disappearance of rotating internships. While some general surgery graduates at the time pursued further clinical training in fields such as cardiac, trauma, or pediatric surgery, there were only a relative handful of surgical fellowships—and they were not always a hot commodity. With the continuing splintering of specializations, a panoply of fellowship training opportunities has emerged: approximately 85% (and climbing) of general surgery residents now pursue fellowship or additional residency training, with a 15% increase from 2018 to 2023. Competition for fellowships has thus increased, and in turn many residents decide to better position themselves to secure a fellowship by completing laboratory years after their second or third year of residency. Following this laboratory training, some residents find their clinical passion in a different branch of surgery altogether, in their third, fourth, or fifth year of residency. While the misalignment of research with their eventual fellowship choice might be rationalized as a "process education," it could alternatively be viewed as a "ticket punching experience" with minimal long-term value. Residents choosing fellowship training have indicated on surveys that they feel less prepared than they would hope after finishing their 5 years of residency. While the current model of surgical residency training has been generally effective in graduating knowledgeable and competent surgeons, the lack of preparation for independent surgical practice reported by residents choosing fellowships indicates a remaining clinical gap in skills following a 5-year general surgery residency.

Another key shift over the last 40 years necessitates new skills training for surgeons: the majority of graduates no longer go into private practice, either solo or in small groups. Between 2001 and 2009, the proportion of surgeons in private practice positions declined from 48% to 33%. The trend continued between 2012 and 2022: the American Medical Association reports that the total count of physicians in private practice decreased by 13% [1]. The fates of these smaller practices vary; some have merged into larger private groups or have been acquired by hospital- or academic-based institutions, while others have closed completely. Many of these physicians are opting to join large health systems, private equity groups, or employed settings. A study conducted by the Medical Group Management Association showed a 75% increase in surgeons employed by hospitals since 2000, and hospital leaders expected to increase surgeon employment over the next years as well [2]. There is no doubt that the financial impact of the COVID-19 pandemic further accelerated the exodus from private practice as revenue losses became unsustainable.

The continuing decline in physician reimbursement has been one of the driving forces that moves physicians out of private practice, while health systems can harness facility reimbursement to attract top talent. The paradigm shift away from private practice is a clear indication that the healthcare landscape is changing and that traditional models of surgical resident education need to be reevaluated. Excellent clinical skills, knowledge, and research acumen remain necessary but will no longer be sufficient as the only predictors of surgical program graduates' future success. The most in-demand surgeons for organizational administration and leadership opportunities will be those who exhibit not only strictly surgical excellence but also the strong analytical and problem-solving skills needed to contend with emerging technological, financial, and healthcare systems challenges across a diverse landscape. Training models that evolve to systematically instill these skills will be key for empowering diverse trainees and institutions to enhance their academics and their reputation by providing and supporting impactful training programs in areas directly related to the changing healthcare environment. These physicians, now and in the future, will find themselves in organizations with increasing numbers of administrators at all levels—empowered with their own graduate training; wielding spreadsheets, statistics, informatics, and educational theories; and all searching the holy grail of "ROI" as the rationale for pursuing (or not) a variety of initiatives which may or may not make sense to clinicians on the ground—but they may not arrive equipped to make counterpoints in language relevant and persuasive to this new and growing clique of administrative experts (Fig. 39.1). For instance, how would the average physician today respond to the statement, "your service line is losing money"? With neither the tools to analyze all sources of revenue and expenses (which might not include downstream revenue) nor the appropriate attributions of financial return to the cost center in question, otherwise-capable surgeons might find themselves out of a job for the wrong reasons. As a result, in addition to clinical excellence, the future of surgery (and, perhaps, the future of all specialties) may well depend on the development of a cadre of surgeon-leaders with further expertise in business, education, engineering, health advocacy, global surgery, informatics, public health, and even law. While all of these skills could be developed outside of the clinical enterprise by non-surgeons, unwillingness to pursue these intellectual skills ourselves will necessarily create ultimate dependencies outside of the profession.

Finally, pursuing an advanced degree during surgical training represents a similar time commitment to that a year or two "in the lab" takes yet provides a durable credential that the surgeon can harness for the rest of their career.

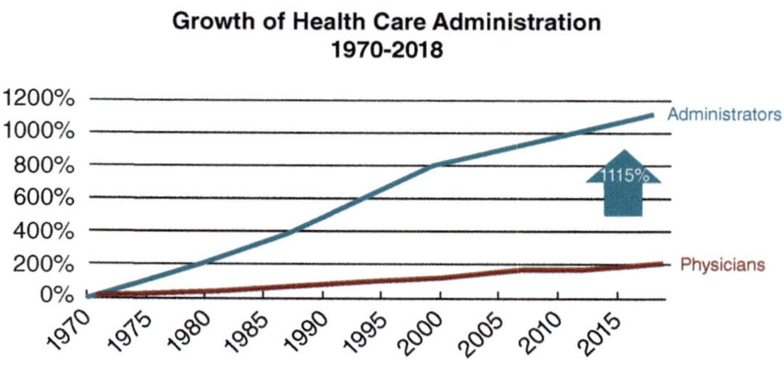

Fig. 39.1 The rise of hospital administrators relative to physician growth [3]

University at Buffalo Approach

In 2016, in response to the growing need for programmatic change, the State University of New York at Buffalo, Jacobs School of Medicine and Biomedical Sciences (SUNY Buffalo) Department of Surgery, developed novel opportunities, integrated into our training model, entitled *Surgery PLUS*. We feel that offering these opportunities in a programmatic fashion, rather than with the scattered or intermittent approach of some programs, not only better prepares our graduates for present day challenges but also embraces the culture of teaching for tomorrow's needs. Surgery PLUS offers our residents and select junior attending surgeons the opportunity to earn durable qualifications fundamentally distinct from dedicated laboratory time by allowing participants to interrupt their surgical residency training to earn a second graduate degree. Manuscripts are often generated in the process, perhaps representing a *new academics*. In our program, these degrees and exceptional experiences have included Master of Business Administration, Master of Science in Biomedical Engineering, an ACGME Residency in Biomedical Informatics leading to board eligibility with an optional Master of Science in Biomedical Informatics, Master of Public Health, Master of Science in Health Profession Education, a global surgery program, and a health advocacy program.

Programmatic Funding Strategy

One of the obvious barriers to developing a program offering multiple degree opportunities for trainees is financing. Unlike in traditional laboratories, where grant funding provides support or where programmatic funding such as T32 training grants can provide salary and benefit support, financing these degree programs is more challenging. Many residents already carry multiple six-figure student loan debt, so adding to that burden is unappealing. An academic "tax" on clinical productivity can certainly help sustain a few of the opportunities but is difficult to sustain over the long haul. We rather sought to develop funding strategies wherever possible, unique to each degree opportunity. For instance, the strategy to fund the MBA program was centered around creating value for the healthcare system. Every hospital system already engages external consultants yearly; building an MBA student capstone team and working on projects as illustrated below represented a cost-effective program to solve relevant and important questions for which internal bandwidth was not available and outside consultation would be prohibitively costly. Our MPH program was funded by the State of New York Empire Clinical Research Investigator Program (ECRIP). This program is designed to produce more clinical researchers, and funding is allocated on a competitive basis. Our applications have primarily concerned themselves with surgical outcomes research. Funding for the informatics program is comparatively straightforward, as this is an ACGME residency training program which provides salary and benefits and includes the opportunity to take additional classes for a Master of Science in Clinical Informatics degree. We sought funding for our MS engineering program by seeking industry partners to the program using the co-op approach, which provided an on-site surgical trainee in the engineering program for 10 months in the research laboratory. To deal with compliance issues, we structured the University's agreement with the industry partner as a scholarship to the School of Engineering and acknowledged that the status of the surgery resident was temporarily transitioned to a non-healthcare engineering student. In addition, the University chose to forgo intellectual property rights, since the co-op approach to the master's degree allowed the director of the industry partner research and development laboratory to be the research supervisor. Unsurprisingly, funding each one of these degrees required a creative and tailored approach to avoid out-of-pocket expenses to the resident for living costs and fringe benefits such as healthcare.

The increasing complexity of healthcare systems has prompted physicians to reevaluate whether excellent clinical education alone is enough to sustain a successful career. Deciding whether to pursue additional degrees is highly dependent on the trainee's goals and on their perception of the value of the degree. Complementing surgery with an additional advanced degree creates extraordinary opportunities, and multiple studies point to benefit of such in advancing one's career. These positive results have been documented with medical students who pursue dual degree programs and with physicians who return to school after a few years of being clinically active, but the literature does not include the impact and outcomes of surgery residents pursuing advanced degrees while completing their surgical residency training.

Master of Business Administration (MBA)

The strategy to fund the MBA was centered around creating and demonstrating value in the healthcare system. For instance, every hospital system engages professional consultants on an almost continuous basis at a high cost. Each new consulting engagement suffers from predictable inefficiencies and drawbacks, e.g., the inherent time required to achieve system familiarization (on the hospital's dime), the temptation to use "cookbook" slide decks and solutions, and a fixed departure date, leaving the report and executive summary behind. We proposed that in return for funding the MBA scholarship for tuition and living expenses equivalent to an NIH PGY3 postdoctoral salary, a custom capstone project mentored by a senior member in the Department of Surgery harnessing four or five senior MBA students (including the surgical resident) for 3 months working on a bandwidth-intensive problem relating to an important aspect to surgical services would be performed. This approach overcomes a number of the inherent limitations to conventional consulting engagements and has provided meaningful insights over the 6-year run of the program so far.

Developing a curriculum for a surgically oriented MBA program which would only extend resident training by 1 year required tight coordination with our school of management. The schedule we devised interweaves school and clinical time: the trainee essentially completes their third (or second) year of training over 2 years, achieving the required 48 clinical weeks in the process. Further complicating the schedule design, the clinical time had to be in meaningful, extended chunks rather than just days on or off the service. The program was approved by the American Board of Surgery 6-year option pathway [4] and is renewed in advance for each new entrant. Another challenge of administering a program of this type is that residents move on and off the Medicare cost report, which tracks and then allocates resources to the hospital where the resident is actually rotating. This choreography initially made avoiding gaps in healthcare benefits a headache. Eventually, however, we recognized that for simplicity's sake, 1 year of clinical work was going to be provided over 2 years, so the healthcare system provided a continuous half-salary with benefits. Lastly, since our long-term goal is to create *surgical* leaders, we chose not to send our residents away for 2 full years; instead, we wove their clinical and school schedules together so residents remained well-integrated into the surgical milieu, reducing the risk of attrition into the business community.

The MBA degree program develops skills essential to strong hospital leadership. Physician leadership in hospitals (i.e., hospitals with a physician president or CEO) has declined significantly over the past 70 years, from 35% down to 4%. This drop can be attributed in part to poor training models and the archaic notion that physicians should "just be clinical." While "efficient healthcare management" is indeed a problem on the radar of newly trained surgeons, many do not know how to effectively address it. They have limited systematic exposure to many critical concepts that are integrated in an MBA program, such as logistics, finance, and economies of scale. The skillset offered by an MBA is not only an asset to a surgeon entering the job market but also an attractive prospect for hospitals seeking an ideally qualified candidate. Surgeons with dual degrees, especially an MBA, are considered ideal candidates for hospital administration roles as surgical leaders—who earn additional administrative stipends on top of their clinical revenues. This is a boon for hospitals that must hire both an administrator and a clinical physician. In addition, studies show that hospitals led by physicians have 25% higher quality scores than those led by executives without medical training. As the healthcare economic landscape continues to evolve, equipping surgical talent with administrative skills and placing the right people in the right roles will create the flexibility to respond to emerging challenges and opportunities.

In order to complete the program, each student must complete a capstone project. MBA students from the entire class were invited to join the surgery capstone to form a five-person consultant team working on health system projects oriented toward a surgical problem. Recent projects include a contribution margin comparison between open, laparoscopic, and robotic inguinal hernias and an analysis of the efficiency of hospital-based screening colonoscopy. These projects culminate with presentations to health system leadership, including the CEO, COO, CFO, and hospital presidents, with specific recommendations for change. So far, seven residents have participated in this program.

Master of Public Health (MPH)

The importance of public health training has become increasingly apparent over the last decade. As public health issues related to an aging population, international travel, and immigration become more prominent, a well-trained workforce, knowledgeable in the social and environmental determinants of health to prevent disease and disability, is essential for healthcare systems. These residents gain skills in addressing community issues, public education, and interdisciplinary collaboration. Such skills include data analysis and interpretation, policy development, and threat assessment. Public health training also includes tracks concerned with outcomes science, epidemiology, and global health. Innumerable major publications harvesting the power of large databases have been prominent in the literature and have informed prospects for optimal care in the future. As a result, scientific organizations interested in advancing health services and outcomes research, such as the Surgical Outcomes Club, have risen to prominence in the *house of surgery*.

Efforts in medical education to equip physicians with the skills to influence care at the community level would help bridge the longstanding gap between medicine and public health. Bridging this gap would enable a broader perspective on serving marginalized populations and improve physician understanding of the health disparities that exist in their own communities. From an academic perspective, the data derived from population medicine is also valuable in its own right. Training physicians to take responsibility for data analysis at local and national levels deepens our understanding of these healthcare issues and improves health outcomes. Four residents are currently enrolled in the MPH program, and one attending surgeon has completed it.

Clinical Informatics Subspecialty Certification (ACGME-Accredited Fellowship Pathway)

The American Medical Informatics Association defines *clinical informatics* as "the application of informatics and information technology to deliver healthcare services." A growing consensus agrees that leveraging bioinformatics and big data can improve clinical decision-making and health outcomes and should therefore be maximized in healthcare and surgical fields. The increasing adoption of electronic health records (EHRs) in hospitals, coupled with high-throughput technologies in clinical labs, requires healthcare professionals trained to understand and interpret data at a high level. The ability to understand how clinical results are generated, to interpret them, and to translate their significance is of great value to both patient and physician. On the other hand, to a surgeon not conversant with this type of information, the complexity and sheer volume of available data can be mystifying rather than illuminating when it comes to making complex clinical decisions. Although bioinformatics expertise can be implemented across many different healthcare domains, our profession will benefit from trainees and practitioners harnessing the power that this form of big data clinical informatics entails.

Clinical informaticists commonly work to optimize the functionality of the EHR. Surgeons clearly have data and information management needs (e.g., image and video storage) that may differ from other specialties. The rapidly growing use of machine learning and artificial intelligence (ML/AI) during video-based surgery will necessitate the incorporation of these analyses into the EHR. Surgical informaticists will be increasingly vital members of healthcare information teams of the future. The pathways to certification for such are through the American Board of Preventive Medicine or the American Board of Pathology [5]. Clinicians in specialties which are members of the American Board of Medical Specialties (ABMS), which includes the American Board of Surgery, may take the certification exam any time after completing an informatics fellowship but will not receive their informatics certification until the primary board certification (e.g., surgery, medicine, pediatrics, OB/GYN, etc.) is achieved. Three of our residents have chosen and completed this *Surgery PLUS* option to date.

Master of Science in Engineering/Engineering Internships

Surgeons are necessarily tool users but can also become toolmakers, iterators, consultants, designers, and device entrepreneurs. By studying and embracing engineering principles, surgeons can apply these skills to solve technical clinical problems from a different angle. Critical thinking and problem-solving skills are common to both surgery and engineering, and this intersection creates the opportunity to develop habits of orthogonal thinking, leading to novel ideas. Surgeons (and others) work diligently to identify unmet needs in patient care, promote patient safety, and ensure quality care. As advances in surgical technology develop medical devices that evaluate anatomy and physiology, the surgeon-engineer is a strategic combination for ensuring higher quality healthcare for surgical patients. We developed two models of programs to encourage this combination. The first program is a combined internship and Master of Science program over 2 years. This format is particularly appealing to our industry partners, as embedding a clinician with engineering skills has created valuable synergistic team enhancement. The second program places surgical residents in engineering organizations working to develop real world surgical devices. Internships range from 1 to 2 years. To date, six surgical residents have been through this program.

Master of Science in Health Profession Education (MSHPE)

Surgical education has become a specialty unto itself. Every aspect, including didactic formatting, simulation, surgical skills training, entrustable professional activities development, and operating room teaching, is undergoing revolutionary change. Our surgical profession needs trained educators who can design curriculum based on the principles of adult learning coupled with intimate task insight. Pursuing this track while in residency gives the surgical resident a real-time view of potential gaps in their current curriculum and the opportunity to facilitate curriculum change to meet healthcare needs. The positive impact of a resident-designed curriculum was highlighted by a Yale University study conducted in 2005–2006 and 2006–2007 that showed that a new curriculum, designed by two chief surgery residents to include a more strategically focused approach to learning, significantly increased the participants' ABSITE scores by an average of 10.2 percentage points.

Curriculum development objectives are derived from academic, technological, and social imperatives to improve training. From simulation to robotics, surgical education is evolving. As the US healthcare system continues to emphasize the importance of quality patient care, cost efficiencies, and merit-based incentive programs, it is imperative that surgical residents be academically equipped to address these growing trends. We have sent our residents and attending to the Master of Science in Health Profession Education (MSHPE) program at the MGH Health Professions Institute. This program includes both on-site and online participation. One unintended benefit of this program is that trainees have provided substantial educational benefits to our training program as they integrate the real-time projects into their coursework. In essence, the excellent return on investment to our educational programs encouraged the Department of Surgery to finance these scholarships directly. To date, three residents and one attending surgeon have gone through this program, and their impact has been remarkable.

Global Health

In 2015, the 68th World Health Assembly recognized that access to surgical care is a basic human right, citing that 11% of the world's diseases can be treated surgically. Focused education on improving surgical care systems worldwide is foundational to achieving global equity through policy, research, and resource building. A 2008 survey of the 253 general surgery residency program directors in the USA regarding their institutions' global health activities showed that 33% (n = 23) of respondents' programs offered educational activities in global health and that 86% (n = 18) of these global health programs offered clinical rotations abroad [6]. The number of programs offering global health instruction has increased since that time: of respondents to a 2021 survey of 258 general surgery residency programs, 62% (n = 28) offered global surgery opportunities, 56% (n = 25) offered clinical rotations, 22% (n = 10) offered research opportunities, and 9% (n = 4) offered advocacy opportunities [7]. Challenges and barriers to establishing these programs remain; in particular, developing these programs requires selecting particularly motivated individuals. We have structured our program using the American Board of Surgery Flexible Pathway, which allowed our resident to accomplish the requirements of the fourth year of surgical training over 2 years. The curriculum incorporated additional rotations that would be useful for surgeons wishing to pursue careers in global surgery, such as obstetrics, neurosurgery, and orthopedic trauma. During this time, three in-the-field experiences in Europe, Africa, and the Middle East were arranged as part of this program and funded by the Department of Surgery.

Advocacy Program

Our profession, to say nothing of the future of healthcare in general, will be shaped by passionate and well-informed advocates. There are multiple outlets for this energy, three of the most obvious being advocacy on behalf of our communities, our patients, and our profession. For instance, our field increasingly recognizes that the social determinants of care have measurable impacts on patient outcomes. Government and private funding are inadequate to meet the total cost of care for vulnerable patients, many of whom require (measurable but unreimbursed) additional services. Medical schools and residency programs across the country currently teach health advocacy through didactic lectures and sporadic events, embodying a "check the box" approach to curricular design that rarely results in meaningful change. Surgical residents with an interest in effecting change on a larger scale understand that advocacy should be part of professional action. Accordingly, we believe these activities should be given the same level of academic credit as traditional academic productivity, teaching, and administration. Our current plan is a four-part approach for surgical residents who are passionate about policy (economic, accessibility, or otherwise) to partner with University at Buffalo's law and management schools to create a healthcare policy "microcredential" coupled with three internships: congressional, major surgical, and medical society. These experiences will position these talented and motivated surgical residents for roles in major societies such as SAGES and the American College of Surgeons. Intentional preparation during surgical training will develop the kinds of young leaders and advocates that every subspecialty will need moving forward.

Discussion

Our Surgery PLUS program provides durable credentials and meaningfully transformative experiences that will inform the entire arc of our trainees' professional careers. Thus far, they have matched in excellent fellowships and secondary residencies. Early graduates from the program are already serving in dual roles that are often both clinical and administrative. These clinical-adjacent healthcare specialties are characterized by custom, hybrid lexicons which, spoken by the surgeon, create implicit credibility in all the arenas we must master in the future.

Conclusion

Preparing surgical residents for the future requires more than imparting an excellent clinical, technical, and basic science knowledge base; it has become an opportunity to make significant contributions to surgical care and the formation of future leaders in healthcare. The University at Buffalo Surgery PLUS program strives to inspire and create tomorrow's surgical leaders, today.

SAGES Takeaway

- Postgraduate surgical education has evolved, requiring surgeons to navigate technological advances, shifts away from private practice, and the imperative for analytical, problem-solving, and leadership skills, in addition to clinical excellence.
- The University at Buffalo's Surgery PLUS program integrates various graduate degrees into surgical residency. The program's unique funding strategies support degrees such as MBA, MPH, clinical informatics, engineering, health profession education, and global health.
- Creating tomorrow's healthcare leaders requires surgical residents to actively engage in health advocacy, including a healthcare policy "microcredential," and diverse internships that can prepare them for impactful roles to address societal challenges in surgical care.
- Providing valuable durable credentials and transformative experiences facilitates excellence in dual clinical and administrative roles, preparing future surgical leaders for tomorrow's healthcare system.

References

1. Kane C. Policy research perspectives—recent changes in physician practice arrangements: shifts away from private practice and towards larger practice size continue through 2022. American Medical Associa-

tion; 2023. https://www.ama-assn.org/system/files/2022-prp-practice-arrangement.pdf.
2. Muoio D. Physicians' departure from private practice has accelerated since 2018, AMA says. Fierce Healthcare; 2021. https://www.fiercehealthcare.com/practices/physicians-departure-from-private-practice-has-accelerated-since-2018-ama-says.
3. Drum K. Join me on a dive down the rabbit hole of health care admin costs. Mother Jones; n.d. https://www.motherjones.com/kevin-drum/2019/06/join-me-on-a-dive-down-the-rabbit-hole-of-health-care-admin-costs/. Accessed 24 Oct 2023.
4. Leave policy—general surgery | American Board of Surgery. n.d. https://www.absurgery.org/default.jsp?policygsleave. Accessed 24 Oct 2023.
5. Informatics: research and practice | AMIA—American Medical Informatics Association. n.d. https://amia.org/about-amia/why-informatics/informatics-research-and-practice. Accessed 28 Nov 2023.
6. Jayaraman SP, Ayzengart AL, Goetz LH, Ozgediz D, Farmer DL. Global health in general surgery residency: a national survey. J Am Coll Surg. 2009;208(3):426–33. https://doi.org/10.1016/j.jamcollsurg.2008.11.014.
7. Rosenberg A, Jayaram A, Still M, Hauser B, Dworkin M, Faktor K, Petroze R. Global surgery opportunities for general surgery residents: are we making progress? J Surg Res. 2022;279:436–41. https://doi.org/10.1016/j.jss.2022.06.043.

Part IX

Leading Systems—Healthcare Delivery

Health Policy and Advocacy 40

L. Renee Hilton and Ross Goldberg

Background and Significance: How Are Medical Laws Made

Having never been taught about healthcare policy and advocacy in either medical school or residency, many surgeons do not realize how much of a daily impact both the legislative and regulatory side of medicine can have on their daily practices. Each side works in its own separate way, yet they remain interconnected on how they ultimately impact the everyday surgeon. Adding to the frustration is that many of these impacts change over time, as new laws or new regulations are enacted or previous ones altered. Understanding

L. R. Hilton (✉)
Bariatric Surgery, Center for Obesity and Metabolism, Augusta University Medical Center, Augusta, GA, USA

Digestive Health Center, Augusta University Medical Center, Augusta, GA, USA

Department of Surgery, Medical College of Georgia at Augusta University, Augusta, GA, USA
e-mail: lhilton@augusta.edu

R. Goldberg
Department of Surgery, Jackson Health System, University of Miami, Miami, FL, USA
e-mail: Ross_goldberg@dmgaz.org

S. M. Johnson et al. (eds.), *The SAGES Manual of Strategy and Leadership*, https://doi.org/10.1007/978-3-031-62359-2_40

how these two areas work allows a surgeon to navigate the process to ensure that they can provide high quality care to their patients.

Surgeons usually know more about the legislative process, that is, the more visible of the two. A legislature, either state-based or federally based, has broad impact as it is the policymaking branch of the government by creating, debating, and ultimately enacting laws. It also oversees the implementation of those laws and can conduct studies that it uses to help enact laws. These laws cover a broad range of topics, healthcare being one of the major areas that they focus on.

Those that make up these legislative bodies come from a variety of backgrounds, with varying expertise on these numerous topics. With such a large range of topics to cover, it is impossible for an individual legislator to be an expert on all topics, so they rely upon their staff and subject matter experts to help shape their opinions and ultimately whether they support or vote against any legislation. A legislator's staff is more robust on the federal level, leaving many of the state legislators more dependent on outside subject matter experts to help craft their views on a topic.

When dealing with healthcare-related topics, there are few healthcare practitioners in elected office when compared to the general population of these legislative bodies. That means the majority of those debating and voting on healthcare issues are approaching it from the viewpoint of either a patient or a patient's family. While this viewpoint is an important one that is needed in any healthcare legislative debate, it is still a limited view of how the healthcare system works. Legislators need the perspective of those "on the ground" taking care of patients to get a broader view on how the healthcare system works, many of which do not have that personal experience to draw from. Some of the healthcare topics that legislatures frequently cover include physician payment issues, insurance/patient access issues, health information technology, graduate medical education (GME), scope of practice, workforce, and healthcare-related research.

What is also important to understand is that most times the legislative process is a slow process. Any legislator can introduce legislation, but there is a process in which any legislation is evaluated, vetted, and voted upon before it becomes a new law. This is a deliberate process, as it is difficult to undo a law, even a "bad" one once it has been enacted. This process is to ensure that any new legislation is thoroughly researched, debated, and altered as needed as it makes its way through the legislative process. While this is the exact opposite of how surgeons evaluate and treat ongoing healthcare issues, it is important to understand why this process is in place and why it is designed the way it is. With the ability of a legislature to redefine a surgeon's job with just one vote, it is imperative that a process is in place to ensure that no undue damage is done by any single piece of legislation.

The other side of this equation, the regulatory side, has an equally important and impactful role in a surgeon's practice. While the legislatures enact the laws, many times it falls to the regulatory bodies to interpret and implement them. Many regulatory rules that are written have a bigger impact on a surgeon's practice, and these can be unilaterally decided by such a body. Such areas of interest include physician and facility payments, both through government bodies and private insurers, quality and value-based care, patient safety, telemedicine, and digital health.

At times there can be disagreement between those that worked on enacting the laws and those who oversee implementing them. One recent example of this is the *No Surprises Act*, passed by the Congress in 2020. The Centers for Medicare and Medicaid Services (CMS), under the supervision of the US Department of Health and Human Services (HHS), produced a rule on how billing disputes would be handled between health insurances and physicians, as directed to by the new law. The administration's interpretation on how to enact that law differed from those who lobbied for and helped craft the law, leading to numerous lawsuits to try and resolve the dispute [1, 2]. This is also a clear example on how the interpretation of a law can have significant impact on the daily surgical practice.

Who Determines How We Get Paid?

One example of a complex and important regulatory process is the rules that CMS publishes to establish or modify the way the agency administers its numerous programs, which includes the Medicare Physician Fee Schedule, which is the basis on which most physicians are reimbursed for the care they provide. Beginning in 1992, Medicare payments use the resource-based relative value scale (RBRVS) to calculate the way it pays for physician services [3–5]. The concept behind the RBRVS is that physician payments should vary with the resource costs for providing those services, being designed to improve and stabilize the payment system while providing the physicians themselves a way to continuously improve it [3–5]. In essence, payments are determined by evaluating three components to all services provided: physician work, practice expense, and professional liability insurance [3–5]. Payments are ultimately calculated by multiplying the combined costs of a service from the three above components, times a conversion factor, a monetary amount that is determined by CMS on an annual basis, and finally adjusting for geographical differences in those resource costs [3–5].

Understanding the Relative Value Unit (RVU)

The relative values to the three components are updated annually and are based on recommendations from the American Medical Association (AMA)/Specialty Society Relative Value Scale Update Committee (RUC) [3–5]. Formed in 1991, this group makes recommendations to CMS on the relative values that should be assigned to new or revised codes in the Current Procedural Terminology (CPT®) code book [3–6]. The RUC is designed to represent the entire medical profession, with 22 of the 32 members appointed by major national medical specialty societies, including those that represent surgeons [7]. While the RUC provides recommendations to CMS, ultimately CMS decides whether to follow those recommendations or make changes on their own [3–5].

This is a clear example of how the legislative and regulatory processes interact with one another. It was the Congress who passed the Social Security Act that required CMS to establish payments based on national uniform relative value units (RVUs) and the Omnibus Budget Reconciliation Act of 1989 that required Medicare to switch to a RBRVS payment schedule [3–5]. It was then up to HHS and CMS to determine how those payments were to be calculated, regulated, and evaluated from year to year, with the Congress still having the ability to pass legislation that directly impacts how CMS implements the law.

Regulatory issues go far beyond physician reimbursement. There are numerous agencies under the Department of Health and Human Services that are involved with regulation, including such groups as the Food and Drug Administration (FDA), Centers of Disease Control and Prevention (CDC), Health Resources and Services Administration (HRSA), and the National Institute for Occupational Safety and Health (NIOSH), to name a few. All these bodies can impact the surgeon's daily practice, and coordinating efforts to be aware of and address regulatory issues that arise are vital in maintaining the surgical practice.

Surgeon Advocacy: How Do I Get Involved?

Now that you have an understanding of how policy is made and changed from both the legislative and regulatory side of medicine, let's discuss how you, the surgeon, can become involved and advocate for your patients and impact change. As with most things in medicine, there is a learning process to advocacy; mentorship has as vital of a role here as it does in clinical practice. If you have never partaken in advocacy efforts and are looking for a how to advocate step by step guide, then the remainder of this chapter is for you. Much of this advice is expert opinion and from leaders in advocacy since such processes are not often founded in evidence, but rather years of experience, successes, and failures.

Society Membership

Reading and education about the process is a great first step. Prior to participating in any advocacy efforts, physicians should take advantage of the many resources provided by national and/or state/local societies. These valuable tools can be found through many resources; most professional societies such as the Society for

Advanced Endoscopy and Gastrointestinal Surgery (SAGES), the American Society of Metabolic and Bariatric Surgery (ASMBS), the American Medical Association (AMA), and the American College of Surgeons (ACS) have access to care or advocacy committees [8–10]. Maintaining membership and a presence in national and local societies will be very helpful to any physician looking to participate in advocacy efforts. Through membership in these societies, you will receive monthly newsletters, join and take part in meetings, and have access to advocacy toolkits which include white sheets for education during trips to your state and national capitols, opportunity for grant funding for travel, CME education at annual meetings, and most importantly mentorship from physicians who have done advocacy work [8]. Presenting data and evidence when advocating is important; most of this data is already collected and ready for you to use in these online toolkits. There are so many resources available through these societies that it is impossible to list them all. It is not necessary to join every society mentioned here; if you are already a member of a national medical society, inquire about an advocacy committee and society resources.

How to Advocate the Right Way

Is there a right way to advocate? The simple answer is yes. While reading and education are great introductions to advocacy, learning about advocacy will not take the place of real life experience and mentorship. We have a powerful voice as physicians, and we should take caution to use it appropriately when educating legislators, governors, lay persons, and patients regarding medical care and treatment options. This is where mentorship is invaluable. You should learn how to meet with and speak to a medical director of an insurance company or legislation members; understand that the individuals you are speaking with are very intelligent, but their background may be in business, law, or something else nonmedical. Use language that they can understand. Speak to them with respect and also come at the discussion from a place of listening as much as talking. Know how much time you will be allotted to speak, and compress the information into a manageable delivery allowing for time for questions.

Listed here are important and key talking points for your initial meeting:

- Define the problem for which you are meeting that day. We recommend keeping this very focused. Example: The state of X does not currently offer x surgery for patients with Medicaid.
- Define what the surgery/medication/service is that you are advocating for in lay person terminology. Example: Bariatric surgery is removing part of the stomach or rearranging the stomach and bowel to allow for a patient to lose weight.
- Tell them why the surgery/medication/service should be covered. Example: Metabolic and bariatric surgery has been shown to increase life expectancy by treating comorbidities such as hypertension and diabetes.
- If applicable, tell them what groups are already covering the surgery/medication/service. Example: We are one of only three states not offering this to our Medicaid patients.
- Suggest what change you would make to the current policy. Example: We recommend including metabolic surgery as a treatment option for obesity for patients with Medicaid.

We recommend leaving a single page handout with these talking important talking point and any references used to make your points with the policymakers. If you would like to use a handout already created, then we recommend accessing these through the already mentioned society advocacy toolkits. Always leave a written out form of contact in case they require additional information or meetings. You want to make it easy for them to contact you and follow up if needed. Clear communication and forming good relationships with those making the policies will be helpful for future discussions.

How to Discuss Costs

Be patient, and understand that the person you are speaking to may really want to help you; however, funding is a very important aspect for providing access. If there is no money in the bank account, they cannot write the check. Medical care is expensive; as physicians who talk a lot about advocacy, we tend to also talk about financial implications. What will be the ROI, return on investment; is it "worth it" from a cost savings standpoint to offer the patient surgery or medical care. Most of us practicing medicine would argue that caring for a human being is always worth the cost; however, there are limited funds available for healthcare, and policymakers decide where such funding will go. One example specifically is bariatric and metabolic surgery; as bariatric surgeons, we face many obstacles, none more so than the weight bias seen in our specialty. Obesity not being recognized by major carriers as a disease is beyond frustrating. Seeing a disease that you care for daily be attributed to bad patient decision-making that now needs cosmetic or elective care is maddening. We know this is not the case; however, many people are not educated about the disease process of obesity. It is not as simple as telling that patient to eat less or exercise more. This is why I encourage any physician who will be discussing any disease process or need for policy change to open the discussion with a simple question, "What do you know about this disease?" Educate first about the medical problem and how it is impacting your patient. Discuss how the proposed management would impact the individual patient, the disease process, or an entire patient population or community. We as physicians are not the experts in financial return of investment; we are the experts in medicine, the core of the discussion, the most important part of the discussion, which is how can we help patients and improve their health.

Where Should I Start?

Advocate locally. Trips to Washington DC may not fit into your practice schedule, and that is okay. Advocate locally within your own hospital, community, and state. The first advocacy experience can be and probably should be something within your own hospital system. If new guidelines from a professional society are published, then start trying to make policy change within your own hospital. Meet with your hospital leadership, and find out who can help you change the policy to include new guidelines and the most up to date treatment recommendations.

Contribute to organized advocacy groups. Many professional societies rely on membership and donations to political action committees (PACs) to make advocacy happen. The seats at the table for AMA and RUC and many other important committees discussed previously in this chapter are determined by the number of members not just in that society but also in the AMA. Paying the annual fee to join not just your preferred medical society but also the AMA is vital for increasing your specialty's representation. Some physicians will prefer this option; if you are short on time and feel that donating to a group to advocate for your cause is your best way of advocating, then do this. There are a number of PACs available to donate through in nearly every national surgical or medical organization; several are listed here: AMA AMPAC, ASMBS ObesityPAC, and ACS ACSPA-SurgeonsPAC [10–15]. AMPAC is the bipartisan political action committee of the American Medical Association and helps involve more physicians personally in politics by offering advocacy workshops; workshops are available for sign up for physicians on their website [13]. Another option is to donate to medical foundations which not only fund research but also advocacy efforts.

Summary

In summary, healthcare advocacy is a complex but vital part of patient care. Passion is the most important characteristic needed in anyone wanting to participate in advocacy. Advocacy is time-consuming, and at times it can be frustrating for surgeons who are often used to seeing immediate results. The effort and challenge associated with the process is small in comparison with the reward that comes when you as a surgeon see a policy changed and millions of lives affected due to your involvement and hard work. Lastly, just like any other skill acquired in surgery, practice will lead to improvement. We hope this chapter gives you the resources and encouragement to start advocating today for your patients.

SAGES Takeaway

- Healthcare policy formation is an essential process and requires physicians to understand and engage in advocacy efforts.
- Key strategies for effective advocacy include defining specific healthcare problems, articulating the necessity of the proposed surgery or service, and suggesting policy changes, all crucial elements when engaging with policymakers.
- Advocacy efforts should focus on how proposed policies directly impact patients; emphasizing the need for surgeries, medications, or services; and explaining their potential benefits, especially in improving patients' quality of life and longevity.
- Healthcare advocacy demands patience and persistence; the eventual impact on policy changes can positively affect millions of lives. Passion and practice are essential in this process.
- Surgeons should feel empowered to engage in advocacy efforts to help shape healthcare policies and improve patient outcomes.

References

1. Cass A. Lawsuits and logjams: a No Surprises Act timeline. Becker's Healthcare; 2023. https://www.beckershospitalreview.com/finance/lawsuits-and-logjams-a-no-surprises-act-timeline.html.
2. Henry TA. Court: No Surprises Act final rule favors insurers, must be revamped. American Medical Association; 2023. https://www.ama-assn.org/delivering-care/patient-support-advocacy/court-no-surprises-act-final-rule-favors-insurers-must-be.
3. Centers for Medicare & Medicaid Services. Calendar Year (CY) 2023 Medicare physician fee schedule final rule. Centers for Medicare & Medicaid Services; 2022. https://www.cms.gov/newsroom/fact-sheets/calendar-year-cy-2023-medicare-physician-fee-schedule-final-rule.
4. RBRVS overview. American Medical Association. 2023. https://www.ama-assn.org/about/rvs-update-committee-ruc/rbrvs-overview.

5. Medicare physician payment schedule. American Medical Association. 2023. https://www.ama-assn.org/practice-management/medicare-medicaid/medicare-physician-payment-schedule.
6. CPT purpose & mission. American Medical Association. https://www.ama-assn.org/about/cpt-editorial-panel/cpt-purpose-mission.
7. Composition of the RVS Update Committee (RUC). American Medical Association. 2023. https://www.ama-assn.org/about/rvs-update-committee-ruc/composition-rvs-update-committee-ruc.
8. Access to care toolkit. ASMBS. https://asmbs.org/state-chapters/access-to-care-toolkit.
9. Advocacy and health policy. SAGES. https://www.sages.org/leadership/committees/committee-descriptions/.
10. Access to care. AMA. https://www.ama-assn.org/health-care-advocacy/access-care.
11. About obesity PAC. ASMBS. https://asmbs.org/obesitypac.
12. Access to care AMPAC. American Medical Association. https://www.ama-assn.org/health-care-advocacy/access-care/ampac.
13. AMPAC candidate workshop. American Medical Association. https://www.ampaconline.org/political-education/ampac-candidate-workshop.
14. ACSPA-SurgeonsPAC. ACS. https://www.facs.org/advocacy/get-involved/surgeonspac/.
15. Surgeons PAC. ACS. https://www.surgeonspac.org/.

Ensuring Quality Surgical Care

41

Juliane Bingener-Casey
and Haris Khwaja

Surgeons globally strive to provide high quality care to their patients; patient safety, patient experience, and effectiveness of care are important elements of quality in healthcare [1]. The World Health Organization (WHO) reports the global crude mortality rate after major surgery at 0.5–5%, with postoperative complications as high as 25%, half of which are considered preventable by the WHO [2].

To ensure quality surgical care, surgical leaders can seize opportunities to shape surgical care for the future. Here, we present definitions of quality in health and surgical care as well as describe how quality can be measured on a system level, through healthcare access and quality indices, and measurement of long-term and short-term treatment outcomes and patient reported measures and patient satisfaction. In addition, we reflect on the methods to enable quality improvement and maintain gains achieved.

J. Bingener-Casey (✉)
Department of Surgery, Mayo Clinic College of Medicine and Science, Rochester, MN, USA
e-mail: BingenerCasey.Juliane@mayo.edu

H. Khwaja
Chelsea and Westminster Hospital & Imperial College, London, UK
e-mail: Haris.khwaja@ibcclub.org

S. M. Johnson et al. (eds.), *The SAGES Manual of Strategy and Leadership*, https://doi.org/10.1007/978-3-031-62359-2_41

Definitions

Quality Surgical care

The World Health Organization (WHO) and the Institute of Medicine (IOM) have defined quality care as safe, effective, efficient, patient centered, timely, and equitable care (Table 41.1). The WHO includes care integration as an additional component [2].

The WHO-World Bank-Organization for Economic Co-operation and Development (OECD) report, "Delivering Quality Health Services," highlighted the need for action across multiple stakeholders at all health system levels [3]. This report stated that the provision of quality services requires adequate governance; a skilled and competent health workforce that is supported and motivated; financing mechanisms that enable and encourage quality care; information systems that continuously monitor and learn to drive better care; medicines, devices, and technologies that are available, safe, and appropriately regulated; and accessible and well-equipped healthcare facilities [3].

Surgeons in the USA are used to assessing the safety of their care through morbidity and mortality conferences, where we analyze and compare complications and death as defined by surgeons

Table 41.1 Components of safe surgical care as defined by the IOM and WHO

IOM criteria	Description
Safe	Absence of preventable complications, injury, and death
Effective	The care/procedure is evidence based, improves the patient's condition and/or quality of life
Efficient	The care/procedure is provided with the least waste and burden possible
Patient centered	The care/procedure is centered on the patient's needs, preferences, and values
Timely	Care/procedures are delivered in a timely way to prevent additional disease burden or harm to the patient
Equitable	Care is accessible to all patients, regardless of their background

and experienced by our patients [4]. The WHO and IOM definitions are broader and emphasize patient centeredness. Traditional surgical quality metrics may not always emphasize patient centeredness as illustrated by patient stories:

- Patients in a bariatric surgery trial may have no mortality, low morbidity, and superior weight loss due to a very restrictive procedure but experience a significant decline in quality of life due to persistent nausea and vomiting.
- A patient survives a postoperative heart attack with expedient intervention and is compliant with all rehabilitation efforts. She now describes a very low quality of life as the many well-intended rehabilitation appointments (burden of treatment) have destroyed her social life and purpose.

In both situations, the care is safe; however, patient centeredness and effectiveness may have room for improvement, and no statement can be made whether the care was efficient, timely, and equitable.

Healthcare Systems

Surgical care is not delivered in a vacuum; rather, it is delivered within a local, regional, or national healthcare system [4]. In a working model developed by human factors engineers, a system is comprised of care teams, the physical environment, organizational conditions, tools and technologies, as well as tasks that accompany the patient on their health journey [5] (Fig. 41.1). The complexity of this journey is illustrated by a patient example: a 78-year-old widowed patient with an artificial mitral valve presents to a rural emergency department with a large bowel obstruction. Imaging is consistent with an obstructing mass and the patient is referred to a tertiary care facility. Additional diagnostic steps are taken, a colon cancer diagnosis is established, and the patient receives operative care and requires rehabilitation upon discharge and oncology follow-up, which is not available at the rural healthcare facility.

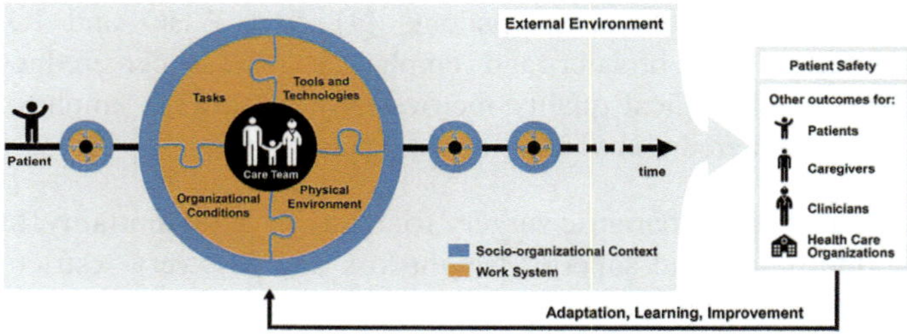

Fig. 41.1 SEIPS 3.0 model—sociotechnical systems approach to patient journey and patient safety

All of the facilities, care teams, tasks, organizational conditions, etc. make out that particular healthcare system taking care of the patient. The number of points where this routine healthcare journey can come off the evidence-based track and an error occur is significant. By adding external stressors on the system, such as a facility damage, an infectious disease epidemic, or a ransomware attack on the electronic health record, the quality of care can soon become significantly compromised. Systems that can recover errors and provide safe quality care under stress are termed *resilient* [6].

Measuring Quality on a System Level

Measuring quality and healthcare access has become an increasingly important priority in global health policy. There is greater emphasis on the use of amenable mortality, deaths from causes that should not occur in the presence of effective medical care, to approximate national levels of quality and personal healthcare access [7–12]. Amenable mortality metrics are thought to provide an indicator of what should be addressed by the delivery of effective healthcare and thus the performance on overall quality and healthcare access. Combining such measures with those capturing preventable health outcomes can provide a more complete set of potential pathways for improving health [13, 14]. The Nolte and McKee list of causes amenable to healthcare remains the most widely used framework to quantify national levels of healthcare access and quality based on amenable mortality [7, 11, 12]. This is particularly relevant for the USA, Europe, the OECD, and other countries such as Brazil, China, and Mexico [10, 15–19].

Globally, especially in low- and middle-income countries (LMIC), data depicting surgical safety are scarce, and mortality and excess death may be some of the few available data points [20]. The Global Burden of Diseases (GBD) collaborative has developed the Healthcare Access and Quality (HAQ) index to track improvements and gaps in quality and healthcare access in 195 countries and territories over time [21, 22].

The HAQ index reflects many factors that affect service access and quality allowing for broader investigation of trends in personal healthcare and quality. The HAQ index uses age-standardized, risk-standardized mortality rates for 32 causes of death that timely and effective healthcare could potentially prevent. The extensive cause-of-death standardization processes that occur as part of GBD allows for better comparisons across locations and over time. Furthermore, risk-standardizing death rates for environmental and behavioral risk factors help isolate differences in healthcare access and quality from variations in death rates due to background risk exposure.

In addition to excess mortality attributable to lack of access to care, including high quality surgical care, complications from operative care result in 11% of total disease burden in the USA, of which nearly half is estimated to be preventable [23]. This creates not only significant patient suffering but also financial liabilities for the healthcare systems. Measuring quality is a necessary tool to ensure quality care.

In the USA and other high-income countries, the recent decades have seen the introduction of national surgical quality databases to compare and benchmark surgical care across institutions and assist surgeons in risk prediction for our patients. There are numerous databases available to measure surgical quality outcomes, including the American College of Surgeons devised programs NSQIP and TQIP and cancer treatment databases. They are mirrored by MBSAQIP, SESQIP, hospital-based data, payor-based data (e.g., SCIP measures, PSI), and data collated by health quality interest group such as LEAP Frog [24]. These databases often do not directly measure access to care or the lack thereof.

Patient reported outcome (PRO) measures inform on other domains of patients' well-being, such as overall quality of life; physical, social, mental, and spiritual functioning; and how it is influenced by surgical care. In the USA and the UK, the PROs measure health benefits in patients undergoing surgery, such as hip or knee replacement, varicose vein, or hernia surgery based on preoperative and postoperative questionnaires. This has helped collect information on the effectiveness of care delivered (did it make the patient feel and function better) as reported by the patients themselves. PROs also allow for the assessment of the clinical quality of elective procedures for clinicians, managers, and commissioners benchmarking, regulators, and clinical audit and for patients and general practitioners exercising choice. More recently efforts are underway to add patient reported outcomes to some national level databases (e.g., TQIP) to ensure care is effective and patient centered.

A further important indicator of quality of care is patient satisfaction which can be captured via multiple methods. For example, the Patient Satisfaction Questionnaire Short Form (PSQ-18) contains 18 items involving the 7 dimensions of medical care satisfaction including general satisfaction, technical quality, interpersonal manner, communication, financial aspects, time spent with clinician, accessibility, and convenience [25].

The Consumer Assessment of Healthcare Providers and Systems (CAHPS) survey in the USA assesses healthcare from the patient's experience perspective [26]. The aim of the survey is to monitor healthcare quality and help consumers select providers and for quality improvement. Different versions of CAHPS surveys have been developed to assess the experiences with ambulatory care (e.g., health plan, physician group, and individual physician) and healthcare facilities (e.g., hospitals, nursing homes, and dialysis centers). They are developed using a rigorous process that includes stakeholder input, focus groups, cognitive interviews, and field testing of draft surveys with patients.

Some of the data sets are administrative in nature and have somewhat low fidelity in the clinical setting. Clinician driven data usually have higher fidelity but require more resources as they involve dedicated data abstractors with surgical expertise. Many of those data sets are reported back to healthcare systems, and it is rare that only one data set is provided.

Underlying many of these databases is the Donabedian model of quality assurance, which preceded the SEIPS systems concept. The Donabedian model measures quality in terms of structure (e.g., nurse to patient ratio, number of procedures performed in a hospital/by a surgeon), process (prophylactic antibiotics given on time, sepsis protocol followed in a timely manner), or outcome (anastomotic leak rate, wound infections, survival, etc.) [27]. Composite measures may use two or more of these measures in combination. In addition, measurements are often driven by what is measurable and by what measures are relevant:

High risk procedures with high frequency of complications lend themselves to have outcomes measured (e.g., leak after colectomy), whereas high risk, low frequency procedures may be better served by structure measures (e.g., volume for pancreatectomies). A frequently performed procedure with low infection rate will not benefit from having the surgical site infection (SSI) rate collected as the events are too rare to be actionable. Thus, knowing that relevant antibiotics have been administered in time is an appropriate proxy quality and safety measure in that setting. A low frequency procedure with low risk (e.g., laparoscopic spigelian hernia repair) may not ever yield enough data to make a statement or improvement; thus, data collection may be an ineffective effort.

An additional useful concept for measuring quality surgical care at the system level is safety I and safety II (Table 41.2). Safety I is defined as the relative absence of adverse events and describes a more reactive posture. Safety II is the ability to successfully perform under varying stressors, including in the everyday clinical work [6]. Both components are important to acknowledge.

Surgical leaders must determine on which data and efforts to focus; they must keep in mind what is important to patients, healthcare teams, and the healthcare system.

Table 41.2 Safety concepts

Safety I	Safety II
Absence of adverse events	Successful system performance despite stressors
Reactive	Proactive
Examines what went wrong (i.e., adverse event), when safety is absent	Examines conditions for things going well, when safety is present

Implementing QI: Enabling Quality Improvement

The first step in quality improvement is recognizing that there may be a problem. Leaders will have to decide what is important and what aligns with the institution's goals and vision. What is feasible right now, and what will have to wait for later? Are there any champions that can lead an improvement effort?

If internal or external data suggest the quality of care should be improved, communicating data and vision to the affected team members in a way that gets their buy-in for quality improvement efforts is of utmost importance.

Communicating Quality Measures

Communicating outstanding quality measures will enforce a sense of mastery and pride for many surgeons. Communicating those results provides an opportunity to recognize the efforts by all team members for excellence in patient care and showcases the importance of quality surgical care. Not communicating quality data denotes that quality is not important. Those verbal and non-verbal communications delineate the organizational culture, beliefs, values, and norms that are shared by healthcare staff and are expressed by who and what is rewarded, supported, expected, and accepted on the level of the work unit, the department, the organization, or the system. A culture of safety supports patient safety and safe practices and can be assessed by AHRQ Surveys on Patient Safety Culture™ (SOPS®). In addition to communication openness and communication about errors, the surveys assess organizational learning, response to error, staffing, management support, teamwork, work pressure, and pace. Better SOPS® scores have been found to correlate with lower surgical site infections and adverse events [28].

Sometimes, quality data are not as good as expected. For some surgeons, being alerted to less-than-optimal quality data will be a reason to strive for better and engage in the improvement process. For others, the same data may be perceived as an offense, an affront to their level of mastery, and may be rejected. In that case, connecting to a group's other professional goals may provide a path for collaboration (see vignette). More information on getting buy-in is available in Chap. 36.

COMMUNICATING RESULTS AND GETTING BUY-IN (EXAMPLE)

A quality officer approaches a successful surgical group with data from multiple sources describing an above average return to the OR (ROR) for bleeding among the group's patients.

The quality officer is dismissed by the chair of the group, stating the officer doesn't understand the groups practice and patient complexity including patient anticoagulation.

Later, the officer learns that the group is interested in being publically ranked highly. The officer then presents to the group how the desired ranking is linked to the number of take backs for bleeding. Now the group engages, analyzes data, devises a checklist, improves ROR and ranking, and is awarded for quality improvement success.

Quality Improvement Strategies

Implementing quality improvement (QI) leans heavily on successful change management. A group of capable leaders (e.g., quality committee) should be enabled to lead and sustain the efforts and report results to governing boards and healthcare participants [29]. It is important to prioritize projects and deliver an early win to build momentum. While at times multiple quality data reports may be not satisfactory and indeed carry a negative financial impact for the health system, discussion of who should lead and be accountable for which project and in which order breaks the needed work down into feasible tasks. Empowering quality champions with additional learning opportunities will be helpful (e.g., quality academy, academic meetings, visits to other institutions, seminars in human factors engineering, or system design), as is collaboration with others inside and outside the institution to gain insight into their tools and experiences [30].

Ensuring the quality champions have sufficient support is part of the culture of safety. The support should be embedded in the system (protected time, financial support, rituals and routines and space that signal importance, position within the power structure).

To operationalize quality improvement, different pathways or strategies can be used; a few are outlined below (safety I):

DMAIC: Define, Measure, Analyze, Improve, Control

A surgical quality problem is defined so it can be measured, data are then analyzed, a protocol for improvement is developed and instituted keeping possible constraints and unintended effects in mind, and longer-term surveillance controls whether the project was successful. For example, thromboembolic (VTE) occurrences (define) after a surgical procedure may be high as outlined by a quality database (measure). The group analyzing the data realizes that tired admitting residents on call not infrequently forget to order VTE prophylaxis for postoperative patients. An electronic order set with options is instituted (improve). VTE occurrence continues to be measured (control). If they improve, measurement continues; if they do not improve, the cycle is repeated.

Other QI tools include PDSA cycles (plan, do, study, act), the model for quality improvement, six sigma, and Kazen (originally used in Japanese manufacturing) [31].

A preventative analysis model is the failure mode analysis (safety II). Its purpose is to identify how a process will work well and how it might possibly fail, ideally to prevent the failure. Failure mode analysis can be applied to processes, equipment, and systems [32]. For example, a hospital plans to introduce a new electronic health record. Quality leaders review the implementation process and realize that during the introduction of the new electronic health record, processes will be slowed down compared to the normal successful flow and in crisis situations (e.g., resuscitation) may initially be inadequate. They devise and communicate possible temporary workarounds until the new environment is fully functional to decrease the risk of failure.

It is helpful if the health system can provide access to the QI tools (i.e., a description how they work, examples) to all healthcare staff interested in QI. A QI learning environment (online or in person) paired with the expectation for health system employees to understand QI processes enables collaboration and dissemination and contributes to the culture of safety.

In the future, there may be additional technologies to assist us in ensuring quality surgical care, such as computer augmented human intelligence, through video or predictive data analysis [33].

The collaboration of surgeons, allied health staff, operations managers, and human factors engineers with the surgical black box tool already enables deeper insights, given that financial, staffing, and time resources are available to define the problems, analyze the existing data and processes, and design an improvement strategy [34].

With all the well-intentioned quality improvement, it is important to be cognizant of possible constraints and countermeasures to avoid untoward outcomes of QI. A powerful example of good intentions leading to problematic outcomes is the prior focus on improving patient pain measures. Decades ago, many patients suffered from undertreated postoperative pain. Nationwide QI provided measurements via the visual analog scale (VAS) and patient satisfaction scores, benchmarks, and financial incentives to improve those patient centered pain outcomes. Unfortunately, an overprescription of narcotic pain medications was among the unintended consequences, contributing to an opioid addiction epidemic and preventable mortality. This example illustrates the gap that can exist between work-as-intended (WAI) by management and policymakers and work-as-done (WAD) at the front line. WAI and WAD are not necessarily the same for many different reasons [6]. A failure mode review (what could possibly go wrong) may be helpful to anticipate negative effects [32].

Maintaining Gains of Systems-Based Improvement

Your team has worked hard and is delivering outstanding results. As noted above, delegating the acknowledgement of such successes to low level subordinates unfortunately signals that quality care is "not a big deal." Now it is important to maintain the gains made and keep the forward momentum. To visualize the gains maintained, reviewing a dashboard of selected metrics in regular intervals will be necessary.

Not infrequently, quality improvement is achieved through significant individual discretionary effort. To maintain continued excellent patient outcomes, integration of those changes into a straightforward day to day workflow is needed. Key patient care processes should be simplified and appropriately standardized (see vignette) [32].

Simplify patient care processes (example):

MRSA infections for high-risk class 1 wounds were decreased in a health system through staph aureus eradication. The initial system involved a nasal swab ordered by allied health staff in the outpatient setting, the patient presented to the lab to have the nasal swab done, a RT-PCR was run, the results forwarded to the care team who then called patients with positive test results, ordered mupirocin ointment, either for pick- up or shipment to the patient. Ointment was then self-administered. This process effectively decreased the rate of MRSA infections.

An alternative process involved standard iodine nasal decontamination for all patients with high-risk class 1 wounds when they presented for surgery. This process was included in the standard order set for surgical procedures. The process decreased the infection rate by the same amount and eliminated multiple process steps, making it easier for patients and teams to comply and increasing the likelihood of maintaining success, in addition to being less costly.

Simplification and standardization contribute to easing the cognitive workload of the care team, decreasing the likelihood of errors. In a review of human factors associated with sentinel or never events, cognitive errors are a large contributor to "never events" [35]. Repetitive cognitive work can often be automated (e.g., electronic order sets) to decrease the likelihood of critical items being forgotten. Effective team functioning, communication, and embracing the culture of safety are of utmost importance. To err is human, and working together we can assist each other in making sure errors don't reach our patients.

Further thought should be given to keeping the teams engaged in continuous improvement and quality care. As others have described, individuals are more likely to remain actively engaged if their purpose aligns with the purpose of the organization, they have the appropriate degree of autonomy to fulfill their work, or they are able to achieve a sense of mastery and belonging to the team [36] (see figure). Those factors in turn are affected by how the health system communicates its mission and vision, what policies and procedures it sets, how professional development and awards are structured, and the overall diversity and culture of the workforce and management.

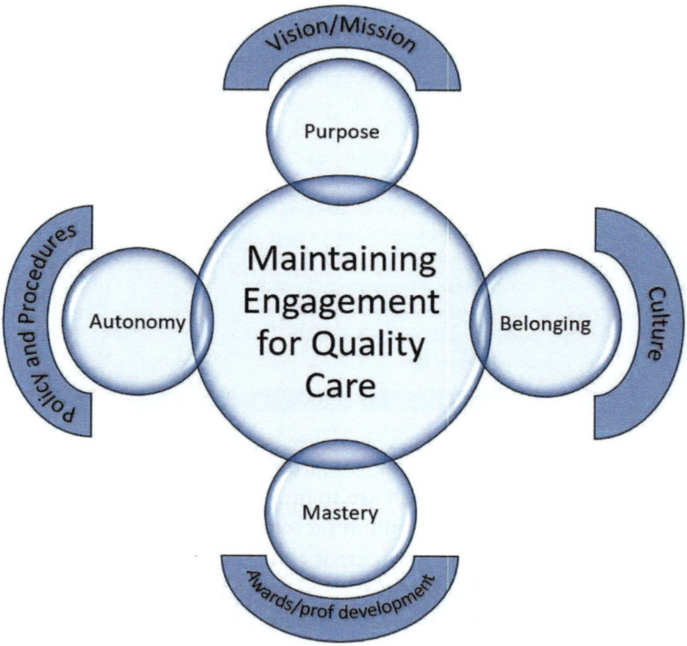

In conclusion, enabling quality surgical care requires more than the absence of harm, and system level leadership will benefit from taking people, data, processes, and the environment in which the patient and healthcare meet into account.

SAGES Takeaway
- Quality surgical care is defined by the IOM and the WHO as more than the absence of harm such as morbidity and mortality and includes patient centered, efficient, effective, timely, and equitable care.
- Quality outcomes should be measured and any improvement strategies integrated into effective and efficient workflows to maintain gains.
- Human factors, technology, data, policies and procedures, awards, and organizational culture all play a role in providing high quality surgical care.

References

1. Secretary of State for Health. High quality care for all: NHS next stage review final report. Stationery Office; 2008.
2. World Health Organization & WHO Patient Safety. The second global patient safety challenge: safe surgery saves lives. Geneva: World Health Organization; 2008.
3. World Health Organization, OECD, and International Bank for Reconstruction and Development/The World Bank. Delivering quality health services: a global imperative for universal health coverage. World Health Organization; 2018.
4. Weiser TG, Porter MP, Maier RV. Safety in the operating theatre—a transition to systems-based care. Nat Rev Urol. 2013;10(3):161–73. https://doi.org/10.1038/nrurol.2013.13.
5. Carayon P, Wooldridge A, Hoonakker P, Hundt AS, Kelly MM. SEIPS 3.0: human-centered design of the patient journey for patient safety. Appl Ergon. 2020;84:103033. https://doi.org/10.1016/j.apergo.2019.103033.
6. Hollnagel E, Braithwaite J, Wears RL, editors. Delivering resilient health care. Routledge; 2019.
7. Nolte E, McKee M. Measuring the health of nations: analysis of mortality amenable to health care. BMJ. 2003;327(7424):1129. https://doi.org/10.1136/bmj.327.7424.1129.

8. Mackenbach JP, Hoffmann R, Khoshaba B, et al. Using 'amenable mortality' as indicator of healthcare effectiveness in international comparisons: results of a validation study. J Epidemiol Community Health. 2013;67(2):139–46. https://doi.org/10.1136/jech-2012-201471.
9. Gay J, Paris V, Devaux M, de Looper M. Mortality amenable to health care in 31 OECD countries: estimates and methodological issues. 2011. OECD Health Working Papers 55.
10. Mackenbach JP, Hu Y, Artnik B, et al. Trends in inequalities in mortality amenable to health care in 17 European countries. Health Aff (Millwood). 2017;36(6):1110–8. https://doi.org/10.1377/hlthaff.2016.1674.
11. Nolte E, McKee M. Does healthcare save lives? Avoidable mortality revisited. Research report. 2004.
12. Nolte E, McKee M. Variations in amenable mortality—trends in 16 high-income nations. Health Policy. 2011;103(1):47–52. https://doi.org/10.1016/j.healthpol.2011.08.002.
13. World Health Organization. The World health report: 2000: health systems: improving performance. World Health Organization; 2000.
14. Schmidt H, Gostin LO, Emanuel EJ. Public health, universal health coverage, and Sustainable Development Goals: can they coexist? Lancet. 2015;386(9996):928–30. https://doi.org/10.1016/s0140-6736(15)60244-6.
15. Archive: Amenable and preventable deaths statistics. https://ec.europa.eu/eurostat/statistics-explained/index.php?title=Archive:Amenable_and_preventable_deaths_statistics.
16. Weber A, Clerc M. Deaths amenable to health care: converging trends in the EU? Health Policy. 2017;121(6):644–52. https://doi.org/10.1016/j.healthpol.2017.03.017.
17. Gusmano MK, Rodwin VG, Wang C, Weisz D, Luo L, Hua F. Shanghai rising: health improvements as measured by avoidable mortality since 2000. Int J Health Policy Manag. 2015;4(1):7–12. https://doi.org/10.15171/ijhpm.2015.07.
18. Radley D, McCarthy D, Lippa J, Hayes S, Schoen C. Aiming higher: results from a scorecard on state health system performance, 2014. The Commonwealth Fund; 2014.
19. Secretaría de Salud. La Mortalidad en México, 2000–2004. Muertes Evitables: magnitud, distribución y tendencias. Secretaría de Salud; 2004.
20. Luan A, Mghase AE, Meyers N, Chang J. Are we curing by cutting? A call for long-term follow up and outcomes research in global surgery interventions—perspective. Int J Surg. 2021;87:105885. https://doi.org/10.1016/j.ijsu.2021.01.011.
21. GBD 2015 Healthcare Access and Quality Collaborators. Healthcare Access and Quality Index based on mortality from causes amenable to personal health care in 195 countries and territories, 1990–2015: a novel analysis from

the Global Burden of Disease Study 2015. Lancet. 2017;390(10091):231–66. https://doi.org/10.1016/s0140-6736(17)30818-8.
22. GBD 2016 Healthcare Access and Quality Collaborators. Measuring performance on the Healthcare Access and Quality Index for 195 countries and territories and selected subnational locations: a systematic analysis from the Global Burden of Disease Study 2016. Lancet. 2018;391(10136):2236–71. https://doi.org/10.1016/s0140-6736(18)30994-2.
23. Plerhoples T, Morton J. Creating a surgical dashboard for quality. In: Tichansky D, Morton J, Bones D, editors. The SAGES manual of quality, outcomes and patient safety. Springer; 2012. p. 25–33.
24. Gonzalez A, Osborne N. Evaluating hospital quality for vascular surgery. Semin Vasc Surg. 2015;28(2):63–7. https://doi.org/10.1053/j.semvascsurg.2015.10.002.
25. Marshall GN, Hays RD. The Patient Satisfaction Questionnaire Short Form (PSQ-18). RAND Corporation; 1994.
26. Cleary PD, Crofton C, Hays RD, Horner R. Advances from the Consumer Assessment of Healthcare Providers and Systems (CAHPS®). Project. Introduction. Med Care. 2012;50(Suppl):S1. https://doi.org/10.1097/MLR.0b013e31826ec0cb.
27. Yu J, Massarweh NN. Surgical quality improvement: working toward value or a work in progress? J Surg Res. 2019;235:160–6. https://doi.org/10.1016/j.jss.2018.09.086.
28. What is patient safety culture? Agency for Health Care Research and Quality. 2022. https://www.ahrq.gov/sops/about/patient-safety-culture.html. Accessed 3 Aug 2023.
29. Machell S, Gough P, Naylor D, Nath V, Steward K, Williams S. Putting quality first in the boardroom: improving the business of caring. The King's Fund; 2010. https://www.kingsfund.org.uk/publications/putting-quality-first-boardroom.
30. Waljee JF, Birkmeyer NJ. Collaborative quality improvement in surgery. Hand Clin. 2014;30(3):335–43, vi. https://doi.org/10.1016/j.hcl.2014.05.003.
31. Lavin JM, Ida JB. Quality improvement methodology. Otolaryngol Clin N Am. 2022;55(6):1301–10. https://doi.org/10.1016/j.otc.2022.07.008.
32. Tezak B, Anderson C, Down A, et al. Looking ahead: the use of prospective analysis to improve the quality and safety of care. Healthc Q. 2009;12 Spec No Patient:80–4. https://doi.org/10.12927/hcq.2009.20972.
33. Eppler MB, Sayegh AS, Maas M, et al. Automated capture of intraoperative adverse events using artificial intelligence: a systematic review and meta-analysis. J Clin Med. 2023;12(4):1687. https://doi.org/10.3390/jcm12041687.
34. Al Abbas AI, Sankaranarayanan G, Polanco PM, et al. The operating room black box: understanding adherence to surgical checklists. Ann Surg. 2022;276(6):995–1001. https://doi.org/10.1097/sla.0000000000005695.

35. Thiels CA, Lal TM, Nienow JM, et al. Surgical never events and contributing human factors. Surgery. 2015;158(2):515–21. https://doi.org/10.1016/j.surg.2015.03.053.
36. Pink D. DRiVE: the surprising truth about what motivates us. Riverhead Books; 2011.

Surgical Quality Considerations in the United Kingdom

42

Michael G. Fadel, Matyas Fehervari, and Haris Khwaja

Introduction

Quality in healthcare can be defined as the application of medical science and technology to maximize its benefits to health without correspondingly increasing its risks [1, 2]. Surgical quality should ensure that the healthcare provided is safe, timely, effective, efficient, person-centered, and equitable [3]. It should be provided to those who need it, tailored to each individual's preferences and values, while avoiding harm. Waiting times should be reduced as much as possible to avoid any delays in treatment, and care should be provided to all gender, ethnicity, geographic location, and socioeconomic status. This necessity across all healthcare systems was highlighted by the World Health Organization (WHO)-World Bank-Organisation for Economic Co-operation and Development report, "Delivering Quality Health Services." This report stated that the provision of quality services requires adequate governance; a motivated, skilled, and competent health

M. G. Fadel · M. Fehervari · H. Khwaja (✉)
Department of Bariatric and Metabolic Surgery, Chelsea and Westminster Hospital, London, UK

Imperial College London, London, UK
e-mail: haris.khwaja@ibcclub.org

S. M. Johnson et al. (eds.), *The SAGES Manual of Strategy and Leadership*, https://doi.org/10.1007/978-3-031-62359-2_42

workforce; information systems that continuously monitor and learn to drive optimal care; financing mechanisms to enable and encourage quality care; medicines, devices, and technologies that are safe and appropriately regulated; and accessible and well-equipped healthcare facilities [4].

Delivering high quality is a multidisciplinary process that can only be achieved through knowledge and efforts to improve patient outcomes and system performance as well as reduce unwanted variation [5]. Quality improvement approaches allow clinicians and healthcare staff to work in a structured manner to identify areas for improvement, explore the options to address, and implement changes to improve patient care [6–8]. There is also an increasing recognition of the importance of organization-wide improvement methods to share learning and experiences across organizations and professions [9, 10].

In the UK, there has been a major shift in the importance of quality and safety in patient care over time. Currently, over 1.5 million major surgical procedures are carried out in the National Health Service (NHS) per year at a cost of around £5 billion [11]. The priorities for quality improvement were outlined by the NHS Operating Framework (2009–2010), which included enhancing access and patient experience and reducing healthcare-associated infections. However, measures of performance on quality indicate that the NHS is finding it difficult to embed continuous quality improvement to some extent [12]. This is aligned with the economic downturn that will result in NHS organizations operating with considerably tighter budgets over the next few years.

In this book chapter, we will outline the measurement and principles of reporting of surgical quality nationally, including quality improvement efforts within surgical training to benefit patients and the healthcare system.

Measuring Surgical Quality in the UK

In 2008, the High Quality Care for All: NHS Next Stage Review report stated that patient safety, patient experience, and effectiveness of care were key components to quality in care [13]. This included ensuring the environment is safe and reducing avoidable harm such as drug errors and healthcare-associated infections, analyzing and understanding patient satisfaction with their own experiences and effectiveness of care. There is also a growing emphasis nationally on the use of amenable mortality, deaths from causes that should not occur in the presence of effective medical care, to approximate levels of quality and personal healthcare access [14–19]. Amenable mortality metrics are thought to provide an indicator of what should be addressed through the delivery of effective healthcare and thus the performance on overall quality and healthcare access in the UK [20, 21].

In addition, the Healthcare Access and Quality (HAQ) index, developed by the Global Burden of Diseases, aims to track improvements and gaps in quality and personal healthcare access over time [22]. The HAQ index reflects many factors that affect service access and quality allowing for broader investigation of national trends in personal healthcare and quality. The HAQ index uses age-standardized, risk-standardized mortality rates for causes of death that timely and effective healthcare could potentially prevent.

Developing meaningful measures of overall health system quality in the UK requires a combination of indicators, including short-term and long-term outcomes, to demonstrate how the system is influenced by the health of the population. Short-term outcomes include excess deaths and outcomes from cancer, stroke, myocardial infarction, and sepsis. Long-term outcome measures include disease burden and life expectancy [5]. An additional important indicator of quality of care is patient satisfaction. For example, the Patient Satisfaction Questionnaire Short Form (PSQ-18) contains 18 items involving the 7 dimensions of medical care satisfaction including general satisfaction, technical quality, interpersonal manner, communication, financial aspects, time spent with clinician, and accessibility and convenience [23].

Patient-reported outcome measures (PROMs) collect information on the effectiveness of care delivered within the NHS as perceived by the patients themselves. For example, preoperative and postoperative questionnaires can be completed by patients on the health benefits of undergoing surgery, such as hip or knee replacement, varicose vein, or hernia surgery based on [24]. PROMs also allow for the assessment of the clinical quality of elective procedures for clinicians, managers, and commissioners benchmarking, regulators, and clinical audit and for patients and general practitioners. The PROMs data specifically provides a measure of patients' self-reported health status before they undergo surgery and explores other indicators for surgery, such as the patients' social situations, medical conditions, and risk of deterioration or complication. PROMs also help support the reduction of health inequalities and disparities.

The outcome of surgery should not be defined entirely by short-term survivorship. As mentioned above, longer-term and additional patient-centered outcomes such as quality of life or disability-free survival are increasingly viewed as important measures of perioperative success by both clinicians and patients [25, 26]. This is particularly important provided the evolving demographics of the surgical population (increasing age and comorbidities) and the rising number of surgical treatments available for previously untreatable conditions. There is also a recognition that not all interventions are in the best interests of patients, and sometimes less invasive approaches may lead to better outcomes and fewer adverse events [27, 28]. Thus, understanding the full implications of a surgical intervention is critical to supporting high-quality patient care and shared decision-making.

Another important assessment of quality in healthcare includes the reporting of preventable healthcare-related harms, or never events. Surgical never events include surgery performed on the wrong body part or patient, wrong surgical procedure performed on a patient, unintended retention of a foreign object in a patient after surgery, or a mismatched blood transfusion [29, 30]. The combination of technical challenges, patient complexity, overworked staff, burnout, and constant stress can result in these unanticipated errors. In the UK, it is predicted that 1 in 20 hospitalizations involve an error, of which 6% are serious [31]. A never events policy and framework is therefore essential with a National Safety Standards for Invasive Procedures (NatSSIPs) policy now in place to increase standardization of safety critical steps in surgery [32].

Surgical Quality Improvement Methods and Approaches

Involvement in quality improvement enables surgical teams to develop clinically relevant practical skills that link directly to the expectations of good surgical practice, such as human factors and interdisciplinary team working and managing complexity. This is a necessary part of the annual review of competence progression (ARCP) for trainees or revalidation requirements and the NHS. The first step in this quality improvement process is to identify the most important areas of improvement within your team and organization to focus on, balancing benefit and risk between allocating resources and benefits to patients. Prioritizing which aspects of surgical care need most improving can be difficult, particularly with complex care provision and pressures to often meet competing targets and requirements. There are an increasing number of data sources and measurement processes that can identify variation in practice or where outcomes fall below good practice. At a national level, performance data such as episode data and the Getting It Right First Time (GIRFT) program are highlighting poor quality and variation in care [33]. Aligning your project with national drivers and priorities can help produce an effective and sustainable improvement process, through continuing engagement, commitment and support from surgical colleagues, and leadership. Local monitoring systems and national clinical audits can also provide more detailed data on performance, as well as patient and staff surveys [34, 35].

An understanding of where the quality improvement fits into the local and national context is essential. There are tools and frameworks that can help with this process, such as the Promoting Action on Research Implementation in Health Services (PARiHS) model [36] which is based on the following:

- **Receptive context**—what are the structures, resources, strategic priorities, and attitudes to the specific area for improvement?
- **Culture**—what is the prevailing culture toward improvement?
- **Leadership**—what is the leadership approach to improvement?

Investigating current practice can also result in an understanding of essential points in a care pathway that needs addressing and improving. Through working within the system, surgical teams have the knowledge of failings in processes and systems, while patients, carers, and families are best placed to observe critical points of failure, such as communication. In addition, a review of the published literature is often required as well as evidence from statutory improvement bodies (e.g., Healthcare Improvement Scotland, the Agency for Healthcare Research and Quality, and NHS Improvement), charities (e.g., the Institute for Healthcare Improvement, the King's Fund, and the Health Foundation), and surgical and academic institutions (e.g., Royal College of Surgeons (RCS), the Healthcare Improvement Studies Institute, Academic Health Science Networks, Collaboration for Leadership in Applied Health Research and Care).

An essential next step of leading quality improvement is agreeing on who needs to be involved and in what way. There should be a core team of individuals from all professional groups, as well as patients, carers, and families. The core team needs to have the appropriate leadership support, collect and monitor data efficiently, and review and act upon results effectively. A platform should continuously be provided for patient voices in order to gain insight into the reality of the care and an understanding of their experiences. The core team will also need to identify any avenues of possible poor communication, motivation, attitude, or behavior. Using change management or behavior models such as the Kübler-Ross model or the behavior change wheel can be helpful in understanding the reasons behind the lack of engagement and developing methods to improve behavior [37]. Communications tools such as SBAR (situation, background, assessment, and recommendation) should be introduced to improve communication among colleagues. When introducing any new processes, it is essential to agree within your team exactly what change you are testing, how you will measure it, and how the change links to your quality improvement objective. These are represented in the model for improvement developed by the Institute for Healthcare Improvement [38]:

- What are we trying to accomplish?
- How will we know that a change is an improvement?
- What change can we make that will result in improvement?

These fundamental aspects cover the four stages of a change cycle, known as the plan-do-study-act (PDSA) cycle [39]:

- **Plan**—build on the evidence and learning to clearly define the test of change linked to measures and a quality improvement goal.
- **Do**—introduce the test for a set period.
- **Study**—review the data.
- **Act**—continue testing to gather further data and expand the test to other areas.

Once the change has been implemented and embedded, the team should ensure ongoing review of measurement data and impact, as well as scaling and integration into broader practice. The Health Foundation's organizational spread checklist and learning report is a useful tool to support integration on an organization-wide level [38]. In addition, it is important to share the successes, failures, and learnings while carrying out the quality improvement activity [40], for example, through open access publications (such as BMJ Open Quality or BJS Open) and the RCS Quality Improvement website. The Standards for Quality Improvement Reporting Excellence (SQUIRE) guidelines also provide a framework for documenting learning from quality improvement [41].

Improving Efforts in Surgical Quality

There is clearly a need to improve structures and processes associated with perioperative care in order to enhance patient outcomes. Numerous national audit and quality improvement initiatives are already operational in the UK, ranging from short-term evaluations of specific clinical areas (e.g., National Confidential Enquiry into Patient Outcome and Death (NCEPOD)) to longer-term continuous national registries and audits (e.g., the National Joint Registry or the National Emergency Laparotomy Audit (NELA)). While these audits are important for national monitoring and quality assurance, the use of data for improvement by clinical teams is variable, despite basic reports of local data being available for review immediately upon electronic data entry. Local teams can often wait for national reports to be published to take action on their local performance, and the lag time between data collection and publication of national results can therefore be a barrier to quality improvement. As a result, the use of data to enhance local quality improvement activity in these different programs varies considerably, driven by culture, resource availability, and clinician engagement [42]. The Perioperative Quality Improvement Programme (PQIP) patient study is a new initiative which is currently underway [43]. It is a multicenter prospective cohort study which recruits patients undergoing major surgery, in order to report and improve patient outcomes, other than mortality and length of stay, from major surgery, other than mortality and length of stay. Feedback will be provided to participating sites on their compliance with evidence-based processes and their patients' outcomes, with the aim of supporting local quality improvement.

Furthermore, the role of management, boards, and organizations setting management by objectives (MBO) plays a key role in quality improvement. A number of themes were published in From Ward to Board [12] including the importance of enabling boards to engage effectively with the clinical quality agenda and ensuring good relationships are combined with robust governance arrangements and strong leadership and clinician engagement. Quality assurance across organizations is essential, along with transparency at surgical board meetings and by valuing and acting on patient experience, including complaints and incidents. Surgical boards must set aside time to develop their capabilities in understanding data, as well as the different methods for quality assurance and quality improvement. This may require additional training and support for board members, particularly nonexecutive directors. Chairs must demonstrate transformational and a proactive style of leadership as well as effective facilitation skills. As laid out by the recommendations in From Ward to Board, there should be a dedicated quality subcommittee to oversee quality improvement and quality assurance and regularly reassure the board that these tasks are being fulfilled effectively.

The definition of quality governance in terms of strategy, processes and structures, capabilities and culture, and measurement has been set out by the Monitor's Quality Governance Framework [44]. Quality should drive the Trust's strategy, and the board should be aware of the potential risks to quality and have the necessary leadership skills and knowledge to ensure delivery of the quality agenda. Furthermore, there should be clear, defined roles and accountabilities in relation to quality governance and procedures in place for escalating and resolving issues. The board should also actively engage with staff, patients, and other key members, and the appropriate quality information should be analyzed and challenged where necessary.

Improvements are also required in monitoring and standardizing quality measures ensuring data completeness, analysis, and utilization for improving patient outcomes in surgery. There is a need to standardize measurement of communication and information transfer. Several reports of studies cite communication breakdown as a common cause of surgical errors and adverse events, and deficits in information transfer ultimately affect processes of care [45]. Effective and standardized communication among all members of the operating team, including the preoperative and postoperative team, should facilitate safe surgery. The rate of postoperative complications is often influenced by effective communication and handover between clinicians [46], and therefore, there should be a particular focus on leadership within surgical training.

The measurement of surgical skills and improvement efforts may be further influenced by artificial intelligence and video analysis in the future. Traditionally, surgical skills have been assessed in the surgical theater through direct observation by mentors and peers, but there is a growing need for a more formal measurement through an established objective validation assessment methodology, for example, performance video analysis by mentors [47]. Process-based feedback may be incorporated into surgical practice, rather than the analysis of morbidity and mortality rates which do not necessarily provide a direct interpretation of why some outcomes are better than others. There is a requirement for an adaptation of new technology and a faster response to changing circumstances in order to improve quality in surgery.

Conclusion

The emergence of surgical dashboards, risk-adjusted benchmarking reports, longitudinal process control charting, clinical registries, and a range of other data initiatives have all helped to establish the field of surgery as a leader in measuring quality. The effort invested in data collection must be matched by similarly robust efforts directed toward improvement, including process improvement, equipment modification or replacement, service redesign, better workflows, and enhanced risk controls.

The resources, professional skills, and expertise required for improvement efforts need to be recognized and supported. Resources vary by local setting but fundamentally include personnel, time, skills and expertise, access to evidence, organizational capacity, and strong leadership to make improvements [48, 49]. In addition, more tools are needed to support the performance of frontline small-scale surgical improvement efforts. Frameworks are essential in providing a systematic approach to enable team members and stakeholders to gain a shared understanding of the effort and objectives. Furthermore, networking and sharing of improvement lessons need to be supported, and there need to be opportunities for collaborative learning and sharing in order to improve patient care in surgery.

SAGES Takeaway

- There is evidence of variability, inefficiencies, and preventable complications in surgical care in the UK.
- Quality improvement efforts are being implemented to enhance patient safety, experience, and access.
- Patient-reported outcome measures provide a useful assessment of the effectiveness of care delivered.
- Improvements are required in monitoring and standardizing quality measures to mitigate the risk of adverse events and further enhance patient outcomes.

References

1. Royal College of Surgeons of England. Good Surgical Practice: a guide to good practice. London: RCS; 2020. https://www.rcseng.ac.uk/standards-and-research/gsp.
2. Royal College of Surgeons of England. Quality improvement in surgery. https://www.rcseng.ac.uk/standards-and-research/support-for-surgeons-and-services/quality-improvement-in-surgery.
3. Institute of Medicine. Crossing the quality chasm: a new health system for the 21st century. Washington, DC: The National Academies Press; 2001.
4. World Health Organisation (WHO). Delivering quality health services: a global imperative for universal health coverage. https://www.who.int/publications/i/item/9789241513906.
5. Batalden PB, Davidoff F. What is 'quality improvement' and how can it transform healthcare? Qual Saf Health Care. 2007;16:2–3.
6. General Medical Council; Academy of Medical Royal Colleges. Generic Professional Capabilities Framework: guidance on implementation. Manchester: GMC; 2017. https://www.gmc-uk.org/education/standards-guidance-and-curricula/guidance/generic-professional-capabilities-guidance-on-implementation.
7. NHS improvement. Developing people improving care. 2016 (updated February 2019). https://improvement.nhs.uk/resources/developing-people-improving-care.
8. Lucas B, Nacer H. The Habits of an Improver: thinking about learning for improvement in healthcare. London: Health Foundation; 2015.
9. Jones B, Horton T, Warburton W. The Improvement Journey: why organisation-wide improvement in health care matters, and how to get started. London: Health Foundation; 2019.
10. Dixon-Woods M, Martin GP. Does quality improvement improve quality? Future Hosp J. 2016;3:191–4.
11. Abbott TEF, Fowler AJ, Dobbs TD, Harrison EM, Gillies MA, Pearse RM. Frequency of surgical treatment and related hospital procedures in the UK: a national ecological study using hospital episode statistics. Br J Anaesth. 2017;119:249–57.
12. Machell S, et al. Putting quality first in the boardroom. 2010. https://www.kingsfund.org.uk/sites/default/files/Putting-quality-first-in-the-boardroom-Sue-Machell-Pippa-Gough-David-Naylor-Vijaya-Nath-Katy-Steward-Sally-Williams-Kings-Fund-April-2010.pdf.
13. Darzi LA. High quality care for all: NHS next stage review final report. Department of Health; 2008. p. 47.
14. GBD 2016 Healthcare Access and Quality Collaborators. Measuring performance on the Healthcare Access and Quality Index for 195 countries and territories and selected subnational locations: a systematic analysis from the Global Burden of Disease Study 2016. Lancet. 2018;391(10136):2236–71.

15. Nolte E, McKee M. Does health care save lives? Avoidable mortality revisited. London: The Nuffield Trust; 2004.
16. Nolte E, McKee M. Measuring the health of nations: analysis of mortality amenable to health care. BMJ. 2003;327:1129.
17. Nolte E, McKee CM. Measuring the health of nations: updating an earlier analysis. Health Aff (Millwood). 2008;27:58–71.
18. Nolte E, McKee M. Variations in amenable mortality—trends in 16 high-income nations. Health Policy. 2011;103:47–52.
19. Mackenbach JP, Hoffmann R, Khoshaba B, et al. Using 'amenable mortality' as indicator of healthcare effectiveness in international comparisons: results of a validation study. J Epidemiol Commun Health. 2013;67:139–46.
20. WHO. The World Health Report 2000—health systems: improving performance. Geneva: World Health Organization; 2000.
21. Schmidt H, Gostin LO, Emanuel EJ. Public health, universal health coverage, and Sustainable Development Goals: can they coexist? Lancet. 2015;386:928–30.
22. Barber RM, Fullman N, Sorensen RJD, et al. Healthcare Access and Quality Index based on mortality from causes amenable to personal health care in 195 countries and territories, 1990–2015: a novel analysis from the Global Burden of Disease Study 2015. Lancet. 2017;390:231–66.
23. Marshall GN, Hays RD. The Patient Satisfaction Questionnaire Short Form (PSQ-18). Santa Monica, CA: RAND Corporation; 1990.
24. Prodinger B, Taylor P. Improving quality of care through patient-reported outcome measures (PROMs): expert interviews using the NHS PROMs Programme and the Swedish quality registers for knee and hip arthroplasty as examples. BMC Health Serv Res. 2018;18(1):87.
25. Boney O, Moonesinghe SR, Myles PS, Grocott MP. Standardizing endpoints in perioperative research. Can J Anaesth. 2016;63:159–68.
26. Myles PS, Grocott MP, Boney O, Moonesinghe SR. Standardizing end points in perioperative trials: towards a core and extended outcome set. Br J Anaesth. 2016;116:586–9.
27. Skou ST, Roos EM, Laursen MB, et al. A randomized, controlled trial of total knee replacement. N Engl J Med. 2015;373:1597–606.
28. Kise NJ, Risberg MA, Stensrud S, Ranstam J, Engebretsen L, Roos EM. Exercise therapy versus arthroscopic partial meniscectomy for degenerative meniscal tear in middle aged patients: randomised controlled trial with two year follow-up. BMJ. 2016;354:i3740.
29. Zaslow J, Fortier J, Bowman C, de Gorter R, Tsai E, Desai D, O'Neill P, Mimeault R, Garber G. Defining healthcare never events to effect system change: a protocol for systematic review. PLoS One. 2022;17(12):e0279113.
30. Thomas EJ. The harms of promoting 'Zero Harm'. BMJ Qual Saf. 2020;29(1):4–6.

31. Brennan PA, De Martino M, Ponnusamy M, White S, De Martino R, Oeppen RS. Review: Avoid, trap, and mitigate—an overview of threat and error management. Br J Oral Maxillofac Surg. 2020;58(2):146–50.
32. Tagar H, Devine M, Obisesan O. How to create local safety standards for invasive procedures (LocSSIPs) by engaging the team in patient safety. Br Dent J. 2019;226:144–51.
33. Aspinal F, Ledger J, Jasim S, Mehta R, Raine R, Fulop NJ, Barratt H. Implementation of the national Getting it Right First Time orthopaedic programme in England: a qualitative case study analysis. BMJ Open. 2023;13(2):e066303.
34. Dixon-Woods M, Leslie M, Tarrant C, Bion J. Explaining Matching Michigan: an ethnographic study of a patient safety program. Implement Sci. 2013;8:70.
35. Bate P, Robert G, Fulop N, et al. Perspectives on Context: a selection of essays considering the role of context in successful quality improvement. London: Health Foundation; 2014.
36. Rycroft-Malone J. The PARIHS framework—a framework for guiding the implementation of evidence-based practice. J Nurs Care Qual. 2004;19(4):297–304.
37. Michie S, van Stralen MM, West R. The behaviour change wheel: a new method for characterising and designing behaviour change interventions. Implement Sci. 2011;6:42.
38. The Improvement Journey: why organisation-wide improvement in health care matters, and how to get started. 2023. http://reader.health.org.uk/the-improvement-journey/.
39. Reed JE, Card AJ. The problem with Plan-Do-Study-Act cycles. BMJ Qual Saf. 2016;25:147–52.
40. Heath C, Heath D. Switch: how to change things when change is hard. Waterville, ME: Thorndike Press; 2011.
41. Ogrinc G, Davies L, Goodman D, Batalden P, Davidoff F, Stevens D. Squire 2.0 (Standards for Quality Improvement Reporting Excellence): revised publication guidelines from a detailed consensus process. Am J Crit Care. 2015;24(6):466–73.
42. Allwood D. Engaging clinicians in quality improvement through national clinical audit. Healthcare Quality Improvement Partnership; 2014.
43. Moonesinghe SR, McGuckin D, Martin P, Bedford J, Wagstaff D, Gilhooly D, Santos C, Wilson J, Dorey J, Leeman I, Smith H, Vindrola-Padros C, Edwards K, Singleton G, Swart M, Baumber R, Sahni A, Warnakulasuriya S, Vohra R, Ellicott H, Bougeard AM, Chazapis M, Ignacka A, Cripps M, Brent A, Drake S, Goodwin J, Martinez D, Williams K, Singh P, Bedford M, Vallance AE, Samuel K, Lourtie J, Olive D, Taylor C, Tucker O, Aresu G, Swift A, Fulop N, Grocott M, PQIP Project team and Clinical Reference Group. The Perioperative Quality Improvement Programme (PQIP patient study): protocol for a UK multi-

centre, prospective cohort study to measure quality of care and outcomes after major surgery. Perioper Med (Lond). 2022;11(1):37.
44. Quality Governance in the NHS—a guide for provider boards. National Quality Board. 2021. https://www.sth.nhs.uk/clientfiles/File/Enclosure%20O3%20-%20NQB%20-%20Quality%20Governance%20in%20the%20NHS%20-%20Guide%20for%20Provider%20Boards.pdf.
45. Kripalani S, LeFevre F, Phillips CO, Williams MV, Basaviah P, Baker DW. Deficits in communication and information transfer between hospital-based and primary care physicians: implications for patient safety and continuity of care. JAMA. 2007;297(8):831–41.
46. Cevasco M, Ashley SW. Quality measurement and improvement in general surgery. Perm J. 2011;15(4):48–53.
47. Reznick RK, MacRae H. Teaching surgical skills—changes in the wind. N Engl J Med. 2006;355(25):2664–9.
48. Ko CY, Martin G, Dixon-Woods M. Three observations for improving efforts in surgical quality improvement. JAMA Surg. 2022;157(12):1073–4.
49. Stephens TJ, Beckingham IJ, Bamber JR, Peden CJ. What influences the effectiveness of quality improvement in perioperative care: learning from large multicenter studies in emergency general surgery? Anesth Analg. 2022;134(3):559–63.

Social Determinants of Health in Surgery

43

Wendy Greene and Michael A. Edwards

Introduction

Social determinants of health (SDoH) are the conditions in which people are born, grow, live, work, and age, including the wider set of forces and systems shaping the conditions of daily life. These conditions include factors such as social and economic status, education, housing, transportation, access to healthcare, environmental factors, insurance status, and race/ethnicity. SDoH can significantly impact the likelihood of developing certain diseases and an individual's health outcomes, including surgical outcomes.

In this chapter we recognize race as a social construct used to describe social political influences on people and the structural inequities and discrimination that produce health disparities. According to the National Institutes of Health (NIH) National Human Genome Research Institute, "race" was constructed as a hierarchal human-grouping system, generating racial classifica-

W. Greene
Department of Surgery, Emory University, Atlanta, GA, USA
e-mail: Wendy.ricketts.greene@emory.edu

M. A. Edwards (✉)
Division of Advanced GI and Bariatric Surgery, Department of Surgery, Mayo Clinic, Jacksonville, FL, USA
e-mail: Edwards.michael@mayo.edu

S. M. Johnson et al. (eds.), *The SAGES Manual of Strategy and Leadership*, https://doi.org/10.1007/978-3-031-62359-2_43

tions to identify, distinguish, and marginalize some groups across nations, regions, and the world. Race divides human populations into groups often based on physical appearance, social factors, and cultural backgrounds (https://www.genome.gov/genetics-glossary/Race). The Human Genome sequencing project in the early 2000s provided scientific evidence to support we have "one human race" and that 99.9% of the genetic variation was the same across all individuals, regardless of their race or ethnicity (https://www.nature.com/articles/nature15393) [1].

In surgery, SDoH play an increasingly significant role in shaping patient outcomes. This chapter will explore the impact of SDoH on surgical outcomes and the mechanisms associated with it. It will also highlight potential interventions to reduce the impact of SDoH on surgical outcomes and mitigate surgical disparities.

Impact of Social Determinants of Health in Surgery

While advances in surgical techniques and technology have improved surgical outcomes, disparities in surgical care persist, with disadvantaged groups impacted by SDoH and experience worse outcomes than their advantaged counterparts. These SDoH include five primary domains and several associated variables [2] and are detailed in Table 43.1. Research has shown that patients of lower socioeconomic status; who are uninsured, less educated, and frailer; and from minority racial/ethnic groups are at higher risk of experiencing adverse surgical outcomes [3–7]. Patients living in areas with higher levels of poverty had a higher risk of surgical complications and readmissions, according to a study by Diaz and Pawlik [8]. Patients living in neighborhoods with lower levels of education had a higher risk of complications following surgery, according to a study by Bonner et al. [9].

Insurance status is another significant predictor of surgical outcomes, with uninsured patients experiencing worse outcomes than insured patients. Additional studies by Downing et al. [10] revealed uninsured trauma patients had a higher mortality rate

Table 43.1 Social determinants of health domains and variables

Domains	Economic stability	Education access and quality	Health care access and quality	Neighborhood and built environment	Social and community context
Variables	• Income • Poverty level • Affordable housing • Nutritional service	• Graduation rates • Higher education • Language development • Literacy	• Health literacy • Healthcare access • Primary care access • Health tools access	• Crime and violence • Housing quality • Healthy food access • Environmental conditions • Transportation • Walkability score • Internet access	• Discrimination • Incarceration • Social cohesion • Civic participation

than those with private insurance, even after controlling for injury severity and demographic factors. Lack of access to preventive care and delayed presentation to the hospital may contribute to these disparities.

Another crucial factor that impacts surgical outcomes is health literacy. Patients with low health literacy may struggle to understand surgical instructions, manage their medication regimens, and communicate effectively with healthcare providers [11]. This can lead to complications, longer hospital stays, and increased healthcare costs. In addition, frailty is a condition characterized by decreased physiological reserve, reduced mobility, and increased susceptibility to adverse health events [12, 13]. Older adults and those with chronic conditions are at higher risk of developing frailty, and frailty has been associated with increased risk of complications following surgery.

Race/ethnicity has been shown to be a predictor of surgical outcomes, with non-white patients experiencing worse outcomes than white patients. In a study conducted by Ingram et al. [14], non-white children undergoing appendectomy had a higher risk of postoperative complications, longer hospital stays, and higher costs compared to white children. Similarly, in a study by Groenewald et al. [15], racial and ethnic minorities were less likely to receive surgical procedures than whites and, when they did, had higher rates of complications and mortality. These disparities may be driven by a variety of factors, including reduced access to healthcare, lower health literacy, and implicit bias on the part of healthcare providers. These disparities can increase surgical complications, length of stay, and healthcare costs.

Mechanisms Through Which SDoH Affect Surgical Outcomes

Several mechanisms have been proposed to explain the relationship between SDoH and surgical outcomes. These mechanisms include differences in access to healthcare, differences in the quality of care, and biases in clinical decision-making.

Access to Healthcare

One of the main mechanisms through which SDoH affect surgical outcomes is differences in access to healthcare. Disadvantaged groups may face barriers to accessing healthcare, such as lack of insurance, lack of transportation, and lack of providers in their area. These barriers may result in delayed presentation to the hospital, delayed diagnosis, and delayed treatment, all of which can negatively impact surgical outcomes. In addition, patients who lack access to healthcare services may face financial barriers to care, including high out-of-pocket costs and limited insurance coverage, which can further exacerbate healthcare disparities [16].

Improving access to healthcare is an important strategy for reducing healthcare disparities and improving surgical outcomes. This can be accomplished through a variety of approaches, including expanding insurance coverage, increasing the availability of healthcare services in underserved areas, and improving transportation options for patients who live in rural or remote areas. Several studies have demonstrated the positive impact of increased access to healthcare services on surgical outcomes. A study of patients undergoing elective colorectal surgery found that patients who lived in areas with a higher density of healthcare providers had lower rates of postoperative complications and shorter hospital stays [17]. Another study of patients undergoing elective spine surgery found that patients who had insurance coverage had lower rates of postoperative complications and shorter hospital stays compared to uninsured patients [18, 19]. Additionally, a study of patients undergoing elective joint replacement surgery found that those who had insurance coverage had lower rates of complications and were more likely to receive rehabilitation services compared to uninsured patients [20].

Improving access to healthcare services can also help to address disparities in surgical outcomes among different racial/ethnic groups. A study of patients undergoing cardiac surgery found that African-American patients were less likely to receive timely surgical intervention compared to white patients, which was associated with higher mortality rates [21]. Similarly, a study of patients undergoing cancer surgery found that African-American patients were less likely to receive appropriate surgical treatment and had lower survival rates compared to white patients [22, 23].

To address these disparities, efforts have been made to improve access to healthcare services for underserved populations. For example, the Affordable Care Act (ACA) expanded insurance coverage and provided funding for community health centers and other healthcare providers in underserved areas. These efforts have been associated with improved access to healthcare services and better health outcomes for underserved populations [24].

Quality of Care

Differences in the quality of care may also contribute to SDoH-related disparities in surgical outcomes. Disadvantaged groups may receive lower-quality care due to a lack of resources, such as staffing, equipment, and facilities, in their local healthcare facilities. They may also receive care from providers who have less experience or who are not up to date on the latest care pathways, decision-making, surgical techniques, and technologies.

Cloyd et al. [25] conducted a study that demonstrated the impact of differences in the quality of care on surgical outcomes among disadvantaged groups. The study found that patients from low-income neighborhoods were more likely to experience surgical complications, including infections, bleeding, and blood clots, compared to patients from higher-income neighborhoods. The researchers also found that patients from low-income neighborhoods were more likely to receive care from hospitals with lower nurse staffing levels, which may have contributed to the higher complication rates [26]. Additionally, a lack of access to specialized surgical care may also contribute to disparities in surgical outcomes. For example, rural or remote areas may have limited access to specialized surgical services, which can result in delays in diagnosis and treatment and a higher risk of complications.

Overall, differences in the quality of care can significantly impact surgical outcomes and contribute to disparities among disadvantaged groups. It is important to address these disparities by improving access to high-quality care and ensuring that all patients receive the same level of care, regardless of their socioeconomic status or geographic location.

Clinical Decision-Making

Research has shown that biases in clinical decision-making in surgery can significantly impact surgical outcomes, leading to disparities in care and patient outcomes [27].

A study published in 1999 by Bach et al. in the *New England Journal of Medicine* (NEJM) found that implicit bias among surgeons may contribute to racial disparities in the treatment of patients with early-stage lung cancer. The study found that black patients were less likely to receive surgical treatment for early-stage lung cancer compared to white patients, even after controlling for other factors such as age, sex, and comorbidities. The authors suggested that implicit bias may be a contributing factor to these disparities [28].

Implicit bias can lead to disparities in surgical care, with certain patient populations, such as women, minorities, and older adults, being at higher risk for receiving suboptimal care. Addressing implicit bias among surgeons may be an important strategy for improving surgical outcomes and reducing disparities [29].

Gender bias may contribute to disparities in surgical outcomes for women. Women undergoing coronary artery bypass graft surgery (CABG) were less likely to receive arterial grafts, which are associated with better long-term outcomes, compared to men. The authors suggested that gender bias may be a contributing factor to these disparities [30]. These studies demonstrate the significant impact of biases in clinical decision-making on surgical outcomes and highlight the need for addressing implicit bias and promoting equitable care in surgery.

Interventions to Reduce SDoH-Related Disparities in Surgical Care and Outcomes

Improve Healthcare Access

There are several interventions that may help mitigate disparities in surgical outcomes. One approach is to improve access to healthcare for underserved populations. This may include expanding Medicaid coverage, increasing funding for community health clinics, and implementing telehealth services to improve access to specialty care [31]. Patient navigation programs are designed to help patients navigate the healthcare system and access needed services. These programs typically involve a trained healthcare professional who works with patients to coordinate their care and address any barriers to accessing healthcare services. Patient navigation programs have been shown to be effective in improving access to care and reducing healthcare disparities [32, 33].

Improve Communication and Health Literacy

Another approach is to improve communication between patients and healthcare providers. This may involve providing health literacy education to patients, training healthcare providers to communicate effectively with patients from diverse backgrounds, and implementing strategies to reduce implicit bias in the delivery of healthcare services [34]. Health literacy programs are designed to help patients better understand their medical conditions and the healthcare system. These programs may include workshops, educational materials, and one-on-one counseling sessions with healthcare providers. By improving health literacy, patients are better equipped to understand surgical instructions, manage their medication regimens, and communicate effectively with healthcare providers [35]. Patient education programs are designed to help patients better understand their medical conditions and the healthcare system [36, 37].

In addition to improving access to healthcare, healthcare literacy, and reducing implicit bias, there are several other strategies that can be employed to help mitigate disparities in surgical outcomes and are discussed in the following paragraphs.

Preoperative Optimization Program

Preoperative optimization programs are designed to help patients prepare for surgery and reduce their risk of complications. These programs typically involve a multidisciplinary team of healthcare providers who work with patients to optimize their medical conditions prior to surgery. This may include optimizing chronic medical conditions, improving nutrition, and increasing physical activity. Preoperative optimization programs have been shown to be effective in reducing postoperative complications and improving surgical outcomes in high-risk patients [38].

Cultural Humility and Competency Training

Cultural humility and cultural competency are both approaches aimed at promoting understanding and respectful interactions across diverse cultures. While they share some similarities, they differ in their emphasis and underlying principles. Cultural humility is a framework that emphasizes self-reflection, openness, and a willingness to learn from others. It recognizes the limitations of one's own cultural knowledge and seeks to address power imbalances by actively listening to and valuing the experiences and perspectives of others. Cultural humility encourages a lifelong commitment to learning about different cultures and challenging personal biases [39].

Cultural competency refers to the ability to understand, appreciate, and effectively interact with individuals from different cultural backgrounds. It involves acquiring knowledge about diverse cultures, including their values, beliefs, and practices, and applying this knowledge to deliver culturally appropriate care or services. Cultural competency focuses on developing specific skills and knowledge to bridge cultural gaps and reduce disparities in healthcare, education, and other fields [40, 41]. By improving cultural humility and competency, healthcare providers are better equipped to communicate effectively with patients, reduce implicit biases, and improve patient outcomes [40, 41].

Collaborative Care Models

Collaborative care models involve a multidisciplinary team of healthcare providers who work together to coordinate the care for patients. These models are designed to improve communication between healthcare providers and to ensure that patients receive comprehensive care that addresses all their medical needs. Collaborative care models have been shown to be effective in improving patient outcomes and reducing healthcare costs [42].

Community-Based Interventions

Community-based interventions are designed to address SDoH that impact surgical outcomes. These interventions may include improving access to healthy foods, increasing opportunities for physical activity, and providing transportation to healthcare services. By addressing these SDoH, community-based interventions can improve health outcomes and reduce healthcare disparities [43].

Health Equity Initiatives

Health equity initiatives are designed to promote equity in healthcare by addressing the root causes of healthcare disparities. These initiatives may include improving access to healthcare, addressing implicit bias in the healthcare system, and increasing funding for research on healthcare disparities. By promoting health equity, these initiatives have the potential to reduce healthcare disparities and improve patient outcomes [44, 45].

Reduce Implicit Bias

Implicit bias, also known as unconscious bias, is a type of bias that occurs when people hold attitudes and beliefs that affect their judgment and decision-making without being aware of it. Implicit bias has been identified as a significant factor that affects health disparities and surgical outcomes. Implicit bias can influence healthcare providers' perceptions of their patients' symptoms, decision-making processes, and even their likelihood of receiving certain treatments [46]. The following sections will discuss how implicit bias affects SDoH and surgical outcomes and provide some ways to address this issue.

Impact of Implicit Bias on SDoH and Surgical Outcomes

Implicit bias can affect SDoH in various ways. For instance, healthcare providers may make assumptions about a patient's education, socioeconomic status, and financial resources based on their race or ethnicity. These assumptions can lead to differences in the quality of care that patients receive. Studies have shown that implicit bias affects patient-provider communication, which can affect patient satisfaction, trust in the healthcare system, and adherence to treatment plans [47, 48].

In the context of surgical care, implicit bias can affect the quality of care that patients receive. For example, studies have shown that implicit bias can affect the referral of patients to surgical specialists, the use of surgical interventions, and the quality of care that patients receive [49]. Moreover, implicit bias can affect the decision-making process in surgical care, which can lead to disparities in surgical outcomes. For instance, a study found that uninsured patients with pelvic fractures were less likely to receive diagnostic imaging than their insured counterparts [50].

Addressing Implicit Bias in Surgical Care

Addressing implicit bias in surgical care is essential to reducing health disparities and improving surgical outcomes. One way to address implicit bias is to increase awareness among healthcare providers. Providers need to be educated about the impact of implicit bias on health disparities and surgical outcomes. Training programs can be developed to help healthcare providers recognize and address their implicit biases. These programs can use simulations and role-playing exercises to help providers become more aware of their implicit biases and develop strategies to overcome them [6, 7].

Another strategy to address implicit bias is to implement policies and practices that promote equity in healthcare. Policies can be developed to address disparities in access to care and treatment. For example, policies can ensure that patients receive the same level of care, regardless of their race or ethnicity. Practices can also be implemented to reduce the impact of implicit bias on decision-making. Decision support tools can be developed to help providers make objective decisions based on evidence-based guidelines [51].

Conclusion

The impact of social determinants of health (SDoH) on surgical outcomes is a complex issue that requires a multifaceted approach. SDoH factors such as race, ethnicity, insurance status, income, education, and housing have been shown to impact surgical outcomes. The mechanisms through which SDoH affects surgical outcomes include differences in access to healthcare, differences in the quality of care, and biases in clinical decision-making.

Interventions and strategies to improve access to care, address biases in clinical decision-making, and improve the quality of care provided can mitigate SDoH-related disparities in surgical care and outcomes and contribute to achieving health equity. Additional initiatives such as preoperative optimization programs, health literacy, cultural humility training, patient navigation education programs along with collaborative care models, community-based intervention are also important strategies that may contribute to mitigate disparities in surgical outcomes achieving health equity.

SAGES Takeaway

- Social determinants of health significantly shape surgical results, extending beyond medical advancements.
- Despite medical progress, disadvantaged groups face worse outcomes due to factors like income, race, and education.
- Surgical results are impacted by factors such as race, insurance

status, and housing, leading to disparities in access, quality, and clinical biases.

- Disparities stem from differences in healthcare access, care quality, and biases in clinical decisions, emphasizing the complexity of SDoH's influence.
- Addressing disparities requires improving healthcare access, addressing biases, and enhancing overall care quality, vital for reducing healthcare disparities and improving outcomes for disadvantaged groups.

References

1. Nurk S, et al. The complete sequence of a human genome. Science. 2022;376(6588):44–53.
2. Bakefield WS, Ammar N, Olusanya OA, Shaban-Nejad A. An urban population health observatory system to support COVID-19 pandemic preparedness, response, and management: design and development study. JMIR Public Health Surveill. 2021;7(6):1–15.
3. Greene WR, Oyetunji TA, Bowers U, Haider AH, Mellman TA, Cornwell EE, et al. Insurance status is a potent predictor of outcomes in both blunt and penetrating trauma. Am J Surg. 2010;199(4):554–7.
4. Bennett KM, et al. Patient socioeconomic status is an independent predictor of operative mortality. Ann Surg. 2010;252(3):552–8.
5. Kiran RP, et al. Impact of resident participation in surgical operations on postoperative outcomes: National Surgical Quality Improvement Program. Ann Surg. 2012;256(3):469–75.
6. Haider AH, et al. Racial disparities in surgical care and outcomes in the United States: a comprehensive review of patient, provider and systemic factors. J Am Coll Surg. 2013a;216(3):482.
7. Haider AH, et al. Disparities in trauma care and outcomes in the United States: a systematic review and meta-analysis. J Trauma Acute Care Surg. 2013b;74(5):1195.
8. Diaz A, Pawlik TM. Social determinants of health and surgical care. Curr Probl Surg. 2023;60(4):101300.
9. Bonner SN, et al. Neighborhood deprivation and Medicare expenditures for common surgical procedures. Am J Surg. 2022;224(5):1274–9.
10. Downing SR, et al. The impact of insurance status on actuarial survival in hospitalized trauma patients: when do they die? J Trauma Acute Care Surg. 2011;70(1):130–5.
11. Oliveira D, Gildasio S, et al. The impact of health literacy in the care of surgical patients: a qualitative systematic review. BMC Surg. 2015;15:1–7.

12. Revenig LM, et al. Too frail for surgery? Initial results of a large multidisciplinary prospective study examining preoperative variables predictive of poor surgical outcomes. J Am Coll Surg. 2013;217(4):665–70.
13. Wahl TS, et al. Association of the modified frailty index with 30-day surgical readmission. JAMA Surg. 2017;152(8):749–57.
14. Ingram M-CE, et al. Systematic review of disparities in care and outcomes in pediatric appendectomy. J Surg Res. 2020;249:42–9.
15. Groenewald CB, et al. Racial and ethnic differences in pediatric surgery utilization in the United States: a nationally representative cross-sectional analysis. J Pediatr Surg. 2022;57(8):1584–91.
16. Scott JW, et al. Lifting the burden: state Medicaid expansion reduces financial risk for the injured. J Trauma Acute Care Surg. 2020;88(1):51–8.
17. Lu PW, et al. The distribution of colorectal surgeons in the United States. J Surg Res. 2020;251:71–7.
18. Alosh H, Riley LH III, Skolasky RL. Insurance status, geography, race, and ethnicity as predictors of anterior cervical spine surgery rates and in-hospital mortality: an examination of United States trends from 1992 to 2005. Spine. 2009;34(18):1956–62.
19. Badin D, et al. Disparities in elective spine surgery for Medicaid beneficiaries: a systematic review. Glob Spine J. 2023;13(2):534–46.
20. Freburger JK, et al. Disparities in post-acute rehabilitation care for joint replacement. Arthritis Care Res. 2011;63(7):1020–30.
21. Cook NL, et al. Differences in specialist consultations for cardiovascular disease by race, ethnicity, gender, insurance status, and site of primary care. Circulation. 2009;119(18):2463–70.
22. Trivedi AN, Sequist TD, Ayanian JZ. Impact of hospital volume on racial disparities in cardiovascular procedure mortality. J Am Coll Cardiol. 2006;47(2):417–24.
23. Morris AM, et al. Understanding racial disparities in cancer treatment and outcomes. J Am Coll Surg. 2010;211(1):105–13.
24. Behr CL, et al. Geographic access to federally qualified health centers before and after the affordable care act. BMC Health Serv Res. 2022;22(1):385.
25. Cloyd JM, et al. Predictors of readmission to non-index hospitals after colorectal surgery. Am J Surg. 2017;213(1):18–23.
26. Ball JE, et al. Post-operative mortality, missed care and nurse staffing in nine countries: a cross-sectional study. Int J Nurs Stud. 2018;78:10–5.
27. Ayanian JZ. Determinants of racial and ethnic disparities in surgical care. World J Surg. 2008;32:509–15.
28. Bach PB, et al. Racial differences in the treatment of early-stage lung cancer. N Engl J Med. 1999;341(16):1198–205.
29. Cykert S, et al. Factors associated with decisions to undergo surgery among patients with newly diagnosed early-stage lung cancer. JAMA. 2010;303(23):2368–76.

30. Maynard C, et al. Gender differences in the treatment and outcome of acute myocardial infarction: results from the Myocardial Infarction Triage and Intervention Registry. Arch Intern Med. 1992;152(5):972–6.
31. Lesher AP, et al. Development and evolution of a statewide outpatient consultation service: leveraging telemedicine to improve access to specialty care. Popul Health Manag. 2020;23(1):20–8.
32. Wells KJ, et al. Patient navigation: state of the art or is it science? Cancer. 2008;113(8):1999–2010.
33. Wells KJ, et al. Comparing clinical and nonclinical cancer patient navigators: a national study in the United States. Cancer. 2022;128:2601–9.
34. Pérez-Stable EJ, El-Toukhy S. Communicating with diverse patients: how patient and clinician factors affect disparities. Patient Educ Couns. 2018;101(12):2186–94.
35. der Giessen V, Jeanine AM, et al. Effect of a health literacy training program for surgical oncologists and specialized nurses on disparities in referral to breast cancer genetic testing. Breast. 2021;58:80–7.
36. Berkman ND, et al. Health literacy interventions and outcomes: an updated systematic review. Evid Rep Technol Assess. 2011;199:1–941.
37. Sentell T, Braun KL. Low health literacy, limited English proficiency, and health status in Asians, Latinos, and other racial/ethnic groups in California. J Health Commun. 2012;17(Suppl 3):82–99.
38. Levett DZH, et al. Preparing the patient for surgery to improve outcomes. Best Pract Res Clin Anaesthesiol. 2016;30(2):145–57.
39. Tervalon M, Murray-Garcia J. Cultural humility versus cultural competence: a critical distinction in defining physician training outcomes in multicultural education. J Health Care Poor Underserved. 1998;9(2):117–25.
40. Betancourt JR, Green AR, Carrillo JE. Cultural competence in health care: emerging frameworks and practical approaches, vol. 576. New York: Commonwealth Fund, Quality of Care for Underserved Populations; 2002.
41. Hook JN, et al. Cultural humility: measuring openness to culturally diverse clients. J Couns Psychol. 2013;60(3):353.
42. Sinkler MA, Furdock RJ, Vallier HA. Treating trauma more effectively: a review of psychosocial programming. Injury. 2022;53:1756–64.
43. Hillier-Brown FC, et al. A systematic review of the effectiveness of individual, community and societal level interventions at reducing socioeconomic inequalities in obesity amongst children. BMC Public Health. 2014;14(1):1–18.
44. Braveman P. Health disparities and health equity: concepts and measurement. Annu Rev Public Health. 2006;27:167–94.
45. Braveman P. What are health disparities and health equity? We need to be clear. Public Health Rep. 2014;129(1_Suppl 2):5–8.
46. FitzGerald C, Hurst S. Implicit bias in healthcare professionals: a systematic review. BMC Med Ethics. 2017;18(1):1–18.

47. Maina IW, et al. A decade of studying implicit racial/ethnic bias in healthcare providers using the implicit association test. Soc Sci Med. 2018;199:219–29.
48. Hagiwara N, et al. Detecting implicit racial bias in provider communication behaviors to reduce disparities in healthcare: challenges, solutions, and future directions for provider communication training. Patient Educ Couns. 2019;102(9):1738–43.
49. Torain MJ, et al. Surgical disparities: a comprehensive review and new conceptual framework. J Am Coll Surg. 2016;223(2):408–18.
50. Bolorunduro OB, et al. Disparities in trauma care: are fewer diagnostic tests conducted for uninsured patients with pelvic fracture? Am J Surg. 2013;205(4):365–70.
51. Johnson TJ, et al. The impact of cognitive stressors in the emergency department on physician implicit racial bias. Acad Emerg Med. 2016;23(3):297–305.

The Fundamentals of Leadership Development Curriculum

44

Education Based Implementation of Diversity Initiatives

Jenny M. Shao and Yewande Alimi

The Importance of Diversity, Equity, and Inclusion in Leadership

Diversity, equity, and inclusion (DEI) are key components of effective surgical leadership. Diverse teams are more innovative, creative, and productive than homogeneous teams. They are also better able to understand and respond to the needs of a diverse patient population and enable us as physicians to deliver optimized patient care. While many leadership development courses exist, diversity, equity, and inclusion are often added as a small component of the course and are not wholly incorporated throughout, giving leaders little opportunity to recognize how big of a role DEI plays in everyday actions and decision-making. The goal of developing the

J. M. Shao (✉)
Department of Surgery, University of Michigan, Ann Arbor, MI, USA
e-mail: jmshao@med.umich.edu

Y. Alimi
Department of Surgery, Georgetown University School of Medicine, Washington, DC, USA
e-mail: Yewande.r.alimi@gunet.georgetown.edu

S. M. Johnson et al. (eds.), *The SAGES Manual of Strategy and Leadership*, https://doi.org/10.1007/978-3-031-62359-2_44

Fundamentals of Leadership Development curriculum (FLD) is to recognize that effective leadership cannot flourish without understanding and utilizing a diverse and inclusive mindset.

Fostering DEI in surgical culture goes beyond just assessing diversity metrics and meeting the appropriate numbers—at the heart of it all, the goal is to create an environment where all team members feel valued and respected, regardless of their background, identity, physical attributes, or personal characteristics. It is a commitment to providing equal opportunities for all team members to develop their leadership skills, advancing the pipeline of diverse leaders, and advocating for and mentoring early-career surgeons from underrepresented groups. This emphasizes on identifying the inequities that exist on a systems level and then using the power and influence gained in leadership positions levels the playing field for those whom we are leading.

These positive changes cannot exist in isolation and without holding leaders accountable for the surgical culture that they create at their institutions and organizations. This means setting clear goals for diversity and tracking progress toward those goals. It also means providing resources and support to leaders who are working to achieve diversity goals. The Fundamentals of Leadership Development curriculum is geared toward surgical leaders or those stepping into leadership roles and seeks to foster leadership that is mindful, inclusive, diverse, and equitable. It also seeks to provide leaders with concrete, positive action tools to improve upon their surgical culture.

Goals and Visions of FLD

The Fundamentals of Leadership Development (FLD) curriculum is designed to help surgeons develop the skills and knowledge they need to be effective leaders in a diverse environment. The curriculum is based on the following goals and visions:

- To increase the number of surgeons from underrepresented groups in leadership positions
- To create a more inclusive and equitable healthcare environment for all patients

- To develop surgeons who are skilled in conflict resolution and negotiation while being mindful of DEI issues

The FLD curriculum is designed to be interactive and engaging. It includes a variety of learning activities, such as case studies, role-playing exercises, and group discussions. The curriculum also includes a strong focus on self-reflection and personal development.

The basis of the curriculum was designed around several key competencies targeted at multiple levels of leadership development: self, teams, and systems. At each level, participants are expected to master different competencies to obtain key leadership skills necessary to succeed (Table 44.1). These were designed by asking the question, "What key leadership qualities would we expect to see from a mindful, inclusive, and equitable leader?". At each level, participants will engage in reading materials, video, and interactive components to learn about their leadership style, communication strategies, and how to problem solve difficult situations. These competencies will then be employed in a small group setting for didactic discussion scenarios.

Table 44.1 Fundamentals of Leadership Development competencies

Mastery level	Competency
Novice	**Self** Self-awareness Mindfulness Emotional intelligence Communication Commitment to social justice
Intermediate	**Team** Recruitment/retention Navigating conflict management Creating cultural competency and safety
Advanced	**System** Social determinants of health Improving diversity pipeline Innovation

Education and Awareness Can Lead to Systemic Change

Influencing surgical culture change on a systemic level is difficult to accomplish. Surgical leaders nationally and institutionally may employ different strategies to meet these goals. Some methods may include recruitment and retention of diverse individuals, creating pathways to promotion, formalizing mentorship and sponsorship, formation of diversity and inclusion committees, recognizing opportunities for better healthcare equity and delivery, and commitment to leadership development and education, just to name a few.

The FLD curriculum falls under leadership development and education; increasing the knowledge, awareness, and mindfulness of department leaders can then lead to a trickle-down effect for the whole department, system, and institution. The curriculum provides a framework for understanding the importance of diversity and inclusion, and it offers strategies for creating a more inclusive and equitable environment on multiple levels. While diversity training widely exists on basic levels at most institutions, there is much evidence to show that many of these programs can have the opposite intended effect and fall short. Data indicates that diversity programs focused on "controlling behavior," grievances, performance ratings, and hiring tests created more bias as leaders rebelled against rules threatening their autonomy and self-perceptions. Instead, successful programs focused on engaging leaders in problem-solving, encouraging social accountability, and exposing leaders to diverse people [1].

The implementation of a dedicated curriculum for surgeons also needs to consider surgeon specific factors such as availability, time constraints, and accessibility. To address potential issues, the curriculum was designed to improve ease of accessibility so that it could be completed on a surgeon's own time. For instance, modules were broken down into short sections, and modules that can be completed in 10–15-min stretches are designed well for downtime between cases or between meetings. These self-guided learning modules were a mixture of different formats including reading, lecture, videos, interactive components, and online discussion forums to help participants better engage with the material.

The second portion of the course is a case-based small group didactic discussion session. This format was chosen based on literature demonstrating that optimally effective leadership training programs should provide an intimate setting, promote speak-up culture, be customized for surgeons, and involve interactive activities [2]. This case-based problem-solving format would also allow participants to interact with individuals who had different perspectives and strategies for problem-solving. Ultimately, the combination of problem-solving and interactions with diverse teams would provide a strong foundation for taking these learned positive actions and solutions back to real everyday life in the clinical and administrative setting.

Recruitment, Retention, and Promotion of Diversity Within Surgical Departments

One of the main focal points of the FLD curriculum focuses on teaching leaders how to improve recruitment, retention, and mentorship in surgery. This is crucial for promoting diversity within the field and by actively working to attract and retain a diverse group of surgeons. This allows healthcare organizations to enhance cultural competence, reduce health disparities, and provide more equitable access to surgical care. The curriculum spends less time defining the "pipeline problem" but specifically focuses on solutions and how individuals can serve as better mentors and letter writers and how to mitigate bias in surgical promotion and advancement. On a team level, the curriculum discusses how team leaders can improve recruitment and retention in surgery, enhance diversity by widening the recruitment pool, and implement mentorship and sponsorship strategies for underrepresented in medicine individuals. On a systems level, FLD discusses how these strategies can be implemented on an institutional level and how to create buy-in among key stakeholders and leadership.

This section of the curriculum focuses on how actively recruiting from underrepresented groups on the resident and faculty level surgical programs can tap into a larger pool of talented individuals who bring diverse perspectives and experiences. Literature has demonstrated that despite almost equal gender enrollment in medical school, advancement of women in surgery remains disparate and lags dramatically behind expected numbers. Only 10% of women faculty become full professors of surgery, and less than 5% of department chairs in surgery are female [3, 4]. This disparity applies not only to women but also affects underrepresented in medicine individuals and those who are less "traditional" or have multiple points of intersectionality.

Improving the diversity of our departments is not just a numbers game, but gender and racial/ethnic diversity within surgical departments positively influences patient outcomes and satisfaction, leading to better patient outcomes and a more inclusive healthcare environment [5]. Additionally, diversity in the surgical workforce can help address healthcare disparities experienced by marginalized populations. Research has shown that minority patients are more likely to receive culturally competent care and have better health outcomes when treated by physicians from similar backgrounds. By diversifying the surgical workforce, we can improve patient trust, communication, and outcomes. These findings are supported by additional studies which show that patients who were treated by a surgeon of the same race or ethnicity had lower mortality rates than patients who were treated by a surgeon of a different race or ethnicity and that patients who were treated by a team that included a diverse range of professionals had better surgical outcomes than patients who were treated by a team that was less diverse [6–8].

Ultimately, surgeons from diverse backgrounds bring unique perspectives and cultural knowledge, which can improve patient-centered care and help address cultural biases in healthcare delivery. By fostering a diverse surgical workforce, healthcare organizations can ensure that patients' cultural, linguistic, and social needs are better understood and addressed. A diverse workforce can help to improve communication between patients and providers, reduce implicit bias, and improve overall decision making. A systematic review by Dogra et al. highlighted the importance of diversity and cultural competence in medical education and healthcare delivery, and this ultimately starts by taking care to educate and recruit our surgeons and surgical leaders [9].

Recruitment of diverse individuals to bolster our surgical culture without additional mentorship and sponsorship is not enough to ensure success. Mentorship programs that actively engage diverse surgeons can help address barriers faced by underrepresented individuals and provide guidance and support throughout their surgical careers. Multiple studies have emphasized the importance of mentorship in diversity and inclusion in academic surgery and helping pave pathways for success and promotion [10] indicating that once diverse and talented individuals have been recruited, methods to ensure retention are also necessary.

Diversity Builds and Improves Healthcare Equity

The second major theme of the FLD curriculum is promotion of healthcare equity and delivery. While many other leadership curricula have centered on upscaling leaders' knowledge and awareness of diversity, equity, and inclusion, few curricula have focused directly on the clinical aspect of healthcare equity. The health equity domain of the curriculum serves to provide a framework to incorporate healthcare equity in the clinical work environment. Using the didactic small group discussions, the FLD curriculum uses clinical scenarios with DEI themes to help learners develop practical and evidence-based solutions. Specifically, the curriculum tasks the novice learner to explore how stories that are internalized affect the care of their patients. It urges the intermediate learner to explore culturally appropriate care and address health inequities within their institution.

FLD explores the importance of delivering culturally competent care and how ensuring this in our health systems is impactful in the outcomes of our patients. Understanding and delivering culturally competent care requires leaders to understand the patient's cultural background and how it may affect their health beliefs and practices. By exploring these concepts, we create a framework for leaders to understand that delivering culturally competent care and embedding it within our healthcare system can help to reduce health disparities. Additionally, outside of culture alone, leaders explore how different social determinants of health including ethnicity, race, income, education, food security, and distressed indices can impact the way in which our patients interact with our healthcare systems. FLD challenges the master learner to understand how diverse patient populations may encounter obstacles within the healthcare systems structure and how they can advocate for and effect change. The collaborative nature of the curriculum also allows for learners to lean on colleagues to explore varied structures within the healthcare system and to discuss and exchange ideas at a leadership level.

In addition to cultural competency and concepts of social determinants of health, FLD also focuses on the systemic inequities embedded into our healthcare system since its inception. For instance, the historical context in which creatinine (Cr) and estimated glomerular filtration rate (eGFR) are reported for black patients and white patients comes from an erroneous assumption that black patients have higher muscle mass, therefore higher Cr and an adjusted eGFR [11]. This impacts how doctors have been taught to practice medicine for years and has downstream consequences on patients such as delay in care that is needed or perhaps even lifesaving interventions such as listing for transplant. Other instances of race and gender based medicine include clinical research, which is mostly conducted on white males, and effectively underrepresenting how interventions, drugs, and other therapies can affect the broader and general population [12, 13]. Learning to understand and question our healthcare systems is the first step to improving and adopting evidence-based medical practices that can start to mitigate disparities.

Identifying and finding implementable solutions to advance systemic healthcare equity is important, and finding individuals and leaders who are attuned to these issues again reiterates the need for diversity in the workforce. Recruitment and retention of a diverse workforce including the hiring of racial and ethnic minorities, persons with disabilities, and LGBTQ+ individuals is integral in creating a work environment that can address healthcare challenges equitably. Additionally, collecting and using data on ethnicity, race, and language preference with our patients can facilitate delivering culturally competent care and provides data for systems to better identify health disparities.

The Impact of Cultural Competency and Mindfulness on Conflict Resolution and Negotiation for Surgical Leaders

The last major topic that the FLD curriculum addresses is conflict negotiation and tensions within the space of DEI. While many studies have identified the competitive advantage of diverse teams, a decrease in implicit bias, and improvement in healthcare outcomes within an inherently biased system, there are others who may still need convincing or suffer from diversity fatigue [14]. The difference in approaches and viewpoints about strengths of diverse teams and practices may lead to conflict and possible challenging scenarios to navigate. An adept leader will need to navigate these delicate situations and employ appropriate conflict management solutions and demonstrate the appropriate emotional intelligence to succeed. At the individual level, learners will focus on understanding their own conflict resolution styles and gain insight into how they as leaders may approach difficult situations [15]. On a teams and mastery level, leaders will learn how to navigate and manage others within conflicts in the DEI setting, addressing micro and macro aggressions effectively, and how to influence systems and institutions to decrease biases in large scale settings. This portion of the curriculum provides surgical leaders concrete tools and positive actions to tackle divisive situations well.

On many levels, conflict resolution and negotiation are a combination of self-understanding of conflict management styles, insight into motivators for others, appropriate communication, and understanding strategies to better advocate for a specific outcome. While these leadership skills have not traditionally been discussed in the context of DEI, they are not mutually exclusive. As clinical, academic, and administrative leaders, everyone operates within a larger systemic context that is inherently biased and affords privilege toward certain individuals. Recognizing these power imbalances and acting on them to influence and change culture to allow for additional diversity, inclusion, and equity can be difficult to accomplish. An example, on a more individual level, would include how to recognize, intervene, and be an upstander/ally to combat micro and macro aggressions. This is communication and conflict negotiation in its most basic form, and the FLD curriculum seeks to teach how to navigate these situations in a thoughtful manner to educate and inform rather than humiliate and shame.

Scaling these important negotiation and conflict management strategies to employ them in a larger context as a surgeon leader is also important in creating lasting cultural and institutional change. During negotiations, oftentimes, leaders fail to take into context appropriate cultural, background, gender, and other personal contexts that may sway and inform how they approach situations. For instance, studies have shown that women were more effective at negotiating on behalf of others rather than for themselves and that gender differences in negotiation lessened with additional negotiating experience and education [16]. Additionally, cultural context can also influence situations and approaches to negotiation and potentially lead to misunderstandings between doctor-patients, colleagues, and institutions if these factors are not understood or recognized [17]. Creating mindfulness, understanding, and practicing best strategies for success in these situations will not only allow surgeon leaders to be better clinicians but will also allow them to negotiate more effectively at the C-suite level.

National Implementation Strategies of Surgical Culture Change

These leadership curriculum and diversity initiatives are strategies and tools to educate surgical leaders to effect the dissemination of positive surgical culture change. Institutional change lies with those in leadership positions and creates a trickle-down effect that leads to positive improvements in the DEI space for patients, faculty, trainees, and overall culture [18, 19]. Ultimately, our basis for implementation of DEI initiatives need to center on reaching those who have the ability and power at higher administrative and clinical levels to be able to lead by example and be positive role models. Instead of focusing on just implicit bias training, diversity metrics, and numbers alone, the discussion should seek to answer, "As surgical leaders, how can we educate ourselves and influence others to create a safe space that encourages diversity of thought, practices inclusion, and seeks to bring healthcare equity to all?".

An educational curriculum like FLD is just the start to implement national surgical culture change. Currently the course is being offered to SAGES members at the annual SAGES meeting, and those who are interested in furthering their leadership skills are invited to learn more about the course and register at https://www.sages.org/fld-sign-up/. Future directions from the course will include data collection from participants and gathering additional data driven implementation plans and strategies, with attention to identification of barriers and facilitators to success. This data will be necessary to understand optimal methods of content delivery and drivers of change. The systemic inequities have already been identified, and now it's time to focus on practical solutions that can improve and move the needle in a positive direction. These changes will not occur overnight; it will take time, effort, and reimagination of how we have previously addressed DEI in leadership and a focus on continual revision of how institutions and national organizations improve and change healthcare delivery.

SAGES Takeaway

- Effective leadership requires a diverse, equitable, and inclusive mindset in order to flourish, and intentional steps need to be taken to teach surgical leaders the right skills to succeed.
- The Fundamentals of Leadership Development curriculum focuses on three key areas of surgical leadership development: increasing diversity in surgical leadership, healthcare equity, and conflict negotiation.
- Education and awareness among key stakeholders in surgical

leadership is necessary to create the necessary culture change and influence actions of others.

- Data collection to identify facilitators and barriers to behavioral and culture change specific to implementation of DEI curriculums will be important to better understand education efforts.

References

1. Dobbin F, Kalev A. Why diversity programs fail. 2016. https://hbr.org/2016/07/why-diversity-programs-fail. Accessed 24 June 2023.
2. Gauly J, Court R, Currie G, et al. Advancing leadership in surgery: a realist review of interventions and strategies to promote evidence-based leadership in healthcare. Implement Sci. 2023;18:1–25. https://doi.org/10.1186/s13012-023-01274-3.
3. Bevilacqua LA, Siena NM, Gardner CA, et al. Gender disparities among leadership in academic surgical publishing over the past decade. Am J Surg. 2022;223:47–52. https://doi.org/10.1016/j.amjsurg.2021.07.038.
4. Sexton KW, Hocking KM, Wise E, et al. Women in academic surgery: the pipeline is busted. J Surg Educ. 2012;69:84–90. https://doi.org/10.1016/j.jsurg.2011.07.008.
5. Girod S, Fassiotto M, Grewal D, et al. Reducing implicit gender leadership bias in academic medicine with an educational intervention. Acad Med. 2016;91:1143. https://doi.org/10.1097/ACM.0000000000001099.
6. Britton BV, Nagarajan N, Zogg CK, et al. US surgeons' perceptions of racial/ethnic disparities in health care: a cross-sectional study. JAMA Surg. 2016;151:582–4. https://doi.org/10.1001/jamasurg.2015.4901.
7. Haider AH, Dankwa-Mullan I, Maragh-Bass AC, et al. Setting a national agenda for surgical disparities research: recommendations from the National Institutes of Health and American College of Surgeons summit. JAMA Surg. 2016;151:554. https://doi.org/10.1001/jamasurg.2016.0014.
8. West MA, Hwang S, Maier RV, et al. Ensuring equity, diversity, and inclusion in academic surgery: an American surgical association white paper. Ann Surg. 2018;268:403. https://doi.org/10.1097/SLA.0000000000002937.
9. Dogra N, Reitmanova S, Carter-Pokras O. Twelve tips for teaching diversity and embedding it in the medical curriculum. Med Teach. 2009;31:990–3. https://doi.org/10.3109/01421590902960326.
10. Dossett LA, Waljee JF, Dimick JB. Ensuring equal access to mentorship and sponsorship for surgeons through structured team-based mentoring. Ann Surg. 2020;272(6):939–40. https://doi.org/10.1097/SLA.0000000000004500.

11. Eneanya N, Brooks K. Filtering bias out of kidney testing—Penn Medicine. 2021. https://www.pennmedicine.org/news/publications-and-special-projects/penn-medicine-magazine/winter-2021/filtering-bias-out-of-kidney-testing. Accessed 24 June 2023.
12. Jin X, Chandramouli C, Allocco B, et al. Women's participation in cardiovascular clinical trials from 2010 to 2017. Circulation. 2020;141:540–8. https://doi.org/10.1161/CIRCULATIONAHA.119.043594.
13. Nazha B, Mishra M, Pentz R, Owonikoko TK. Enrollment of racial minorities in clinical trials: old problem assumes new urgency in the age of immunotherapy. Am Soc Clin Oncol Educ Book. 2019:3–10. https://doi.org/10.1200/EDBK_100021.
14. Smith JL, McPartlan P, Poe J, Thoman DB. Diversity fatigue: a survey for measuring attitudes towards diversity enhancing efforts in academia. Cultur Divers Ethnic Minor Psychol. 2021;27:659–74. https://doi.org/10.1037/cdp0000406.
15. Sinskey JL, Chang JM, Shibata GS, et al. Applying conflict management strategies to the pediatric operating room. Anesth Analg. 2019;129:1109–17. https://doi.org/10.1213/ANE.0000000000003991.
16. Mazei J, Hüffmeier J, Freund PA, et al. A meta-analysis on gender differences in negotiation outcomes and their moderators. Psychol Bull. 2015;141:85–104. https://doi.org/10.1037/a0038184.
17. Gunia BC, Brett JM, Gelfand MJ. The science of culture and negotiation. Curr Opin Psychol. 2016;8:78–83. https://doi.org/10.1016/j.copsyc.2015.10.008.
18. Evans MN, Thomas ME. The trickle-down effect of positive leadership on diversity and inclusion. J Bus Ethics. 2018;149:179–92.
19. Joshi AM, Jackson MJ. The role of leadership in diversity and inclusion. Acad Manag Perspect. 2016;30:27–44.

Global Leadership and Practice Considerations

45

Linda P. Zhang, Sahle Griffith, and Wesley P. Francis

Introduction

The field of global surgery addresses the immense unmet surgical needs of low- and middle-income countries (LMICs) to improve health outcomes for individuals and communities. To address the substantial burden of surgical diseases and disabilities, global surgery requires a comprehensive approach that involves strengthening healthcare systems, expanding surgical infrastructure, enhancing access to affordable surgical services, improving surgical training and workforce capacity, and prioritizing surgical care as part of the national and international health policy. Global surgery can promote health equity, encourage research and innovation, and foster partnerships for sustainable impact.

L. P. Zhang (✉)
Department of Surgery, Icahn School of Medicine at Mount Sinai, Mount Sinai Hospital, New York, NY, USA
e-mail: linda.zhang@mountsinai.org

S. Griffith
Department of Surgery, Faculty of Medical Sciences, University of the West Indies, Cave Hill Campus, Queen Elizabeth Hospital, Barbados, Bridgetown, Barbados

W. P. Francis
Department of Surgery, UWI School of Clinical Medicine and Research, Princess Margaret Hospital, Nassau, Bahamas

S. M. Johnson et al. (eds.), *The SAGES Manual of Strategy and Leadership*, https://doi.org/10.1007/978-3-031-62359-2_45

Leadership in global surgery is critical in improving surgical outcomes worldwide. It requires vision, strategic planning, collaboration, advocacy, and cultural humility. This chapter explores the pivotal role of leadership in global surgery, the qualities of effective leaders, strategies that can be employed to address the challenges facing leaders in global surgery, ethical considerations, and how to build a career in global surgery leadership. By implementing effective leadership principles, surgeon leaders can foster sustainable solutions, drive innovation, and empower change in global surgery.

Defining Leadership in the Context of Global Surgery

Leaders in global surgery are tasked with a unique role that can seem daunting at times but can be tremendously impactful when properly executed. Being a leader in global surgery means driving initiatives that promote equitable access to safe, timely, and affordable surgical care. Addressing the unmet surgical needs of LMICs, surgeon leaders need to have the vision and strategic thinking to push forward an agenda that is aligned with stakeholders, mobilize resources, and collaborate with diverse stakeholders. In addition, leaders in global surgery must prioritize capacity-building and long-term sustainability. They design programs that strengthen surgical systems and provide high-quality surgical services to individuals and communities. Focusing on programs with lasting impact, leaders promote programs that can be integrated into existing healthcare systems.

Sustainable Development Goals

Leaders in global surgery play a crucial role in achieving the Sustainable Development Goals (SDGs) set by the United Nations [1–3]. The SDGs provide a comprehensive framework for addressing global challenges, including those related to healthcare and surgical care. Specifically, leaders can achieve better health and well-being for a population by reducing the burden of surgical conditions and preventing disabilities while also promoting economic growth by addressing health-related impoverishments caused by untreated surgical conditions. In addition, by fostering research and technological advancements, leaders in global surgery can support development of context-specific solutions, leading to surgical efficiency and efficacy.

Healthcare Equality

Leadership in global surgery is instrumental in driving the agenda for healthcare equity globally. Leaders work toward overcoming geographical, socioeconomic, and cultural barriers that limit access to surgical services, particularly for vulnerable populations. Global surgery leaders are keenly aware of the social determinants of health and the inequalities inherent within a healthcare system. They design programs that promote gender equality by ensuring that women and girls have equitable access to essential care, especially in maternal and gynecological health. They advocate for programs that address barriers related to cultural norms. By advocating and implementing equitable interventions, leaders can reduce disparities in access to surgical care and promote social justice on a global scale.

Qualities of Effective Leader in Global Surgery

Vision and Strategy

An effective leader in global surgery must have a vision and strategy that promote equitable access to timely and safe surgical care in LMICs. There are a few principles of global surgery that should be included in the strategic planning of a surgeon leader in global surgery.

1. *Universal access to essential surgical care*: The strategy should involve expanding access to basic surgical procedures,

such as basic general surgery procedures (appendectomy, cholecystectomy, and hernia repair), trauma-related injuries, cesarean sections, cataract surgeries, and many other surgical interventions deficient in LMICs [4–7].

2. *Integration into existing healthcare systems*: In order to have sustainability, programs should be designed for integration and collaboration with existing healthcare systems. This involves strengthening health systems, establishing referral networks, and ensuring that surgical services are coordinated and aligned with primary care, emergency services, and specialized care.
3. *Capacity-building*: It is essential that programs prioritize development of a skilled surgical workforce to enhance the surgical infrastructure. The strategic planning should include training programs and mentorship to build local surgical capacity. In addition, programs also need to focus on building the surgical infrastructure, including operating theaters, anesthesia services, and surgical equipment.
4. *Context-specific solutions*: All programs in global surgery fundamentally requires context-specific solutions. No two healthcare environments are the same, and solutions must be tailored to the specific needs of each setting. Local disease burden, sociocultural norms, and available resources must be considered when designing a program. Engaging the community and collaborating with local stakeholders in the decision-making processes are essential in developing context-specific strategies.
5. *Research and innovation*: In the past, research has fallen to the wayside as global surgery programs prioritize surgical care delivery. Leaders of global surgery need to foster a culture of research and innovation in all their global surgery programs. Program design and outcomes should be data-driven, clearly showing an impact to the community. They should promote technological advancements to create innovative solutions for better healthcare delivery.
6. *Health equity, advocacy, and social justice*: Leaders in global surgery should prioritize reducing disparities in accessing surgical care, especially for vulnerable populations, such as women, children, rural communities, and marginalized groups.

Collaborative Partnerships

Collaborative partnership in global surgery brings together diverse stakeholders, leverage expertise and resources, promote local ownership, strengthen health systems, and enable scaling up of interventions. It can involve government and nongovernmental organizations (NGOs), academic institutions, healthcare professionals, and local communities. Recognizing the value of working together, collaborative partnerships can achieve greater impact, sustainability, and equity in improving surgical care in LMICs.

Successful global surgery programs require a comprehensive and multidisciplinary approach. By establishing collaborative partnerships, programs can pool the knowledge, skills, and resources from multiples entities, to collectively strategize in achieving common goals. In addition, partnerships can coordinate action among various stakeholders to align their efforts, avoid duplication of interventions, and maximize efficient use of resources. Through collaborative partnerships, best practice interventions can be then scaled up and replicated. As such, collaborations facilitate dissemination of evidence-based interventions, supporting context-specific adaptations and spread of innovative solutions.

The sustainability of any initiatives is dependent on local buy-in of the community. Collaborative partnerships that involve local stakeholders, such as healthcare providers, community organizations, and government agencies, will promote local ownership. Proposed initiatives should involve local partners throughout the design, implementation, and evaluation process of the program. This will ensure that interventions are contextually appropriate, culturally sensitive, and responsive to local needs. By partnering with local stakeholders, programs are also strengthening the healthcare system in that community. Partnerships can address challenges frequently seen in LMICS, tackling shortcomings in healthcare infrastructure, workforce development, supply chain, and data collection systems. Furthermore, collaborative partnerships can allow for knowledge sharing and capacity-building, leading to development of a skilled surgical workforce. Through sharing best practices, experiences, and lessons learned from different contexts, the exchange of knowledge strengthens the capacity of individuals and institutions involved in global surgery. This exchange is reciprocal, as both low-resource and high-resource entities can gain distinct knowledge and expertise through this exchange. Lastly, through collaborative partnerships, leaders in global surgery can amplify the collective voice, advocate for policy changes, and call greater attention to surgical care on national and international agendas.

In sum, leaders in global surgery use a collaborative approach to ensure that investments in surgical care are integrated into broader health system strengthening efforts, leading to long-term impact and sustainable surgical care improvements. Partnerships are mutually beneficial for all involved entities and are vital in fostering ownership and longevity of the program.

Advocacy and Policy

Leaders in global surgery are advocates for health equity, social justice, and high-quality surgical care for all. These leaders raise awareness about the unmet surgical needs of communities and its socioeconomic and health impact on vulnerable individuals. They engage with policymakers, funders, and the public to promote global surgery initiatives and investment in surgical infrastructure and workforce. Leaders advocate for policy changes, resource allocations, and health system reforms to embed surgical care as an essential component of universal health coverage and global health. By uniting a diverse set of stakeholders, leaders in global surgery can influence policy decisions and resource allocation, leading to greater attention and additional strategies to improve surgical services.

Cultural Humility

By incorporating cultural humility into their practice, leaders in global surgery can foster culturally sensitive and patient-centered care, enhancing the surgical experience and outcomes of patients from diverse cultural backgrounds. They promote a more inclusive and respectful healthcare system that considers the diverse cultural backgrounds and beliefs of individuals and communities. Particularly in global surgery, it is crucial to both understand and acknowledge the cultural context in which surgical care is delivered. Cultural sensitivity builds trust and rapport between providers and patients by acknowledging that patients possess valuable knowledge about their own cultural beliefs, preferences, and goals of care. Healthcare providers should adapt their approach to minimize barriers to surgical care, including addressing language barriers, socioeconomic factors, and cultural norms. Providers need to be aware of their own communication style and engage in a shared decision-making process that is both culturally appropriate and acceptable. Furthermore, providers should recognize their own cultural biases and assumptions, and they should engage in self-reflection to identify and challenge these biases.

By demonstrating respect, empathy, and cultural sensitivity, leaders in global surgery can establish alliance based on mutual trust and understanding. They are keen to understand the cultural dynamics at play and develop contextually appropriate interventions that are responsive to the needs and priorities of the community.

Strategies Employed by Effective Leaders in Global Surgery

Building and Strengthening Local Surgical Systems

The provision of quality surgical care in a timely and affordable manner is the goal of global surgery. It is therefore a key component in achieving the United Nations Sustainable Development Goals 2030 (SDGs) [8]. However, these lofty ideals while universally agreed do require far greater effort to accomplish as we move from high- to lower-income jurisdictions. To this end, the global surgical leader must be cognizant of the various barriers to provision of quality surgical care most notably in low- to middle-income countries (LMICs) and low-income countries (LICs).

These jurisdictions almost routinely have significant deficits in the system that hamper achievements of the SDGs, whether they be deficiencies in physical infrastructure and skilled manpower, financial constraints, or administrative/institutional bias [9, 10].

In order to strengthen these surgical systems, innovative thought is required. As Niccolo Machiavelli so succinctly surmised in his political treatise, The Prince, "And it ought to be remembered that there is nothing more difficult to take in hand, more perilous to conduct, or more uncertain in its success, than to take the lead in the introduction of a new order of things, because the innovator has for enemies all those who have done well under the old conditions, and lukewarm defenders in those who may do well under the new." To this end, not only must the global leadership respect the customs of the jurisdiction, but there must be acute awareness that in many of these LMICs and LICs, traditional hierarchies do still significantly impact on local surgical leadership and administration. Often the decision-makers in those environments are chosen not based on a culture of specific training in surgical leadership or a history of fostering evidence-based innovative practice, but more so on political affiliations, clinical acumen, and seniority [11]. None of which necessarily pairs well with developing novel care delivery pathways. To this end, partnerships with established programs in HICs and the input of respected leaders from those environments may go a long way in helping to build out robust strategies for success.

As a direct caveat to this model, it becomes necessary to arrange for the identification of dynamic surgical leaders in these LMIC states who may already be on the ground fighting for the necessary levels of "buy-in" for novel or expanded surgical delivery platforms and offer them support in terms of both mentorship and also lobby, as often these locales are hostile to change. The local surgical lead paired with supportive global leadership is a powerful combination. The local leader has in-depth knowledge of the deficiencies in the environment and the logistics of that space. These can be quite significant and range from service provision in small, isolated communities, technique modifications necessary for resource poor settings, and political affiliations of the power brokers. It can also be as simple a matter as vagaries in power supply from the grid that necessitates the use of surge protection on valuable equipment. This expertise is invaluable to the global surgical leader as they attempt to strengthen local systems from outside.

Surgical Training and Education

A direct corollary that results from this is the training of manpower and other skilled personnel to foster the delivery of an expanded suite of services. This can initially be achieved by the creation of memoranda of understanding between the surgical leaders in jurisdictions with established training programs for the service that is to be offered and the local institutions who are seeking to expand their services with this new procedure. This allows for the establishments of regular workshop and skill sharing sessions, in conjunction with the refinement of the techniques on lists dedicated to addressing that surgical skill, thus allowing the entire system at that institution to benefit not only in skill acquisition by live testing performance but in addition allowing any logistic or technical faux pas to be identified and addressed under the direct supervision of skilled mentors. Once the basic skill sets have been mastered, the use of cheaper, readily available technology can allow for expert preceptorship of previously trained mentees via distance mentorship.[12,13,1415]

It is well recognized that certain complex surgical procedures require more in-depth training algorithms. This clearly has been identified by some global surgical leaders, with the resultant creation of global disparity fellowships at major training centers in the HICs, thus exposing qualified surgeons from LMICs to advanced techniques that hopefully can then allow for capacity-building in their home jurisdictions. As discussed earlier, there must concomitantly exist the desire to support these nascent programs in their infancies, as obstacles to change may seem insurmountable and result in outward migration of these highly trained surgeons from the LMICs, and ultimately little of the long-term benefits would be accrued [16–18].

Research and Innovation

One of the great tragedies of global surgery is the paucity of robust research emerging from LMICs and LICs. This results in two significant impairments of progress in these locales: a sluggish approach to the adoption of evidence-based management strategies, under the guise that "this evidence may not be reproducible in our environment," and secondly a relative absence in the global discussions on the contribution of diversity in ethnicity and culture on the epidemiology and outcomes for many surgical pathologies. Global surgical leadership can be of paramount importance in forging inroads into reversing this phenomenon. Poor access to widespread electronic medical records (EMRs) across the global south makes the creation of robust databases extremely challenging. Yet again, this produces possible opportunities for robust partnerships. Surgical leaders in the global north may be able to lobby for the creation of "open source" or shared EMR facilities that allow affiliated centers in the LMICs and LICs to enter patient information while still maintaining some level of proprietary control on their datasets, thus allowing for robust data collection, analysis, and ultimately publication, in this way encouraging a culture of evidence-based surgery to emerge. Ultimately this would make the innovation of healthcare systems not only more readily accepted but also more accurately targeted to real as opposed to perceived needs.

Innovations in safe instrument reprocessing are one way in which traditionally LMICs and LICs have led the world. Necessity is the mother of invention and innovation, so in areas with sparse resources, ingenuity is working overtime. As concerns mount over the impact of single use devices and their impact on the environment, the time has come for the entire global surgical community to practice the most sustainable options possible [19, 20].

Mobilization of Resources and Finances

Global surgical leadership requires recognition of fundamental truths. Many LMICs and LICs have very meager resources to spend on healthcare; in fact, across Latin America and the Caribbean, the average public health expenditure is around 4% of gross domestic product (GDP), much lower than the 8% allocated to this same parameter by the countries of the Organisation for Economic Co-Operation and Development (OECD) [21]. Statistics from the same region have documented that about 30% of the population of the region have no access to healthcare because of financial constraints [22]. Admittedly the complexities of healthcare financing are beyond the scope of this paper; however, it is imperative for global surgical leadership to lobby for the creation of safe, robust, and cost-efficient approaches to providing quality surgical care to the majority of the world's populace. This may in some instances require the establishment of private-public partnerships [9]. In others, partnering with centers in HICs, such that decommissioned but functional, surgical equipment could be sent to areas in need. The power of building up a lobby from within the public should not be underestimated. The ability of the voice of the electorate to change the tide of political discourse is enormous. Surgical leadership should always attempt to forge robust partnerships with the public we serve, as they are our most powerful ally for change.

Community Engagement and Empowerment

Whether it's a Level 1 facility in a rural LIC or a tertiary facility in a HIC, community engagement and support are an invaluable adjunct in the fight for surgical innovation. A focused emphasis on free public educational lectures or educational content on social media can secure public engagement on the need for expanded or innovative surgical services. By making the community stakeholders in this process, public engagement can not only allow for lobbying of increased public funding for such ventures but also can result in individuals from the community donating their time and resources to the development project itself.

Workforce and Capacity-Building

Capacity-building can only begin where the administration and surgical leadership identify a unified direction of growth. The traditional method of selecting surgical leaders based on seniority or political affiliations may not result in the type of leadership that fosters growth. It is imperative that formal training in management and leadership be made widely available and that surgical leaders in key administrative positions be selected only from personnel who have had formal managerial training. The significant downstream effects of this approach will be innumerable in terms of capacity-building.

Example of Global Surgery Programming

There are various programs through surgical societies that provide surgical services to underserved areas, implemented in a manner that exemplifies concepts considered in this chapter. One such example is the outreach program of The Americas Hepato-Pancreato-Biliary Association (AHPBA), where a well-designed and appropriately implemented program successfully provided complex hepatobiliary surgery to patients in Honduras while building the surgical capacity of the local workforce and healthcare infrastructure.

The AHPBA made outreach missions a part of its strategic plan, and the first mission to Honduras was led by Dr. Gazi Zibari (former president of AHPBA). Evaluating the existing surgical infrastructure, resources, and healthcare systems in the target region is crucial. Once conceptualized, we identified a local surgeon who was able to assist with a needs assessment in Honduras by identifying the local community needs, prevalent health issues, barriers to healthcare access, and resource challenges. This assessment guided the development of appropriate strategies to improve surgical care capacity and effectiveness [23, 24].

After identifying the need, the planning stage involved gathering stakeholders to assist in the execution of the mission. Collaborations with local and international organizations, healthcare professionals, governments, and nonprofits were vital. We were able to secure supplies, sutures, staples, and instruments from industry partners. Once the team had mobilized the needed human resources and the necessary supplies, all details for execution of the mission were clarified and communicated to all stakeholders involved. Networking helped in leveraging expertise, sharing resources, and creating synergies to address global surgical challenges [25].

The local team was actively engaged in the ground logistics of the mission, including providing the full spectrum of surgical care. All cases were seen by the outreach team and discussed preoperatively. Appropriate indications for each case were determined and resource allocation addressed, especially ensuring that postoperative care did not exceed the capabilities of the local team or cause any undue strain on existing limited resources. The team was able to carry out complex surgical procedures in hepatobiliary, surgical oncology, and minimally invasive general surgery procedures with close follow-up of outcomes.

Sustainable change involves establishing long-term solutions that endure beyond individual initiatives. This includes training local healthcare providers, building local capacity, and integrating global surgery practices into the existing healthcare systems [26]. In addition to providing direct surgical care, this program improved the capacity of the local workforce by providing specialty training to a local surgeon. Through the relationship built from this mission, the local surgeon was then afforded fellowship training in hepatobiliary surgery in Canada and subsequently returned to his home country to continue practicing in his community. This relationship developed through the mission continues today.

The blueprint for such an initiative encapsulates the mission and vision of global surgery leadership. While many other surgical societies have similar programs, this kind of outreach can serve as an entry for surgeons interested in entering this space. This initiative was a collaborative effort by members of a surgical society with local surgeons on the ground, supplementing their human and infrastructural resources to effect tangible and objective advancement to the community.

Ethical Considerations

Resource Constraints and Infrastructure Gaps

The resources available across the global surgical environment are significantly varied. It is common for LMICs to lack the capacity to dedicate large proportions of their annual budgets to healthcare [22]. Ultimately that means that the resources available for surgery, intensive care, and acute care are all far more meager than within most HICs. This has bearing not only on the kinds of cases that can be undertaken, simply based on what equipment is available in the environment. Furthermore, if a skill exists in the environment but the resources expended to achieve a particular outcome using those skills on one patient affect the ability to provide service to many patients, the ethics of offering that therapeutic option to one patient should be considered and discussed among healthcare personnel. This is also true for visiting global experts who may be tempted to offer a procedure as a part of an itinerant surgical team brought in to train local clinicians. The global team must consider the resource constraints of the local infrastructure and avoid teaching/performing procedures that require postoperative clinical and infrastructural support that is too taxing to the host institution.

Another ethical challenge facing global surgery is the temptation to either lower standards of care in LICs or to accept lower standards as global leaders attempt to expand services. We must be ever vigilant in guarding against this inclination. For instance, the use of mosquito netting for inguinal hernia repair has been proposed and practiced at various LMICs, sometimes initiated by global teams from HICs. While the lack of prosthetic material is apparent in many LMICs, the safety of mosquito netting and its long-term effects are not well-known. Such an approach calls into question the ethical dilemma of lowering the standard of care in LMICs in an attempt to expand surgical services. The risks and benefits of mosquito-net hernia repair should be weighed against a primary tissue hernia repair. Global leaders and local institutions need to undergo a full discussion and disclosure of these risks and benefits prior to implementation.

Practice Considerations

Global surgery is an emerging field that addresses the disparities in surgical care and access to surgical services on a global scale. Incorporating global surgery into one's surgical practice requires a strategic and multidimensional approach. In developing a vision for a global surgery practice, a surgeon should aspire to improve surgical care access, outcomes, and equity on a global scale. This could include providing surgical services to underserved populations, training local healthcare professionals, building sustainable surgical infrastructure, and fostering research to inform evidence-based practices [22].

Incorporating global surgery in one's surgical career can vary widely, depending on one's time availability and level of commitment. In the past, most global surgery endeavors have focused on providing purely direct surgical care to underserved populations, in the format of short term mission-type trips. While participation in these programs offers insight into the field of global surgery, they have limited impact on capacity-building of the local workforce and infrastructure. Despite this, some surgeons in HICs have limited time availability to devote to global surgery, and this venue may be a feasible option to contribute to the field of global surgery.

Alternatively, as the focus in global surgery shifts forward sustainability, surgeons have built their global surgery practice to emphasize training at the host institution, building sustainable surgical infrastructure and fostering research. This includes a well-designed and organized program, from conception to implementation, which incorporates many of the key concepts discussed in this chapter. These programs are established at an institutional level or at a national surgical society level, and surgeons committed to global surgery contribute at varying levels of engagement.

One critical component that is often lacking for surgeons interested in incorporating global surgery into their career is funding support for performed work. Identifying and securing funding sources are fundamental for sustainable global surgery initiatives. Surgeons need to explore grants, philanthropic organizations, governmental aid, and partnerships to support their vision. Despite significant interest for social equity, especially from the newer generation of surgeons, funding support for global surgery is severely lagging behind. This is unfortunately the case on an individual institutional level, public and nonprofit grant-funding level, and national/international level. Furthermore, there is currently no uniformed metric or quantitative assessment of professional engagement performed in the field of global surgery [27]. As a result, many surgeons contributing to the field of global surgery are currently performing their role on their own time and expense, with insufficient recognition by their own institutions. To build a sustainable career in global surgery for future generation of surgeons practicing global surgery, significant efforts need to be made now by the current global surgery leaders to rectify this deficiency.

Conclusion

The future of leadership in global surgery necessitates a proactive approach to address the disparities in surgical care globally. Effective leadership is crucial for policy and practice implementation. Leaders must advocate for policy changes that prioritize surgical care, ensuring it is an integral part of universal healthcare systems. This should encompass a focus on securing and effectively allocating resources to improve surgical infrastructure, workforce training, and access to surgical services. L.D. Britt in his charge to the surgical community said, "there is no quality without access,"—sustainable development can only be achieved by building capacity through improving the human resources as advancements are made to change infrastructure. There must be aligned efforts to improve access to patients, or these initiatives will be met with frustration and limited success. Policies should incentivize healthcare professionals to undergo specialized training in global surgery and facilitate collaboration between nations, promoting not only the exchange of best practices and innovations in surgical care, but provide training opportunities for surgeon from LMICs [22, 26].

In summary, leadership in global surgery requires a multifaceted approach that encompasses a clear vision, understanding of global health challenges, collaborations, resource assessment, funding identification, cultural humility, and a focus on creating sustainable and impactful change. Utilizing existing research and collaborating with experts in the field are crucial for effective implementation and success in the global surgery arena.

SAGES Takeaway

- Leadership in global surgery requires a proactive approach to tackle disparities and advocate for policy changes that prioritize surgical care within universal healthcare systems.
- Effective leaders should focus on securing and allocating resources wisely to enhance surgical infrastructure, workforce training, and access to services, recognizing the essential link between quality and access in surgical care.
- Leadership in global surgery necessitates a multifaceted approach, including collaboration, specialized training, and a focus on sustainable change, leveraging existing research and expertise for successful implementation and impact.

References

1. Roa L, Jumbam D, et al. Global surgery and the sustainable development goals. Br J Surg. 2019;106(2):e44–52.
2. Eckert N, Rusch G, et al. Sustainable development goals and risks: the yin and the Yang of the paths towards sustainability. Ambio. 2023;52(4):683–701.
3. Asma S, Lozano R, et al. Monitoring the health-related sustainable development goals: lessons learned and recommendations for improved measurement. Lancet. 2020;395(10219):240–6.
4. Saluja S, Mukhopadhyay S, et al. Quality of essential surgical care in low- and middle-income countries: a systematic review of the literature. Int J Qual Health Care. 2019;31(3):166–72.
5. Price R, Makasa E, et al. World health assembly resolution WHA68.15: "strengthening emergency and essential surgical care and anesthesia as a component of universal health coverage"—addressing the public health gaps arising from lack of safe, affordable and accessible surgical and anesthetic service. World J Surg. 2015;39(9):2115–25.
6. Blair K, Paladino L, et al. Surgical and trauma care in low- and middle-income countries: a review of capacity assessments. J Surg Res. 2017;210:139–51.
7. Forrester JD, Forrester JA, et al. self-reported determinants of access to surgical care in 3 developing countries. JAMA Surg. 2016;151(3):257–63.
8. Meara JG, Leather AJ, et al. Global surgery 2030: evidence and solutions for achieving health, welfare, and economic development. Surgery. 2015;158:3–6.

9. Ward E, Fox K, et al. A review of hospital care in Jamaica: morbidity and mortality patterns, resource allocation and cost of care. West Ind Med J. 2001;50(S2):21.
10. Wilson CB, Cawich CO, et al. Starting a laparoscopic surgery Service in a Rural Community Hospital in Jamaica: successes and challenges of the Percy Junor hospital experience Caribbean. Med J. 2014;76(1):8–11.
11. Machiavelli N. The Prince (W. K. Marriott,Trans.). PROJECT GUTENBERG EBOOK (Original work published 1532); 1998.
12. Cawich SO, Harding HE, et al. Leadership in surgery for public sector hospitals in Jamaica: strategies in the operating room. Perm J. 2013;17(3):121–5.
13. Cawich SO, Griffith S, et al. Distance mentoring in advanced minimally invasive surgery in the Caribbean: a model for low-resource environments. Curr Med Res Prac. 2021;11(3):125–8.
14. Cawich SO, Mencia M, et al. Trauma surgery via distance mentoring: a model inspired by the 2020 pandemic. Trop Dr. 2021;52(1):102–3.
15. Asfaw Z, Todd R, et al. Use of virtual platform for delivery of simulation-based laparoscopic training curriculum in LMICs. Surg Endosc. 2023;37(2):1528–36.
16. Dugger CW. Small developing lands hit hardest by brain drain. New York, NY: New York Times. p. A9.
17. Negron R. Personal networks and migration decision: the case of Jamaican brain drain. J Identity Migration Stud. 2012;6(1).
18. Johnson N. Analysis and assessment of the brain drain phenomenon and its effect on Caribbean countries. Florida Atlantic Comparative Studies Journal. 2009;11:1–16.
19. Cunha MF, Pellino G. Environmental effects of surgical procedures and strategies for sustainable surgery. Nat Rev Gastroenterol Hepatol. 2023;20:399–410.
20. Shoham MA, Baker NM, et al. The environmental impact of surgery: a systematic review. Surgery. 2022;172(3):897–905.
21. PAHO. Health in the Americas: health financing in the Americas. 2017. https://www.paho.org/salud-en-las-americas-2017/uh-financing.html.
22. Sullivan R, Alatise OI, Anderson BO, et al. Global cancer surgery: delivering safe, affordable, and timely cancer surgery. Lancet Oncol. 2015;16(11):1193–224.
23. Farmer PE, Kim JY. Surgery and global health: a view from beyond the OR. World J Surg. 2008;32(4):533–6.
24. Shrime MG, Bickler SW, Alkire BC, Mock C. Global burden of surgical disease: an estimation from the provider perspective. Lancet Glob Health. 2015;3:S8–9.
25. Ozgediz D, Roayaie K, Debas H, et al. Surgery in developing countries: essential training in residency. Arch Surg. 2005;140(8):795–800.

26. Ng-Kamstra JS, Greenberg SLM, Abdullah F, et al. Global surgery 2030: a roadmap for high income country actors. BMJ Glob Health. 2016;1:e000011.
27. Peck GL, Garg M, et al. The American College of Academic International Medicine 2017 consensus statement on international medical programs: establishing a system of objective valuation and quantitative metrics to facilitate the recognition and incorporation of academic international medical efforts into existing promotion and tenure paradigms. Int J Crit Illn Inj Sci. 2017;7(4):201–11.

International Medical Graduates: Strategies to Mitigate Challenges in Medical Education

46

Carolina Torres Perez-Iglesias, Fariha Sheikh, and Daniel B. Jones

Leaders are directly responsible for ensuring a diverse and welcoming work environment. Surgical educators need to understand the unique challenges of different learners and appreciate the value they bring to the healthcare team. International medical graduates (IMGs) represent an important pillar of the healthcare system, representing a quarter of all licensed physicians in the USA [1]. IMGs are defined as individuals who receive their basic medical degree from a medical school located outside the USA and Canada [2]. The reasons for choosing to pursue training in the USA can be professional, educational, and/or personal. They bring aspirations of advancing their professional careers through specialty training in a nation renowned for its cutting-edge medical systems, including the potential for better opportunities,

C. Torres Perez-Iglesias (✉)
Department of Surgery, Beth Israel Deaconess Medical Center, Boston, MA, USA
e-mail: ctorresp@bidmc.harvard.edu

F. Sheikh · D. B. Jones
Department of Surgery, University Hospital, Rutgers New Jersey Medical School, Newark, NJ, USA
e-mail: sheikhf@njms.rutgers.edu; dj477@njms.rutgers.edu

S. M. Johnson et al. (eds.), *The SAGES Manual of Strategy and Leadership*, https://doi.org/10.1007/978-3-031-62359-2_46

high-quality education, networking, research, and personal growth through immersion in a different culture. Currently, IMGs comprise approximately a fifth of all first-year residency positions annually [3]. Besides helping address the physician shortage in the country and enriching the diversity of the medical workforce [4, 5], IMGs also fill an important role working in medically underserved areas [6, 7]. Patient outcomes for those treated by IMG physicians have been shown to be equivalent and, in some cases, superior, attributed to the culturally competent care provided to those with similar ethnicities and languages [8–10].

Prior to practicing medicine in the USA, IMGs must take the US Medical Licensing Examination (USMLE) tests and become certified by the Educational Commission for Foreign Medical Graduates (ECFMG), a process that takes many years and costs multiple thousands of dollars [11, 12]. Unfortunately, despite the increase in training positions over the last decade, the percentage of IMG-filled positions decreased in 2022, and match rates for non-US citizen IMGs remain lower than 50% [3, 13]. Before residency, IMGs are commonly separated from family and friends, move into a new country, and deal with complex legal and immigration policies [14–16]. Specifically in the surgical specialties, IMGs will commonly be primarily considered for non-designated preliminary residency positions, a 1-year contract without any guarantee to be able to stay in the country and continue training after it. Multiple studies have shown that less than half of IMGs in preliminary positions will find a categorical spot to complete residency training [17–20].

In addition, the challenges faced by IMGs extend into the training years. A study by Moore and Rhodenbaugh demonstrated that IMGs are commonly perceived as less desirable and capable than local graduates. Almost 90% of polled members of the Association of Program Directors of Surgery preferred offering positions to USMG over IMGs despite having equal qualifications [21]. More than half also reported purposefully avoiding IMGs, in part because of the perceived potential for language barriers, the concern for substandard quality and abilities compared to USMG, and the lack of familiarity with educational standards at non-US medical schools. The short term that these residents may spend in programs sometimes can lead to the perception that preliminary residents are disposable or temporary, potentially affecting the willingness of faculty or peers to dedicate time to their learning and training. The decreased perceived investment of senior members of the department or program in preliminary residents can lead them to feel unsupported and isolated [22]. Similarly in fellowship training, only a third of MIS programs are willing to accept and sponsor visas for IMG applicants [23]. Although new studies have presented a more balanced perspective, recognizing the value of IMGs in terms of diversity and patient care benefits, negative perceptions persist [24]. The challenge lies in recognizing and addressing these perceptions to level the playing field for IMGs. Finally, often preliminary IMG residents will not report negative experiences, such as discrimination, abuse, etc., due to fear of appearing weak or problematic. This stigma is reminiscent of the expectations placed on foreign workers, who are frequently expected to work diligently without complaining [25].

Challenges faced by IMG during residency training [26]
Separation from family and friends
Learning medical terminology in a foreign language
Discrimination based on race, ethnicity, education, etc.
Changing immigration policies and restrictions [27]
Learning new cultural norms and language
Adaptation of communication skills into a different culture
Limited availability of categorical positions
Lack of familiarity of programs and staff with visa sponsorship and conditions
Lack of access to moonlighting or other income opportunities under visa sponsorship
Adaptation to a foreign medical health system
Navigating a foreign culture and medical healthcare system

To mitigate these challenges, proactive strategies are imperative. Recognizing the unique needs and challenges of IMG residents offers an avenue for tailored support. IMGs confront challenges during training that can adversely impact their educational experience and career progression. The strategic implementation of initiatives such as specialized mentorship can offer tailored support and bridge the gap between challenges and success. At Beth Israel Deaconess Medical Center, a general surgery program with a high representation of IMGs, a specialized mentorship program was developed with the goal of supporting IMGs during the first years of residency. Faculty and residents serve as mentors, and educational sessions are hosted throughout the year on topics such as technical skills, communication skills, cultural dexterity, ABSITE, immigration, and else. Establishing specialized mentorship which aims at recognizing and understanding the nuances of the experiences of IMG residents can help the program foster a stronger sense of belonging and support. IMGs also highly benefit from cross-mentorship by members of the department highly invested in their success and well-being despite not being IMGs themselves. Moreover, this kind of initiative not only benefits the mentees but also empowers mentors to recognize their biases and learn from diverse members of the medical workforce, as well as participate in community-building activities. Mentors do not need to be IMGs or have background experience in visas, immigration, ECFMG certification, or else.

Similarly, a special program was created with dedicated time toward mentoring and guiding preliminary surgery residents at Rutgers New Jersey Medical School toward success. The program was developed based on the experience of faculty who themselves are IMGs and now want to pay forward the support they received when they were residents. With over 15 preliminary residents both PGY 1 and PGY 2 level, several of which are IMGs, the goal is to find every person a categorical position by the close of the academic year. Residents receive support to complete necessary visa paperwork, meet with residency leadership since the beginning of the year to create a detailed plan along a strategic timeline, are encouraged to share personal statements for review, are scheduled for mock interviews, are offered opportunities in professional societies, and are assigned an additional faculty mentor to ensure a multifaceted support system and broader networking opportunities. Throughout the year, the residents maintain close communication with residency leadership regarding their progress and potential applications, receiving tailored support in the process until each resident has obtained a position for the following academic year, ideally a categorical position. The support is evident for IMGs throughout the application process, and residents are matched based on merit.

Surgical societies can support IMGs by increasing opportunities in committees and positions of leadership, where they are currently underrepresented [28]. For junior residents, these can help them network, improve research productivity, and increase visibility when they apply for categorical positions. Other societies, like the Latino Surgical Society, can help pair IMGs with mentors who understand their backgrounds and challenges. Many medical institutions and organizations have already recognized the importance of mentorship and are working toward being more inclusive. The American Medical Association released a toolkit in 2022 for international medical graduates who are already licensed to practice in the USA or seeking licensure with topics such as types of visas required to practice medicine in the USA, academic and clinical opportunities, mentorship, financial planning, and else [29].

Leaders need to recognize the value that IMGs bring to the healthcare system, and addressing the obstacles they face will not only enrich the diversity of the medical workforce but also enhance patient care and outcomes. As the medical community strives for inclusivity and excellence, understanding the unique challenges that minority groups are facing, designing interventions tailored to address any unintended inequalities, and empowering IMGs through targeted strategies are essential steps toward achieving these goals.

Strategies to support IMG during residency training
Conduct an individual needs assessment of IMG trainees [30]
Peer mentorship [31]
Faculty mentorship
Recognition for their hard work and contribution to the healthcare system
Recognition for the cultural and contribution to diversity of the workforce
Create more opportunities/positions for preliminary residents (increase positions, increase funding, etc.)
Mental health and emotional support
Increased funding and research opportunities for IMGs

Strategies to support IMG during residency training
Increase leadership opportunities for IMGs in academic societies
Remunerate physicians who can provide care in multiple languages
Unconscious bias and cultural competence training for faculty, residents, and other staff (i.e., nurses)
Support training for programs into visa and immigration conditions for trainees
Implement fair, unbiased recruitment strategies for all residency/fellowship applicants

SAGES Takeaway

- **Surgical educators and leaders must ensure a diverse and welcoming environment**. Leaders in healthcare are directly responsible for creating a diverse and inclusive work environment. This includes understanding the unique challenges faced by different learners, such as international medical graduates (IMGs), and recognizing the value they bring to the healthcare team.
- **IMGs play a vital role in the healthcare system**. IMGs make up a significant portion of licensed physicians in the USA, addressing physician shortages and enriching workforce diversity. They also contribute to healthcare in medically underserved areas, often providing culturally competent care to patients with similar backgrounds.
- **IMGs face unique challenges in training and practice**. IMGs encounter obstacles in the process of becoming licensed physicians in the USA, including complex exams, legal and immigration issues, and lower match rates. In surgical specialties, they may initially hold non-designated preliminary positions, facing uncertainty in continuing their training.
- **Proactive strategies are crucial for supporting IMGs**. To address the challenges faced by IMGs, specialized mentorship programs and initiatives tailored to their needs are essential. These programs can provide critical support, foster a sense of belonging, and empower both mentors and mentees to learn from diverse experiences in the medical workforce. Additionally, surgical societies and institutions should actively work toward increasing opportunities and representation for IMGs in leadership roles.

References

1. American Medical Association. How IMGs have changed the face of American medicine [WWW Document]. 2021. https://www.ama-assn.org/education/international-medical-education/how-imgs-have-changed-face-american-medicine. Accessed 19 Aug 2023.
2. Educational Commission for Foreign Medical Graduates, ECFMG Certification Overview [WWW Document]. 2023a. https://www.ecfmg.org/certification/#:~:text=Who%20is%20an%20IMG%3F,determines%20whether%20they%20are%20IMGs. Accessed 19 Aug 2023.
3. National Resident Matching Program. Charting outcomes in the match. International Medical Graduates; 2020.
4. American Medical Association. Backlog of H-1B visas for physicians affects patients in need [WWW Document]. 2018. https://www.ama-assn.org/education/international-medical-education/backlog-h-1b-visas-physicians-affects-patients-need. Accessed 14 May 2023.
5. Norcini JJ, van Zanten M, Boulet JR. The contribution of international medical graduates to diversity in the U.S. physician workforce: graduate medical education. J Health Care Poor Underserved. 2008;19:493–9. https://doi.org/10.1353/hpu.0.0015.
6. Torrey EF, Torrey BB. The US distribution of physicians from lower income countries. PLoS One. 2012;7:e33076. https://doi.org/10.1371/journal.pone.0033076.
7. Traverso G, McMahon GT. Residency training and international medical graduates: coming to America no more. JAMA. 2012;308:2193. https://doi.org/10.1001/jama.2012.14681.
8. Hing E, Lin S. Role of international medical graduates providing office-based medical care: United States, 2005-2006. NCHS Data Brief. 2009:1–8.
9. Norcini JJ, Boulet JR, Dauphinee WD, Opalek A, Krantz ID, Anderson ST. Evaluating the quality of care provided by graduates of international medical schools. Health Aff Proj Hope. 2010;29:1461–8. https://doi.org/10.1377/hlthaff.2009.0222.
10. Tsugawa Y, Jena AB, Orav EJ, Jha AK. Quality of care delivered by general internists in US hospitals who graduated from foreign versus US medical schools: observational study. BMJ. 2017;356:j273. https://doi.org/10.1136/bmj.j273.
11. Educational Commission for Foreign Medical Graduates. Fees Overview [WWW Document]. ECFMG. 2023b. https://www.ecfmg.org/fees/. Accessed 19 Aug 2023.
12. Pinsky WW. The importance of international medical graduates in the United States. Ann Intern Med. 2017;166:840–1. https://doi.org/10.7326/M17-0505.
13. Educational Commission for Foreign Medical Graduates. ECFMG News | Match Day Adds 7,500+ International Medical Graduates to U.S. GME Programs [WWW Document]. ECFMG. 2021. https://www.ecfmg.org/

news/2021/03/19/match-day-adds-7500-international-medical-graduates-to-u-s-gme-programs/. Accessed 14 Aug 2023.

14. Chen PG-C, Curry LA, Bernheim SM, Berg D, Gozu A, Nunez-Smith M. Professional challenges of non-U.S.-born international medical graduates and recommendations for support during residency training. Acad Med. 2011;86:1383–8. https://doi.org/10.1097/ACM.0b013e31823035e1.
15. Gozu A, Kern DE, Wright SM. Similarities and differences between international medical graduates and U.S. medical graduates at six Maryland community-based internal medicine residency training programs. Acad Med. 2009;84:385–90. https://doi.org/10.1097/ACM.0b013e318197321b.
16. Meghani SH, Rajput V. Perspective: the need for practice socialization of international medical graduates—an exemplar from pain medicine. Acad Med. 2011;86:571–4. https://doi.org/10.1097/ACM.0b013e318212e08b.
17. Rajesh A, Asaad M, Chandra A, McKenzie TJ, Farley DR. Outcomes of non-designated preliminary general surgery interns: a 25-year Mayo Clinic experience. Surgery. 2020;167:314–20. https://doi.org/10.1016/j.surg.2019.09.013.
18. Ritter KA, Anand RJ, Beard K, Edelman DA, Huth L, Namm J, Hope W, Allen S, Joshi A, Hildreth A, Tu C, Seavey CN, Vilchez V, Lipman J. Impact of surgery program characteristics on fate of non-designated preliminary surgery interns. J Surg Educ. 2020;77:e11–9. https://doi.org/10.1016/j.jsurg.2020.06.001.
19. Sarosi GA, Silver MA, Ben-David K, Behrns KE. Training outcomes of preliminary surgical residents in a university and veterans affairs surgical residency. JAMA Surg. 2014;149:1127. https://doi.org/10.1001/jamasurg.2014.2054.
20. Yoo PS, Kozol R, Reilly P, Seashore JH, Duffy A, Chandawarkar R, Longo WE. AVAS best clinical resident award (tied): fate of non-designated preliminary general surgery residents seeking a categorical residency position. Am J Surg. 2009;198:593–5. https://doi.org/10.1016/j.amjsurg.2009.07.024.
21. Moore RA, Rhodenbaugh EJ. The unkindest cut of all: are international medical school graduates subjected to discrimination by general surgery residency programs? Curr Surg. 2002;59:228–36. https://doi.org/10.1016/S0149-7944(01)00644-4.
22. Sullivan MC, Yeo H, Roman SA, Jones AT, Bell RH, Sosa JA. Discrepancies in training satisfaction and program completion among 2662 categorical and preliminary general surgery residents. Ann Surg. 2013;257:1174–80. https://doi.org/10.1097/SLA.0b013e3182718ef1.
23. Romero-Velez G, Rodriguez-Quintero JH, Moran-Atkin E, Lima DL, Malcher F, Camacho DR. Exploring the challenges for international medical graduates pursuing minimally invasive surgery training in the United

States and Canada: a cross-sectional analysis. JSLS. 2022;26(e2021):00084. https://doi.org/10.4293/JSLS.2021.00084.
24. Rajesh A, Asaad M, AlJamal YN, Azevedo RU, Stulak JM, Heller SF, Rivera M, Farley DR. International medical graduates are comparable to American medical graduates as general surgery interns. J Surg Res. 2021;258:239–45. https://doi.org/10.1016/j.jss.2020.08.043.
25. Lambert JR, Akinlade EY. Immigrant stereotypes and differential screening. Pers Rev. 2019;49:921–38. https://doi.org/10.1108/PR-06-2018-0229.
26. Murillo Zepeda C, Alcalá Aguirre FO, Luna Landa EM, Reyes Güereque EN, Rodríguez García GP, Diaz Montoya LS. Challenges for international medical graduates in the US graduate medical education and health care system environment: a narrative review. Cureus. 2022;14:e27351. https://doi.org/10.7759/cureus.27351.
27. Al Awamlh BAH. Alien J-1 physicians in a pandemic. JAMA Intern Med. 2021;181:743–4. https://doi.org/10.1001/jamainternmed.2021.0730.
28. Morris-Wiseman LF, Cañez C, Romero Arenas MA, Hsu C-H, Nfonsam VN. Race, gender, and international medical graduates: leadership trends in academic surgical societies. J Surg Res. 2022;270:430–6. https://doi.org/10.1016/j.jss.2021.09.043.
29. American Medical Association. International Medical Graduates (IMG) toolkit: introduction [WWW Document]. American Medical Association; 2022. https://www.ama-assn.org/education/international-medical-education/international-medical-graduates-img-toolkit-introduction. Accessed 14 Aug 2023.
30. Kehoe A, McLachlan J, Metcalf J, Forrest S, Carter M, Illing J. Supporting international medical graduates' transition to their host-country: realist synthesis. Med Educ. 2016;50:1015–32. https://doi.org/10.1111/medu.13071.
31. Odebunmi T, Jennifer MS, Erayil SE, Wongjarupong N. A trainee-led way to help international medical graduates meet the challenges of a U.S. residency. Acad Med J Assoc Am Med Coll. 2021;96:484–5. https://doi.org/10.1097/ACM.0000000000003797.

Enhancing the Surgical Value Chain Through Partnership with Industry

47

Sharona B. Ross

Introduction

Partnerships between the medical technology industry and surgeons can be both productive and disruptive, oftentimes to benefit stakeholders along the entire surgical value chain. Industry provides an active gateway for introducing the newest technologies that benefit operating rooms and laboratories, as well as enhance a surgeon's diagnostic support and clinical practice. Access to the most innovative and revolutionary technologies can assist a surgeon in improving patient outcomes, increasing their productivity, and enhancing the care team experience. This chapter is written in support of, "appropriate and equitable" industry partnerships with surgeons, together with certain caveats intended to safeguard the surgical community.

The industry-surgeon partnership should embrace a symbiotic dynamic whereby the industry can access surgeons for their creative design input, real-world operational insights, and user-experience feedback. Surgeons can enjoy access to the most disruptive and efficacious surgical technologies as they become available. Far too often, however, these partnerships are one-sided. Surgeons are far too ready to "give up" their rights to intel-

---

S. B. Ross (✉)
Digestive Health Institute, AdventHealth Tampa, Tampa, FL, USA

S. M. Johnson et al. (eds.), *The SAGES Manual of Strategy and Leadership*, https://doi.org/10.1007/978-3-031-62359-2_47

lectual property developments without the proper attribution, remuneration, and operational feedback. Consequently, industry often gains from these imbalanced relationships by utilizing the surgeon feedback on their products and offerings without providing substantive value back to participating surgeons. When these partnerships are set up appropriately and equitably, much can be gained on both sides in the pursuit of improved patient care and increased surgical productivity.

Going back to an era when all operations were performed "open," surgical instrument companies worked with surgeons to develop better vascular clamps, bowel clamps, needle holders, and so on. Industry functioned like a guild of skilled metal workers, conjuring up an image of modern-day blacksmiths. Industry did not need consultations with many surgeons in this period because the efforts in designing and manufacturing new instruments were quite rudimentary.

With the introduction of more advanced instrumentation, such as in the field of laparoscopy, the landscape of the surgeon-industry interface dramatically changed. Producers of laparoscopic equipment scrambled to interact with surgeons utilizing this emerging approach. From new visualization and imaging equipment to energy instruments to graspers, scissors, needle holders, complex stapling instruments, and accessories, laparoscopy initiated an entirely new surgical paradigm that would reshape how many procedures would be performed. Often, if not always, changes or advancements in instrumentation resulted from conversations and extensive observations in the operating rooms between industry and surgical team members. While widely acknowledged that the evolution and enhancement of surgical instrumentation have been dynamic fields, there have been instances where the engagement of academic and research thought leaders from the American surgical community might not have been as frequent. Traditionally situated in academic realms, these individuals sometimes operated on different innovation timelines. The private sector, however, was perceived as being both quick and nimble and eager to embrace change in favor of improved outcomes and greater productivity.

In the early days of the development and use of laparoscopic instruments, industry was often cited to be the motivating force behind the adoption of this emerging technology among hospitals and its surgeons. The acceleration of the adoption of laparoscopic technology was advanced by the enduring need for hospitals to capture greater surgical market share from their competitors. Industry often shared with their surgical counterparts that nearby competing hospitals were already adopting new minimally invasive surgical (MIS) approaches because patients preferred it, productivity (revenue) increased, and patient outcomes improved. As a result, surgeons were eager not to be left behind and pushed their hospitals to embrace change. This dynamic helped to give rise to the initial type of productive and symbiotic industry-surgeon relationship advanced in this chapter.

With the emergence of the laparoscopic innovation cycle, industry understood that they could control who attended and who could teach their "product-safety" courses. Surgeons were funneled into courses sponsored by industry to learn various laparoscopic techniques utilizing their own industry-specific products. In contrast, SAGES has played a crucial role in providing independent, balanced, and comprehensive training to surgeons, particularly evident in the laparoscopic cholecystectomy training programs conducted in the 1990s. These programs, operated in collaboration with the industry, maintained its focus on educational integrity, patient safety, and surgeon proficiency, ensuring surgeons were equipped with the necessary skillset without being bound by industry obligations [1].

With the advent and emergence of the robotic platform, however, the pressure from industry to adopt a new robotic innovation cycle became less formidable perhaps because there were (and still are) fewer surgical robotic companies than there were in the field of laparoscopy and perhaps because the value of adoption of minimally invasive technology had been much more established as both a market need and patient efficacy issue. While surgical outcomes with robotic surgery have been notably positive, it's crucial to acknowledge the accompanying challenges and critiques, such as cost-effectiveness, potential malfunction or disruption on the platform, and accessibility, to ensure a balanced perspective on its global emergence and impact. That is why it is now imperative to structure the industry-surgeon partnership in the most "appropriate and equitable" manner that ultimately benefits all stakeholders in the surgical value chain, including industry, the surgeons, their hospitals, and, above all, our patients.

Identifying at least six major types of relationships between surgeons and industry where guidance is needed, it's imperative to note that the perspectives and recommendations herein are formulated from an individual, comprehensive standpoint and require further discussion and consensus within the wider professional community:

1. Industry's support of continuing medical education (CME) programs and events
2. Industry's role in producing real-world evidence and publishing medical literature
3. Industry's support for local or "outside" (i.e., away from home) speaking, proctoring, and/or mentoring engagements.
4. Industry-sponsored consulting and design agreements
5. Industry-provided food, gifts, and travel for outside activities marginally or unrelated to medicine (in its broadest definition), such as fishing trips, dinners, golf outings, meetings in exotic places, etc.
6. Industry promoting surgeons as innovators in peer-to-peer events for the self-serving benefits of both parties

Industry Support of CME Programs and Events

Industry spends great sums on reaching out to physicians and patients, expecting a return on their expenditures. Pharmaceutical and other healthcare-related companies spent approximately $12–15 billion per year ($8000–15,000 per year, per physician) on marketing a decade ago [2]. That has now risen to $30 billion [3]. Today, Big Pharma shells out $20 billion yearly to endear physicians, not a trivial sum [3, 4]. The pharmaceutical industry in the USA spent $6.88 billion on direct-to-consumer advertising in 2021. The expenditure remained stable compared to 2020, when $6.86 billion was invested into Big Pharma ads. In 2020, television ad spending of the pharma industry accounted for 75% of the total ad spent on television. These ads often encourage patients to ask their providers about particular drugs or procedures; thereby, the companies influence the use of industry's products [3].

In a more direct approach, both pharmaceutical and medical device companies play pivotal roles in financially supporting continuing medical education (CME) programs [2, 5–7]. Many physicians commonly regard CME courses as their most valuable source for clinical information. In fact, they are well attended and highly sought after. Yet, there's a looming concern: the potential influence of sponsors over the content, which may sometimes reflect the interests or perspectives of these funding entities. In recent years, support for CME activities has increased tremendously. Historically, between 1992 and 2001, industry support of medical school-sponsored CME quintupled [9]. Ten years ago, 17% of CME funding came from industry, and according to the 2017 ACGME Annual Data report, pharmaceutical companies and medical device companies combined accounting for 28% of continuing medical education funding in 2017; today, their joint contribution hovers around 40% [5, 6]. Organizations that conduct CME programs claim that without financial support from industry, CME programs must rely on registration fees, which, when combined with travel and housing expenses, would make the programs unaffordable for many participants and could discourage attendance [3]. Physicians have expressed that they are not willing to pay higher registration fees, which may necessitate that CME activities require commercial support from pharmaceutical companies [7]. Interestingly, only 42% of physicians are willing to pay increased registration fees if it meant commercial support would be less or nonexistent [7].

However, evidence suggests that CME programs sponsored by industry are more biased (in favor of the sponsoring companies' products) than programs not sponsored by industry [6, 8] and may influence physicians' professional behavior (e.g., increased use of the sponsor's mechanical staplers) [4, 10, 11]. These findings raise the ethical concern of industry's influence on physicians who participate in industry-sponsored CME programs. It is, therefore, important for surgeons to be vigilant when developing program agendas. The agendas must be unbiased and data-driven and provide full disclosures. It is important to acknowledge the level of contribution of all supporting industry. Industry does not have to be discouraged from supporting CME programs, but full disclosure is essential for the program's integrity. If disclosure requirements are perceived as too burdensome or stringent, it may discourage industry participation, potentially impacting viability of beneficial educational programs. Clearly, balance is necessary without sacrificing integrity.

My own relationship with industry partners has been very productive and equitable. It has allowed me to develop and continue what has become an annual international surgical symposium to support women in surgery—the International Women in Surgery (WIS) Career Symposium. Industry support has been key to advancing and supporting women who aspire to become surgeons, as well as for surgeons in training, to attend the conference with minimal to no registration fees. Thousands of prospective surgeons have benefited from industry support, while, in turn, the industry sponsors have created strong brand recognition and furthered their corporate citizenship goals and commitment to surgical excellence. Of course, all conflicts of interest are clearly stated and published at each conference, and CME credits are not available for all presentations.

Industry's Role in Producing Real-World Evidence and Publishing Medical Literature

In recent years, a variety of published articles dealing with important broad-reaching topics of societal interest that impact medicine and patient care have been published. Topics included, among many, ideal physician behaviors and, germane to this article, institutional conflicts of interest (COIs), as well as a journal's approach to publication of industry-sponsored clinical research [2–12].

The legitimacy of interactions among industry sponsors of research, investigator-authors who communicate the information to medical journals, and the journals/editors who review and ultimately determine whether to publish the material is of paramount importance. In this age of transparency, disclosure of COIs has assumed great prominence in medical journals, but there is room for improvement, especially given the abundance of new online "journals." Transparency is not always clear, disclosure policies are varied, and their disclosure policy implementation (by journals and medical societies) is sometimes asymmetric and biased. Furthermore, it seems that not enough transparency has been required of authors [13]. In this context, it's important to note the guidelines set by SAGES regarding their Policy on Commercial Support and Conflict of Interest. These guidelines represent an effort by medical societies to establish clear standards for managing conflicts of interest and ensuring ethical conduct in industry-sponsored research. The SAGES policy also provides a framework for management and disclosure of COIs and ultimately is a step toward addressing challenges posed by the abundance of new online "journals," where transparency and disclosure policies can be varied or asymmetrically applied [14].

Occasionally, industry will hire professional writers (termed ghostwriters) to draft papers concerning clinical trials sponsored by industry and invite academic physicians to accept authorship of the articles (without acknowledgment of the compensated writer) to increase their credibility. These "guest" authors supposedly made little contribution to the research, analysis, interpretation of the data, and writing of the manuscript, an unacceptable practice [13]. Authorship criteria of the ICMJE (International Committee of Medical Journal Editors) state that "Authorship credit should be based on:

1. Substantial contributions to conception and design, acquisition of data, or analysis and interpretation of data.
2. Drafting the article or revising it critically for important intellectual content.
3. Final approval of the version to be published.
4. Agreement to be accountable for all aspects of the work, including accuracy and integrity of any part of the work.

5. Authors should meet conditions 1, 2, 3, and 4. All individuals who meet the first criterion should have the opportunity to participate in the review, drafting, and final approval of the manuscript."

A conflict of interest (COI) has been defined as "a set of conditions in which professional judgment concerning a primary interest (such as a patient's welfare or the validity of research) tends to be unduly influenced by a secondary interest (such as financial gain)." COIs do not necessarily indicate the occurrence of any improper behavior, much less scientific misconduct, analogous to a state of potential energy. In 2001, the ICMJE published a policy/editorial, "Sponsorship, Authorship, and Accountability," that specified principles for investigators working with industry to ensure investigator access to study data and control of the decision to publish study results. It is not difficult to understand the degree of extra scrutiny of industry-sponsored research by reviewers and editors, but the extent and the method of doing so are important to ensure that work deserving publication is not censored. However, as surgeons, we must retain the trust and confidence of patients and the public.

One journal has taken a different approach to preventing ghostwriting and guest authoring. *Neurology* announced in 2008 a new policy wherein anyone who writes the first draft of a manuscript accepted for publication will be a named author [13]. The writer may not merit authorship per ICMJE criteria. Authorship is two-faceted: it provides credit and recognition for work done before publication, and it assigns responsibility to explain and defend the work after publication.

1. Medical writing is a valuable, accepted function that can assist in the timely, well-organized, clear communication of scientific studies.
2. Medical writing or editorial assistance that does not merit named authorship should be acknowledged.
3. The source of funding support for all work should be noted.

4. We would be taking the battle against COI to the extreme if we adopted a policy in which we discounted expert opinion solely because of a *potential* conflict of interest.

All policies on COI should involve all faculty, part-time faculty, postgraduate residents in training, and all fellows, staff, students, and trainees. Essentially, everyone employed or utilizing facilities of the institution should subjugate to these policies. Surgeons, by nature, are very busy and all help will be appreciated by them, but the caveats are obvious.

Industry Support in Local or "Outside" (i.e., Away from Home) Speaking, Proctoring, and/or Mentoring Engagements

Industry seeks surgeons to profit from their knowledge, their reputation, and their skills. Usually, such surgeons are busy clinicians with a positive firsthand experience with specific devices. They generally hold leadership positions in their institutions and beyond and are willing to share their experiences and train other surgeons. It is important that surgeons be aware of the communication of Special Fraud Alert which was issued by the Department of Health and Human Services on November 16, 2020. This Special Fraud Alert was to comment on company-sponsored events at which a physician or other healthcare professional makes a speech or presentation to other healthcare professionals about a drug or device or a disease state on behalf of the company. From 2017 to 2020, it is estimated that such events cost industry $2 billion. These events may violate "kickback" statutes [15].

Their fraud alert was issued to highlight certain inherent risks of remuneration related to speaker programs. Drug and device companies and healthcare professionals should consider these risks when assessing whether to offer, pay, solicit, or receive remuneration related to speaker programs. This Special Fraud Alert was not intended to discourage meaningful healthcare professional training and education; it just pointed out the need to be careful, transparent, honest, and open.

Industry-Sponsored Consulting and Design Agreements

Consulting arrangements with industry can favorably impact a surgeon's productivity, improve patient care and teaching methods, as well as benefit the entire surgical field. As a consultant, surgeons have an opportunity to develop a more productive and equitable relationship with industry together with securing greater access to new technologies, engaging in direct collaboration with engineers, and providing critical data and empirical feedback to hone product development.

A cautionary note. Surgeons who enter into consulting agreements should thoroughly understand and adhere to policies of their employer. Furthermore, it's crucial to align with the Accreditation Council for Continuing Medical Education (ACCME) Standards for Integrity and Independence, especially when it comes to managing financial relationships in consulting roles [16]. Moreover, SAGES has previously outlined some considerations regarding consulting fees, which may offer valuable insights for surgeons entering consulting agreements [17]. The SAGES White Paper further explores these relationships, which may encompass grant support, salary, speaker honoraria, consultant fees, ownership interest, and their proper disclosure and management for maintaining ethical standards in consulting engagements [18]. If there are no policies, an IRB review and approval should be obtained. It is important that agreements with industry do not interfere or conflict as a matter of law, policy, or practice with the requirements established by the employer.

Guidelines on Accepting Industry-Provided Perquisites and Participating in Outside Activities

These topics should be self-evident. While striving for an appropriate and equitable relationship with industry, it's important to exercise discernment in accepting gifts or favors that could potentially tarnish your reputation or that of your employer. For instance, while modest meals or refreshments provided during professional interactions may be acceptable, extravagant gifts or favors should be avoided as they can create a perception of undue influence or bias, making surgeons beholden to industry to some extent. This, in turn, could lead to partiality toward certain industry sponsors. If uncertain, it's advisable to perform due diligence, seek guidance from your department director and human resources, or even consult with an attorney to ensure compliance and professional integrity.

Surgeons as Innovators in Peer-to-Peer Events with Industry Support: The Impact on Healthcare

I hope to convey this story with accuracy and fairness. During the cold war, Felicien Steichen and Mark Ravich, two surgeons from the USA, traveled to Moscow to attend a medical meeting. They were both of Eastern European descent and both spoke Russian. The exact purpose of their travel is shrouded in some mystery and mystique beyond the scope of the story I need to tell. Some suggest that they were agents involved in covert activities, acting as informants during a tense political period. While in Moscow, they encountered the first stapling devices modeled for human use. They wanted to bring some of these staplers back to the USA but were forbidden to leave Russia with Russian intellectual property. Their guide, a medical student, took them to a local shop that produced these staplers, allowing them to purchase several units. It's worth pausing here to acknowledge the ethical dilemmas posed by transporting these staplers out of Russia, given the intellectual property laws of the time. Upon returning to the USA, Steichen and Ravich, after making some improvements to the design and functionality of the staplers, formed the US Surgical Corporation, now a precursor to a division of Medtronic, with Mr. Leon Hirsch. This story, while demonstrating the potential for surgeons to catalyze paradigm shifts in healthcare and surgery, especially in collaboration with the industry, also highlights the complex and sometimes ethically challenging paths innovations can traverse. "Opportunity favors the prepared mind," but it also requires an awareness and navigation of ethical boundaries.

Since its inception, the US Surgical Corp., and its corporate successors, has stood as an early example of how a productive and equitable industry-surgeon partnership might be established. They have worked in many ways to improve the field of surgery with its introduction of surgical staplers to skin closure staplers to staplers used in anastomoses and beyond. Along the way, the US Surgical Corp. trained thousands of surgeons to utilize their products safely and efficiently, a great service to healthcare, patients, and surgeons. It led the revolution into laparoscopy, training thousands of surgeons on the safe utilization of laparoscopes, laparoscopic instruments, clip appliers, and more. Practicing surgeons were often the inspiration for progress and the source for innovation. Both parties, surgeons and the US Surgical Corp., prospered greatly by their synergistic relationship. Surgeons were a vital partner in the success of the US Surgical Corp. and vice versa. Specifically, surgeons profited by contractual financial support, support for professional societal meetings, research support, educational grants, and many other ways. The US Surgical Corp. profited in their relationship with surgeons by having broad-based exposure to their customers and by the expertise the surgeons brought to the relationship. The relationship between surgeons and the US Surgical Corp. represents a true "win-win" relationship that hopefully can be emulated and replicated into the future. In our efforts to curtail conflicts of interest, we as providers and surgeons cannot exclude industry except at our own peril and that of our patients.

In reflecting on industry-surgeon partnerships, my relationship with Intuitive Surgical, Inc. provides a timely, current example of an appropriate and equitable industry-surgeon partnership, particularly in the domain of robotic surgery over the last decade, with tremendous educational and clinical support from Intuitive Surgical, Inc. This involvement has facilitated various opportunities, such as mentorship, access to the latest technologies, and networking with global surgical peers. However, sharing this experience is not an endorsement, but a depiction of one instance of such collaboration. It's important to highlight the overarching and universal takeaway that transcends individual experiences: the committed adherence to principles of transparency, mutual benefit, and ethical guidelines in all industry-surgeon interactions. Throughout my journey, maintaining transparency about my partnership and acknowledging potential perceptions of conflict of interest have been critical to ensuring that collaborations are conducted ethically and with integrity. It is important to state that our partnership has notably been a "two-way street."

In Summary

The relationship between surgeons and industry should exist as an appropriate and equitable partnership. A surgeon's partnership with industry can be (and should be) extremely productive and rewarding. Of course, great care must be given to how these relationships develop so that surgeons don't give away their intellectual property rights and are fairly compensated for their efforts. Surgeons should never be in a position to generate a manuscript with an undue (or inappropriate) level of industry aid and input, particularly if they don't know how the data was compiled and can't speak to or defend the content of the manuscript. Once again, care and utmost attention must be given to avoid potential conflicts of interest and hospital/institutional policy violations.

This document has been drafted in support of furthering and fine-tuning industry-surgeon partnerships and not to discourage developing relationships with industry in general. Working with industry can be fun, exciting, and very rewarding. Just let everyone and anyone in positions of responsibility and beyond know, preferably in advance, what you are doing, with whom you are doing it, under what terms and circumstances, and to what end. Be transparent.

SAGES Takeaway

- Collaborations between the medical technology industry and surgeons offer opportunities to introduce innovative ideas, enhance diagnostic support, and improve patient outcomes.
- For a successful partnership, a symbiotic dynamic should exist, where the industry gains creative design input and operational insights from surgeons.
- The history of industry-surgeon collaborations evolved from basic surgical instruments to more complex technologies which help to reshape surgical practices in efforts to improve patient outcomes.

- While industry support is important for continuing medical education and innovation, surgeons should approach industry collaborations with transparency.
- Surgeons should avoid conflicts of interest, ensure fair compensation, and acknowledge potential pitfalls and complexities to maintain the integrity of the surgeon-industry relationship.

References

1. SAGES. Guidelines for the clinical application of laparoscopic biliary tract surgery. https://www.sages.org/publications/guidelines/guidelines-for-the-clinical-application-of-laparoscopic-biliary-tract-surgery/.
2. Blumenthal D. Doctors and drug companies. N Engl J Med. 2004;351:1885–90.
3. Mole B. Big Pharma shells out $20B each year to schmooze docs, $6B on drug ads. https://arstechnica.com/science/2019/01/healthcare-industry-spends-30b-on-marketing-most-of-it-goes-to-doctors/.
4. Schhwartz LM, Woloshin S. Medical marketing in the United States, 1997-2016. JAMA. 2019;321:80–96.
5. Relman AS. Separating continuing medical education from pharmaceutical marketing. JAMA. 2001;285:2009–12.
6. Wazana A. Physicians and the pharmaceutical industry: is a gift ever just a gift? JAMA. 2000;283:373–80.
7. Industry sponsored CME: controversies surrounding pharma funding. 2019. https://www.cmelist.com/industry-sponsored-cme-controversies-surrounding-pharma-funding/.
8. Packer S, Parke DW II. Ethical concerns in industry support of continuing medical education: the con side. Arch Ophthalmol. 2004;122:773–6.
9. Leichter SB. Continuing medical education in diabetes: the impending crisis (the business of diabetes). Clin Diabetes. 2004;22:174–7.
10. Davis DA. CME and the pharmaceutical industry: two worlds, three views, four steps. Can Med Assoc J. 2004;171:149–50.
11. Wilson FS. Continuing medical education: ethical collaboration between sponsor and industry. Clin Orthop Relat Res. 2003;412:33–7.
12. Holmer AF. Industry strongly supports continuing medical education. JAMA. 2001;285:2012–4. Erratum in: JAMA. 2001;285:2451.
13. Hirsch LJ. Conflicts of interest, authorship, and disclosures in industry-related scientific publications: the tort bar and editorial oversight of medical journals. Mayo Clin Proc. 2009;84(9):811–21. https://doi.org/10.1016/S0025-6196(11)60491-6.

14. Society of American Gastrointestinal and Endoscopic Surgeons (SAGES). Policy on Commercial Support and Conflict of Interest. https://www.sages.org/accme/policy-commercial-support-conflict-interest/.
15. Special fraud alert: speaker programs. Washington, DC: Office of the Inspector General.
16. ACCME. Standards for integrity and independence in accredited continuing education. https://accme.org/accreditation-rules/standards-for-integrity-independence-accredited.
17. Chekan EG, Muryama K, Provost D, et al. Society of American Gastrointestinal Endoscopic Surgeons (SAGES) guidelines on continuing medical education and financial relationships. Surg Endosc. 2006;20:1168–70. https://doi.org/10.1007/s00464-006-0077-5.
18. Shadduck P, Sylla P, Schwarz E, Reinke C, Denk P, Ginsberg S, Asbun H, Pryor A. SAGES perspective: professional medical associations, commercial interests, and conflicts of interest. Surg Endosc. 2023;37(4):2517–27. https://doi.org/10.1007/s00464-023-09897-9. Epub 2023 Mar 14.

Diversity, Equity, and Inclusion: Transparency, Measures, and Accountability

48

Shaneeta M. Johnson and Henry Lin

What Is Diversity?

Diversity has been defined as the "presence of different human characteristics in a group of people" [1]. There are two basic categories of these characteristics: immutable (primary characteristics) and mutable (secondary characteristics). Primary characteristics include "race, color, ethnicity, national origin, sex assigned at birth, sexual orientation, age, mental and physical abilities" [2]. Secondary characteristics "may vary in importance at different points in life," including socioeconomic status/income, nationality, education, language skills, profession, religion, work or military experience, work style, political beliefs, some physical characteristics, marital status, family and parental status,

S. M. Johnson (✉)
Department of Surgery, Morehouse School of Medicine, Atlanta, GA, USA

Satcher Health Leadership Institute, Morehouse School of Medicine, Atlanta, GA, USA
e-mail: shajohnson@msm.edu

H. Lin
Medical Corps, US Navy, Canton, CN, USA

S. M. Johnson et al. (eds.), *The SAGES Manual of Strategy and Leadership*, https://doi.org/10.1007/978-3-031-62359-2_48

communication styles (including language (different dialects) and speech), learning styles, and geographic location [2].

Equity vs. Equality

Equity has been defined as equal opportunity with appropriately adjusted resources for historical disadvantages while maintaining quality standards for high performance with efficient and successful fulfillment of individual potential [1]. On the other hand, equality most often refers to everyone having equality of opportunity, i.e., "everyone has a right to apply for a position regardless of their race, ethnicity, sexual orientation, gender identity, or social status" [3]. Equity of the healthcare workforce differs from but is related to the healthcare equity of patients. Health equity has been prioritized for accrediting bodies like the Joint Commission and payors like Medicare [4, 5].

Inclusivity

Inclusivity is the "practice of providing equal access to resources and support to all members of a group, regardless of their background or individual characteristics" [1]. Furthermore, inclusivity or "inclusion exists when traditionally marginalized individuals and groups feel a sense of belonging and are empowered to participate in majority culture as full and valued members of the community, shaping and redefining that culture in different ways [2, 6]." Inclusivity does not exclude the previously traditional dominant stereotype.

Inequities in Medicine

DEI in Academic Medicine

Medical school faculty are predominantly male and white. As leadership progresses higher in academic ranks there is a widening of the gap of achievement of rank and tenure for women and underrepresented in Medicine (URiM) minorities. In 2017, women accounted for just 11% of full professors in surgery [7]. Asian women represented 1.3% of full professors [7]. There were 10 African-American women as full professors (0.26% of full professors), 5 LatinX female full professors (0.13% of full professors), and 318 full professor white women (8.2%) [7]. AAMC data on leadership in academic medicine demonstrated that while 54.6% of medical school matriculants in 2023 were women, only 23% of clinical department chairs and 27% of medical school deans were women [8–10]. 18% of medical school deans were under represented in medicine faculty [11]. Further data demonstrated that only 8% of surgery department chairs were women; thus far, there have been three African-American women surgical chairs [12, 13].

There is a significant lack of diversity in the surgical workforce, including URiM physicians, female surgeons, LGBTQ surgeons, and rural surgeons [14]. Female general surgeons, African-American surgeons, and LatinX surgeons account for a minority of surgeons. African-Americans account for 5% of physicians, while LatinX physicians account for 4% of the physician population [14].

Data demonstrates that black and LatinX residents have lower matriculation rates but experience higher rates of adverse actions [9, 15]. National data shows that 70% of black, 46% of Asian, and 25% of LatinX surgical residents report they have experienced discrimination compared to 13% of white residents [16]. URiM learners cite discrimination, prejudice, and feelings of isolation as causes related to their ethnicity that contribute to adverse experiences in medical school [17, 18]. Additionally, non-white self-identification is an independent predictor of a lower likelihood of being selected for surgical residency interviews [19].

In 2009, the LCME set standards to increase institutional diversity and pathway programs (LCME) [20]. Meanwhile, medical schools targeted a more holistic admissions process with a greater focus on the applicant's potential to contribute to the learning environment and less reliance on test scores and grades [21].

However, the question remains, are we moving the needle? Have these DEI programs served their intended purposes to increase the diversity of the healthcare workforce? Are we ensuring that our programs are not merely window dressing but, indeed, are achieving DEI?

Studies demonstrate a persistent failure to improve diversity. After 40 years, a study in the *New England Journal of Medicine* revealed that we have, in fact, not moved the needle. While black male medical students accounted for 3.1% of the national student body in 1978, they represented only 2.9% in 2019 [22]. Without the four HBCU medical schools, that percentage would be 2.4% [22]. Native Americans accounted for less than 1% of the medical student body in 2019 [22]. While African-Americans account for 30% of the U S population and the Latinx population accounts for approximately 18%, they account for 5% and 4% of our physician population [14]. Unfortunately, the trend we are seeing is in the wrong direction. In response, the AAMC released two reports addressing the current paradigm—"Reshaping the Journey: American Indians and Alaska Natives in Medicine" and "Altering the Course: Black Males in Medicine [14]." Recent data also demonstrate higher rates of adverse actions on underrepresented trainees during residency, including dismissal [15, 23]. This is particularly concerning considering the lack of diversity in the medical workforce pipeline. Haruno et al demonstrated that female residents had a higher relative risk of attrition than their male counterparts, and URiM trainees had a significantly higher relative risk of attrition than non-URiM trainees. African American residents had the highest attrition rates of 10.6% [23].

DEI in Research Funding

URiM faculty have lower grant funding rates by NIH and other funding agencies [7]. It is critical to increase the percentage of research and funding of URiM faculty to improve the diversity of the surgical workforce.

Diverse Workforce Impact

A diverse healthcare workforce is essential and has demonstrated significant benefits. However, few ethnic minority patients share race or ethnicity with their physicians. The diverse workforce shortage is a significant contributor. Congruence of race or ethnicity of patient and healthcare provider has been associated with improved health outcomes. These include a 50% decrease in the mortality rate for black newborns if cared for by black physicians, improved adherence to treatment regimens, and potential impact on cardiovascular outcomes for black men cared for by black physicians [24–26]. Further study has demonstrated that female patients were more likely to survive a myocardial infarction if their emergency physician was also female [27].

Additionally, underrepresented minorities are more likely to serve disadvantaged and underserved communities [28, 29]. These include low-resource, Medicaid, non-English, and under-/uninsured communities [28, 29].

How Do We Achieve Equity?

DEI Initiatives Within Medical Organizations

Several recent concerted initiatives by medical and surgical institutions have been directed toward increasing diversity, equity, and inclusion within these organizations. Recognizing the need for increased diversity and inclusion, the LCME introduced new standards (LCME Element 3.3) in 2009 to increase institutional diversity and pathway programs [20]. Similarly, medical schools adopted a more holistic admissions process, relying less on grades and considering further the applicant's potential addition to the medical school class [21]. Unfortunately, these efforts have not shown great success as recent studies demonstrate fewer African-American males entering medical school than 40 years ago and fewer African-American male surgical residents today [22, 30]. Similarly, other ethnic groups such as Native Americans and LatinX populations also show little advances in diversity within the medical workforce [14].

We must critically evaluate our environments, evaluating for the presence of implicit and explicit biases, structural racism, stereotyping, unequal and unfair promotion practices, lack of inclusion, and adverse actions. Data demonstrates that non-white faculty have lower promotion rates than white faculty and face racism and bias from peers, superiors, and patients [14].

It is impossible to outlaw bias. The typical approach is a classic command and control approach to introducing diversity and equity [31]. Diversity training may be window dressing or ineffective unless participation is voluntary. While grievance procedures may provide an avenue to highlight or expose biases, they may also worsen bias by unfairly exposing the complainant. Additionally, minorities have been shown to be rated lower on performance readings ratings, and among the almost 90,000 discrimination complaints to the EEOC in 2015, nearly 45% included a charge of retaliation [32].

Mindset and culture change are complex. It is a slow, methodical process that requires a shared desire for change, assessment of institutional culture, and climate capacity for diversity and inclusion.

The 2021–2022 medical school admission cycle demonstrated significant gains in diversity and inclusion. There was a 21% rise in African-American students, an 8.3% rise in Asian students, and a 7.1% rise in LatinX student applications. More applicants were non-white, and there was a corresponding rise in LatinX and African-American matriculants (12.7% from 12.0% and 11.3% from 9.5%, respectively). Women accounted for 56.8% of applicants, 55.5% of matriculants, and 52.7% of total enrollment [33].

There are undoubtedly several possible reasons for these gains. First, the global pandemic of COVID-19 may have increased interest in the field of medicine. Second, there were reduced costs related to decreased travel requirements during this application cycle. Finally, we have seen an increased awareness of social inequities in the past several years. This increased awareness has brought about a significant response from institutions and organizations, including SAGES, the Southeast Surgical Congress, the American Surgeon Journal, the American College of Surgeons, and the American Board of Surgery [34–37]. Implementation of diversity and inclusion curriculums and implicit bias training is imperative to improving the cultural competencies of the surgical department.

Many surgical organizations have implemented DEI initiatives to increase representation and inclusivity. These include the following:

Diversity and Antiracism Task Forces

In 2020, the American College of Surgeons convened a task force on racial issues to develop antiracism guidelines [38]. The American Board of Surgery also conducted a structured retreat to provide insight into racism within the field of surgery [37].

Increased Inclusion in Committee and Organizational Leadership

Many organizations, including SAGES, have made concerted efforts to increase diverse participation in their committee and executive leadership [39, 40]. Additionally, the creation of speaker bureaus such as the SAGES Speaker Bureau may lead to increased representation of diversity among program participants.

Creation of Diversity and Inclusion Committees

Many organizations have adopted diversity and inclusion committees to provide a voice and ensure the inclusion of all groups within the organization. In 2017, SAGES developed the We "R" SAGES committee as its diversity committee.

The committee has developed several initiatives, including leadership development programs, climate surveys, and diversity leadership retreats [41].

Climate Surveys

SAGES and other organizations have utilized membership climate surveys to obtain critical feedback to improve diversity, equity, and inclusion within the organization [41].

Journal Symposiums

Journals such as *The American Surgeon* have composed symposiums on increasing surgical diversity and inclusion [36].

Mentorship and Leadership Development Programs

To increase diversity and inclusion practices within leadership, surgical organizations such as the American College of Surgeons, Association of Women Surgeons, Southern Surgical Association, and SAGES have introduced mentorship and leadership development programs such as the Fundamental of Leadership Development Course and the Southern Surgical Association Leadership Development Program [34, 35, 42].

Examination of Fair Journal Practices

In response to a call for increased diversity within editorial practices, the current and former editors-in-chief of *JAMA* issued a call to action for surgical journals to increase their diversity within the editorial process. The call was very successful, with more than 50% agreement by the editors of surgical journals [43].

Additional efforts will be required to improve DEI within surgical organizations further. These include strategic direct contact (SDC) , which incorporates mentorship and exposure to representative organizations.

Solving the Diversity, Equity, and Inclusion Dilemma: Justice, Equity, Diversity, and Inclusion (JEDI) and Strategic Directed Contact (SDC)

We should include strategic directed contact (SDC) to achieve our DEI ideals (Fig. 48.1). SDC comprises directed engagement of younger generations, mentoring, increased strategic contact and exposure to underrepresented and minority organizations, and accountability of organizations.

It is imperative to engage diverse populations early. Increased engagement may decrease the leaks in the pipeline which have been shown to provide significant obstacles to providing a diverse healthcare workforce. Pathway programs such as Nth Dimension

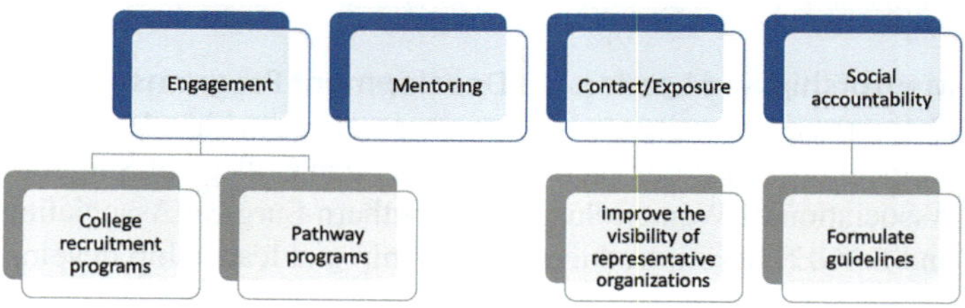

Fig. 48.1 Strategic directed contact

and MSM Surgery Reach have demonstrated success in reaching young, diverse populations in high school and college to improve the visibility of representative organizations and provide guidance and a pathway to medical and scientific fields [44, 45].

Mentorship is necessary to reduce bias, engage leaders, and increase leadership diversity [31]. Formal mentorship has been shown to increase diversity in leadership within organizations. Approximately only 10% of firms have mentoring programs. While white men tend to find mentors independently, women and minorities more often require help from formal mentorship programs.

We need to further our collaborations and support organizations supporting women, minorities, and other underrepresented surgeons, such as the Association of Women Surgeons, the Society of Black Academic Surgeons, the National Medical Association, the Society of Asian Academic Surgeons, the Society of Out Surgeons, and the Latino Surgical Society. Increased representation is vital to improving the pipeline of diverse surgeons. Recent studies have demonstrated that only 8% of department chairs of surgery are female [46]. There have been only three African-American female surgery chairs [12]. It is important to avoid tokenism in hiring practices and ensure the presence of women, minorities, and other diverse populations in positions of power.

With our JEDI efforts, we must include SDC and culture change. The social justice movement has proven what is possible with increased awareness. SDC has been proven to be successful in improving diversity and inclusion efforts. We must implement policy changes and guidelines to ensure the longevity of our actions and desired outcomes.

Transparency and Accountability

How to Create Effective Diversity Structures vs. Window Dressing

Transparency, inclusion, and accountability are critical to developing effective organizational diversity infrastructures. The commitment of the organization's leadership to tackle challenges of diversity that arise and implement diversity, equity, and inclusion as core values is imperative. The leadership's willingness to be open, inclusive, and responsive is vital. Four pillars for success are outlined in "Why Greater Transparency is Key to a Winning DEI Strategy" [47]. These include using data and metrics to inform strategy, alignment of DEI objectives with organizational goals, clear and transparent communication, and commitment to continuous improvement.

Leadership and Organizational Commitment to a Culture of Inclusion

The organizational or institutional leadership must demonstrate a commitment to a culture of inclusion. This commitment is more profound than the climate surveys, vision statements, and development of diversity committees. It requires an organizational culture shift. Leadership must demonstrate intent to develop a culture of inclusion and build institutional capacity for change, including recruiting allies and change agents [48].

SAGES leadership has held meetings to further the understanding and initiatives of diversity and inclusion within its membership and foster transparency and accountability within the organization. This organizational flexibility is needed to institute long-standing values of inclusion within any organization. Other surgical organizations have created liaisons from the diversity committee to all committees to ensure that, at every level, diversity, equity, and inclusion are considered and that these tenets are embedded as a part of the organization's infrastructure.

Metrics, Accountability, and Transparency

Climate Survey

In 2017, the We R SAGES committee, the predecessor to the present SAGES Diversity, Leadership & Professional Development (DLPD) committee and led by Dr. Dana Telem, sent out climate surveys to more than 700 committee members in the second largest surgical organization in the USA. With a response greater than 50%, overall satisfaction was 8.1/10, and 93.6% did not experience bias within the organization [41]. There were, however, three areas of concern noted: 1) transparency of advancement within the organization, 2) value, and identity of the organization that had transitioned minimally invasive techniques into mainstream general surgery practice, and 3) concerns for biases further than gender and ethnicity and incorporating age, surgical specialty, non-surgeon status, international membership, and private vs. academic practice [41]. With these areas identified, SAGES leadership enacted several approaches to improve diversity and inclusion, including mentorship development programs, participation in formal leadership development programs with other surgical societies, transparency and clarity on committee member onboarding, and development of the SAGES CV, which details a member's contribution to the organization in a transparent manner [49]. Additional efforts included adding programs (such as health policy and advocacy) and committees for groups that may have historically felt excluded (e.g., acute care surgeons and private practice), evaluation of the website for inclusivity, unconscious bias training for SAGES leadership, the institution of a strategic retreat for planning and proactively ensuring diversity within SAGES committees, and meeting session chairs and speakers [49].

Diversity, Equity, and Inclusion Indices

Another method to achieve transparent healthcare equality is via indices such as the Health Equality Index [2] and the SAGES DEI Index. Accepted and validated metrics are needed to measure success and identify areas of weakness.

SAGES DEI Index

The SAGES DEI Index, led by Dr. Shaneeta Johnson and the DLPD Committee, is being developed to comprehensively evaluate the DEI values of healthcare organizations and to allow for the implementation of initiatives to impact surgical outcomes. The DEI Index will address the following tenets:

1. There is a knowledge gap within organizations regarding the effective implementation of diversity, equity, and inclusion (climate assessment).
2. Lack of diversity and inclusion has been shown to impact provider satisfaction.
3. Surgical outcomes and patient experience are impacted by a lack of diversity and inclusion.

The index will target healthcare organizations, academic training programs, surgical societies, accrediting bodies, patient advocacy groups, insurers, and payors. The data will evaluate the socioeconomic factors, social determinants of health within the patient population, diversity of leadership within the organization, hiring practices, comparison of demographics of providers, patients, and leadership, as well as outcomes, partnerships, and collaborations.

The internal pilot has focused on three areas:

1. Leadership—review of the leadership body and structure of the SAGES organization
2. Membership—evaluation of the diversity makeup of the SAGES membership via recent demographic survey
3. Scholarship—determination of gender and other diversity of conference speakers and presentations via gender representation study underway

A critical view of an organization's commitment to diversity, equity, and inclusion is vital to addressing gaps and improving strengths.

SAGES Initiatives to Address Diversity, Equity, and Inclusion

SAGES has initiated several programs and initiatives to address diversity, equity, and inclusion. These include the following:

Organizational Climate Survey

SAGES Climate Survey, first launched in 2017, has been relaunched. The results will be compared to the initial survey discussed above and utilized to determine areas of improvement and areas to be addressed.

Social Justice and Health Equity Award

In 2021, SAGES launched the Social Justice and Health Equity Award. This award recognizes individuals who have worked to personally address healthcare inequities due to long-standing systemic racism or social injustice. The awardees have represented significant health equity champions. A noted tenet of organizational culture change is the use of awards and other tokens to reinforce and reward culturally appropriate and desired behaviors.

Increased Gender and URIM Representation

SAGES has increased its efforts and proactively sought and addressed diverse representation in its leadership and membership. Since its inception in 1981, the leadership has been predominately white men. However, in recent years, there has been increased diversity of gender and ethnicity represented in the board and committee leadership of the organization (Figs. 48.2, 48.3, 48.4, 48.5, 48.6, and 48.7). There have been four female presidents -Jo Buskye (2010), Aurora Pryor (2019), Liane Feldman (2021), and Patricia Sylla (2023). There have been two African-American presidents - Kenneth Forde (1983) and Patricia

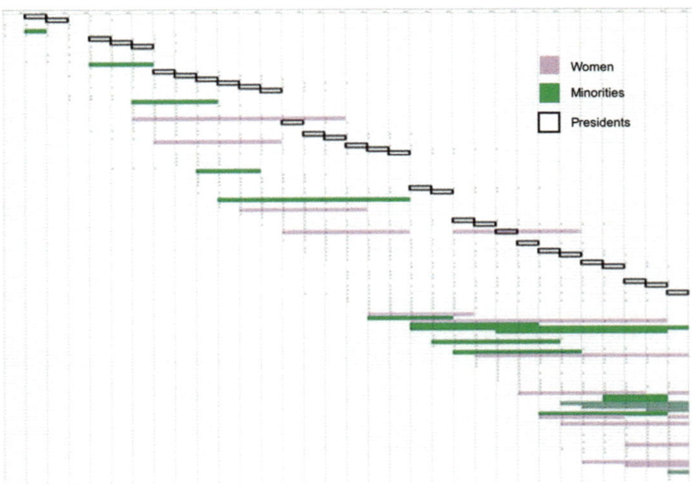

Fig. 48.2 SAGES leadership gender diversity. SAGES leadership from 1987 to 2018. Each row represents a surgeon and their time on the board by year. The black outlines represent the presidents [50]

Sylla (2023), one African-American female president - Patricia Sylla (2023), and one Hispanic president - Horacio Asbun (2021) within SAGES.

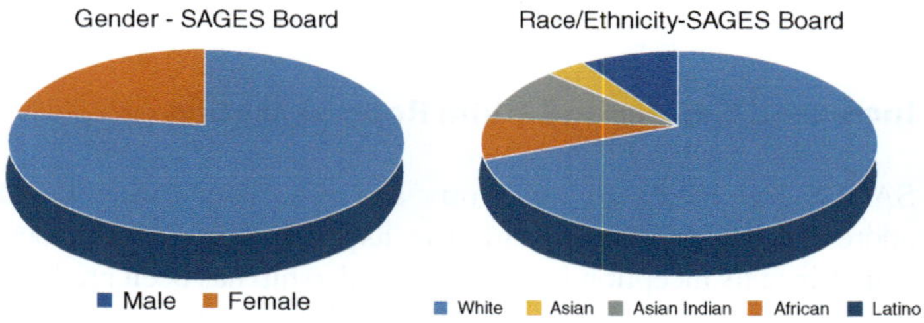

Fig. 48.3 SAGES leadership gender diversity. SAGES Board of Governors representation by gender and race [50]

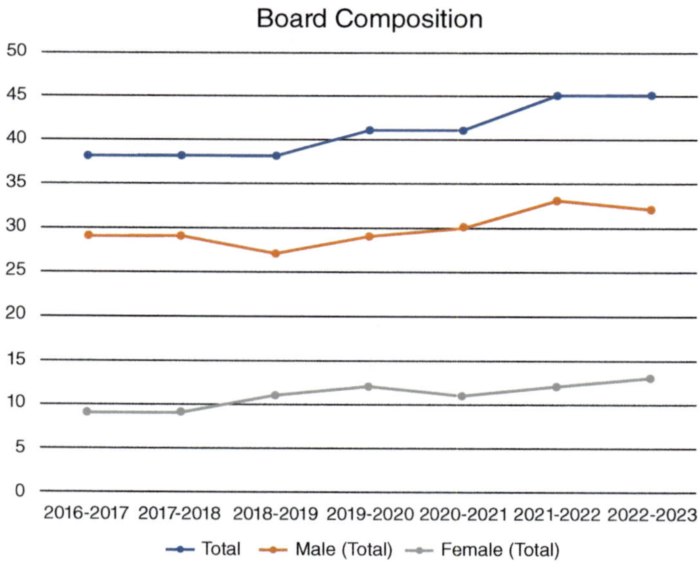

Fig. 48.4 Gender composition of SAGES Board

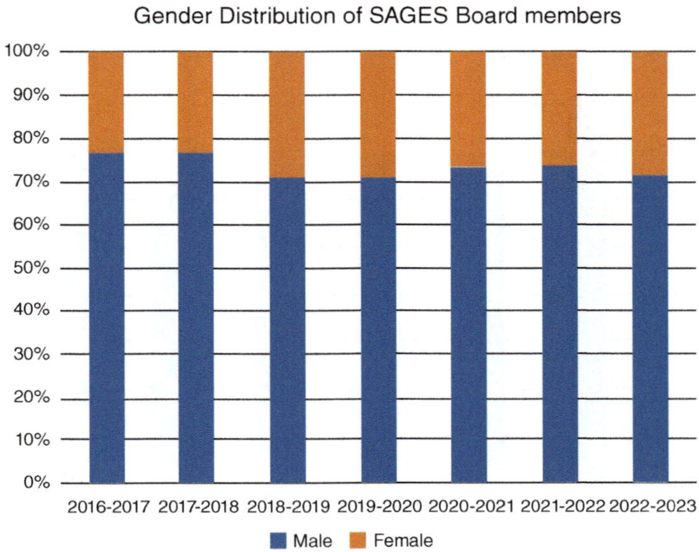

Fig. 48.5 Percent gender representation on SAGES Board

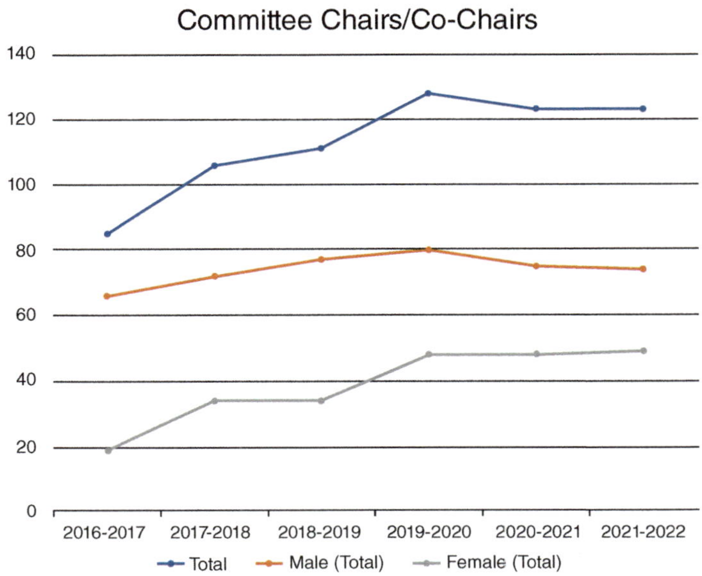

Fig. 48.6 Gender composition of SAGES committee chairs and cochairs

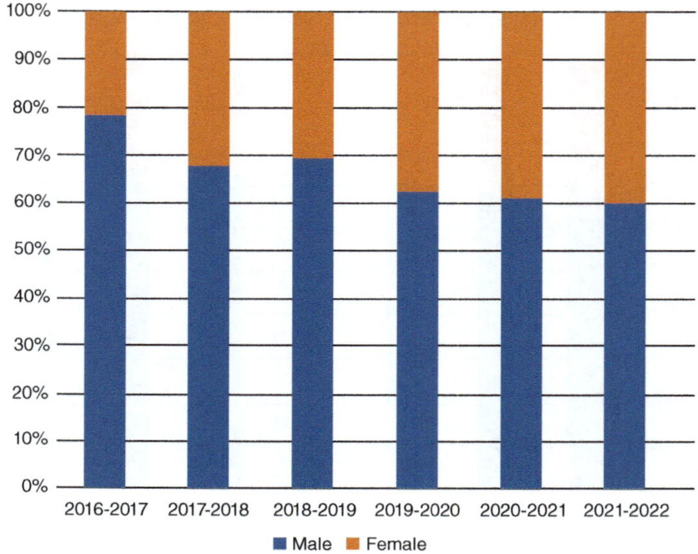

Fig. 48.7 Gender representation of SAGES committee chairs and cochairs

Likewise, gender representation within SAGES committee chairs and cochairs has demonstrated increased diversity over the past several years in direct response to initiatives to increase diversity and transparency.

Fundamentals of Leadership Course

SAGES launched this course with support from the American College of Surgeons in 2022 to equip early career surgeons and those with leadership aspirations with knowledge and skills to navigate leadership progression. The course focuses on DEI initiatives and skills for the aspiring leader [51].

Sustainability in Surgical Practices (SSP) Task Force

The surgical operating room plays a significant role in the impact of healthcare on the global carbon footprint. Surgeons can make changes within their operating practices, healthcare organizations, and broader communities to impact sustainability. Diverse populations are more greatly affected by non-sustainable practices and the impact of these practices on climate change and the carbon footprint (https://www.sages.org/sustainability-in-surgical-practice/) [52].

Gender Representation Study

This study will review the gender diversity representation of SAGES speakers at the annual meeting to determine diversity within the conference. Prior studies have shown increasing gender diversity within SAGES speakers over the past several years (Fig. 48.8).

Demographic Survey

SAGES has launched a demographic survey to attain an accurate view of the makeup of its membership with regard to gender, ethnicity, practice type, geography, specialty, and other areas. This information will allow the organization to better serve the needs of its membership and leadership. The survey results demonstrated a variety of practice types and years of practice. There was a predominance of male members as well as white surgeons. The highest number of surgeons considered themselves general/MIS surgeons, followed by bariatric surgery, acute care surgery, and colorectal surgery.

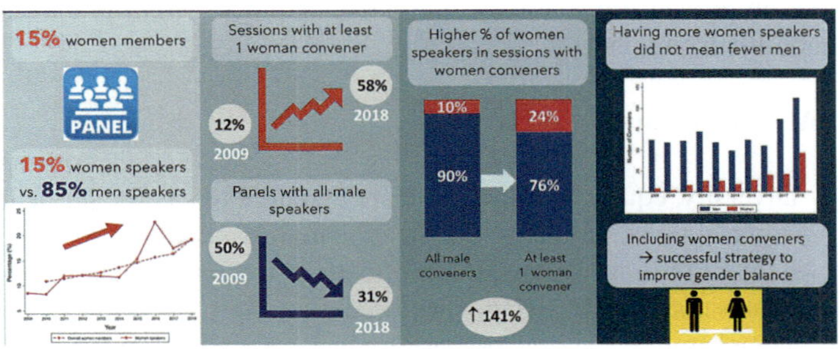

Fig. 48.8 Gender distribution of speakers on panels at the SAGES annual meeting from 2009 to 2018 [39].

SAGES Speaker Bureau

The SAGES speaker bureau allows members to place a profile on the SAGES website showcasing their areas of expertise. The bureau will then allow the membership and organization to increase diversity and utilization of the strengths, skills, and expertise of all members (https://www.sages.org/speaker-catalog/) [53].

DEI Index

The DEI Index, as previously discussed in this chapter, will allow SAGES to lead in assessing the current DEI state of healthcare organizations and provide resources for improvement and education.

Conclusion

Diversity, equity, and inclusion are essential for any surgical practice, society, or healthcare organization. The impact of lack of DEI is significant and includes an impact on patient outcomes and a substantial effect on healthcare providers and diverse communities. Diversity within the healthcare workforce has significant benefits and outcomes for patients [24, 28, 29]. The surgeon and organization can employ numerous initiatives to improve DEI and achieve favorable results. These include utilizing data and metrics, improved transparency, and accountability within practices and organizations.

SAGES Takeaway

- Diversity, equity, and inclusion are essential tenets for surgical organizations, practices, and healthcare organizations.
- Lack of DEI has significant implications for patient health outcomes and the physician workforce.
- Transparency and accountability are critical to ensure the achievement of DEI goals and improve DEI practices.

- Methods to improve DEI include the implementation of metrics such as the DEI index, climate surveys, mentorship, and increased collaboration and representation with underrepresented organizations to increase the pipeline of underrepresented in medicine groups within medicine.

Acknowledgments John Mellinger MD FACS, Ruchir Puri MD FACS, DLPD Committee.

References

1. Peres-Iglesias CT, Johnson S, Jones DB, Gangadharan, Diversity, equity, and inclusion. In Jones DB, Pocket Surgery, 3rd ed, Wolters Kluwer, 2024.
2. Advance Geo Partnership. A primer on diversity. In: Resources. 2019. https://serc.carleton.edu/advancegeo/resources/what_diversity.html.
3. Masterclass Website. https://www.masterclass.com/articles/equity-vs-equality.
4. CMS. CMS framework for health equity. https://www.cms.gov/about-cms/agency-information/omh/health-equity-programs/cms-framework-for-health-equity.
5. Joint Commission Health Care Equity. https://www.jointcommission.orghttps://www.jointcommission.org/our-priorities/health-care-equity/.
6. Gettysburg. Glossary of terms—diversity & inclusion—Gettysburg.edu. https://www.gettysburg.edu/offices/diversity-inclusion/resources/.
7. Berry C, et al. A call to action: black/African American women surgeon scientists, where are they? Ann Surg. 2020;272(1):24–9.
8. AAMC https://www.aamc.org/data-reports/faculty-institutions/report/faculty-roster-us-medical-school-faculty
9. https://www.aamc.org/news/press-releases/new-aamc-data-diversity-medical-school-enrollment-2023
10. https://www.aamc.org/data-reports/faculty-institutions/data/us-medical-school-deans-trends-type-and-gender
11. https://www.aamc.org/data-reports/faculty-institutions/data/us-medical-school-deans-trends-type-and-race-ethnicity
12. Association of Women Surgeons. https://www.womensurgeons.org/page/FemaleSurgeryChairs.
13. Kennedy GE, Bergstresser SL, Rakestraw SL, Novak Z, Corey B, Chen H, Sutzko DC. Does chair of surgery gender influence divisional or residency program director gender diversity? J Surg Res. 2021;267:224–8.
14. Association of American Medical Colleges. Diversity in medicine: facts and figures 2019. 2021.

15. AMA Innovations in Medical Education Webinar Series. Focusing on diversity: promoting mission-aligned medical school admission and residency selection processes. Webinar June 2020_Diversity_ALL (ama-assn.org). 2020. https://community-files.ama-assn.org/image/authenticated/s%2D%2DQlTfmWHS%2D%2D/Webinar-June-2020_Diversity_ALL-3.pdf.
16. Yuce T, Turner P, Glass C, et al. National evaluation ofracial/ethnic discrimination in US surgical residency programs. JAMA Surg. 2020;155:526–8.
17. Dyrbye LN, et al. Race, ethnicity, and medical student well-being in the United States. Arch Intern Med. 2007;167(19):2103–9.
18. Collins KS, et al. Diverse communities, common concerns: assessing health care quality for minority Americans. New York: Commonwealth Fund; 2002.
19. Jarman BT, Kallies KJ, Joshi ART, et al. Underrepresented minorities are underrepresented among general surgery applicants selected to interview. J Surg Educ. 2019;76:e15–23.
20. Liaison Committee on Medical Education. Liaison Committee on Medical Education (LCME) Standards on Diversity. https://health.usf.edu/~/media/Files/Medicine/MD%20Program/Diversity/LCMEStandardsonDiversity1.ashx?la=en.
21. Glazer G, Danek J, Michaels J, et al. Holistic admissions in the health professions: findings from a National Survey. Washington, DC: Urban Universities for HEALTH; 2014.
22. Morris DB, Gruppuso PA, McGee HA, Murillo AL, Grover A, Adashi EY. Diversity of the national medical student body—four decades of inequities. N Engl J Med. 2021;2021(384):1661–8.
23. Haruno LS, Chen X, Metzger M, et al. Racial and sex disparities in resident attrition among surgical subspecialties. JAMA Surg. 2023;158(4):368–76. https://doi.org/10.1001/jamasurg.2022.7640.
24. Greenwood BN, et al. Physician-patient racial concordance and disparities in birthing mortality for newborns. Proc Natl Acad Sci USA. 2020;117(35):21194–200.
25. Alsan M, Garrick O, Graziani G. Does diversity matter for health? Experimental evidence from Oakland. Am Econ Rev. 2019;109(12):4071–111.
26. Evans MK, et al. Diagnosing and treating systemic racism. N Engl J Med. 2020;383(3):274–6.
27. Greenwood BN, Carnahan S, Huang L. Patient–physician gender concordance and increased mortality among female heart attack patients. Proc Natl Acad Sci. 2018;115(34):8569–74.
28. Moy E, Bartman BA. Physician race and care of minority and medically indigent patients. JAMA J Am Med Assoc. 1995;273(19):d1515–20. https://doi.org/10.1001/jama.1995.03520430051038.
29. Marrast LM, Zallman L, Woolhandler S, Bor DH, McCormick D. Minority physicians' role in the care of underserved patients: diversifying the

physician workforce may be key in addressing health disparities. JAMA Intern Med. 2014;174(2):289–91.

30. Keshinro A, Butler P, Fayanju O, Khabele D, Newman E, Greene W, Ude Welcome A, Joseph KA, Stallion A, Backhus L, Frangos S, DiMaggio C, Berman R, Hasson R, Rodriguez LM, Stain S, Bukur M, Klein MJ, Henry-Tillman R, Barry L, Oseni T, Martin C, Johnson-Mann C, Smith R, Karpeh M, White C, Turner P, Pugh C, Hayes-Jordan A, Berry C. Examination of intersectionality and the pipeline for black academic surgeons. JAMA Surg. 2022;157:e217430. https://doi.org/10.1001/jamasurg.2021.7430. Epub ahead of print.
31. Harvard Business Review. https://hbr.org/2016/07/why-diversity-programs-fail.
32. Elvira M, Town R. The effects of race and worker productivity on performance evaluations. Indust Relat J Econ Soc. 2001;40(4):571–90.
33. Boyle P. Medical school applicants and enrollments hit record highs: underrepresented minorities lead surge. AAMC; 2021. https://www.aamc.org/news-insights/medical-school-applicants-and-enrollments-hit-record-highs-underrepresented-minorities-lead-surge.
34. American College of Surgeons. https://www.facs.org/member-services/yfa/mentor/annual.
35. American College of Surgeons. ACS to host discussion on DEI and antiracism. https://www.facs.org/publications/bulletin-brief/061521/retreat.
36. Johnson SM, Stewart JH 4th. 21st century lens on diversity, equity, and inclusion in surgery antiracism symposium. Am Surg. 2021;87(11):1701–3. https://doi.org/10.1177/00031348211038589. Epub 2021 Aug 17.
37. Stewart JH, et al. Acknowledgment, reflection, and action: the American Board of Surgery Leans into antiracism. Ann Surg. 2021;273(4):619–22.
38. American College of Surgeons. Taskforce reports on how the ACS can confront racism in surgery. Bulletin; 2021.
39. Dumitra T, Lee L, Mueller CL, Fried GM, Jones DB, Feldman LS. Gender distribution of speakers on panels at the SAGES annual meeting. Surg Endosc. 2020a;34(9):4140–7.
40. Dumitra T, Alam R, Fiore JF Jr, Mata J, Fried GM, Vassiliou MC, Mueller C, Lee L, Feldman LS. Is there a gender bias in the advancement to SAGES leadership? Surg Endosc. 2020b;34(1):458–63.
41. Telem DA, et al. SAGES climate survey: results and strategic planning for our future. Surg Endosc. 2018;32(10):4105–10.
42. Perez et al. SSA Program Supports Next Generation of Inclusive Leadership. ACS Bulletin. 2023. https://www.facs.org/for-medical-professionals/news-publications/news-and-articles/bulletin/2023/may-2023-volume-108-issue-5/.

43. Kibbe MR, Freischlag J. Call to action to all surgery journal editors for diversity in the editorial and peer review process. JAMA Surg. 2020;155(11):1015–6. https://doi.org/10.1001/jamasurg.2020.4549.
44. Nth Dimensions. https://www.nthdimensions.org.
45. MSM Surgery Reach. https://www.msm.edu/Education/surgery/Reach/index.php.
46. Lautenberger DM, Dandar VM. The state of women in academic medicine 2018–2019: exploring pathways to equity. Association of American Medical Colleges; 2020.
47. Fast Company. Why greater transparency is key to a winning DEI strategy. 2022.
48. Marcelin JR, Siraj DS, Victor R, Kotadia S, Maldonado YA. The impact of bias in healthcare: how to recognize and mitigate it. J Infect Dis. 2019;220(220 Suppl 2):S62–73. https://doi.org/10.1093/infdis/jiz214.
49. Qureshi AP, Johnson SM, Sylla P, Pryor AD, Telem D, Jones DB, Bingener-Casey J, Feldman LS, Mellinger J. Leaning in and moving forward: a call to action and review of diversity initiatives in SAGES. Surg Endosc. 2024;38(8):4095–103. https://doi.org/10.1007/s00464-024-10814-x.
50. Pryor AD, Bader A, Talamini M. Minorities in leadership: are we moving the needle? Surg Endosc. 2019;33(12):3875–9. https://doi.org/10.1007/s00464-019-07122-0.
51. Fundamentals of Leadership Development. https://www.sages.org/fld-sign-up/.
52. Sustainability in Surgical Practice. https://www.sages.org/sustainability-in-surgical-practice/.
53. Sages Speaker Bureau. https://www.sages.org/speaker-catalog/.

Sustainable Surgery

49

Jonathan Vandenberg,
Shaneeta M. Johnson,
Emmanuel Gabriel, and Patricia Sylla

Introduction

The term climate change has gained attention in the news in recent decades. Climate change involves the release of greenhouse gases (GHGs) through the burning of fossil fuels. GHGs include carbon dioxide, methane, and nitrous oxide, among several others. Fossil fuels include coal, oil, and natural gas, which are burned to generate power in the form of electricity. The energy created by fossil fuels helps power facilities, manufacture products, and provide transportation. GHGs enter the atmosphere and act as a blanket over Earth, trapping solar radiation and resulting in increasing temperatures. The Earth's surface absorbs the excess heat, with 90% of this heat being absorbed by the Earth's oceans [1, 2]. As oceans slowly heat up, glaciers melt, ocean levels rise, and

J. Vandenberg · E. Gabriel
Department of Surgery, Mayo Clinic Florida, Jacksonville, FL, USA
e-mail: Gabriel.Emmanuel@mayo.edu

S. M. Johnson (✉)
Department of Surgery, Morehouse School of Medicine, Atlanta, GA, USA
e-mail: shajohnson@msm.edu

P. Sylla
Division of Colorectal Surgery, Mount Sinai, New York, NY, USA
e-mail: Patricia.sylla@mountsinai.org

S. M. Johnson et al. (eds.), *The SAGES Manual of Strategy and Leadership*, https://doi.org/10.1007/978-3-031-62359-2_49

extreme weather events become more common. These effects contribute to coastal flooding, property loss, societal disruption, pollution, the spread of infectious disease, exacerbation of acute and chronic illnesses, and resource shortages. Figure 49.1 further characterizes the health effects of climate change.

The healthcare system is facing significant challenges due to climate change via the vectors of rising temperatures, increasing natural disasters, rising sea levels, and air pollution. The World Health Organization has declared climate change as the most significant public health threat facing humanity [3]. Studies have shown that the negative impacts on patient health are increasing due to temperature-related morbidity and mortality, air pollution-related health effects, and frailty caused by respiratory and cardiovascular impacts from heat and weather events. Climate change has also been associated with increased adverse birth outcomes. Urbanization, exposure to increased heat levels, and exposure to natural disasters and extreme weather events also lead to higher levels of injury and mortality, increased trauma burden on the healthcare system, and increased demand on its capacity (Fig. 49.2). Unless significant action is taken to reduce carbon emissions and curb climate change, the impact on global health will be tremendous. All populations globally are impacted by climate change. However, low-income, disadvantaged, and vulnerable populations are most at risk from the effects of climate change. These populations include children, the elderly, areas with weak health infrastructure, migrant communities, minoritized commu-

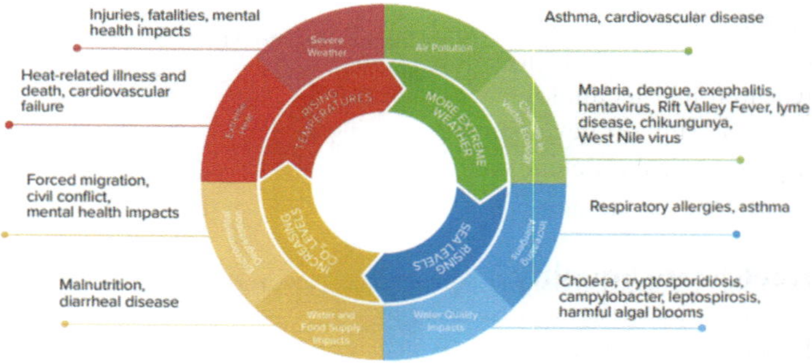

Fig. 49.1 Climate change health impacts. (Healthcare Without Harm)

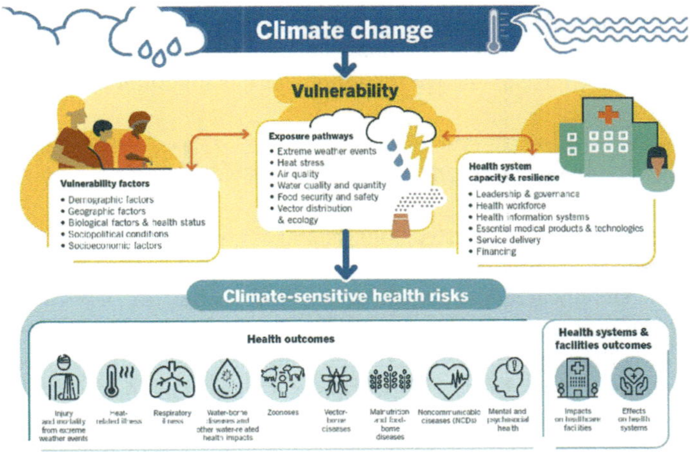

Fig. 49.2 Climate change impacts. (World Health Organization)

nities, those with chronic diseases, women, and low socioeconomic communities. Social, political, and ecological inequities in vulnerable populations worsen these impacts and create significant health inequities.

The Earth has already started to experience the catastrophic effects of climate change. The last 8 years have been the warmest ever recorded in Earth's history [1]. Record-setting storms, floods, droughts, and wildfires are increasing in frequency across the world. The World Health Organization estimates that climate change is expected to cause approximately 250,000 additional deaths per year from the impacts of malnutrition, malaria, diarrhea, and heat stress alone. Additionally, the direct damage costs to health are estimated to be between US$2 and 4 billion annually by 2030 [3]. By the end of the twentieth century, new data showed that human activity was principally responsible for the GHG emissions and climate changes. Globally there was a realization that there was a dire need for international action to address climate change. Governmental panels were created, eventually leading to The Paris Climate Agreement in 2015. The agreement was an international treaty with a goal of limiting the global average temperature increase to 1.5 °C above preindustrial levels [4]. Global emissions must be reduced by 50% by 2030 to meet this goal. As the detrimental effects of climate change become evident, sectors worldwide have to change for a more sustainable future.

Healthcare, Surgery, and Climate Change

The healthcare industry significantly contributes to climate change due to its high energy expenditure and resource utilization. Healthcare is estimated to be responsible for 4.4% of all greenhouse gas emissions worldwide [5]. The U S healthcare system is the most energy-intensive healthcare system in the world and would rank 13th in the world for total GHG emissions if the healthcare system itself was considered a country [6]. Nationally, the U S healthcare sector is responsible for 8.5% of greenhouse gas emissions [7]. The operating room (OR) is the top energy consumer and waste producer in the hospital, accounting for almost one-thirf of the waste produced [8]. The need for sterility, ventilatory requirements, 24/7 availability, and advanced technology renders the surgical field a top contributor to the healthcare sector's carbon footprint. However, surgery's carbon footprint is complicated and extends well beyond the doors of the OR.

The Greenhouse Gas Protocol created a widely accepted framework for categorizing GHG emissions in the early 2000s. The framework divides GHG emissions into three scopes: scopes 1, 2, and 3 [9]. Our focus will be relating the scopes to emissions generated by healthcare centers and surgery as represented in Fig. 49.3. Scope 1 emissions are directly released by the healthcare facility and include on-site vehicles and anesthetic gases released into the atmosphere. Scope 2 emissions are indirect emissions from purchased energy sources used to power the healthcare facility including electricity, air-conditioning, and heating. Scope 3 are indirect emissions from supply chain production including transport, disposal waste, chemical, foods, devices, and equipment [10]. Scope 1 and 2 comprise 7% and 11% of the GHG emissions, respectively. Scope 3 produce the largest share of GHG emissions at 82% [10]. Scope 3 encompass the healthcare supply chain and the emissions produced in the manufacturing of medical goods.

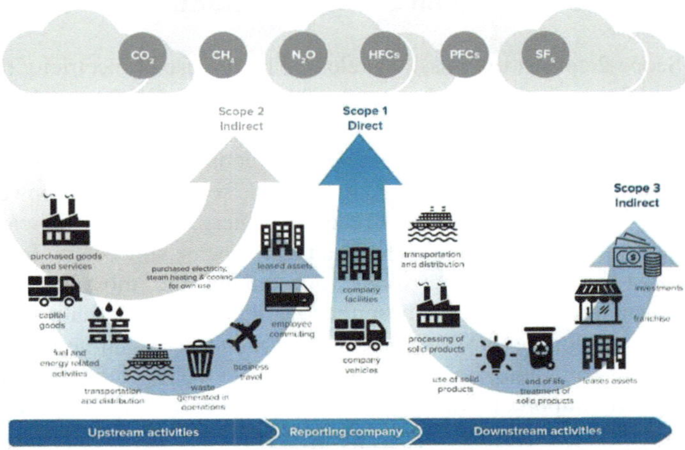

Fig. 49.3 Scopes of GHG emissions. (Healthcare Without Harm)

Surgery's Impact on Climate Change

Anesthetic Gases

Scope 1 emissions in the OR consist of volatile anesthetics, including desflurane, isoflurane, sevoflurane, and nitrous oxide and their direct release into the atmosphere. These are commonly used anesthetics in the operating room which are hundreds to thousands of times more potent greenhouse gases than CO_2. It is estimated that anesthetic gases contribute at least 0.6% of healthcare's global climate impact [11]. When used in the OR, only a small percentage of these gases are metabolized by the patient. The rest of the gas is evacuated by the HVAC system in the OR and released into the atmosphere [12]. Desflurane and nitrous oxide are particularly potent, leading the American Society of Anesthesiologists to advocate for avoiding these inhaled anesthetics and using regional and intravenous anesthesia when appropriate [13].

OR and Supply Chain Energy Expenditure

Scope 2 consist of emissions released by the use of electricity by healthcare facilities and comprise 11% of total GHG emissions. Currently, 60% of all electricity is still produced from burning fossil fuels. As of 2023, 21% of US power is being generated by renewable energy sources such as wind, solar, and hydropower [14]. Although the amount of renewable energy sources is increasing, the energy powering the healthcare sector still comes from fossil fuels. Operating rooms are among the most energy-consumptive units in the hospital. OR lights, heating, ventilation, air-conditioning (HVAC) systems, and monitors are all necessary high-energy requirements during surgery. HVAC systems are particularly important due to government regulations requiring minimum air circulation rates, particulate removal, and positive pressure within ORs for ventilation safety. Older hospitals with outdated, inefficient energy infrastructure result in more emissions being released and cost hospitals thousands of dollars annually.

The medical supply chain is the largest emitter of GHGs in healthcare and surgery. Scope 3, which consist of the indirect emissions from the supply chain, account for approximately 80% of GHG emissions. For example, a company that produces the suction tubing used during an operation has a facility where they manufacture their product. Scope 3 include all the power required to power that facility as well as the transportation emissions to ship these products to the hospital. As one can imagine, this requires a significant amount of energy to manufacture, ship, and dispose of the hundreds of products available for daily use in the OR (Fig. 49.4).

Waste Management: Reduction, Recycling, and Reuse

Waste is an unavoidable by-product of healthcare, especially in the OR. The US healthcare system produces approximately four million tons of waste per year [15]. It is estimated that operating rooms contribute 20–33% of all waste in the hospital, with some

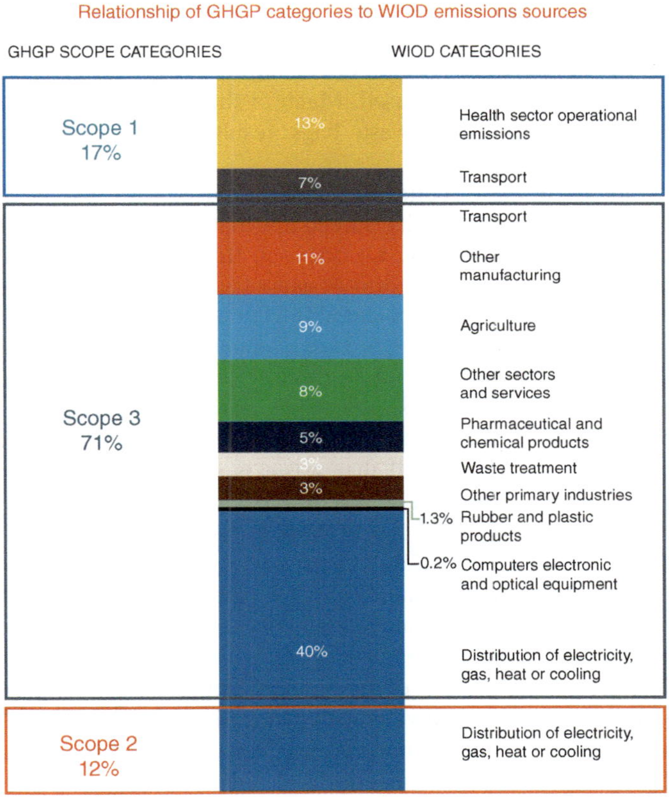

Fig. 49.4 Health care greenhouse gas (GHG) emissions by GHG Protocol Scope and World Input-Output Database categories. (Healthcare Without Harm)

institutions reporting upward of 70% [16, 17]. Waste in the OR includes biohazard waste, sharps, pharmaceuticals, radioactive, and general waste. Approximately 80% of waste in the OR is generated before the patient rolls into the room [18]. Most waste produced are disposable supplies including plastic wrapping, blue sterile wrap, drapes, gowns, gloves, sponges, and basins [19]. An essential step in waste reduction is reducing overage. Overage is waste which is opened in surgical packs and trays and discarded at the end of the case without ever being used because it is no longer sterile. Surgical packs and trays are typically standardized and not designed for specific operations or surgeon preferences, so many materials go unused. Much of this trash is mistakenly placed in red biohazard waste bags, resulting in emissions and wasted money.

Biohazard waste, defined as medical waste saturated in the blood or other potentially infectious materials, is commonly placed in a red waste bag for disposal. Red bag waste requires special treatment in the form of autoclaving, microwaving, or incineration as it poses a potential infectious health risk. Medical waste treatment centers require large amounts of energy, primarily fueled by fossil fuels, leading to GHG emissions when compared to general waste disposal. Institutional studies have found that up to 90% of the waste placed in red biohazard bags is incorrectly placed, meaning all that waste is undergoing unneeded energy-intensive disposal [2, 20]. Red bag waste also costs seven to ten times the disposal cost of general waste, costing hospitals hundreds of thousands of dollars per year.

Similarly, pharmaceutical waste is another costly form of waste both for the environment and hospital finances. Drugs prepared at the beginning of surgical cases in case of emergency typically go unused 50% of the time [21]. Intravenous (IV) bags, syringes, ampoules, and vials with medication must be discarded in hazardous waste and undergo specialized incineration, autoclaving, or chemical decontamination.

Data on OR recycling is lacking, and it is unclear if a majority of institutions have a recycling infrastructure. Challenges to recycling in the OR include understaffing and resources to sort, store, and collect recyclables. Staff may often lack knowledge or education on how waste should be stratified into recycling, biohazard waste, or general waste. The composition of OR waste has been evaluated, and an estimated 30% is plastic, and 30% is paper or cardboard. Of the plastic waste, approximately 80% is recyclable [22]. One source of plastic waste in the OR is the blue sterile polypropylene wrap that covers surgical instruments. This wrap has been found to comprise 19% of the total waste in the OR [23].

Single-use products are used routinely in the OR. Most of these products, including gowns, drapes, basins, and instruments, are discarded as waste during or after the case. However, in recent decades, there has been an increased drive for reprocessing medical devices in hospitals and surgery centers. Approximately 25% of US hospitals were using reprocessing of single-use surgical devices in 2010 with this number likely increasing over the last decade [24]. A barrier to reuse has been sterility concerns of the reprocessed item and patient safety. In 2008, a report was released by the US Government Accountability Office which concluded reprocessed devices do not pose an increased health risk when compared with new devices [25]. Medical device reprocessing has been increasing to help cut costs and emissions. Reprocessing companies report total annual savings for hospitals using their services as high as 138 million dollars, with over four million pounds of waste saved [24].

Future Directions

Education

Climate change education must be included in medical education. Globally, younger generations are conscientious, passionate, and leaders in climate change movements. As these individuals become healthcare professionals, the dynamic between healthcare, health, and climate change is emerging in discussions. This is evident by the surge in sustainability-focused healthcare publications over the last two decades. Medical societies such as the Medical Society Consortium on Climate and Health, Practice Greenhealth, and Healthcare Without Harm are spreading awareness of healthcare's impact on the climate. These leading advocacy groups have a mission to create a more sustainable future for healthcare. They produce educational material on sustainability, provide information on how to start projects, distribute current research, and arrange national conferences. Surgical organizations such as the Society of American Gastrointestinal and Endoscopic Surgeons (SAGES) and the European Association of Endoscopic Surgeons (EAES) have also begun to evaluate surgical practices and provide education [26, 27]. Additionally, social media has contributed to education on climate change with well-known surgical podcasts such as Behind the Knife producing content on sustainability in surgery. Increased awareness about the impact of surgery on climate change will help to guide change.

Collaboration

Change is not possible without multisector collaboration. Surgery has many stakeholders who contribute to the indirect and direct causes of GHG emissions. Prominent stakeholders such as the federal and state governments control policies that can influence climate-friendly healthcare changes. Recently, the federal government has collaborated with healthcare systems to drive change. In 2022, the Department of Health and Human Services announced a Health Sector Climate Pledge for health organizations to commit to decreasing their GHG emissions by 50% by 2030 and net zero emissions by 2050 [28]. Over 116 organizations encompassing 872 hospitals have signed the pledge as of April 2023. SAGES was the 2nd surgical organization signatory of this pledge and was recognized at the UN COP conference in 2023. Within the healthcare system, hospitals have hired sustainability consultants to help identify areas of high GHG emissions to reduce their carbon footprint. Collaboration within the hospital is essential for quality improvement projects to help reduce emissions. Environmental services, custodial staff, engineers, device representatives, nurses, surgical technicians, anesthesiologists, nurse anesthetists, and surgeons are all crucial team members involved in daily decisions that impact OR energy use, waste, recycling, and product use. Multidisciplinary sustainability teams should be created with individuals from these fields to bring specialized viewpoints and resources together. Many of the publications cited in this chapter arise from nurses, surgeons, and anesthesiologists who have collaborated with their colleagues to make meaningful changes to help reduce emissions in the OR. In May 2021, The National Academy of Medicine launched the Action Collaborative to Decarbonize the U.S. Health Sector which is comprised of a private-public sector partnership to address the carbon footprint of the health sector [29].

Sustainability Initiatives

The first step to reducing emissions with a climate mitigation strategy is collecting data to determine an institution's current carbon footprint as many healthcare corporations do not track their impact on the climate. Healthcare Without Harm, one of the medical societies whose mission is to reduce healthcare's impact on the environment, has created a climate impact checkup calculator that institutions can use to measure their GHG emissions [30]. The calculator analyzes scopes 1, 2, and 3 and allows institutions to implement changes to reduce these emissions. With this data, hospitals can track and mitigate their progress on quality improvement projects. We will discuss several of these simple changes which can be made in the OR to significantly reduce emissions.

Anesthetic Gases

Anesthetic gases, including nitrous oxide, sevoflurane, isoflurane, and desflurane, are potent GHGs that are a part of scope 1 emissions in the OR. Most of these gases will be released into the atmosphere rather than metabolized by the patient. Obtaining current baselines of anesthetic gas use in the OR will allow anesthesiologists to evaluate the impact their practices have on the environment. Anesthetic gases can be replaced by parental anesthetics when feasible. Reductions of these gases should be tracked, and future goals be set to reduce emissions. The American Society of Anesthesiologists is leading the movement by creating an Inhaled Anesthetic 2023 Challenge to reduce inhaled anesthetic carbon emissions by 50% in 2023 [31]. They have created a sustainability checklist that can be used in ORs worldwide to help reduce direct emissions from anesthesia.

OR and Supply Chain Energy Expenditure

The largest share of GHG emissions from surgery comes from the energy used to power the OR and the manufacturing process of OR devices and materials. The transformation of the national energy grid from fossil fuels to renewables is in progress but will not occur overnight. Healthcare facilities are responsible for reducing their energy use. Institutions can start by analyzing their energy use to identify energy reduction strategies. Energy reduction strategies include updating HVAC systems and installing light-emitting diode (LED) and motion-sensing lights. LED lights are more energy efficient and have a 30–50 times longer lifespan, saving hospitals energy and money [20]. Motion-sensing lights can turn off ORs that are not in use saving electricity and money. Hospitals can also invest in renewable energy sources such as solar and wind to power their facilities. Practice Greenhealth has resources for hospitals on best practices in energy efficiency to assist them in reaching net zero carbon emissions [32].

Health systems nationally and globally have begun to address and mitigate their carbon footprint with sustainability and cost-saving impacts. The New York Presbyterian Hospital experienced almost $2 million in annual savings by installing energy-saving LED lighting and variable frequency drives, replacing outdated cooling systems with more efficient equipment, and other improvements on air handler units and boiler economizers. Similarly, the Cleveland Clinic adjusted its ventilation to meet guidelines, reduced the system's energy use, and saved approximately $250,000 annually. They also decreased the number of air exchanges when operating rooms are unoccupied, reducing energy use and saving $2 million per year [33].

The supply chain is responsible for approximately 40% of healthcare's emissions. Hospitals should prioritize purchasing from companies with sustainable commitments who manufacture climate-friendly products which can be reused or recycled. Additionally, working with companies to repurpose and reuse products is a significant step toward reducing scope 3 emissions in healthcare. Industry representatives and collaborations may be utilized to maximize sustainable research and design practices with surgical devices.

Waste Management Reduction, Recycling, and Reuse

The OR produces more waste than any other area in the hospital. Tracking waste produced in the OR is necessary to identify areas for improvement. Red biohazard bags are an area for improvement as up to 90% of the trash placed in them is not biohazard waste and therefore incurs additional energy costs for disposal. Biohazard waste reduction strategies include educating OR staff members that only waste with saturated blood or bodily fluids is placed in red bags. Quality improvement projects focusing on red bag waste have used tactics such as having more general waste containers available, posting signs over red bag waste containers, or not opening red bags unless there is visible blood or bodily fluid soiled waste. These actions have helped reduce red bag waste at some institutions by 50% and saved the hospital tens to hundreds of thousands of dollars annually [34, 35].

Due to the sterile requirements of the OR, many materials and devices are designed for single use. Surgical packs are generic and contain materials that go untouched during the case and then are disposed of. Audits of surgical packs and trays to limit the overage in ORs will reduce the amount of waste produced. Collaboration with suppliers who design surgical packs or the creation of custom packs by OR central supply in accordance with surgeon preference cards are two ways that may help reduce overage [36]. Hospital systems that have performed surgical pack audits have reduced surgical waste by five tons and saved over $100,000 annually [37]. Reusable surgical linens, including drapes and gowns, comprise much of the OR waste. Switching to reusables has been shown to have prevented hundreds of thousands of pounds of waste and saved the hospital $38,000 annually [37]. Reusable gowns and drapes are estimated to have at least a 100-use lifetime, and making the switch could reduce surgical waste volume by over 50% [38, 39]. Blue sterile wrap is a common item found in the waste bins after surgery, given the sterile instruments it packages. Institutions have created projects to recycle the blue sterile wrap to be repurposed into other retail products and prevented several tons of recyclable plastic from entering the landfill. Other recyclable products in the OR include forced air-warming blankets, saline and sterile water plastic bottles, IV bags, oxygen masks and tubing, and suction tubing [22]. Most of these items are thrown in general waste. The opportunity to educate and organize a recycling program and reduce thousands of tons of waste represents a simple but impactful change.

Conclusion

Climate change has been identified as the number one public health threat to patients this century. While the healthcare field has imparted significant good for the well-being of patients, it has also contributed significantly to the detrimental impact of climate change. The surgical field is particularly energy-intensive and highly waste-producing. Until recently, little attention was centered on the effect of surgery on the environment. Given what we now know about the dangers of climate change, we owe it to our patients to adopt sustainable surgical practices to reduce emissions and prevent the catastrophic effects of climate change. Through data collection, education, collaboration, and action, we can create a more sustainable future for the field of surgery.

SAGES Takeaway

- Climate change is a serious public health threat.
- The healthcare industry is a significant contributor to the global carbon footprint.
- Surgery is an energy- and resource-intensive field with a significant impact on the carbon footprint.
- Surgeons are equipped to make sustainable changes in their practices and organizations that can lessen their impact.

References

1. World Meteorological Organization. Past eight years confirmed to be the eight warmest on record. 2023. https://public.wmo.int/en/media/press-release/past-eight-years-confirmed-be-eight-warmest-record#:~:text=The%20warmest%20eight%20years%20have,contributed%20to%20record%20global%20temperatures. Accessed 31 May 2023.
2. National Centers for Environmental Information. Ocean heat content rises. 2021. https://www.ncei.noaa.gov/news/ocean-heat-content-rises. Accessed 31 May 2023.
3. World Health Organization. Climate change and health. 2021. https://www.who.int/news-room/fact-sheets/detail/climate-change-and-health. Accessed 3 Aug 2023.

4. United Nations Framework Convention on Climate Change (UNFCCC). Paris Agreement TIAS No. 16-1104. 2015.
5. Pichler PP, Jaccard IS, Weisz U, et al. International comparison of health care carbon footprints. Environ Res Lett. 2019;14(6):064004.
6. Eckelman MJ, Sherman J. Environmental impacts of the U.S. health care system and effects on public health. PLoS One. 2016;11(6):1–14.
7. Commonwealth Fund. How the US Health Care System Contributes to Climate Change. 2022. https://www.commonwealthfund.org/publications/explainer/2022/apr/how-us-health-care-system-contributes-climate-change. Accessed 4 Aug 2022.
8. MacNeill AJ, Lillywhite R, Brown CJ. The impact of surgery on global climate: a carbon footprinting study of operating theatres in three health systems. Lancet. 2017;1(9):e381–8. https://doi.org/10.1016/S2542-5196(17)30162-6.
9. Ranganathan J, Corbier L, Pankaj B, et al. The greenhouse gas protocol: a corporate accounting and reporting standard. WBCSD; 2004. p. 1–116.
10. Eckelman MJ, Huang K, Lagasse R, et al. Health care pollution and public health damage in the United States: an update. Health Aff Millwood. 2020;39(12):2071–9.
11. Karliner J, Slotterback S, et al. Health care's climate footprint: how the health sector contributes to the global climate crisis and opportunities for action. 2019. pp. 1–40.
12. Vollmer MK, Rhee TS, Rigby M, et al. Modern inhalation anesthetics: potent greenhouse gases in the global atmosphere. Geophys Res Lett. 2015;42:1606–11.
13. Devlin-Hegedus JA, McGain F, Harris RD, et al. Action guidance for addressing pollution from inhalational anaesthetics. Anaesthesia. 2022;77:1023–9.
14. U.S. Energy Information Administration (EIA). What is U.S. electricity generation by energy source. 2023. https://www.eia.gov/tools/faqs/faq.php?id=427&t=3. Accessed 31 May 2023.
15. Health Care Without Harm. Waste management: the issue. 2010. https://noharm-uscanada.org/issues/us-canada/waste-management. Accessed 31 May 2023.
16. Goldberg ME, Vekeman D, Torjman MC, et al. Medical waste in the environment: do anesthesia personnel have a role to play. J Clin Anesth. 1996;8:475–9.
17. Tieszen ME, Gruenberg JC. A quantitative, qualitative, and critical assessment of surgical waste. Surgeons venture through the trash can. JAMA. 1992;267:2765–8.
18. Donaldson K. Save the planet: recycling in the OR. In: Infection control today. 2020. https://www.infectioncontroltoday.com/view/save-planet-recycling-or. Accessed 31 May 2023.
19. Conrardy J, Hillanbrand M, Myers S, Nussbaum GF. Reducing medical waste. AORN J. 2010;91(6):711–21.

20. Laustsen G. Greening in healthcare. Nurs Manag. 2010;41(11):26–31.
21. Atcheson C, Spivack J, Williams R, et al. Preventable drug waste among anesthesia providers: opportunities for efficiency. J Clin Anesth. 2016;30:24–32.
22. Wyssusek KH, Keys MT, van Zundert AAJ. Operating room greening initiatives—the old, the new, and the way forward: a narrative review. Waste Manag Res. 2019;37(1):3–19.
23. Environmental Protection Agency. Reusable totes, blue wrap recycling and composting. 2002. https://19january2017snapshot.epa.gov/www3/region9/waste/p2/projects/hospital/totes.pdf. Accessed 31 May 2023.
24. Kwakye G, Pronovost PJ, Makary MA. Commentary: a call to go green in health care by reprocessing medical equipment. Acad Med. 2010;85:398–400.
25. United States Government Accountability Office. Report to the committee on oversight and government reform, house of representatives. Reprocessed single-use medical devices: FDA oversight has increased, and available information does not indicate that use presents an elevated health risk. Washington, DC: United States Government Accountability Office; 2008.
26. Pietrabissa A, Sylla P. Green surgery: time to make a choice. Surg Endosc, 2023;37(9):6609–6610. https://doi.org/10.1007/s00464-023-10229-0.
27. https://www.sages.org/sustainability-in-surgical-practice/.
28. U.S. Health and Human Services. Health sector commitments to emissions reduction and resilience. 2023. https://www.hhs.gov/climate-change-health-equity-environmental-justice/climate-change-health-equity/actions/health-sector-pledge/index.html#:~:text=Specifically%2C%20pledge%20signers%20committed%20to,on%20this%20goal%20every%20year. Accessed 31 May 2023.
29. Dzau VJ, Levine R, Barrett G, Witty A. Decarbonizing the U.S. health sector—a call to action. N Engl J Med. 2021;385(23):2117–9.
30. Health Care Without Harm. Climate impact checkup. In: Health care climate action. 2023. https://healthcareclimateaction.org/checkup. Accessed 31 May 2023.
31. American Society of Anesthesiologists. Inhaled anesthetic 2023 challenge. 2023. https://www.asahq.org/about-asa/governance-and-committees/asa-committees/environmental-sustainability/inhaled-anesthetic-challenge. Accessed 31 May 2023.
32. Practice Greenhealth. Best practices in energy efficiency. 2023. https://practicegreenhealth.org/tools-and-resources/best-practices-energy-efficiency. Accessed 31 May 2023.
33. Hegwer. How Cleveland clinic saved millions through smarter energy use. 2018. https://www.hfma.org/operations-management/cost-reduction/59381/#:~:text=Cleveland%20Clinic%20also%20uses%20an,save%20%242%20million%20a%20year. Accessed 4 Aug 2023.

34. Kwakye G, Brat G, Makary M. Green surgical practices for health care. Arch Surg. 2011;146:131–6.
35. Stonemetz J, Pham JC, Necochea AJ, et al. Reduction of regulated medical waste using lean sigma results in financial gains for hospital. Anesthesiol Clin. 2011;29(1):145–52.
36. Kagoma YK, Stall N, Rubinstein E, Naudie D. People, planet and profits: the case for greening operating rooms. CMAJ. 2012;184(17):1905–11.
37. Choiniere D, Ayers C, Moyle J. Greening the OR: guidance documents. 2013. https://practicegreenhealth.org/sites/default/files/upload-files/gor_checklist_r5_web.pdf. Accessed 31 May 2023.
38. Brennan B. Greening the OR: an Australian perspective. Todays OR Nurse. 1994;16:25–32.
39. Stall NM, Kagoma YM, Bondy JN, et al. Surgical waste audit of 5 total knee arthroplasties. Can J Surg. 2013;56:97–102.

Index

A
Academic health systems (AHS), 525
Academic leader, 501, 502
Academic leadership ladder, 480
Academic pathways, 478, 479
Academic surgeons (AS), 477, 478
Academic surgery
  barriers, 25
  clinical practice, growth and propagation, 27
  clinical productivity, 23
  cross-sectional survey, 23, 24
  factors, 26
  faculty recruitment, 27
  formal mentorship program, 24
  institution's promotion and tenure process, 26
  leadership, 26, 27
  promotion and tenure processes, 25
  salary and benefits, 25
  surgical education and provision, 24
  surgical position, 24, 25
Accountability, 268, 553, 556, 692, 708, 711
  challenges, 444, 445
  definition, 443
  distribution, 442
  effective communication, 445
    active listening, 445
    barriers, 450–452
    continuous improvement, 453, 454
    in high-pressure environment, 446
    integration, 447, 448
    interdisciplinary collaboration, 453
    patient-centered models, 453
    technological advancements, 452
    tools and techniques, 446, 447
    verbal and non-verbal communication, 445
  historical perspective, 443
  leadership, 449, 450
  mentorship and training, 449, 450
Accountable Care Organization (ACO), 528
Accreditation, 495
Accreditation Council for Continuing Medical Education (ACCME), 694

S. M. Johnson et al. (eds.), *The SAGES Manual of Strategy and Leadership*, https://doi.org/10.1007/978-3-031-62359-2

Active listening, 319, 439
Adoption, 237
Advocacy, 576, 581, 585–588, 660
Advocate, 585, 588
Affiliative style, 255
Agreement, 311
American Medical Association (AMA), 184
Anesthetic gases, 727, 733
Annual Procedure Volume, 245
Annual review of competence progression (ARCP), 615
Anxiety, 521
Areas of conflict, 312
Artificial intelligence (AI), 390
Assertive and controlling personality, 298
Assessment bias, 355
Attraction-selection-attrition theory, 279
Augmented intelligence (AI), 173
Authoritative style, 255
Authorship, 372, 692
Autocratic leader, 252
Autonomy in decision making, 317
Awareness, 644

B

Bariatric Surgery team/program, 238
Basic science research, 344
Behaviors, 235
Benchmark institutions, 335
Bench research, 344
Bicultural audit, 278
Bidirectional communication, 493, 497
Biostatistics, 361
Blame-oriented atmosphere, 303
Blinding/masking, 355
Bolman & Deal's four frames, 515, 516, 519
Brandeis Health Leadership Program (BHLP), 461
Budgeting, 494
Burnout, 200, 301, 302

C

Capacity building, 658, 665
Career advancement
  fellowship training, 205, 206
  marketing, 210, 211
  promotion
    in academic settings, 208, 209
    private practice, 209, 210
    revenue generation and, 207, 208
  wellness, 207
Career-development awards, 352
Career promotion
  criteria for, 116–119, 121
  institution's promotion track, 113–116
  package preparation, 121–124
  process and timeline, 124, 125
Case-control studies, 356
Case Mix Index (CMI), 335
Certainty within workplace, 324
Change management, 321, 322, 547, 548
Changes, 323
Checking, 257
Clinical research, 345
Cluster group designs, 354
Coaching sessions, 238
Coaching style, 255
Collaboration, 732
Collaborative care models, 633
Collaborative endeavors, 484
Collaborative partnership, 659, 660
Collective intelligence, 547
Communicating quality measures, 600
Communication, 197, 236, 237, 254, 261, 317, 485, 487, 497
  breakdown, 322
  plan, 339
Community engagement, 665
Compassion, 247
Compassion fatigue and emotional exhaustion, 302
Comprehensive analysis of leading departments, 335

Conflict in workplace, 310
Conflict of interest (COI), 690–693
Conflict resolution, 196, 197
Confusion, 521
Consolidated Standards of Reporting Trials (CONSORT), 369
Consulting arrangements, 694
Continuing medical education (CME), 95, 96, 174, 688–690
Continuous assessment, 433
Continuous improvement, 453, 454
Contract negotiation
  bargaining power, 46
  call requirements and pay, 40, 41
  compensation and benefits, 42–44
  contract review, 42, 46
  malpractice insurance, 45, 46
  payors' panels, 41
  physician contracts, 46
  reduced hours/reduced compensation, 41
  responsibilities and services, 40
  restrictive covenants, 44, 45
  termination, 41, 42
Coronary artery bypass graft surgery (CABG), 631
Correlated variables and multicollinearity, 367
COVID-19, 146–148, 385
Critical Care Support and Training for Patient Safety, 245
Critical tendencies, 299
Crossover trials, 354
Cultural competence, 320, 437, 438
Cultural development, 323
Cultural humility, 633, 656, 660
Cultural Iceberg model, 272, 273
Culturally competent care, 646–649
Culture, 234, 246
Current Procedural Terminology (CPT) codes, 184
Customer-centric culture, 238
Cybersecurity, 149, 150

D
Database development, 359, 360
Data Review and Identifying Deficiencies, 246
Defense Health Agency (DHA), 87
Deming Cycle of continuous quality improvement, 255
Democratic style, 255
Demographics changing, 512
Department of Highly Fundable Esoterics, 287, 294
Descriptive Statistical Tests, 362, 363
Descriptive statistics, 362
Developmental changes, 323
Difficult personalities, 297
  causes and motivations, 301
  emotional reactions, 300
  forms, 298
  in healthcare workplace, 298
  negative experiences, 302
  subordinate positions, 299
  types, 303–305
Disagreement, 311
Diversity, 321, 701, 703, 705, 709
Diversity, equity, and inclusion (DEI), 6, 287, 290, 294, 318, 436, 460, 641
  fostering, 642
  implementation, 651
  positive improvements, 650
Document management, 351
Dominance, Influence, Steadiness, and Conscientious (DISC) assessment, 224–226
Donabedian model, 430–432
Doximity Residency Navigator Tool, 335

E
Education, 644, 645
Electronic health records (EHR), 572
Electronic medical records (EMRs), 60, 664

Emotional intelligence (EI), 192, 394, 492, 541
Empire Clinical Research Investigator Program (ECRIP), 568
Employee skill growth, 322, 323
Employment, 49–52
Empowered patients, 512
Engineering internships, 573
Enhancing the Quality and Transparency of Health Research (EQUATOR) network, 370
Environmental assessment, 333
Equity, 321, 702, 705, 709
  in retention and promotion, 319
Estimated Glomerular Filtration Rate (eGFR), 648
Excitement, 521
Executive coaching, 313
External relationships, 486
External Resources Sharing Agreement (ERSA), 93
External stressors, 302

F

Faculty member, 498, 499
Fair market value (FMV), 61
Focus groups and seek feedback, 324
Formal leadership training, 313
Frustration, 521
Fundamentals of Leadership Development Curriculum (FLD), 642–644, 647, 649, 650
Fundraising, 497

G

Geographic and demographic assessments, 239
Getting it Right First Time (GIRFT), 615
"Glass half empty" mentality, 299
Global Burden of Diseases (GBD), 597
Global health, 575
Global health engagement (GHE), 104
Global surgery, 566, 567, 657, 668, 669
  leadership, 656, 657
  qualities of effective leader, 657–659, 661
  strategies employed, 662, 663
Global Surgery Programming, 666, 667
Goal implementation
  strategic plan
    adaptability, 412
    benefits, 413
    career changes/ advancement, 409
    challenges, 408
    change management, 411, 412
    communication, 410–412
    interpersonal skills, 411
    judgment/laying blame, 412
    PDCA method, 408, 409
    progress and performance, 408
    reasonable expectations, 411
    resources
      and collaboration, 410
    SMART, 409
    strategic thinking, 411, 412
    tasks, resources, and resource, 409
    team management and leadership, 410
Good change management, 323
Governance, 553
  effectiveness and efficiency, 555
  equity and inclusive, 557
  participation and consensus orientation, 554
  principles, 558–560
  responsiveness, 555
  strategic vision, 555
Graduate Medical Education (GME), 89, 90, 582

Greenhouse gases, 723
Gross domestic product (GDP), 664–665
Group practice, 56–57

H

Harvard Leadership Development Program, 462
Healthcare, 249, 724, 726
Healthcare Access and Quality (HAQ), 613
Healthcare disparities, 629, 632, 634, 646
Healthcare equality, 657
Healthcare leadership, 261
Healthcare marketing
  burnout, 136, 137
  HIT, 134–136
  licensure, credentialing, and insurance, 129, 130
  payor contracts, 130–132
  practice management
    office space and equipment, 132, 133
    office staff, 133, 134
  surgical practice types, 127–129
  trend-watching and diversification, 137, 138
Health care organization (HCO), 468, 470–472
Healthcare quality, 251
Healthcare system, 595, 611, 612
  leadership development
    cultural competence, 437, 438
    implementation science, 432–434
    innovative strategies, 434, 435
    opportunities, 438
    prioritizing recruitment efforts, 436, 437
    quality improvement approach, 430–432
    sustainability, 438, 439
  mission, vision, and core values, 429, 430
Healthcare workforce, 702, 704, 708
Health equity, 658
Health equity initiatives, 634
Health information technology (HIT), 134–136
High-performance team, 260
Historical controlled trials, 354
Historical financial biases, 336
Historically-controlled studies, 354
Hofstede's model, 269, 270
Holistic review, 320
Hospital based practice, 58
Hospital leadership, 332
Human relations approach (HRA), 418, 419
Human relationships
  characteristics, 195
  Covey's concept, 193
  emotional intelligence, 192
  leadership, 191
  mission statement and goals, 191, 192
  reflection, feedback, and practice, 194
  self-awareness, 192, 193
  social skill, 194, 195
Human resource frame, 519
Human resource management
  aspects, roles, and responsibilities, 419, 420
  assumptions, 419
  benefits, payroll and any grievance, 420
  commitment, skills, and knowledge, 418
  emotions, feelings, and social needs, 419
  financial reward, 418
  Hawthorne Studies, 419
  policies, 418
  selection technique, 420
  skilled and diverse workforce, 420
Human talent, 496
Humble inquiry, 310
Hypothesis testing, 361

I

Iceberg culture model, 272–273
Ideation process, 336
Inclusion initiatives, 321
Inclusivity, 702, 706, 711
Industry, 686–691, 693–696
Inequities, 703, 704, 706, 713
Inferential Statistical Tests, 364–365, 367
Inferential statistics, 362, 367
Innovation, 686, 687, 695, 696
Integration
  credentialing and privileging
    competency, 179–181
    definition, 179
    institution, 182, 183
    maintenance of skills, 184
  device representatives, 174
  quality improvement, 177, 178
  surgical technology
    augmented intelligence (AI), 173
    growth of, 171, 172
    machine learning (ML), 173
    technological advancement, 172, 173
  systematic process, 174–177
Integrity, 253
Intelligence, 557
Internal relationships, 485
International Medical Graduates (IMGs), 675, 680
Intrinsic personality traits, 301

K

K-awards, 352
Kotter's 8-Step Process for Leading Change, 324
Kotter's model, 515
Kotter's steps, 517–518

L

Laissez-faire leadership, 252
Leadership, 154, 235, 250, 449, 450, 536, 540, 607, 615, 702, 707, 710, 711, 716
  and communication styles and preferences, 313
  vs. management, 257, 258
  pathways, 483
  skills, 253–254
  styles, 251–253, 261, 538
Leadership challenges in 2023, 309
Legislation, 582
Length of Stay (LOS), 528
Lewin's Change Management Model, 324
Light-emitting diode (LED), 734
Listening, 311
Locum tenens (LT)
  healthcare insurance and retirement, 58
  overview, 31, 32
  positions for surgeons
    compensation, 35
    factors, 33, 34
    features, 33
    identification, 32, 33
    licensing, 34, 35
    malpractice coverage, 35, 36
    position details, 36, 37
Low- and middle-income countries (LMICs), 655–657, 659, 661, 662, 664

M

Machine learning (ML), 173
Malpractice insurance, 45, 46
Managed Services Provider (MSP), 33
Management, 254
  definition, 417
  human resources
    aspects, roles, and responsibilities, 419, 420
    assumptions, 419
    benefits, payroll and any grievance, 420
    commitment, skills, and knowledge, 418
    emotions, feelings, and social needs, 419
    financial reward, 418

Hawthorne studies, 419
policies, 418
selection technique, 420
skilled and diverse workforce, 420
skills
conflict resolution, 196, 197
human relationships, 191–195
leveraging strength, 198–200
prioritization, 198
talent management, 425
benefits, 424
definition, 423
elements, 424, 425
negotiation, 421–423
physician-leaders, 424
TMALDA, 425
Manuscript preparation for peer-review and publication, 368
Manuscripts, 368
Marketing availability and costs, 239
Master of Business Administration (MBA), 569, 570
Master of Public Health (MPH), 571
Master of Science in Health Profession Education (MSHPE), 574
Mckinsey 7S framework, 271, 272
Measurable goals, 324
Measuring quality, 596–599
Medical laws, 581–583
Medical practice adaptation, 150
crisis
cybersecurity breaches, 149, 150
internal adaptation, 146–148
residency coordinator, 144–146
leadership behavior, 142
leadership responsibility, 142, 143
residency programs, 141, 142
Memorandum of Agreement (MOA), 94
Memorandum of Understanding (MOU), 94
Mentorship, 157, 158, 678, 679
for general surgery residents, 374
training and, 449, 450
Metabolic and Bariatric Surgery (MBS) Committee, 241–243
Metabolic and Bariatric Surgery Accreditation and Quality Improvement Program (MBSAQIP) criteria, 239
Methods section, 369
Metrics, 711
Military health system (MHS)
academic medicine and research, 99–101
administrative leadership, 96, 97
agreements, 93–96
clinical practice, 91–93
clinical skills, 89
deployment, global health, and operational assignments, 102–105
initial job and location assignment, 89–91
memorandums, 93–96
military career and command, 105–107
military-civilian partnerships, 93–96
professional development and education, 97–99
structure, 88
Military treatment facilities (MTF)
clinical practice, 91–93
initial job and location assignment, 89
Minimally Invasive Surgical (MIS), 687
Minorities, 500, 501
Mission of clinical, education, and research excellence, 335
Mission statement, 331, 332
Mobilization, 665

Modern management
in healthcare, 254
Multidisciplinary team (MDT), 240, 349–350
Myers-Briggs Type Indicator (MBTI), 226, 227

N

National Emergency Laparotomy Audit (NELA), 618
National Health Service (NHS), 612
National Institute for Occupational Safety and Health (NIOSH), 585
National presence, 488–490
National Quality Measures Clearing House, 250
National Safety Standards for Invasive Procedures (NatSSIPs), 614
Natural experiment, 356
Negotiations, 49–52
Networking, 154, 484
Neutral zone, 521
New beginning stage, 522
"New Investigator" (NI) status, 353
NIH R01 awards, 353
Noncompliance, 292
Normal distribution of a data set, 366
North American Locum Tenens Organization (NALTO), 32, 33
Nostalgia, 521

O

Objectives and Key Results (OKRs), 234
Off duty employment (ODE), 95
Operationalization
  abstract concepts, 233
  institutional commitment at the highest level, 239
  observations and quantifiable data, 233
Oppositional and undermining personality, 300
Optimal leadership, 483
Organizational culture, 540
  core values, 272
  cultural strength, 276
  defined, 265, 266
  elements, 266, 268
  intangible aspects, 267–269
  leadership style, 272
  merger process, 278
  qualities, 277
  shared values, 272
  strength, 275
  strengthening and maintaining, 278
  tangible aspects, 267
Organizational culture models, 269, 270
Organizational Environmental Assessment, 333, 334
Organizational missions and goals, 336
Organizational norms, 301
Organizational policy, 289
Organizational procedures, 290
Organizational socialization, 279, 280
Organizational subcultures, 270
Orientation, 236
Outcomes, definition, 235

P

Pacesetting style, 255
Partnership, 685, 686, 688, 696, 697
Passive-avoidant leadership style, 253
Patient care, 343
Patient reported outcome (PRO), 598
Patient-reported outcome measures (PROMs), 613
Perioperative Quality Improvement Programme (PQIP), 618
Personal career goals, 347
Personality traits, 301

Persuasion, 543
Physician burnout, 513
Physician Leadership Academy (PLA), 459, 460
Plan-do-check-act/adjust (PDCA), 255, 257, 408, 409
Planning, 256
Policy, 288, 289, 581, 585, 588, 590
Political action committees (PACs), 589
Political frame, 519
Practice types
  group practice, 56–57
  HMOs, 57
  hospital based practice, 58
  locum tenens, 58
  private practice, 55, 56
Pre-employment, 50
Preferred Reporting Items for Systematic Reviews and Meta-Analysis (PRISMA), 369
Preliminary resident, 677–679
Preoperative optimization programs, 632
Presentation and publication, 367
Primary care physicians (PCPs), 526
Primary care providers (PCPs), 530
Prioritization, 198
Private medical practice
  advantages, 13–15
  career advancement, 209, 210
  career choice
    business plan development, 20
    finance management, 21
    patient care, 20, 21
    professional help, 20
  challenges, 17–19
  definition, 11
  disadvantages, 15–17
  financial aspects
    assets and liabilities, 62
    call, holiday, vacation schedules, 59, 60
    community, 60
    due diligence, 63
    EMR, 60
    financial structure and benefits, 60, 61
    FMV, 61
    leadership, 59
    non-compete clause, 62
    office/support staff, 60
    post-closing items, 62
    purchase price, 61
    purchase/self agreement, 61
    tax issues, 62
    transition structure, 61
    valuation, 62
    warranty and representations, 61
    work culture, 60
    work life balance, 59, 60
  group practice, 12, 13
  healthcare cost, 55
  revenue cycle, 64–66
  risk tolerance, 13
  salaried/employed positions, 13
  solo practice, 11, 12, 56
Proactive change, 513, 514
Processes and policies development, 238
Productive research career, 346
Productive working rapport, 313
Productive working relationship, 313
Professional military education (PME), 106
Program director (PD), 481, 482
Programmatic funding strategy, 567, 568
Project management models, 350
Promising Leaders Program, 460, 461
Promotion, 483
Public policy, 289

Q

Quality governance, 619
Quality improvement (QI), 246, 336, 346, 600, 602, 604, 612, 615–617

Quality of care, 250
Quality surgical care, 594, 595

R

Randomization, 354
Randomized controlled trials (RCTs), 354
Reactive change, 513, 514
Receptive context, 615
Recognition, 484
Recruitment, 320, 645, 647
Recycling, 735
Red flags, 49–52
Reinforcement of values, 237, 239
Relative value units (RVUs), 42, 43, 584
Request for applications (RFA), 357
Research, 664
Research funding, 351–353
Research mentorship, 373, 374
Research package, 347–349
Research projects, 350
Research tracks, 344–349, 351, 352
Resident and Associate Committee of the American College of Surgeons (RAS-ACS), 154
Resistance, 322, 521
Resource constraints, 667, 668
Resources, 549
Responsiveness, 555
Retention, 645
Return on investment (ROI), 529
Royal College of Surgeons (RCS), 616

S

SAGES Foundation Excellence in Medical Leadership Award, 461
SAGES Manual of Strategy and Leadership, 329, 332, 334, 336, 337, 339, 341
Satisfactory performance, 324
Scientific manuscript writing, 371
Scope of practice
  macro-contextual factors, 164
  macro factors, 165, 168, 169
  micro factors, 164
    costs and benefits, 167, 168
    degree of specialization, 166
    non-monetary rewards, 168
    personal competitive advantage, 167
    personal context and goals, 166
    work-life balance, 167
  SWOT analysis, 165
Self-awareness, 319
Self-Management for Managers, 306
Servant leadership, 252
Simplification, 605
Situational leadership model, 538
Social determinants of health (SDoH), 625, 636
  access to healthcare, 629, 630
  addressing implicit bias, 635, 636
  clinical decision-making, 631
  community-based interventions, 634
  health equity initiatives, 634
  impact, 626, 628
  implicit bias, 634, 635
  improve communication, 632
  improve healthcare access, 631
  quality of care, 630
Socialization
  bandwidth and time, 156
  collaboration, 155, 156
  mentorship, 157, 158
  networking, 154, 156
  opportunities, 155
  physicians and allied health professionals, 155–156
  sponsorship, 157, 158
  team dynamics, 155
Social skill, 194, 195
Society membership, 585, 586

Society of American Gastrointestinal and Endoscopic Surgeons (SAGES), 707, 711, 712, 716–718, 731
 Facebook™ groups, 5
 leadership and strategic skills, 4
 overview, 1–4
"Specific Aims" page, 357, 358
Specific-measurable-attainable-result oriented-time (SMART), 256, 409
Sponsorship, 157, 158, 692
Stakeholders, 527, 542
Standardization, 605
Steering committee, 330
Steering committee meetings, 332
Strategic directed contact (SDC), 708, 709
Strategic planning, 329, 331, 337–340, 460, 495, 543
Strategic thinking
 basics, 535, 536
 leadership and management, 537, 538
 leadership styles, 538, 539
 organizational culture, 540
Strategic vision, 553, 555
Strengthening the Reporting of Observational Studies in Epidemiology (STROBE), 369
Strengths, weaknesses opportunities, threats (SWOT) analysis, 165, 223, 224, 334, 542
Structural frame, 519
Study design, 353
Substantive unconscious bias training, 320
Successful grant writing, 356
Supply chain energy expenditure, 728
Surgeon compensation, 348
Surgeon credentialing, 244, 245
Surgeon disengagement, 322
Surgery, 676, 678
Surgical administration
 mission and vision, 468–470
 priorities
  best practices of healthcare, 472, 473
  clinical care and delivery, 472, 473
  cost management, 474
  HCO leadership, 471, 472
  hospital administrators, 471
  information sharing and coordination, 471
  patient safety, 471
  patient satisfaction and outcomes, 471, 472
  personnel management, 474
  regulatory requirements, 472, 474
  roles, 470, 471
  Veterans Administration, 473
 skills and qualities, 468
Surgical education
 associates, 381
 direct reports, 382
 environmental opportunities, 382, 383
 environmental threats, 382
 job demands, 382
 leadership characteristics
  clinical and technical competence, 386, 387
  emotional intelligence, 386
  forward thinking, 385, 386
  honesty and truthfulness, 385, 386
  humility and modesty, 386
  inspirational, 385, 386
  surgical residency training, 384
 leadership styles, 387, 388
 organizational factors, 381
 regional and national educational teams, 383, 384
 supervisors, 382
 teaching modalities and resources, 389–391
 team growth and effective teamwork, 388, 389

Surgical leadership, 641
Surgical training, 566, 576, 663
  applying for practice, 78, 79
  board exam preparation, 81
  clinic participation, 74
  during internship, 70, 71
  excelling in clinical duties, 76
  fellowship, 79, 80
  as junior resident, 71–73
  letters of recommendation, 80
  memory, cognition, and patient communication, 77–78
  operative experience building, 76, 77
  operative feedback, 73
  operative opportunities/clinical duties, 82
  practice laparoscopic/robotic skills, 74
  presentations/lectures, 78
  program, attendings, or colleagues, 82
  as senior resident, 74, 75
  surgical residency, 81
  work-life balance, 81
Sustainability, 438, 439
Sustainability initiatives, 733
Sustainable Development Goals (SDGs), 656
Sustainable surgery, 723, 725
Symbolic frame, 519
Systematic long-term follow-up after obesity surgery, 245
Systems thinking, 496, 545

T

Talent management
  benefits, 424
  definition, 423
  elements, 424, 425
  negotiation, 421–423
  physician-leaders, 424
The Talent Management and Leader Development Academy (TMALDA), 425
Team assessment
  adaptability and flexibility, 229
  DISC assessment, 224–226
  evaluation, 219–223
  feedback, 228
  goal alignment, 228
  individual assessment, 216, 217
  issues, 229–231
  legal and ethical standards, 229
  life cycle, 218
  MBTI, 226, 227
  measurable data points, 218
  objectives and expectations, 227, 228
  overview, 217
  performance improvement plans, 228, 229
  performance metrics, 228
  recognition and rewards, 228
  self-assessment, 219, 220, 228
  surgical setting, 217, 218
  SWOT analysis, 223, 224
  360-degree feedback, 220
Team building, 325, 349, 350
Team culture, 246
Team development, 315, 316
Team dynamics, 317, 318
Team effectiveness, 460
Team huddles/meetings, 318
Team management
  challenges, 400–402
  detail-oriented/evaluator, 400
  emotional intelligence, 394
  emotionally-oriented/harmonizer, 400
  execution of processes, 257
  forming stage, 258
  hierarchy, 394, 395
  idea-oriented/energizer, 400
  leadership styles
    affiliative style, 396
    authoritative style, 396, 397
    coaching style, 397
    coercive style, 395
    democratic style, 396

medical education leaders, 397, 398
pacesetting style, 396, 397
performances, 397, 398
logical/advancer, 400
mentor and mentee relationship, 399
norming stage, 259
storming stage, 259
strategies, 394, 395
stress management, 394, 395
Team meetings, 318
Team structuring, 325
Teamwork, 261, 315
Technological advances, 512
Thromboembolic (VTE), 602
Time management, 486, 487, 492, 541
Training investment, 324
Transactional leadership, 251
Transformational leadership, 251
Transformations, 511, 513
Transformative changes, 323
Transitional changes, 323
Transition model, 520, 523, 532
Translational research, 344
Transparency, 556, 709, 711
Tribal culture, 273–275
Tribal leadership, 275
Trust and respect between team members, 316
Trusting your team members, 317

U
Uncommunicative and unresponsive personality, 300
United Nations Development Programme (UNDP), 553
Universal Reporting Guidelines, 370
USU, 99, 100

V
Value-centric paradigm, 512
Value model, 237
Veteran affairs (VA), 93
Virtual reality (VR), 390
Vision, 253
Vision balancing with practicality, 339, 340
Vision casting, 542
Vision statement, 331, 332
Visual analog scale (VAS), 604
Vulnerability, 234

W
Waste management, 730, 731
Waste management reduction, 735
Work-as-intended (WAI), 604
Working relationships with difficult people, 314, 315
Workplace dynamics, 298
Workplace toxicity, 298
Writing good policy, 291
Writing good procedure, 293
Writing policies, 290, 291
approval and implementation, 292, 293
date, 292
prewriting stage, 292
and procedures, 293
purpose statement, 291
statement of policy, 292
Writing procedures, 294

GPSR Compliance

The European Union's (EU) General Product Safety Regulation (GPSR) is a set of rules that requires consumer products to be safe and our obligations to ensure this.

If you have any concerns about our products, you can contact us on ProductSafety@springernature.com

In case Publisher is established outside the EU, the EU authorized representative is:

Springer Nature Customer Service Center GmbH
Europaplatz 3
69115 Heidelberg, Germany

Batch number: 10732632

Printed by Printforce, the Netherlands